Diagnosis and Management of Ocular Motility Disorders

Diagnosis and Management of Ocular Motility Disorders

Alec M. Ansons
Consultant Ophthalmic Surgeon
Manchester Royal Eye Hospital
Oxford Road
Manchester

Helen Davis
Senior Lecturer in Orthoptics
Department of Ophthalmology and Orthoptics
Royal Hallamshire Hospital
University of Sheffield
Sheffield

**Blackwell
Science**

© 1986, 1991, 2001 by
Blackwell Science Ltd
Editorial Offices:
Osney Mead, Oxford OX2 0EL
25 John Street, London WC1N 2BS
23 Ainslie Place, Edinburgh EH3 6AJ
350 Main Street, Malden
    MA 02148-5018, USA
54 University Street, Carlton
    Victoria 3053, Australia
10, rue Casimir Delavigne
    75006 Paris, France

Other Editorial Offices:
Blackwell Wissenschafts-Verlag GmbH
Kurfürstendamm 57
10707 Berlin, Germany

Blackwell Science KK
MG Kodenmacho Building
7–10 Kodenmacho Nihombashi
Chuo-ku, Tokyo 104, Japan

First published 1986
Reprinted 1987
Second edition 1991
Reprinted 1992, 1994
Third edition 2001

Set by Graphicraft Limited, Hong Kong
Printed and bound in Great Britain by
Redwood Books, Trowbridge

The Blackwell Science logo is a
trade mark of Blackwell Science Ltd,
registered at the United Kingdom
Trade Marks Registry

For further information on
Blackwell Science, visit our website:
www.blackwell-science.com

DISTRIBUTORS

Marston Book Services Ltd
PO Box 269
Abingdon, Oxon OX14 4YN
(*Orders*: Tel: 01235 465500
          Fax: 01235 465555)

USA
Blackwell Science, Inc.
Commerce Place
350 Main Street
Malden, MA 02148-5018
(*Orders*: Tel: 800 759 6102
          781 388 8250
          Fax: 781 388 8255)

Canada
Login Brothers Book Company
324 Saulteaux Crescent
Winnipeg, Manitoba R3J 3T2
(*Orders*: Tel: 204 837 2987)

Australia
Blackwell Science Pty Ltd
54 University Street
Carlton, Victoria 3053
(*Orders*: Tel: 3 9347 0300
          Fax: 3 9347 5001)

A catalogue record for this title
is available from the British Library

ISBN 0-632-04798-4

Library of Congress
Cataloging-in-publication Data

Ansons, Alec M.
    Diagnosis and management of ocular
    motility disorders.—3rd ed. /
Alec M. Ansons, Helen Davis.
        p. ; cm.
    Rev. ed. of: Mein, Joyce. Diagnosis and
management of ocular motility disorders /
Joyce Mein and Roger Trimble. 2nd ed. 1991.
    Includes bibliographical references and index.
    ISBN 0-632-04798-4
    1. Eye—Movement disorders.
I. Davis, Helen.
II. Mein, Joyce. Diagnosis and
management of ocular motility disorders.
III. Title.
    [DNLM: 1. Ocular Motility Disorders—diagnosis.
2. Ocular Motility Disorders—therapy.
3. Eye Movements.
4. Oculomotor Muscles—physiopathology.
WW410 A622d 2000]
RE731 .A57 2000
617.7'62—dc21
DNLM/DLC   00-023115
for Library of Congress

Contents

Preface to the Third Edition

It is a privilege to be given the opportunity to prepare the Third Edition of this book. Joyce Mein had the original concept for this work, and we have been fortunate to have had her help and advice in this edition.

It is with very great regret that we record the death of Roger Trimble who contributed so much to the Second Edition. His passing is a great loss to British ophthalmology.

In this edition we have maintained the basic framework of the book, which was presented so well previously, and added an extra chapter on an 'Introduction to concomitant strabismus'. Other chapters have been thoroughly revised and brought up to date. To reflect the expanding role of the Orthoptist an attempt has been made to be more explicit in regard to management and treatment recommendations. As far as possible the indications, contraindications and dangers of each recommendation are fully discussed.

It is hoped that the authors' experience and expertise as presented will allow the reader to deal competently with most areas of strabismus and ocular motility they are likely to encounter.

We would especially like to thank Lynne Mallinson for the references and secretarial help, Robin Farr for the additional photographs and illustrations, Alison Firth and Alison Spencer for proof reading and the valuable help from many colleagues in Manchester and Sheffield.

Alec M. Ansons
Helen Davis

Preface to the First Edition

Our aim in writing this book has been to give guidance on the diagnosis and management of ocular motility disorders, based largely on our own clinical and teaching experience, rather than to provide a comprehensive textbook on this far-ranging subspecialty of ophthalmology. We have emphasized the practical aspect throughout the book. We have attempted to indicate in some detail the problems which may arise in clinical practice and the precautions which can be taken to avoid them, stressing those methods which we have found to be appropriate for each of the conditions discussed. It is hoped that the style we have adopted, using headings, subheadings and tabulation, will make the text easy to read and understand. There is no section on anatomy and physiology. These subjects are referred to only when we have considered more detailed knowledge essential to understanding of the text, as in the chapters on the principles of surgery and on supranuclear disorders. The book is deliberately little illustrated. We have assumed familiarity with standard equipment and have not included pictures of apparatus in most general use. To have provided photographs to illustrate all the ocular motility disorders we discuss would have been a daunting and perhaps impossible task which we reluctantly decided not to undertake. Static photography of what are essentially movement disorders is rarely satisfactory, especially where the more obscure incomitant conditions are concerned. Video-recordings are of greater value, both in diagnosis and in teaching. Neither have we provided a comprehensive list of the numerous excellent publications on all aspects of strabismus: the references we have given are simply intended as a guide to further reading or to the source of relatively new knowledge on some subjects. We confess to a slight bias towards subjects in which we have or have had a particular interest.

The book is divided into three sections. Section I deals in sequence with the assessment of the patient. The questions which it attempts to answer are whether the ocular motility disorder, using the term in its widest sense, is the result of neurological, ocular, muscular or orbital disease; whether defective vision is due to pathological processes or to amblyopia and whether the defect can be treated to achieve a functional cure or, failing that, satisfactory cosmetic improvement. Section II covers in detail the principles and methods of non-surgical treatment, optical, orthoptic and pharmacological, emphasizing practical value and limitations. The principles of surgical management cover relevant aspects of anaesthesia, as well as the pre- and post-operative care of the patient, including the management of complications. Surgical procedures are described, illustrated and evaluated. Botulinum toxin injection as an alternative to muscle surgery is included in this section. Finally, Section III discusses the application of conservative and surgical methods to specific non-paralytic and paralytic conditions and to nystagmus. We have attempted to give an overall picture of the methods available but have put the emphasis on those which we have found most likely to succeed. We hope we have communicated our conviction that meticulous observation and equally careful recording of the findings are central to the management of strabismus and associated disorders. Detailed descriptions of ocular motility disorders are bedevilled by problems of nomenclature. Universal agreement on terms and their meanings is rarely attained. We have tried to use terminology which is in general use. Alternative or synonymous terms have been added where indicated.

This book could not have been written without the help and advice of our friends and colleagues. Our thanks go to all of them. Our special gratitude goes to Anne Gelder for her admirable secretarial work and for the very many hours she devoted to preparation of the book on our behalf; to Bruce Noble FRCS, Consultant Ophthalmologist at the General Infirmary at Leeds, for his meticulous illustrations in the surgery section, drawn with the informed eye of a surgeon as well as an artist; to Michael Geall, medical photographer and illustrator, for his careful preparation of some illustrations; to Andrew Fox, orthoptic teacher and source of much useful information and to Margaret Harcourt for her patience, support and forbearance.

I
ASSESSMENT

1
History

Patients with ocular motility disorders present for one or more of the following reasons:
- manifest strabismus;
- defective ocular movement;
- nystagmus;
- abnormal head posture;
- defective vision;
- subjective symptoms.

An accurate and detailed history must be recorded to aid diagnosis, assist in planning management and arrive at a correct prognosis. This first contact with the patient, or the parents if the patient is a child, gives the examiner an opportunity to assess cooperation, to establish a good relationship with the patient and to gain his confidence.

General principles

The reason for attendance must first be established. Subsequent questions depend largely on whether the patient is a child or an adult. Greater emphasis is placed on the obstetric history and developmental milestones in children, whereas the medical history can be of paramount importance in adults.

Children

It is important to involve the child in the history taking as much as possible: surprisingly young children are aware of the questions being asked; they can supply helpful information while allowing the examiner to form an impression of their intelligence and capabilities.

Because so many disorders of vision and ocular motility are associated with developmental anomalies, hereditary disorders or diseases of childhood, the patient must be considered as a whole, whatever the reason for presentation, and a full medical, obstetric, family and social history should be recorded.

Medical history

The following information should be obtained:
- The child's general development, including milestones and his progress at nursery or school.
- Details of any significant or recent illness and its treatment.
- Any trauma, especially to the head or face.

Obstetric history

Enquiries should be made about:
• The mother's health during pregnancy.
• The child's birth weight and gestational age if known.
• The neonatal history, especially if there were post-natal problems with resuscitation and/or the child was admitted to a neonatal intensive therapy unit.

Family history

Particular reference should be made to a family history of any of the following disorders:
• Strabismus, which is frequently familial. Its presence in other family members makes it more likely that the child has a true rather than an apparent strabismus and he should be kept under observation even if the squint is not apparent at the first visit. There may be social problems if more than one child requires treatment.
• Refractive error.
• Severe visual defects, which are frequently hereditary if present in early childhood. Parental consanguinity should be noted.

Social history

The examiner should enquire into relevant social background which may affect the future management of the child. It is, for example, necessary to know if he is in residential care rather than living with his parents.

Adults

Adults are more likely to present with symptoms, particularly diplopia. In many cases the symptoms are due to acquired eye movement defects, comprising neurogenic palsies, myogenic palsies and mechanical restriction of ocular movement. It is essential to find and treat the underlying cause if this is unknown. A detailed medical history should be taken in all cases.

Medical history

The examiner should question the patient on:

• Past and current illnesses.
• Current medication: the drug history is a good guide to the state of the patient's health and may provide a clue to the cause of an acquired motility disorder. The patient may say that he is in good health but on questioning may admit to being on regular treatment with, for example, insulin or digitalis. Some drugs, notably anticonvulsants, can be the cause of defective ocular movement.
• Trauma affecting the head or face.
• Other symptoms and signs: examples are unsteadiness of gait, weight loss or gain, or change in appearance noted by the patient's family.
• Ophthalmic history: this may include visual problems, a childhood squint or previous episodes of diplopia.
• Hereditary factors.

Social history

The patient's occupation should be noted and he should be asked how it has been affected by the complaint. He should be questioned specifically about alcohol consumption and smoking, as both are relevant to recognized motility disorders. Alcoholism can lead to Wernicke's syndrome, which is a rare condition, and cigarette smoking can be the cause of the paraneoplastic syndromes, which are more common.

Manifest strabismus

History taking is discussed below in general terms. Points relating to specific types of strabismus are referred to in subsequent chapters.

Children

The majority of patients attending with manifest strabismus are children. Most will have concomitant deviations but children with congenital and acquired defects of ocular movement can present in this way. In all cases it is necessary to ascertain:
• The direction of the strabismus.
• The age at which it was first noticed.
• Who noticed it.
• Whether the onset was sudden or gradual. A history of sudden onset is usually reliable, whereas a

gradual onset probably implies a longer duration than that stated. A sudden onset of esotropia should always suggest the possibility of an acquired sixth nerve palsy.

• Whether the squint is constant or intermittent. A constant deviation with a variable angle is often mistaken for an intermittent strabismus.

• When the squint is seen, for example on looking up from a book or on lateral gaze. An apparent increase on lateroversion suggests an incomitant deviation but is also a common feature in pseudoesotropia due to epicanthus.

• Whether there has been an increase or a decrease in the angle of deviation since its onset.

• If there are other features which could be related to the strabismus, such as a compensatory head posture. Older children should be asked about symptoms, particularly whether diplopia is present. This is usually but not invariably indicative of recent onset. Signs suggesting possible diplopia in younger children are:

1 increased clumsiness;

2 reluctance to play;

3 covering or closing one eye, although this is also a common diagnostic sign in intermittent exotropia.

In general, a history of occasional exotropia should be believed, whereas an occasional esotropia may be due to epicanthus or another cause of pseudostrabismus. If the esotropia is not seen on initial examination, risk factors should be considered. A family history of squint and/or hypermetropia, or the presence of even a small esophoria, are all reasons for believing the parent's observations and keeping the child under review.

Adults

Adults may present with a manifest strabismus dating from childhood, either because they would like surgery to improve alignment or because the strabismus has become symptom-producing: diplopia may occur if a change in the angle of deviation causes the image to fall outside the suppression scotoma. As much information as possible should be elicited about the type and onset of the strabismus and its subsequent course. The patient should also be questioned about:

• His reason for attendance. A patient who is embarassed by his appearance may complain instead about minor symptoms. It can be helpful if the possibility of strabismus surgery is suggested.

• Recent change in the angle of deviation. Some patients present with consecutive exotropia and should be asked when this was first noticed. Photographs taken over the past few years may help in this respect.

• The treatment already received. Particular attention should be paid to previous strabismus surgery and the patient's records should be obtained if possible.

Defective ocular movement

Children may present because limitation of ocular movement has been noticed by the parents or another observer. Usually the defective movement is marked, congenital in origin and mechanical rather than neurogenic: examples are Brown's syndrome and Duane's retraction syndrome, although the restricted movement in the latter condition is often masked by head movement. Occasionally an overaction secondary to limitation of movement is the presenting sign, for example a marked overaction of an inferior oblique muscle. It is rare for adults to present for these reasons.

The examiner should enquire about:

• The nature of the defective movement.

• How and when it was discovered.

• Any associated signs, particularly an abnormal head posture. It is unusual for symptoms to be present.

Nystagmus

Children

The parents of an infant or young child may describe rhythmic, irregular or 'dancing' eye movements, or the nystagmus may have been detected by a paediatrician or the family doctor.

The parents should be asked:

• The age of onset. The nystagmus may have been present at birth but is more often acquired in infancy.

• Whether they think it is constant or intermittent. They may have noticed an increase in some gaze positions.

• If the movement has remained static or has improved or deteriorated.

- Their opinion of the child's vision, comparing it with that of siblings at the same age if possible.
- If there are associated signs, such as strabismus, involuntary head movement or an abnormal head posture.
- The obstetric and medical history, particularly whether the child is receiving anticonvulsant therapy, as an overdose of a drug such as phenytoin may induce nystagmus. Older children may present with acquired nystagmus (see below).

Adults

Adults with congenital nystagmus occasionally present because their visual acuity is inadequate for their work, hobbies or interests. More usually nystagmus in an adult is acquired, mainly due to cerebellar or labyrinthine damage. Acquired nystagmus is frequently associated with oscillopsia and is incapacitating. Other neurological signs are probable. The patient should be questioned about the onset and duration of the nystagmus, with particular reference to all symptoms and signs and to the general medical history.

Nystagmus is considered in detail in Chapter 23.

Abnormal head posture

A few patients, usually children, may present because of a marked abnormal head posture, adopted to compensate for a congenital ocular muscle palsy, mechanical restriction of ocular movement or congenital nystagmus. Abnormal head posture is discussed in detail in Chapter 2.

Defective vision

A common cause of defective visual acuity without outward sign of strabismus or nystagmus is uncorrected refractive error, especially when one eye is principally affected (anisometropic amblyopia). However, defective vision may be the main reason for attendance in a few patients with strabismus and/or nystagmus. Low vision may be the consequence of either condition, or it may be the underlying cause. The possibility of primary ocular pathology makes differentiation very important.

The examiner should enquire into:
- The nature of the defect.
- How it affects the patient.
- Whether poor vision is a subjective complaint or is deduced from the patient's behaviour. The former applies more to older children and the few adults who present for this reason, whereas the latter applies to young children.
- How the defect was discovered. Monocular low vision in particular is often found through visual screening or by chance.
- Whether vision appears static or is deteriorating.
- Any associated symptoms or signs, including headache or strabismus.
- The patient's medical and family history, particularly one of refractive error.

Subjective symptoms

Symptoms commonly fall into two categories, diplopia, and headache and eyestrain.

Diplopia

Diplopia occurs when the visual axes are not parallel, causing the image of the fixation object to fall on peripheral retina. The image is projected according to the visual direction of the retinal area stimulated.

Diplopia can be a symptom in the following types of strabismus.

Concomitant strabismus. Diplopia is almost invariably horizontal, with uncrossed or homonymous separation of the images in esotropia (i.e. the right-hand image is seen by the right eye), and crossed or heteronymous separation in exotropia. The separation of the images will not alter significantly in different directions of gaze. Diplopia in concomitant strabismus can signify:
- Recent onset.
- Sudden change in the angle of deviation, usually following strabismus surgery.
- Marked improvement in the vision of the squinting eye, for example after cataract extraction and lens implant in exotropia secondary to unilateral cataract.

Decompensated heterophoria and convergence insufficiency. Diplopia is usually transitory and can be fused by blinking or changing fixation in most cases.

The patient may complain of blurred vision rather than diplopia if the images overlap. Most patients will be adults, as decompensation in children usually results in persistent manifest strabismus.

Decompensated congenital ocular muscle palsies. If decompensation occurs in childhood, the outcome is often manifest strabismus with suppression; however, some children complain of diplopia. When decompensation occurs in adult life, diplopia is generally the presenting symptom.

Vertical muscle palsies are most likely to decompensate, therefore the diplopia is often vertical, with the higher eye seeing the lower image. Torsional diplopia is rarely if ever a feature of congenital muscle palsy. The diplopia is usually intermittent with a gradual onset and the patient is often vague about its duration.

Acquired limitation of ocular movement. Diplopia can be horizontal, vertical and/or torsional, depending on the nature of the defect. The separation of the images will decrease in the opposite direction, when fusion may be possible. Diplopia is usually the presenting symptom in children and adults and can be the first sign of serious disease. The onset can be gradual or sudden: patients are usually precise about the onset and the duration. Further information can be found in Chapters 18–22.

Headache and eyestrain

These symptoms can result from decompensating heterophoria and convergence insufficiency, due to the effort required to maintain binocular single vision. Most patients with these complaints will be adults, often those working on exacting visual tasks or who are unwell or excessively tired. In the context of ocular motor disorders, other causes are uncorrected refractive error, ill-fitting spectacles and accommodative anomalies. When taking the history, the examiner should bear in mind the many other causes of headache, a number of them with more serious implications. Heterophoria and convergence insufficiency are discussed in Chapter 16.

All patients should be asked about:
- The nature of their symptoms.
- When they first became apparent.
- When they occur, with particular reference to variation during the day.
- Whether they have remained static, improved or deteriorated.
- How they affect work and hobbies.
- If they can be overcome in any way.
- Relevant trauma—however, care should be taken in attributing the symptoms to the trauma: the injury may be unrelated, or a fall, for example, may be the result of an underlying problem rather than its cause.
- A detailed medical history should be taken, including current medication. The past ophthalmic history should be recorded, with particular reference to childhood strabismus and spectacle wear.

2
Ophthalmic Examination

Introduction

Examination of the patient has two main aims.
• Diagnosing the nature and degree of the ocular motor disorder.
• Detecting other ocular and nonocular disorders and assessing their relationship to the motility problem.

The ophthalmic examination should be carried out with strabismus and ocular movement defects in mind. A concomitant strabismus may be the first outward sign of ocular pathology, and a constant strictly unilateral esotropia or exotropia in a young child should always be suspect; it is well recognized, for example, that a child with optic nerve glioma can present in this way. A sudden onset of a constant esotropia in a child may be due to a sixth cranial nerve palsy and can be a sign of neurological disease, including cerebral tumour. Congenital nystagmus can result from bilateral ocular pathology, particularly albinism and congenital cataract. When ocular pathology and strabismus coexist, the examiner must assess how much of the vision loss is due to primary pathology and how much to associated deprivation. Additional strabismic amblyopia can develop and may respond to occlusion treatment.

Exotropia can follow loss of vision in one eye in an adult patient and must be considered when planning treatment, for example, in traumatic cataract. The ocular signs can point to the aetiology of acquired cranial nerve palsies. Common examples are those due to diabetes and vascular disease. In a few patients defective vision due to ocular pathology can dissociate a heterophoria or a congenital ocular muscle palsy. Symptoms attributable to decompensation, for example diplopia, may be the reason for presentation in such cases.

Ophthalmic examination should be carried out in a logical sequence, using a cycloplegic agent for fundus examination and refraction at the end of the sequence so that it does not interfere with the performance and interpretation of other tests.

Examination is discussed in the following order:
• Assessment of the patient's appearance, including his facial features and head posture.
• Measurement of the uncorrected and corrected visual acuity, assessed after refraction without cycloplegia if necessary.
• Observation of the position and function of the eyelids.
• Observation and measurement of the position of the globe.
• Assessment and measurement of the ocular deviation and ocular movement.
• Examination of the eyes:
1 analysis of pupil size and reaction;
2 examination of the anterior and posterior segments.

Additional examination, which may be indicated from the preliminary findings, includes:
• Refraction with cycloplegia.
• Investigation of other aspects of visual function—measurement of the visual fields, colour vision testing and recording the contrast sensitivity threshold.
• Investigation of binocular function.
• General medical examination.
• Laboratory and radiological investigations.

The assessment and measurement of visual function, refraction, ocular deviation, ocular movements and binocular function are referred to only briefly in this chapter because they are discussed in detail in subsequent chapters.

General appearance

The appearance can provide clues to the patient's general condition and to the ocular motility disorder.

Children

General features

Many easily recognized conditions are associated with a high incidence of strabismus and eye movement problems. These include:

• hydrocephalus
• microcephalus
• albinism
• Down's syndrome
• cerebral palsy
• cranial dysostosis.

Facial features

Strabismus can be simulated by:
• epicanthus;
• a narrow or wide interpupillary distance;
• facial asymmetry.

Disorders of the facial skeleton, such as hypertelorism or Crouzon's syndrome, are associated with strabismus and, in the latter case, with impaired vision.

Facial asymmetry may be a consequence of the branchial arch syndromes: it can be associated with a head tilt of ocular or nonocular origin.

Loss of facial expression is characteristic of Möbius' syndrome.

Both parents' appearance should also be noted since some disorders are familial.

Adults

General features

Signs of congenital abnormality can be present, as described above. Significant acquired neurological signs which are easily seen include:
• facial nerve palsy;
• tremor;
• ataxia;
• deafness (unilateral deafness may be due to an acoustic nerve tumour).

The main signs suggestive of thyroid disease are lid retraction and proptosis in thyrotoxicosis, and myxoedema in hypothyroidism.

Facial features

Loss of facial expression suggests the possibility of myasthenia or muscular dystrophy.

Outward evidence of facial trauma can indicate the possible nature of defective ocular movement, for example:
• Flattening of the zygomatic arch can be associated with a blow-out fracture of the orbital floor.
• Scarring in the region of the trochlea, often from

windscreen glass, can result in trapping of the superior oblique tendon.

Head posture

An abnormal head position may result from nonocular causes or may compensate for an ocular condition, when it can be significant in both diagnosis and management. The underlying condition can be congenital or acquired. The head posture can be observed from approximately six months of age, when an infant can normally sit unsupported. An abnormal head posture may be present all the time or adopted only when needed, especially if it is uncomfortable to maintain.

Components

An abnormal head posture has three possible components, which may be present singly or in combination:
• head tilt to the right or left shoulder;
• face turn to the right or left side;
• chin elevation or depression.

Examination

• Initially nonocular and ocular head postures must be differentiated. The essential differences between them are:

  1 the presence or absence of a strabismus or other ocular abnormality, for example nystagmus, when the head is straightened;

  2 the ability to straighten the head—it should always be possible to straighten the head if the cause is ocular but some patients with nonocular head postures may be unable to do so because of bony changes in the cervical spine or muscle contracture.

• The components of the head posture should be analysed, noting the position in which the eyes are placed. Straightening the head, then allowing it to resume a comfortable position, often simplifies recognition of its different components.

• The head posture should be assessed for near and distance as it may vary significantly from one distance to the other; for example, a patient with a partial sixth nerve palsy may need a face turn only for distance.

• Long-term observation may be needed to see an intermittent head posture. Observation of a child when playing may reveal, for example, the chin elevation seen in esotropia with 'A' pattern, which may be too uncomfortable to maintain all the time.

• A cover test should be performed with the abnormal head posture and with the head straight, noting the difference in the degree of ocular deviation and whether there is recovery to binocular single vision.

• The head posture should be observed when testing the monocular and binocular visual acuity. In some patients it is present only when clear vision is required.

• Early unposed photographs can indicate the duration of the head posture. They should show whether it is consistent and if it has changed with time. An intermittent abnormal head posture may be seen on photographs.

Causes of abnormal head posture

Nonocular head postures

Congenital

Nonocular torticollis ('wry-neck'). This condition is caused by contracture of the sterno-cleido-mastoid muscle in the neck. The typical head posture comprises a head tilt to the affected side, a face turn to the normal side and chin elevation.

Differential diagnosis is made by:
• Attempting to straighten the head, which will be impossible in nonocular torticollis, but easily achieved in ocular torticollis.
• Examination of the ocular posture by cover test. There should be no manifest deviation in nonocular torticollis, but a hypertropia should be detected in ocular torticollis when the head is straight.

Acquired

There are several possible acquired causes of nonocular abnormal head posture.
• Deafness: if this is unilateral, or is more marked in one ear, the patient may turn his face to the more affected side. This is a common cause of face turn, especially in the elderly. It is worth questioning the patient about his hearing if there is an unexplained or atypical head posture.
• Defects of balance.
• Disorders of the cervical spine.

• Habit: although this is commonly cited as a cause of abnormal head posture by parents, it is unlikely to explain a persistent abnormality and other reasons for the head posture should be sought.

Abnormal head posture may be associated with other less common neurological or medical conditions, including brain tumours, stressing the need for thorough investigation. Abnormal head posture may be associated with other less common neurological or medical conditions (Boutros & Al-Mateen 1995).

Ocular head postures

The main reasons for the adoption of an abnormal head posture are:

• To obtain or maintain a field of binocular single vision and place it centrally. This applies to:

1 all forms of congenital or acquired paralytic strabismus, including those with mechanical restriction of movement;

2 'A' and 'V' patterns;

3 a few cases of heterophoria and convergence deficiency;

4 high degrees of anisomyopia (the 'heavy eye' syndrome).

• To obtain better visual acuity and/or centralize the visual field. This applies to:

1 nystagmus with an eccentric null area in which the oscillations are much reduced or absent;

2 gross restriction of ocular movement which prevents foveal fixation in the primary position;

3 visual field defects;

4 ptosis.

A head tilt is seen in some patients with dissociated vertical deviation but the reason for the tilt is not clear.

Abnormal head postures in the ocular conditions referred to above are discussed in the relevant sections of this book.

Head movement

The patient should be observed for abnormalities of head movement. These can take the following forms:

• Movement of the head rather than the eyes in order to maintain binocular single vision. This is often seen in Duane's retraction syndrome, when it can successfully mask the limitation of ocular movement. This sign may be the observer's first indication of the syndrome.

• Head nodding or head shaking is a feature of some types of nystagmus and is commonly seen in spasmus nutans. The rate of head movement does not correlate with the rate of nystagmus.

• Exaggerated head thrusts on attempting to change fixation, which are seen in congenital ocular motor apraxia.

Visual acuity

Visual acuity should be measured monocularly for near and distance, with and without spectacles if worn. If monocular vision is defective, it is advisable to test the acuity with both eyes open. A pinhole can be used to assess how much of the defect can be accounted for by an uncorrected refractive error. Any special features should be noted, such as 'screwing up' of the eyes, an abnormal head posture or head movement. When vision is defective the patient's optimum reading distance and near visual acuity should be recorded in addition to his near vision at 33 cm.

Refraction without a cycloplegic agent may be useful at this stage, both to find the best corrected visual acuity and to ascertain the type and degree of refractive error, which can have a bearing on further investigation as well as on diagnosis.

The assessment of vision may require modification, depending on age and cooperation. Methods suitable for young children are described in Chapter 4.

Eyelids

Palpebral fissures

Variants from the normal palpebral fissure shape or size can result in pseudostrabismus or can be characteristic of certain ocular motility disorders.

Shape

Mongoloid palpebral fissures are typical of Down's syndrome, which has a high incidence of esotropia. The fissure shape is believed to be of aetiological significance in 'A' and 'V' patterns (Urrets-Zavalia *et al.* 1961). Patients with 'A' pattern commonly have mongoloid fissures and those with 'V' pattern may have antimongoloid fissures, therefore these patterns should be looked for when investigating the strabismus (see Chapter 17).

Fissure changes during ocular movement

An increase or decrease in the height of the palpebral fissure can be characteristic of some incomitant conditions, for example:
• Narrowing of the fissure on adduction and widening on abduction are diagnostic features of Duane's retraction syndrome.
• The fissure commonly widens on adduction in Brown's syndrome.
• Widening of the fissure occurs on abduction in some cases of acquired sixth cranial nerve palsy.

Congenital anomalies

Epicanthus

Epicanthus is a fold of skin which arises in the medial portion of the upper eyelid and is inserted into the lower eyelid at the medial canthus. It is usually bilateral and symmetrical. It causes an apparent increase in the intercanthal distance and therefore shortens the palpebral fissure along its horizontal axis.

Epicanthus gives rise to pseudoesotropia and is the most common cause of this condition in young Caucasian children. It can also accentuate an existing esotropia. Epicanthus is physiological and usually disappears by 7 or 8 years of age in Caucasians, as the skin fold is gradually taken up by the developing nasal bridge. If it persists and is marked, oculoplastic surgery may be required.

Blepharophimosis

The features of this condition are:
• marked epicanthic folds;
• partial ptosis;
• epicanthus inversus, which is a much less common form of epicanthus in which the skin fold arises in the lower eyelid and is inserted into the upper eyelid;
• telecanthus, which is a widening of the intercanthal distance.

As a result of these features, the palpebral apertures are slit-like and cosmetically unsightly. The condition can be improved rather than cured by oculoplastic surgery.

Both epicanthus inversus and telecanthus can present without blepharophimosis.

Epiblepharon

This anomaly is characterized by a fold of skin running horizontally in the lower eyelid close to the lash line, usually in both eyes. Occasionally the skin can push against the lower eyelid, causing the eyelashes to come in contact with the cornea, but as the lashes are still soft, little irritation results and surgical correction is not required. The fold of skin usually disappears spontaneously by 12 months of age.

Eyelid position and movement

Abnormalities of eyelid position and eyelid movement are commonly associated with ocular movement disorders and should be carefully noted. Correct assessment of the anomaly can aid the diagnosis of the movement disorder and can indicate its aetiology.

Normal position and movement

The eyelid position is symmetrical on both sides. The height of each palpebral fissure is 9–11 mm and the resting position of the upper eyelid margin is 1–2 mm below the superior limbus. This relationship is normally maintained in the different positions of gaze. Movement of the upper eyelid from down-gaze to up-gaze measures 15–18 mm.

Eyelid anomalies

Eyelid anomalies comprise:
• upper eyelid too low—ptosis or pseudoptosis;
• upper eyelid too high—lid retraction;
• abnormal eyelid movement.

Ptosis

Ptosis can be due to:
• underaction of the levator muscle;
• underaction of Müller's muscle;
• mechanical factors.
  Examination aims to establish:
• the degree of ptosis and whether it is unilateral or bilateral;
• whether it is an isolated defect or is associated with defective ocular movement or other anomaly;

- the reason for ptosis;
- its effect on visual acuity and binocular vision.

Ptosis may be complete, when the upper eyelid obscures the pupil, or partial when some eyelid movement is possible. If the pupil is obscured by the ptosis during childhood, there is a high risk of stimulus-deprivation amblyopia.

Causes of ptosis

CONGENITAL PTOSIS
Ptosis dating from birth or with very early onset can be unilateral or bilateral.

Features
Complete unilateral ptosis is associated with:
- severe stimulus-deprivation amblyopia;
- myopia or myopic astigmatism in the affected eye in some cases;
- congenital third nerve palsy in a few cases;
- a constant strabismus in the affected eye, either secondary to low vision or as an exotropia resulting from a third nerve palsy.

The earliest possible surgical treatment of the ptosis is essential to prevent further stimulus deprivation and to allow treatment of the amblyopia.

Partial ptosis may be bilateral or unilateral and can be associated with the following conditions:
- A partial third nerve palsy, affecting either all the extraocular muscles supplied by the nerve or only the superior rectus and the levator muscles, which are supplied by its superior division. It is believed that the latter is more common because the two muscles arise from the same embryonic mass.
- A congenital Horner's syndrome, in which slight ptosis results from underaction of the smooth Müller's muscle. This condition is far more commonly acquired and is described below.
- The Marcus Gunn phenomenon, in which there is a partial ptosis in the primary position which increases or decreases with movement of the lower jaw (see below).

A compensatory head posture of chin elevation may be adopted to facilitate vision when the ptosis is bilateral or affects the fixing eye.

If the ptosis covers the pupil or there is a manifest strabismus, amblyopia will be present.

ACQUIRED PTOSIS
Involutional (age-related) ptosis
Weakness of the levator aponeurosis can develop with age, causing the upper eyelid to droop. A higher than normal skin crease can be seen. Senile ptosis is usually bilateral but not necessarily symmetrical. Ocular movement is usually normal for age: it is recognized that elevation of the eyes is reduced in the elderly.

Neurogenic ptosis
Third cranial nerve palsy. Damage to the third cranial nerve results in paralysis or paresis of the levator muscle and of all or some of the extraocular and intraocular muscles supplied by the nerve. The degree of ptosis depends on the extent of nerve damage.

Other neurological signs may be present, indicating further investigation. A sudden onset of third nerve palsy with pupil involvement, associated with headache, can be due to aneurysm on the circle of Willis, which may rupture, and is a neurosurgical emergency.

Lid function may improve with time, but if the palsy was due to trauma or an aneurysm in particular, reinnervation of the levator is quite often aberrant (the misdirection syndrome; see below).

Horner's syndrome. Damage to the sympathetic nerve supply to the eye results in the following signs:
- Slight unilateral ptosis.
- Miosis of the affected eye.
- Ipsilateral anhydrosis, resulting in warm, dry, flushed skin on the affected side of the face. This is not an invariable sign.
- Heterochromia iridis, which is sometimes present in the rare congenital cases of Horner's syndrome.

There is no associated ocular motor defect other than the ptosis.

A lesion can affect the sympathetic nerve supply at any point along its lengthy pathway from the hypothalamus. Lesions are most likely to occur in the sympathetic chain, where apical lung tumours are a common cause. If the lesion occurs above the level of the neck, due for example to carotid aneurysm, the third nerve can also be affected but because of sympathetic damage, the pupil will be small. The examiner should be careful not to misinterpret this sign by assuming that absence of the usual pupil dilatation rules out an aneurysm as the cause of the palsy.

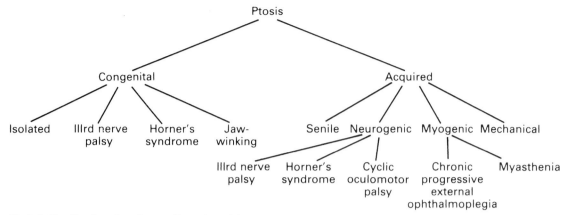

Fig. 2.1 Classification of ptosis according to its aetiology.

Cyclic oculomotor palsy. This condition occurs in childhood and is characterized by unilateral ptosis and limitation of ocular movement during its paretic phase, and by lid retraction during its spastic phase (see Chapter 19). Ptosis is the usual reason for ophthalmic referral.

Myogenic ptosis

Ptosis can be due to disease processes directly affecting the levator muscle:
• Chronic progressive external ophthalmoplegia affecting both eyes is associated with slowly increasing ptosis.
• Myasthenia—the ptosis associated with this disease is usually partial. It may be unilateral and is essentially variable, increasing with fatigue and becoming more marked at the end of the day. There is often limitation of ocular movement and although diplopia is frequently the presenting symptom, myasthenia can present in a variety of other ways.

Myogenic conditions are discussed in Chapter 20.

Mechanical ptosis

Mechanical ptosis is usually due to excessive weight of the upper eyelid, caused by oedema, haematoma or tumour. The ptosis is usually unilateral and is partial in the primary position, but may decrease on down-gaze. Lid closure may be incomplete. It is important to record this sign, which has a bearing on the management of the condition.

The classification of ptosis according to its aetiology is shown in Fig. 2.1.

Pseudoptosis

In pseudoptosis there is drooping of the upper eyelid on clinical inspection but demonstrably normal eyelid function. The causes are:
• Enophthalmos.
• Retraction of the globe in one or more positions of gaze. Duane's retraction syndrome is the main example.
• Hypotropia of the apparently affected eye. The relationship between the upper eyelid margin and the limbus is normal for the down-gaze position, as can be seen when the hypotropic eye is made to fixate in the primary position and the 'ptosis' disappears.

Eyelid retraction

Upper eyelid retraction

Retraction is due to overaction of Müller's muscle, overaction or contracture of the levator muscle, or mechanical factors.

THYROTOXICOSIS

This is the most common cause of lid retraction. Both eyes are usually affected, although often asymmetrically: occasionally the retraction is strictly unilateral. Smooth muscle is believed to be unduly sensitive to sympathetic hormones in thyrotoxicosis, leading to overaction of Müller's muscle. This can result in very variable lid retraction and can also contribute to the lid-lag which is a common feature of this disease (von Graefe's sign).

INFERIOR RECTUS TETHERING
Mechanical restriction of elevation due to tethering of the inferior rectus in thyroid eye disease results in increased drive to the superior rectus in an effort to elevate the eye. As the superior rectus and levator muscles are synergists, equal innervation goes to the levator, resulting in overaction and lid retraction.

LEVATOR SHORTENING
The levator muscle can become contracted in the dry phase of dysthyroid eye disease. This may result in impaired lid closure in addition to lid retraction.

PTOSIS OF THE CONTRALATERAL EYE
When there is a moderate degree of unilateral ptosis, an attempt to raise the affected eyelid is accompanied by synergistic overaction of the contralateral levator muscle (Hering's law), leading to lid retraction of the unaffected eye. This can be particularly obvious when the ptosis is on the side of the preferred eye.

MIDBRAIN DISEASE
Lesions in the upper part of the midbrain can cause unilateral or bilateral lid retraction (Collier's sign). This is commonly associated with Parinaud's syndrome.

POSTOPERATIVE LID RETRACTION
Lid retraction can follow:
• Over-liberal ptosis surgery. Lid closure is also likely to be affected.
• Over-liberal recession of the superior rectus muscle. The anatomical connections between this muscle and the upper eyelid result in retraction.

Lower eyelid retraction
Lower eyelid retraction is relatively uncommon and is usually iatrogenic in origin, caused by recession of the inferior rectus muscle without full division of its palpebral attachments.

Abnormal eyelid movement
Marcus Gunn jaw-winking phenomenon
The jaw-winking phenomenon is a congenital condi-tion in which movement of the jaw results in a change in eyelid position. It is nearly always unilateral.

FEATURES
• There is partial ptosis in the primary position.
• The degree of ptosis increases when the mouth is opened and when the jaw is moved, usually to the affected side. The ptosis then decreases on jaw movement to the sound side, when lid retraction is apparent in some cases. In a few patients the converse occurs, with increased ptosis on jaw movement to the sound side. Rapid change in eyelid position occurs on chewing or sucking, and for this reason the anomaly is often detected early in infancy.
• In a minority of patients there is limitation of up-ward movement of the eye on the affected side, resulting in a hypophoria or, more rarely, a hypotropia.

The phenomenon is believed to be due to a congenital misdirection of the nerve supply to the levator muscle (superior division of the third cranial nerve) and the pterygoid muscles (mandibular division of the fifth cranial nerve). Lyness *et al.* (1988) examined the levator palpebrae superioris in 12 patients with Marcus Gunn phenomenon. They considered that the histological appearance of fibre loss with atrophy and hypertrophy of the remaining muscle fibres was compatible with neurogenic atrophy combined with aberrant reinnervation. Similar changes were also found on the clinically normal side, which they suggested might indicate that the causative lesion was located within the central nervous system.

Many patients learn to disguise the wink in time. The severity of the condition varies greatly. If it is marked, Collin (1984) advises bilateral disinsertion of the levator muscles and bilateral brow suspension.

Aberrant regeneration of the third cranial nerve (misdirection syndrome)
The regrowth of nerve fibres may be misdirected following a third nerve palsy, especially if it is due either to trauma or an aneurysm on the circle of Willis. Misdirection causes elevation of the upper eyelid on down-gaze (pseudo-von Graefe's sign), particularly when the eye is adducted, and can also result in anomalous ocular movement and pupil reaction. Misdirection does not occur in diabetic third nerve palsy. The syndrome is described in detail in Chapter 19.

Facial nerve palsy

Upper or lower motor neurone seventh cranial nerve palsy results in failure of lid closure on the affected side, most noticeable when the patient blinks. The eye elevates if Bell's phenomenon is present, exposing the sclera. The loss of orbicularis tone can also result in ectropion.

Orbicularis tone can be assessed by first asking the patient to close his eyes and keep them closed; the examiner then attempts to raise the upper eyelid, comparing the results in each eye. Slight orbicularis weakness can be detected in this way.

Lid-lag

Lid-lag is characterized by failure of the upper eyelid to follow the downward movement of the globe. This condition commonly occurs in patients with dysthyroid eye disease, when it is usually bilateral, possibly asymmetrical. It can also result from levator resection to correct ptosis.

Examination of the eyelids

Eyelid position

The patient should be on eye level with the examiner and should look straight at him. The eyelid positions should be compared. If the relationship of the lid margin to the limbus appears abnormal, or if asymmetry is present, the height of each palpebral fissure should be measured with a ruler. The comparative height of the eyebrows should be observed: brow wrinkling due to overaction of the frontalis muscle should be noted and may indicate the presence of ptosis. The upper eyelid skin crease should be examined and compared in each eye.

Partial ptosis can result in pseudohypertropia or it can be associated with a strabismus, commonly hypotropia. The eye position in the primary position should be noted. A cover test should show whether or not a true strabismus is present in patients with ptosis or lid retraction.

Eyelid movement

Anomalous eyelid movement may be apparent from observation of the patient when taking the history and on examination of ocular movement.

- The eyelids should be observed as the eyes move into the main positions of gaze, looking for abnormalities of ocular movement as well as eyelid movement. It is important not to raise the upper eyelids when testing on down-gaze, at least initially, otherwise anomalies such as lid-lag and misdirection of nerve fibres can be missed.
- Eyelid closure should be tested. This can be impaired even if ptosis or lid retraction are present, particularly if these are mechanical.

Assessment of ptosis

- Initially true ptosis must be differentiated from pseudoptosis. This is usually easily achieved by observation of enophthalmos and retraction of the globe and by cover test to ensure fixation with the suspected eye.
- The examiner must decide whether a patient with a small degree of upper eyelid asymmetry has mild ptosis of one eye or lid retraction in the other eye. Clues may be obtained from other signs. The presence of ptosis can be confirmed by reduction in the upper eyelid skin crease or slight frontalis muscle overaction. Unilateral miosis suggests ptosis due to Horner's syndrome. Patients with lid retraction may also show lid-lag or other signs of thyroid involvement. Ptosis on one side can result in lid retraction on the other side, as described above, but the ptosis in these cases is usually more obvious.
- Asymmetric bilateral ptosis: if bilateral ptosis affects one eye more than the other, as seen, for example, in some patients with myasthenia, it can be mistaken for unilateral ptosis. The additional innervation required by the levator muscle to elevate the more ptotic eyelid goes equally to the levator in the less affected eye, masking the ptosis or even resulting in apparent lid retraction. The ptosis is made apparent either by covering the more affected eye or by holding up the more ptotic lid.
- Levator function: this should be assessed by preventing the action of the frontalis muscle. The patient first closes his eyes and the examiner holds the eyebrow against the frontal bone. This excludes frontalis contraction when the patient opens his eyes: elevation of the upper eyelid is then due to residual action in the levator and Müller's muscles. Levator function can be

measured by recording the amount of movement of the upper eyelid from down-gaze to up-gaze. The degree of levator function is of great importance in planning ptosis surgery.

• Abnormal head posture: elevation of the chin is the common abnormal head posture, adopted to obtain foveal fixation. If the ptosis is unilateral and is associated with limited upward eye movement, there may also be a head tilt to the affected side to maintain binocular single vision. The degree of head posture should be noted and can be recorded photographically. A marked abnormal head posture may be an indication for early ptosis treatment.

• Further observations which can indicate the possible cause of the ptosis are:

1 Variability, especially an increase in the degree of ptosis as testing proceeds, which suggests the possibility of myasthenia, mainly in adult patients although it cannot be ruled out in children. The patient should be asked to sustain up-gaze for approximately 30 s. The levator muscle fatigues if myasthenia is present and the ptosis will increase.

2 Variable ptosis in a child, which can be part of the Marcus Gunn jaw-winking phenomenon. It is advisable to ask the child to open his mouth wide or give him a sweet to suck to note if the ptosis is influenced by jaw movement.

Assessment of lid retraction

The examiner should note:

• The relationship of the upper eyelid margin to the limbus when the eye is in the primary position.

• The ocular movements, particularly elevation of the eye, observing any change in lid position.

• Lid closure.

Eye position

Interpupillary distance (IPD)

The normal IPD averages 60–65 mm in adult females and 65–70 mm in adult males. An abnormally narrow or wide IPD can result in pseudoesotropia and pseudoexotropia, respectively. Patients with esotropia or esophoria quite often have a narrow IPD, and those with exotropia or exophoria commonly have a wide IPD. The IPD is pathologically wide in some abnormalities of the facial skeleton, for example hypertelorism.

Anomalies of globe position

Displacement of the globe within the orbit can be considered under two headings.

Axial

An axial anomaly is when the eye is displaced forwards or backwards along the line of the anterior-posterior axis. Proptosis (or exophthalmos) results if the globe is pushed forwards, as in dysthyroid eye disease and in some intraconal tumours. Enophthalmos results if the globe sinks back into the orbit, as in orbital floor fractures and some sclerosing orbital tumours, for example metastases from certain carcinomas of the breast.

Nonaxial

A nonaxial anomaly is when the globe is displaced horizontally and/or vertically by tumours arising outside the muscle cone or by trauma; for example, vertical displacement can occur in large orbital fractures in addition to enophthalmos. Binocular single vision may be retained, although there is usually an obvious pseudostrabismus, or a true squint can be present. True and pseudo-strabismus must be differentiated during the examination.

Measurement

Anterior-posterior position

This is measured using an exophthalmometer, an instrument which indicates the position of the cornea with reference to the lateral orbital margin and records the displacement in millimetres. For accurate results the patient should be seated directly opposite the examiner and on eye level with him. To measure the position of the right eye, the left eye should be occluded and the patient should fixate on the examiner's left eye. The procedure is reversed to measure the position of the left eye.

Horizontal position

The distance between the root of the nose in the

mid-line and the centre of each cornea is measured in millimetres using a horizontally held ruler. This method is used for each eye in turn; it does not distinguish between medial displacement of one eye and lateral displacement of the other eye, but clinical features usually indicate the abnormal side.

Vertical position

The vertical position of the two eyes is compared by holding a ruler horizontally across the face so that it is tangential to the inferior corneal margin of one eye. This will show any difference in the vertical position of the eyes, which can be measured using a second ruler held vertically.

When measuring nonaxial displacement the examiner must be on eye level with the patient, who must be looking straight ahead.

Assessment of ocular deviation and ocular movement

Ocular deviation

Preliminary inspection should include comparison of the corneal reflections in the two eyes as the patient fixates a light source at 33 cm. Manifest strabismus measuring 15 Δ or more should be apparent from displacement of the reflection in the squinting eye. A cover test should be used at near and distance to detect the deviation and differentiate manifest and latent strabismus. The prism cover test is the preferred routine method of measurement in suitable cases. Detailed information can be found in Chapter 5.

Ocular movement

Versions should be assessed by asking the patient to follow a moving target, usually a spotlight, from the primary position to the limit of each of the other eight positions of gaze. The movement of the two eyes should be compared and underaction and overaction noted. An alternate cover test should be used to confirm the findings: if ocular movement is limited, there will be an increase in the angle of deviation in the relevant position of gaze. Ductions should be compared with versions: there may be some improvement in excursion on duction if the limitation is due to a neurogenic palsy, but duction and version will be comparable if the cause is mechanical restriction.

The investigation of ocular movement is discussed in Chapter 6.

Examination of the eye

Anterior segment

The patient's pupillary responses, cornea, iris and lens should be examined. Opacities in the media can be detected by observing the red reflex with a direct ophthalmoscope, but detailed examination of the anterior segment requires the use of a slit-lamp microscope. If an anterior segment abnormality is suspected in a young child unable to cooperate with this method, the examination should be carried out under general anaesthesia using the operating microscope. The examiner should look for any defect which could explain reduced vision and should also ensure that there are no other unrelated abnormalities which require treatment.

Pupils

The pupils should first be examined for size and shape.

Normal pupil

The normal pupil is round and its size is the same in each eye, varying according to age. The pupil in infants and very young children is small and does not dilate well. In older children it is highly mobile and varies in size, depending on light intensity and accommodation. The pupil in elderly subjects is often small (senile miosis), making it difficult to assess the light response. The size can be affected by drugs, either those instilled into the conjunctival sac or systemic drugs such as the opiates, which can cause miosis. Both pupils normally constrict simultaneously and equally when light is shone into one eye. A direct reflex occurs in the eye stimulated by the light and a consensual reflex occurs in the unstimulated eye. Both pupils constrict to an accommodative stimulus as part of the near reflex.

Pupil abnormalities
ANISOCORIA

Anisocoria is present when the pupils are of different size. This abnormality can be congenital or acquired.

Congenital anisocoria is quite common and is of no significance provided each pupil responds equally well to a light stimulus. If the light response is abnormal, both congenital and acquired anisocoria can be of considerable clinical importance. Problems sometimes arise in deciding which pupil is abnormal.

MONOCULAR MYDRIASIS
There are several causes of monocular mydriasis.
• Third cranial nerve palsy: the parasympathetic nerve supply to the pupil is carried from the Edinger–Westphal nucleus by the third nerve and may be disrupted in acquired palsies. The pupil is dilated and responds poorly, if at all, to direct or consensual light stimulation. Accommodation is also paralysed or reduced and the near reflex is absent.
• Holmes–Adie tonic pupil: damage to the parasympathetic nerve supply in the ciliary ganglion results in mydriasis and a slow vermiform, or worm-like, response to light, which is the result of sectorial loss of sphincter function. Once the pupil has constricted, it is very slow to dilate again in the dark. Accommodation is also reduced and there is a very slow pupil response to a near stimulus. The sphincter muscle is unusually responsive to weak miotics, due to denervation sensitivity. An acetylcholine analogue such as metacholine chloride can be used to confirm the diagnosis if it is in doubt. Miosis results from instillation of the drug, which would not affect a fixed or dilated pupil due to other causes, although there are exceptions to this rule, for example in some third nerve palsies due to preganglionic lesions. In time the pupil may become smaller but the reduced light response remains.
• Acute glaucoma: the typically oval pupil does not constrict in response to light.
• Trauma: traumatic mydriasis is often associated with sphincter rupture and can be permanent in some patients.
• Mydriatic drugs: unintentional application of a mydriatic can cause consternation in a patient who had presumed an old tube of eye ointment might help his conjunctivitis.

MONOCULAR MIOSIS
This can be due to:
• Horner's syndrome: interruption of the sympathetic fibres results in a small pupil which retains its light response. The diagnosis is established by the presence of slight ipsilateral ptosis and possible facial anhidrosis.
• Anterior segment inflammation: any inflammatory disease which causes iris irritation results in miosis.

BILATERAL MIOSIS
This is associated with the following conditions.
• Argyll Robertson pupils: the pupils are small, fixed and sometimes irregular. They do not respond to a light stimulus but usually show constriction on accommodation. The possibility of underlying syphilis must always be considered but there are a number of other causes. Dissociated pupil responses of this type are a feature of Parinaud's syndrome.
• Accommodative and convergence spasm: miosis is characteristic of this condition.

ABNORMAL PUPIL SHAPE
Abnormalities can occur in association with ocular disease. Common examples are acute glaucoma, in which the pupil is oval, and iritis, in which it is small and irregular due to posterior synechiae.

Pupillary reflexes
EXAMINATION
The pupillary light reflex is tested routinely by shining a small spotlight into each eye in turn, holding the light source just below eye level. It is important to direct the light immediately onto the pupil, especially in young children. If a gradual approach is made, the torch can act as an accommodative target, causing bilateral pupil constriction (the near reflex), which may be mistaken for a light reflex. The test should be repeated two or three times for each eye. The observer should note the speed, quality and symmetry of the direct and consensual responses.

The 'swinging flashlight' test is a more sensitive method. The light is first shone into one eye then rapidly transferred to the other eye and back several times. If there is a partial afferent defect, the pupil of the defective eye will paradoxically dilate as the light is transferred to it, because the direct light reflex is weaker than the consensual reflex (the Marcus Gunn pupillary escape phenomenon). The defect is easily seen as the test is repeated.

The pupil response to accommodation is assessed by presenting a near test type or other detailed target.

ABNORMALITIES OF THE PUPILLARY
LIGHT REFLEX

Abnormalities are caused by lesions affecting either the afferent or efferent pathways.

Afferent pupillary defects

Afferent defects are due to lesions affecting the retina, the optic nerve or the anterior visual pathway, which interrupt or reduce the stimulus reaching the Edinger–Westphal nucleus. As a result, the efferent response from the nucleus to the pupils is correspondingly reduced when the light is shone into the defective eye.

The defect may be complete or partial. If complete, there is no direct or consensual response when light is shone into the defective eye but both pupils constrict normally when the unaffected eye is stimulated. Partial defects, or asymmetrical bilateral defects, can be seen using the swinging flashlight test: the pupil which consistently dilates when stimulated by the light indicates the side of the more defective afferent system.

Efferent pupillary defects

Efferent defects are caused by damage to the parasympathetic nerve supply to the pupil, which is carried in the third nerve from the Edinger–Westphal nucleus to the ciliary ganglion, then via the short ciliary nerves to the sphincter muscle. Both the direct and consensual responses are reduced or lost in the affected eye. Examples of unilateral efferent defects are third cranial nerve palsy, the Holmes–Adie tonic pupil and direct sphincter damage. A bilateral efferent defect is present in Argyll Robertson pupils and in rare cases of bilateral third nerve palsy.

The findings in afferent and efferent pupillary defects are summarized in Table 2.1.

PUPILLARY RESPONSES IN CORTICAL
BLINDNESS

The pupillary light reflex is a subcortical reflex. The pupillary fibres leave the optic tract before reaching the lateral geniculate nuclei. Consequently, even complete bilateral destruction of the cortical pathways posterior to this area will permit normal pupil responses in a blind patient.

Table 2.1 Afferent and efferent pupillary defects (left eye affected).

	Pupillary responses	
	Left eye light stimulus	Right eye light stimulus
Afferent		
Left eye	Defective	Defective
Right eye	Normal	Normal
Efferent		
Left eye	Defective	Normal
Right eye	Defective	Normal

Cornea

The cornea should be examined for size, shape, clarity and sensitivity.

Size

The normal corneal diameter is 11 mm. This measurement remains constant after early infancy and is an indicator of the size of the eye. Abnormalities comprise:

• Microphthalmos, in which the corneal diameter is reduced. This is often associated with other ocular disorders dating from early embryonic life. Examples include congenital cataract and persistence of the primary vitreous.

• An enlarged cornea, which may be an isolated developmental defect (megalocornea) but is more commonly an indication of infantile glaucoma (buphthalmos). The principal signs of buphthalmos are:

1 raised intraocular pressure;
2 corneal oedema, leading to loss of vision;
3 photophobia;
4 splits in Descemet's membrane due to corneal stretching;
5 drainage angle abnormalities;
6 optic disc cupping.

In addition there is a high incidence of refractive errors, usually myopia or myopic astigmatism, and strabismus (Clothier *et al.* 1979).

Shape

The most serious abnormality of shape is keratoconus, in which the cornea becomes progressively conical, leading to irregular astigmatism and gradual visual loss. Vision can be improved in mild cases by a hard contact lens but a corneal graft is indicated when the cone becomes too steep to fit a lens or if central corneal oedema develops.

Clarity

Corneal clarity can be lost due to inflammatory disease, injury or dystrophy. Congenital or early onset opacification can cause severe stimulus-deprivation amblyopia. Corneal clouding is seen in the mucopolysaccharidoses, for example Hurler's syndrome, but these conditions are usually fatal.

Sensitivity

The corneal sensitivity should be tested routinely. Reduced corneal sensation is an important localizing sign of neurological disease, particularly in orbital apex or cavernous sinus lesions. It is also important to test sensitivity in conditions in which the cornea is at risk, particularly when there is corneal exposure, as in Bell's palsy. The combination of exposure and reduced sensitivity greatly increases the risk of corneal ulceration.

Iris

The main iris abnormalities are detailed below.

Aniridia

Congenital absence of the iris can be associated with buphthalmos. In some children malignant kidney tumours (nephroblastoma) can occur.

Coloboma

Congenital sectorial absence of the inferior iris may be isolated or can be associated with coloboma of the choroid and optic disc; vision will be reduced if the macula is involved.

Albinism

Abnormal iris translucency is a diagnostic sign of albinism. It is best seen by observing the undilated iris with retroillumination. Albinism is commonly associated with congenital nystagmus, when vision is likely to be poor.

Heterochromia

A difference in pigmentation, and therefore in the colour of the irides, dating from infancy is usually of no significance although it can occur in congenital Horner's syndrome. If heterochromia is acquired, heterochromic cyclitis is the most common cause: the paler iris is abnormal and keratic precipitates are present.

Lens

Cataract

Lens opacities are one of the commonest problems in ophthalmology. The examiner should assess the type of cataract, the extent to which it has developed and its effect on the patient's vision. Cataract can be congenital or acquired, affecting both eyes or only one.

CONGENITAL CATARACT

The effect of congenital or very early onset cataract on visual acuity depends on the degree of lens opacity. In some types, for example lamellar cataract, vision can be 6/12 or even better, improving still further if the lens has to be removed later. However, if the opacity is dense, severe stimulus-deprivation amblyopia can develop and can be irreversible unless adequate treatment is given in the first weeks of life. Even then the prognosis is guarded, especially in uniocular cataract. Strabismus is common, particularly when both eyes are not equally affected. Nystagmus can develop in untreated, severe bilateral cataract, adversely affecting the outlook. The management of congenital cataract with amblyopia is further discussed in Chapter 10.

ACQUIRED CATARACT IN ADULTS

The examiner should ensure as far as possible that there is no other ocular problem which could adversely affect the outcome of cataract extraction. Any contributory medical cause for the cataract, for example diabetes, should be investigated and treated. The examiner should note the presence of a strabismus, probably an exotropia in an adult patient, which can develop in uniocular cataract that has been present for some months. The exotropia may prevent the restoration of binocular single vision after cataract surgery and can result in diplopia, requiring conservative or surgical treatment.

Cataract extraction with lens implant is indicated in all suitable cases if there is a significant visual problem.

Intraocular pressure (IOP)

IOP should be recorded routinely in patients aged 40 years or more as a screening procedure for glaucoma, irrespective of the reason for presentation. It is recognized that a rise in pressure occurs when ocular movement is mechanically restricted, so that care must be taken to distinguish a false rise (due to restriction) from glaucoma. If the inferior rectus is tight, for example, as it is in some patients with dysthyroid eye disease, even elevating the eye to the primary position in order to measure IOP can cause a rise. The use of duction tensions to differentiate mechanical restriction of ocular movement from neurogenic palsy is described in Chapter 19.

Posterior segment

Fundus

The fundi should be carefully examined in stages, and the following sequence is proposed:

- optic disc;
- macula;
- blood vessels;
- central and peripheral retina.

Examination

Dilation of the pupil for detailed examination of the fundus is mandatory. Either the direct or indirect ophthalmoscope can be used.

DIRECT OPHTHALMOSCOPY

This provides a magnified, erect virtual image of the fundus. Magnification depends on the patient's refractive error, being greater in hypermetropia and less in myopia. Magnification in the emmetrope is $\times 15$, which permits a detailed examination of the fundus but with a small field of view.

INDIRECT OPHTHALMOSCOPY

This gives an inverted image, with less magnification than direct ophthalmoscopy. The field of view is larger and stereoscopic vision results from the use of both eyes. Magnification depends on the strength of the condensing lens, being $\times 2$ with a 30 DS lens and $\times 4$ with a 15 DS lens. The stronger the lens the less the magnification but the larger the field of view. When examining children the illumination should be kept to a minimum to allow tolerance. This method is ideal for examining the peripheral fundus and is the most common method used when assessing infants.

In addition, high-powered lenses can be used in conjunction with the slit lamp, mainly for detailed examination of the disc and macula:

- Volk lens: this is usually a hand-held +90 DS lens which produces a magnified, inverted image of the fundus that the examiner can view stereoscopically. Considerable cooperation is required to maintain a clear view, making this technique unsuitable for very young children. This is the method of choice wherever possible.
- Hruby lens: a strong concave lens gives a very highly magnified image but with a small field of view. This lens is attached to the slit lamp.

Optic disc

The normal disc is pink in colour and slightly oval in shape, with its long axis vertical. The normal disc diameter is 1.5 mm. The disc appears larger in myopia and smaller in hypermetropia when viewed with the direct ophthalmoscope. The oval appearance is exaggerated in astigmatism. The disc margins are usually well defined, but in high degrees of hypermetropia the crowded disc can simulate papilloedema. The disc should be examined for size, colour and swelling or cupping.

ABNORMALITIES
Size

The disc is abnormally small and has a double outline in optic nerve hypoplasia, in which a reduced number of normal optic nerve fibres pass through the optic nerve head. Hypoplasia can be unilateral or bilateral. Except in gross cases, the disc size is not a useful guide in predicting potential visual acuity. Vision can be surprisingly normal in some children while others have only perception of light. Because optic nerve hypoplasia can be associated with midline cortical abnormalities, including septo-optic dysplasia, the advice of a paediatrician should be sought.

Colour

Although the normal disc is pink, there is a considerable degree of individual variation. The disc appears pale in the neonate, and this can be mistaken for optic atrophy. A true atrophic disc is pale or even white, with sharply defined edges, unless the atrophy is secondary to papilloedema.

Swelling (papilloedema)

Swelling can result from:

* raised intracranial pressure;
* raised intraorbital pressure;
* embarrassment of venous drainage, such as central retinal vein occlusion;
* anteriorly sited inflammatory optic nerve lesions (retrobulbar neuritis).

Papilloedema due to raised intracranial pressure is not usually associated with significant vision loss unless the oedema is chronic or the underlying lesion directly affects the visual system. Conversely, profound loss of vision follows retinal vein occlusion or compressive, inflammatory or ischaemic neuropathy.

Children with hydrocephalus may have repeated episodes of raised intracranial pressure due to recurrent valve obstruction, resulting in chronic papilloedema, which leads to optic atrophy. Disc gliosis occurs in optic atrophy and prevents further swelling, therefore in these cases optic atrophy without papilloedema does not exclude raised intracranial pressure, which may cause further loss of vision. Sixth nerve palsy is relatively common in hydrocephalus and results in a persistent esotropia. This may be the only sign of raised pressure and is an indication for immediate treatment.

Cupping

The disc has a physiological cup, with a cup to disc ratio ranging from 0.3 to 0.7. The cup is increased in glaucoma with concomitant loss of visual field and eventual loss of visual acuity. Coloboma results in a large but nonprogressive cup, which may be associated with a static field defect.

Retinal vessels

Common abnormalities of the retinal vessels are:

* Arteriolar sclerosis, usually as a consequence of old age or hypertension. The arterioles appear silvery, and nipping of the veins occurs in hypertension: if it is severe, exudates and even papilloedema may be seen.
* Variation in the calibre of the veins, which is an early sign of diabetes. Later signs include microaneurysms, microinfarcts (cottonwool spots), exudates and haemorrhages. New vessels are seen in the proliferative stage. Hypertension and diabetes are common causes of neurogenic oculomotor palsies therefore these signs can indicate the aetiology of palsy.
* Neovascularization, particularly in the temporal periphery. This sign is characteristic of retinopathy of prematurity (retrolental fibroplasia). Fibrosis causes shrinkage of the temporal retina with traction on the retinal vessels, causing them to straighten. Lateral displacement of the macula follows and gives rise to a marked positive angle kappa and pseudoexotropia. A true strabismus may also be present.
* Diminution in arteriolar diameter occurs in the advanced stage of pigmentary retinal degeneration.

Central and peripheral retina

In examining the central and peripheral retina, the following signs should be noted:

* Abnormal pallor, seen in albinism and in some types of chorioretinal degeneration. It may be difficult to differentiate the normal pallor of the infant fundus from albinism, but iris transillumination defects provide supporting evidence. The retina is pale and swollen in the acute stage of retinal artery occlusion.
* Abnormal pigmentation, which is seen in pigmentary retinal degeneration, may be associated with ocular myopathy (Kearns–Sayre–Daroff syndrome). The more common retinitis pigmentosa causes loss of peripheral field before loss of central acuity. In contrast, the retina may appear normal despite the severe vision loss associated with congenital retinal blindness (Leber's amaurosis): later in childhood atypical retinitis pigmentosa changes may develop in the equatorial and peripheral retina, usually lacking the classical 'bone corpuscle' appearance.

Rubella retinopathy results in a 'moth-eaten' appearance with fine patchy hyperpigmentation and depigmentation of the retinal pigment epithelium. Vision may not be affected unless the condition is complicated by a secondary disciform maculopathy.

Macula

The macula lies some 3 mm, or two disc diameters, temporal to the disc. The normal foveolar light reflex is not always present in infants, sometimes making it difficult to detect subtle macular abnormalities. Macular dystrophies can affect children and young adults. Macular degeneration is a common cause of vision loss in the elderly. Macular scarring, often bilateral, can result from toxoplasmosis acquired *in utero*. Chorioretinal coloboma may involve the macula.

Additional investigations

Refraction

Cycloplegia is essential for accurate refraction of children, otherwise full correction of the refractive error may not be achieved. It is also indicated in older patients, mainly teenage children and young adults, when it is apparent to the refractionist that accommodation is not completely relaxed or when vision cannot be improved to 6/6 in an apparently healthy eye. Refraction is discussed in Chapter 3.

Further investigation of visual function

Visual fields should be recorded in all patients with suspected neurological disease, head trauma or raised IOP. Colour vision should be tested routinely in those with retinal and optic nerve disease or unexplained low vision. Further discussion of these investigations and contrast sensitivity testing can be found in Chapter 4.

Binocular function

Binocular function comprises retinal correspondence, suppression, sensory and motor fusion and stereopsis. Sufficient information on these components of binocular vision can be gained in many patients from the basic examination already described. Further investigation is indicated when this is not the case, mainly in:

• Constant strabismus—it must be stressed that binocular function cannot be deduced from the alleged age at onset;
• Constant diplopia, to assess if fusion is possible;
• Patients requesting cosmetic strabismus surgery, who are at risk of postoperative diplopia;
• Those with symptom-producing heterophoria, to assess the strength of motor fusion.

The methods used are described in Chapter 7.

Medical, laboratory and radiological investigations

In the context of this book, these investigations are indicated mainly in patients with acquired defects of ocular movement that could be due to systemic or neurological disease. Further investigation may also be advisable when there is a sudden onset of esotropia in a child: a diagnosis of sixth nerve palsy should always be considered, especially if the child is more than 5 years old, when concomitant strabismus is less likely to occur.

References

Boutros, G.S. & Al-Mateen, M. (1995) Non-ophthalmological causes of torticollis. *American Orthoptic Journal* 45, 68–73.

Clothier, C.M., Rice, N.S.C., Dobinson, P. & Wakefield, E. (1979) Amblyopia in congenital glaucoma. *Transactions of the Ophthalmological Society of the United Kingdom* 99, 427–431.

Collin, J.R.O. (1984) *A Manual of Systematic Eyelid Surgery*. Churchill Livingstone, Edinburgh, p. 70.

Lyness, R.W., Collin, J.R., Alexander, R.A. & Garner, A. (1988) Histological appearances of the levator palpebrae superioris in the Marcus Gunn phenomenon. *British Journal of Ophthalmology* 72, 104–109.

Urrets-Zavalia, A., Solares-Zamora, J. & Olmos, H.R. (1961) Anthropological studies on the nature of cyclovertical squint. *British Journal of Ophthalmology* 45, 578–596.

3
Refraction

Refractive errors play an important role in the aetiology of nonparalytic strabismus, and accurate correction of these errors is an essential part of strabismus management.

Refractive state of the eye in infancy

Cook and Glasscock (1951) recorded the cycloplegic refraction of 1000 newborn infants and found that 25% were myopic although only to a small degree; the mean refraction was 2.5 dioptre sphere (DS) of hypermetropia, which gradually decreased with normal development of the eye. Studies using photorefraction have similarly revealed a common incidence of myopia and also of astigmatism among normal infants. Atkinson *et al.* (1984), using cycloplegia, reported 4.5% myopia, mainly of low degree, in a study of 1096 infants aged from 6 to 9 months. Howland *et al.* (1978) reported astigmatism in excess of 0.75 dioptre (D) in 50% of 6-month-old infants, over 2 DS being present in 12%. Astigmatism decreased spontaneously with growth until the incidence at 18–24 months equalled that of

the adult population. Ingram *et al.* (1986) reviewed the refraction of a large series of children aged 1 year and found an incidence of hypermetropia of > 4.00 DS in 2.4% of the population screened, but only 0.27% had more than 4.00 DS myopia. They suggest that the subsequent development of amblyopia was directly related to the degree of hypermetropia.

Factors influencing the unaccommodated refractive state

Refraction depends upon:
- the dioptric power of the cornea;
- the dioptric power of the crystalline lens;
- the axial length of the eye.
    Ametropia results from the incorrect correlation of these three elements.

Population studies

Each of the three factors follows a normal (binomial) distribution in the population. If each component of refraction had a random association with the other two, the total refraction of the eye would then also follow a binomial population distribution. However, this is not the case, as there is a marked excess around emmetropia, indicating that the three refractive elements do not vary from one to the other in a random fashion but tend to correlate, excessive axial length being associated with less marked curvature of the lens and cornea, so that potential refractive errors cancel each other out. High degrees of axial hypermetropia and myopia are, however, in excess of expectations and lie well outside the physiological processes.

Genetic factors

Sorsby *et al.* (1962) studied the three components of refraction in unselected cases of like-sexed dizygotic twins. They found a high degree of concordance, both in the total refraction and in its three components in monozygotic twins, but not in dizygotic pairs or in selected control pairs. These findings indicate that the controlling influences determining ocular refraction are strongly genetic in nature.

Environmental factors

There is some evidence that refraction is influenced by environmental factors, probably related to the clarity of visual input. Experiments have shown that the axial length of the eye increases and myopia develops in young animals deprived of pattern vision (Raviola & Wiesel 1978; Wallman *et al.* 1978). The application of animal studies to humans was questioned by von Noorden and Lewis (1987). They studied 10 patients with unilateral dense congenital cataracts in otherwise normal eyes, and two patients with congenital complete unilateral ptosis. Axial length was measured with biometry. The majority of patients showed an increase of axial length of the affected eye compared with the normal eye, but in three patients with congenital cataract, the affected eye was shorter or the same length as the normal eye. Both the patients with unilateral ptosis had a smaller eye on the side of the ptosis. However, a high incidence of myopia was reported in the affected eye in congenital third cranial nerve palsies with complete ptosis (Hoyt *et al.* 1981). Astigmatism can also be associated with congenital

ptosis, probably caused by the pressure of the drooping eyelid on the cornea.

It is recognized that myopia is especially common in prematurely born infants.

Excessive reading in later childhood has been postulated as a cause of acquired myopia, possibly because prolonged accommodation can raise intra-ocular pressure, which in turn induces axial lengthening. There is as yet no widely accepted scientific confirmation of this.

Methods of refraction

Refraction can be assessed objectively or subjectively. The aim is to assess the unaccommodated refractive state of the eye.

Objective methods

Retinoscopy

A streak retinoscope is preferable as the width and orientation of the linear beam can be changed to facilitate assessment of astigmatism. Other apparatus required consists of:
- a lens trial case;
- trial frames for adults and children;
- a disc occluder.

Principle

The test is carried out in a darkened room. A linear light source is reflected from the retinoscope mirror onto the subject's eye, where it is refracted and reflected back to the examiner. The light beam is moved across the subject's pupil, and the examiner deduces the nature of the refractive error from the direction and extent of movement of the streak in different meridia. A lens is interposed and the lens strength adjusted until movement of the streak is neutralized, when the refractive error can be calculated.

Precautions

Various precautions should be taken when assessing refraction by retinoscopy.
- Accommodation must be excluded; a cycloplegic drug is needed in young children and even in some older children and young adults in order to abolish ciliary muscle tone and establish the total static

Table 3.1 Amount to be subtracted from retinoscopy findings to take into account the working distance.

Working distance (m)	Dioptres to be subtracted
1.00	1.00
0.75	1.33
0.66	1.50
0.50	2.00

refraction. A dilated pupil facilitates refraction by increasing the length of the streak. Adult patients and most older children can simply be asked to fixate a distant target. To assess axial refraction the patient should look directly at the retinoscope light; even infants will usually do so as there is no other object of interest.

• A correctly centred trial frame facilitates refraction. If a young child will not tolerate the frame a lens rack or hand-held lenses can be used instead.

• The light beam should fall on the optic axis of the eye so that the reflection comes from the posterior pole. If the beam enters the eye obliquely, off-axis retinoscopy results in overestimation of hypermetropia, underestimation of myopia and spurious indications of astigmatism.

• In order to make a true assessment of the refractive error, the optical principles of retinoscopy require that the dioptric equivalent of the refractionist's working distance is subtracted from the strength of the lens which neutralizes the movement of the retinoscope streak. This amount is the reciprocal of the working distance in metres (Table 3.1). The distance is usually less than 1.

• Once the movement of the streak is neutralized, the accuracy of refraction can be checked, first by decreasing the distance between the mirror and the eye, when the streak (using a plane mirror system) should move 'with' the movement of the light beam, then by increasing the distance, when the movement should reverse to become 'against' the beam movement.

Special problems of refraction of infants and young children

Infants and young children present certain special challenges for retinoscopic assessment of refraction.

• Cooperation—the ability of the child to fix on the retinoscopy light for a long enough period is the main problem encountered. Infants should be refracted at a time when they are quiet (usually after feeding). Children over 9 months of age are more difficult to refract than younger children. A range of audible and mobile small toys may help to induce fixation. If refraction and ophthalmoscopic examination prove impossible, sedation can be used or the child examined under general anaesthesia, although the latter increases the difficulty of obtaining an on-axis refraction and should be avoided if possible.

• If the lenses used have to be held by hand rather than inserted in a trial frame, the refractionist must gauge the cylinder axis by eye.

• If there is a manifest strabismus, the other eye must be occluded to ensure that the squinting eye is fixing. Eccentric or wandering fixation or gross restriction of ocular movement make accurate refraction difficult in patients of any age.

Drugs used in refraction

Anticholinergic drugs abolish the action of the ciliary muscle and the sphincter pupillae; the resultant dilated pupil also allows a thorough examination of the posterior segment of the eye. The two drugs in common use are cyclopentolate and atropine.

Cyclopentolate

This is dispensed as a hydrochloride salt solution in concentrations of 0.5–2%: the 0.5% strength produces insufficient cycloplegia and the 2% strength is not widely available, so the drug is most often used in 1% strength. The drops should be instilled 2–3 times over a 30 min period: maximum cycloplegia is obtained in approximately 1 h in Caucasian subjects; the effects last for approximately 24 h. Cycloplegia takes considerably longer to become fully established in dark-skinned races. An added advantage of cyclopentolate is that it can be instilled by a trained person in the clinic or consulting room. This is the drug of choice in the majority of cases and is effective provided retinoscopy is timed to coincide with its maximum action.

Atropine

Atropine sulphate 0.5% or 1% is used in the form of drops or ointment, which should be instilled twice daily for three days to produce complete cycloplegia. Drops are easier to use than ointment, especially by an untrained person, because they enter the conjunctival sac as soon as the eye is opened, even if deposited at the medial canthus. The drug is more slowly released in ointment form. Atropine ointment 0.5% may be preferred in infants. Unless at least 2 h have elapsed since the last application of ointment, the smeared cornea makes retinoscopy difficult. The effect of atropine on the ciliary muscle lasts for up to 10 days and the effect on the pupil can last for 14 days.

SIDE-EFFECTS

Atropine irritation
Atropine quite commonly causes a contact dermatitis affecting the eyelids and surrounding skin.

Atropine poisoning
Systemic toxic effects, mainly flushing, fever and restlessness, are less common but can occur, especially in the very young child. Some children suffer night terrors.

Any adverse effects should be recorded in the patient's notes and the future use of atropine should be avoided.

INDICATIONS FOR USE
Although atropine is the only agent guaranteed to produce total cycloplegia, its long action, the problems of instillation and its possible side-effects contraindicate its use unless it is considered essential. The routine use of atropine is to be deprecated as a screening procedure. It may be necessary in heavily pigmented irides when cyclopentolate is often ineffective.

Keratometry
Principle
Keratometry is based on the fact that the anterior surface of the cornea acts as a convex mirror as well as a refracting interface. The size of the reflected image of an object of known size is proportional to the radius of curvature of the cornea.

Method
The subject fixates a target and the observer examines the corneal reflections of illuminated 'mires' through a built-in telescope. The positions of the 'mires' can be adjusted until their reflections overlap, giving the radius of curvature and dioptric power of the cornea in that meridian. The arc can be rotated so that the curvatures in all meridia can be calculated. The greatest and least curvatures are found in meridia at right angles to each other when regular astigmatism is present. In an irregular astigmatism there is no such simple relationship and the curvature varies in a random fashion in a number of different meridia.

Value
Only corneal astigmatism is assessed by this method. Problems arise because young children will not always fixate steadily on the target. Although widely used in continental Europe the method is of limited value and is mainly used in contact-lens practice and for assessing the required power of a lens implant for cataract surgery. This is done in conjunction with measurement of the axial length of the eye with ultrasound. Various formulae are available to compute the desired lens power based on the keratometry and axial length.

Photorefraction
Photorefraction is a technique in which the light from a camera flash is changed by the optics of the eye and reflected back from the retina to form a blur circle. The circle can be seen superimposed on the cornea. The refractive error is determined from the size and shape of the blur circle.

Photorefraction was developed by Howland and Howland (1974), using an orthogonal photorefractor which photographed the eyes through a segmented cylindrical lens. This apparatus was adapted by Howland *et al.* (1979) to produce the isotropic on-axis photorefractor. Kaakinen (1979) developed a different photographic technique employing off-axis photorefraction, using a flash placed a measured distance above the camera. This has since been adapted to use two flashes (Kaakinen *et al.* 1987). Both on-axis and off-axis photorefractors photograph both eyes simultaneously.

Method
The apparatus uses a standard 35 mm single lens reflex camera with a wide-aperture lens.

ON-AXIS (ISOTROPIC) PHOTOREFRACTION

The subject is placed so that his eyes are 75 mm from the camera, on eye level with it. He must look directly at the camera and the photographer must be directly behind the apparatus.

Three photographs are taken with the camera focused at different distances:

- at 75 cm with the eyes in focus;
- at 150 and 50 cm with the eyes out of focus.

Blur circles result from the two defocused photographs, which are examined for size and shape. In hypermetropia the blur circle is smaller than the circle from an emmetropic eye, in myopia it is larger and in astigmatism it is elliptical, with the long axis of the ellipse coincident with the more defocused axis of the astigmatism. The circles are compared with each other and with a computerized prediction of the circle for a given refractive error.

Results

Atkinson *et al.* (1984) reported that infants aged 6–9 months could be screened satisfactorily by this method. Thirty infants could be tested in 3 h by two examiners working together. Cycloplegia was used. Hypermetropia averaged 1–4 DS less than the retinoscopy findings. Astigmatism could be detected and its axis identified. Errors were most likely to occur in high degrees of refractive error, in which the blur is very pronounced.

OFF-AXIS PHOTOREFRACTION (KAAKINEN'S METHOD)

The apparatus is used at 1 m distance, taking the same precautions as in on-axis testing. It was designed for use without cycloplegia. This method produces a red reflex as well as a light reflex, allowing assessment of media clarity. A crescent-shaped light reflex is seen adjacent to the pupillary margin. In hypermetropia the crescent lies above the pupil and in myopia it lies below the pupil. The size of the crescent increases with the degree of refractive error. If one flash is used a reflex is produced only in one axis and astigmatism cannot be measured. The use of two flashes was introduced to remedy this defect. Hsu-Winges *et al.* (1989) modified a commercially available Polaroid camera as an off-axis photoretinoscope. The system compared favourably with other systems and had the advantage of immediate production of the photograph for assessment while the patient was present in the clinic.

Results

Day and Norcia (1988) found that the off-axis method was simple and quicker to use but less accurate than on-axis photorefraction. They reported that variable accommodation caused problems with both types of photorefraction. Cycloplegia increased accuracy. It was found that the quality of the photographs was affected by variation in retinal pigmentation and that eccentric fixation could be a source of error. They considered that photorefraction has considerable potential as a screening method but not until the many problems have been solved.

Autorefraction

Autorefractors have been developed with a view to reducing the time spent by clinicians on refraction. They are of two main types: subjective autorefractors and objective autorefractors.

Subjective autorefraction

The patient is presented with a target and manipulates the lens system until he achieves the combination of lenses which gives the best view of the target. Subjective autorefractors range from the basic concept of the double pinhole disc developed by Scheiner in the 17th century, to the more complex systems based on combinations of astigmatic lenses. More recently Alvarez variable-power lenses have been used.

Subjective autorefraction is complemented by objective autorefraction and this technique is now mainly used in clinical practice.

Objective autorefraction

Objective autorefraction is based on the use of infrared light, which is shone into the eye and reflected back through the optical system. The instrument registers the change in infrared light and can compute the degree and nature of any defect in the optical system of the eye.

A review by Wood (1987) showed reasonable correlation between infrared autorefraction and conventional techniques in straightforward refractive errors.

However, autorefraction could be less accurate in high refractive errors and the data could be invalidated by opacities in the media, commonly found in ophthalmic patients. In Wood's clinical study 25% of patients were found to be unsuitable for autorefraction. The main causes of failure were high refractive errors, astigmatism exceeding 2 D, intraocular lens implants, media opacities and macular pathology.

Refraction as a screening procedure

Cycloplegic refraction at 1 year of age was found to be an effective screening method for potential or existing amblyopia and strabismus by Ingram *et al.* (1979), who reported a significant correlation between 2.5 DS or more of hypermetropia in one or more meridia of either eye diagnosed at 1 year and the eventual identification of amblyopia and/or strabismus. Hypermetropic astigmatism was a common cause of amblyopia in this study. Ingram (1977) earlier reported that 72.3% of some 200 children with esotropia and/or amblyopia had 2 DS or more of spherical hypermetropia in the more ametropic eye or had 1 D or more of spherical or cylindrical anisometropia. He found these factors to be more statistically significant than a family history of strabismus or 'lazy eye'.

Subjective methods

Subjective refraction is used with cooperative patients to verify the findings of objective refraction and to find the best possible optical correction for distance and near vision in terms both of vision and comfort. When a cycloplegic retinoscopy has been carried out, subjective verification must wait until all the effects of the cycloplegic agent have worn off. This subjective verification is commonly referred to as a postmydriatic test (PMT).

Method

The lenses, which fully neutralize the patient's refractive error by objective refraction, are first inserted in the trial frames. Each eye is tested in turn and small adjustments in lens strength or axis are made until the best possible distance vision has been achieved. A Jackson cross-cylinder is especially useful for the subjective verification of cylindrical power and axis. It is advisable to retest the patient with both eyes open and the optimum lenses in place to ensure that he remains comfortable, and to test for reading at the patient's normal reading distance.

Correction of refractive errors

Prescription of spectacles

Certain basic concepts must be considered in relation to each type of refractive error before prescribing spectacles.

Hypermetropia

Traditionally hypermetropia has been subdivided as follows:

- Absolute hypermetropia, which is the amount which cannot be overcome by accommodation. It is assessed by the strength of the weakest convex lens that gives the best level of visual acuity.
- Manifest hypermetropia, which is the amount present when all accommodation is relaxed. It is assessed by the strongest convex lens that gives the same level of visual acuity.
- Facultative hypermetropia, which is the difference between the absolute and the manifest hypermetropia, and so is the amount which can be overcome by accommodation. It is proportional to the amplitude of accommodation and therefore reduces with age.
- Total hypermetropia, which is the hypermetropia diagnosed by using complete cycloplegia.
- Latent hypermetropia, which is the difference between total and manifest hypermetropia, accounted for by the resting tone of the ciliary muscle and amounting to approximately 1 DS.

This classification is now largely considered historical. Patients are regarded as having an overall amount of hypermetropia which becomes more manifest with the loss of accommodation and the onset of presbyopia.

Correction of hypermetropia

Discussion has ranged widely over the past few years as to whether latent hypermetropia, as revealed by cycloplegia, is an entity. Subtraction of 0.5 DS for cyclopentolate or 1 DS for atropine is now considered unnecessary, since the patient should be able to relax his accommodation sufficiently to accept the lenses.

• In accommodative esotropia it is sensible to pre-scribe the maximum power convex lenses which can be tolerated and still give the patient optimum dis-tance vision. If hypermetropia is overcorrected or if the patient is unable to accept the lenses the resulting reduction in vision can be a barrier to fusion and can lead to noncompliance with spectacle wear. The daily instillation of 1% atropine in both eyes may result in better acceptance but is not always successful.
• In exotropia or exophoria moderate or low degrees of hypermetropia can be undercorrected.

Myopia

The weakest concave lens which gives the best cor-rected visual acuity is the measure of the amount of myopia. If the strength of the concave lens is increased the patient can accommodate to overcome the induced hypermetropia and will continue to see the same-sized type clearly until sufficient accommodation can no longer be exerted. There is therefore the risk of over-correcting myopia on subjective testing in patients with good amplitudes of accommodation. Overcorrection can be avoided by the use of a duochrome test and by preventing young patients from looking too intently at the vision chart for a long period.

Correction of myopia

The weakest concave spherical lens giving good dis-tance vision should be prescribed. Myopia should never be overcorrected because this may cause either a latent or manifest esodeviation.

GUIDELINES
• Myopia should be fully corrected in exodeviations, with the precautions described above.
• Patients with esotropia or esophoria should be undercorrected if possible, depending on the amount of myopia and on their tolerance of less good visual acuity.
• Whether small amounts of myopia (up to 1 DS) should be corrected depends very much on the indi-vidual patient, who may or may not tolerate the slight reduction in unaided vision.

Astigmatism

Astigmatism is caused by defects in the curvature of the cornea (corneal astigmatism) and/or of the lens (lenticular astigmatism). It occurs when the radii of curvature of these refracting surfaces differ in various meridia. When the meridia with the least and the greatest curvatures are at right angles to each other, the astigmatism is regular; when there is no such sim-ple relationship the astigmatism is irregular. Astig-matism is commonly seen in infancy (Howland *et al.* 1978) but often resolves spontaneously with growth. Most astigmatic refractive errors are regular, bilateral and fairly symmetrical. They may appear as an iso-lated feature (simple astigmatism) or associated with a spherical refractive error (compound myopic, com-pound hypermetropic or mixed astigmatism).

Irregular corneal astigmatism is usually patholo-gical from distortion of the cornea as a result of scar-ring. Regular corneal or lenticular astigmatism can be fully optically corrected by cylindrical spectacle lenses. Hard contact lenses will correct regular or irregular corneal astigmatism but not lenticular astigmatism.

Correction of regular astigmatism

Subjective refraction provides a means of verifying the axis and strength of the cylinder but it does not neces-sarily indicate the strength of cylinder which should be prescribed.

GUIDELINES
• Adults should be prescribed the strength of cylinder with which they achieve a good level of comfortable visual acuity, even if the cylinder prescribed is signific-antly less than that shown on the retinoscopy.
• Patients with uncorrected astigmatism can some-times achieve reasonable unaided vision along one axis by accommodating and it may take some time before they relax their accommodation and achieve optimum visual acuity when wearing the correction.
• If the patient already has comfortable vision with a cylindrical correction, the axis of the cylinder should not be changed.
• Significant astigmatism should be fully and accur-ately corrected as early as possible in children, since uncorrected astigmatism, or even undercorrected as-tigmatism, can cause meridional amblyopia in one or both eyes, particularly when it is oblique. It is accepted that astigmatism of 1 D or more should be corrected in children over the age of 12 months.

Anisometropia

The examiner should first assess the correction for each eye which gives the best acuity but should then test the patient binocularly, noting:
• The presence of diplopia and whether this is due to an image size difference (aniseikonia) or to a manifest strabismus with the correction.
• The binocular visual acuity for near and distance.
• The patient's binocular function. Unless diplopia is present it is usually sufficient to assess this aspect using stereoacuity tests. The patient may have a significantly better response with the correction than he has without it and will therefore find the prescription of lenses beneficial.

Depending on the findings, it may be necessary to modify the correction, especially in older children and adults who have not previously worn spectacles.

Correction of anisometropia

The principal factors that influence the optical correction of anisometropia are aniseikonia and amblyopia.

GUIDELINES
• Anisometropia should be fully corrected in children in order to prevent or treat anisometropic amblyopia.
• Older children and adults may be unable to tolerate a full correction binocularly and the optical correction of the more ametropic eye may need to be reduced, even if optimum visual acuity is not achieved.
• Large differences in refraction may need correction with contact lenses, which should be considered if:
  1 insuperable aniseikonia is present, when contact lenses should reduce the difference in image size: unilateral aphakia is the classic example of this; in favourable cases binocular single vision can be restored with contact lenses;
  2 there is failure to improve the visual acuity in anisometropic amblyopia in children with a difference in refraction of over 4 DS;
  3 there is significantly better binocular function with trial contact lenses than there is with spectacles.
• Patients with a moderate or marked amount of anisometropic myopia may show a hypophoria in the primary position with a head tilt to the side of the more myopic eye, which helps them to maintain comfortable binocular single vision (the 'heavy eye' phenomenon, Bagshaw 1968).

Table 3.2 Changes in accommodation with increasing age in normal Caucasian subjects.

Age (years)	Amplitude of accommodation (DS)
12	12
32	8
45	3
60	1

Presbyopia

Although this condition is physiological and not a refractive error it is convenient to consider it here. The amplitude of accommodation in normal subjects reduces steadily with age, as is shown in Table 3.2. When it is insufficient for the subject's needs, presbyopia occurs. Typical presbyopia usually develops between 40 and 50 years of age, but there are considerable individual variations, partly dictated by the subject's race and by his occupation and particular needs and also by his refractive error. Presbyopia is corrected by convex lenses for use at near distances, assessed at near refraction.

Near refraction

Correction of presbyopia is assessed subjectively: the subjective distance correction should be placed in trial frames; the patient's probable reading addition, deduced from his age, is added; and he is asked to read a near-vision chart with both eyes open in good illumination. If the distance vision is normal the reading correction should be adjusted until he can read N5 (J2) comfortably at his preferred reading distance.

An alternative method of assessing the near refraction is to correct each eye separately, using a near point rule, adding convex lenses to bring the near point to about 28 cm for normal use, adjusting the strength and distance for the patient's special needs. This method does not reveal the patient's normal reading distance and is less well related to normal conditions, making it unsatisfactory.

GUIDELINES
• The patient should be asked details of his working distance and the correction should be modified accordingly. If necessary he should be prescribed two

pairs of near glasses, one for working distance and the other for a normal reading distance—this could apply, for example, to musicians requiring glasses to read music.

• Once the best near correction is obtained, each eye should be checked separately to ensure that the optimum distance is the same in each eye, otherwise the patient is unlikely to be comfortable.

• Although 33 cm is considered a normal reading distance, many patients read with the print held 5–10 cm further from the eyes; the print should remain clear over a range of a few centimetres nearer and further away from the eyes to either side of the preferred distance.

• If too strong a reading correction is given the patient will find it inconvenient to hold reading matter so close to his eyes: if his convergence is not good, symptoms can result from convergence insufficiency, or this condition may be induced by the lack of need for accommodation.

Correction of presbyopia with associated refractive errors

HYPERMETROPIA

Hypermetropic patients may not require a distance correction while most or all of their error remains facultative. Presbyopic symptoms occur earlier in such cases; initially the patient may be comfortable when reading if only the distance correction is prescribed.

MYOPIA

Patients with a low degree of myopia can read clearly by removing their distance corrections and, depending on the degree of myopia, may continue to do so well into old age.

Aphakia

Aphakia follows treatment for congenital or acquired cataract. It may result from traumatic or spontaneous dislocation of the lens and when a penetrating injury has ruptured the lens capsule in patients whose lens matter is soft enough to be absorbed. It may be unilateral or bilateral.

Unilateral aphakia

Several problems are caused by unilateral aphakia.

• Insuperable aniseikonia of around 20–25% if aphakia is corrected by a spectacle lens (Mills 1979), making this form of treatment impractical.

• A manifest strabismus, usually exotropia in older patients and esotropia in young children, if the cataract or uncorrected aphakia persists for some time.

• Stimulus deprivation amblyopia, possibly with added strabismic amblyopia, is probable in patients with aphakia following surgery in congenital cataract or when aphakia is acquired in childhood. Suppression of the image of the aphakic eye occurs easily in children and is sometimes seen in adults. Both amblyopia and suppression are adverse factors in the prognosis for development or restoration of binocular single vision.

CORRECTION OF UNILATERAL APHAKIA

The correction of unilateral aphakia must be achieved with the smallest possible increase in image size: this can be obtained by the use of an intraocular lens implant or by a contact lens, which should be prescribed as soon as possible after the eye becomes aphakic in order to give the best chance of good visual acuity and binocular single vision. The correction of aphakia using contact lenses in infancy is referred to below. With older children and adults a trial contact lens can be fitted in order to diagnose the presence of a manifest strabismus and to evaluate the patient's binocular vision. Should binocular vision be present, then the possibility of a secondary intraocular lens implant should be considered. It is sometimes difficult to demonstrate convincing fusion of images even when the history is favourable, and the examiner should use his discretion in interpreting the results of this investigation. It is often worth prescribing a permanent contact lens in such cases: some patients are even able to control an exotropia once a properly fitted lens is worn. However, a few patients are seen who appear to have no ability to fuse images although normal binocular single vision had been present before the onset of cataract (Pratt-Johnson & Tillson 1989). Treatment for amblyopia and for a manifest strabismus may be required in children.

Near correction

A near correction of a +2.5 or +3 DS will be required for the aphakic eye if it is to be used for close work.

Bilateral aphakia

Bilateral aphakia can be corrected with spectacle lenses, although there are considerable problems with aberrations and with weight unless plastic lenses are worn: contact lenses overcome these difficulties, as do intraocular lens implants, which have now superseded the other methods of correcting aphakia in adults. Discretion is required in the use of intraocular lenses in children.

PROBLEMS
• If spectacles are prescribed they must be correctly centred and accurately fitted; even a slight displacement can result in diplopia as well as adversely affecting vision.
• Patients with bilateral aphakia sometimes have problems in converging; decentration to produce base-in prism effect may therefore be indicated in reading spectacles.

Near correction
Spheres of +2.50 or +3 DS will be required in both eyes whichever method of correcting the aphakia is used. Bifocal glasses are indicated for children and are also often preferred by adults.

Low vision aids for defective near vision

The magnifying effect of a very strong reading correction can often improve near vision in adult patients of all ages with organically determined visual defects, especially when there are relative central scotomata due to macular or optic nerve disease. Reading matter or detailed objects must be held very close to the eyes when wearing the spectacles, causing severe eye strain or diplopia unless the convergence effort required is compensated by strong base-in prisms. It may be preferable to place a strong reading lens in front of only the better seeing eye, using occlusion on the other spectacle lens. When only one eye is used, a reading correction of up to +10 DS can often be tolerated. Children with defective vision from organic causes gain better vision by holding print very close to the eyes, but because they have such good accommodation they do not often find magnifying lenses helpful. They may be helped by Galilean telescopes.

Association between refractive errors and ocular motility disorders

Uncorrected refractive errors can affect: visual acuity; the development and maintenance of binocular single vision; and the compensation and decompensation of a heterophoria.

Visual acuity
Amblyopia results directly from:
• anisometropia, when one eye sees best at all distances (anisometropic amblyopia);
• high degrees of ametropia (ametropic amblyopia).

In both instances the uncorrected refractive error results in a defocused foveal image. When astigmatism is present, the image in the more ametropic meridian is more blurred, leading to meridional amblyopia. If there is a high degree of anisometropia, the differences in image size and quality constitute severe obstacles to the development and maintenance of binocular single vision and a manifest strabismus may develop in the more ametropic eye, when strabismic amblyopia can further compound the visual loss. Compatible images allow the maintenance of binocular single vision in ametropic amblyopia.

Binocular single vision
When a significant degree of spherical refractive error is present, the development and maintenance of binocular single vision is affected by a disturbance in the accommodation–convergence relationship. In anisometropia the main factor is the difference in image size, which can lead to a manifest strabismus as described above.

Accommodation-convergence relationship
Each chapter of accommodation initiates a convergence response which is referred to as the AC/A ratio which is further described in Chapter 5. This can be affected by hypermetropia or myopia.

Hypermetropia
The influence of hypermetropia depends on its degree:
• Subjects with hypermetropia of less than 2 Δ usually succeed in maintaining binocular single vision unless there is a high AC/A ratio, when an esotropia may develop.

• Subjects with moderate degrees, ranging from +2.5 to +6 DS, can accommodate to see clearly, but because each dioptre of accommodation is normally accompanied by 4–6 DS of convergence, overconvergence will occur (accommodative esotropia) unless the two functions can be dissociated, allowing clear single vision. Accommodative esotropia may be fully controlled once the refractive error is fully corrected, or partially controlled, when the angle of deviation is reduced but a manifest strabismus remains (esotropia with an accommodative element, also known as partially accommodative esotropia).

• Patients with high degrees of hypermetropia (+6.5 DS upwards) usually maintain blurred binocular single vision as they cannot sustain sufficient accommodation to see clearly. The defocused images may result in ametropic amblyopia.

Myopia

The influence of myopia depends largely on whether it is present at birth or is acquired during later childhood.

• High degrees of myopia present at birth can lead to esotropia with onset in early childhood. The infant's far-point lies very close to his eyes and he must view objects at this distance in order to use his optimum visual acuity. Convergence develops so that binocular single vision can be maintained at this distance, but because vision at more remote distances is so poor, convergence is not relaxed on looking further away and in time a constant esotropia is present, with and without the myopia corrected. However, marked esotropia sometimes develops in adult life and it is unlikely that this simple explanation is sufficient to account for the deviation in all cases—other unexplained factors must be involved (see Chapter 12).

• The age at onset of acquired myopia is usually from 10 years upwards: at this age the accommodation–convergence relationship is well established, so that when the patient requires less accommodation to see clearly at a near distance he also converges less, leading to a convergence insufficiency or to an intermittent exotropia of the convergence weakness type (near esotropia). Correction of the myopia is usually sufficient to compensate for the deviation.

Decompensation of heterophoria

Uncorrected refractive errors are a common cause of decompensation of heterophoria. In other cases correction of the error is the decompensating factor.

• Uncorrected errors: hypermetropia will decompensate esophoria and acquired myopia will decompensate exophoria.

• Correction of refractive errors: correction of hypermetropia can decompensate exophoria and correction of myopia can decompensate esophoria.

Modification of spectacle prescription in cases of strabismus

When prescribing spectacles the examiner should consider the type of strabismus and whether the management can be helped by overcorrection or undercorrection of spherical refractive errors. Modification of the correction is mainly considered for functional reasons, for example to promote control of an intermittent deviation.

Principle

The principle of modifying the correction is to relax accommodation to allow the fusional reflex to control an esodeviation, or to exert accommodation to allow it to control an exodeviation. Whether overcorrection or undercorrection is possible and the amount by which the correction can be modified is governed by:

• The strength of the refractive error: the higher this is the less the opportunity to increase or decrease the correction.

• The visual acuity: reduction in visual acuity of one line is tolerable to most patients but more than this is usually unacceptable. Tolerance depends on individual needs: older children require good vision for their school work, and adults need clear distance vision for driving and for many occupations, so that any modification is usually confined to young children.

Hypermetropia

If full correction of hypermetropia does not restore binocular single vision a small overcorrection can be considered, either for all distances or for near work in the form of bifocal spectacles (see below). Undercorrection is not advisable if hypermetropia exceeds +4 DS, as problems may arise from later nonacceptance of spectacles or from overaccommodation. A reduction in lens strength to reduce the angle of deviation in an unsightly consecutive exotropia is contraindicated unless the correction is low and has a disproportionate effect on the strabismus, as can happen if the AC/A ratio is high. The patient will almost certainly require his correction again as he becomes older, and in any case the exotropia is likely to increase, therefore it is preferable to prescribe the optimum correction for visual acuity and comfort and to treat the deviation surgically when the patient's appearance warrants it.

Myopia

Myopia presents more of a problem: undercorrection cannot be achieved without reduction in visual acuity. Overcorrection or minus lenses can be used in the treatment of exotropia. Patients with esotropia or esophoria must be given a correction which results in a reasonable level of vision: 6/9 is usually the minimum which patients with potential 6/5 vision will accept. Low myopes should be encouraged to wear their spectacles as little as possible; bifocal spectacles should be considered for those with esotropia of the convergence excess type, at least until the myopia is stable.

These factors are further discussed in Chapters 12 and 16.

Dispensing spectacles

It is essential that spectacle frames are well fitted and accurately centred and that they are comfortable to wear. It is also important that the spectacles are attractive since the main reason why children (and some adults) will not wear them is that they are teased or feel themselves to be unattractive in their spectacles.

Children's spectacles
Infants

Most infants will wear comfortably fitting spectacles, especially when they produce a marked improvement in vision. Spectacles are best attached to the child using straight side-pieces with an elasticated restrainer that passes round the occiput. This ensures a good fit and prevents the child from snatching off the spectacles in the early stages of wear. The side-pieces should be hinged low down on the frames to fit the infant's low ear position. Separate nose-pads are best avoided; a low-placed, built-up nose-bridge is preferable. Large-aperture lenses should be used in frames which fit the infant's facial contours and are centred for his eye positions; these features differ markedly from those of older children.

Infants' spectacles are rarely attractive and the parents must be motivated to accept that the importance of optical treatment outweighs the short-term cosmetic defect. They should be assured that more attractive spectacles will be dispensed as the child grows older.

Older children

For safety, lenses should be made of toughened material. Plastic lenses scratch easily but must be considered to reduce the weight of spectacles correcting aphakia and other high degrees of ametropia. Curled metal ear-pieces should be avoided as they can cause serious skin irritation.

Bifocal lenses for children

Bifocals are indicated in the following circumstances:
• in aphakia;
• as low vision aids;
• in the treatment of selected cases of accommodative esotropia with convergence excess (see Chapter 12).

The aim is that the reading segments should always be used for near vision, necessitating that they are large and set high. Straight-topped bifocals, known as the 'executive' type, are best fitted so that the top of the reading segment passes just below the middle of the pupil when the eye is in the primary position.

Effects of ill-fitting spectacles

Ill-fitting spectacles influence:
• the patient's willingness to wear the spectacles;
• the muscle balance when binocular single vision is present;
• the visual acuity.

Optical effects
Decentration of lenses

A prismatic effect is induced when the optical centre of the lens and the visual axis are not coincident. The prismatic effect is proportional to the amount of decentration and the power of the lens. Decentration results in:

• reduced visual acuity with high-powered lenses;
• symptoms if a significant heterophoria is induced or an existing heterophoria is increased: vertical decentration is most likely to cause discomfort;
• decompensation of binocular single vision in childhood, or even in adults if the lenses are very strong, as in aphakic spectacles, resulting in a manifest deviation and diplopia.

Tilting of spectacle frames

If the frames are twisted round an anteroposterior axis, vertical decentration results and cylindrical axes will be displaced. If extreme, the subject may look through the distance segment of one bifocal lens and the reading segment of the other. Decentration can cause vertical diplopia and a change in cylinder axis will reduce visual acuity and may induce symptoms of eyestrain.

Tilting of the lenses

Tilting in relation to the plane of the face causes astigmatism of oblique pencils, an aberration leading to reduced visual acuity.

Lenses too far from or too near to the eyes

The distance from the cornea changes the effectiveness and magnification of the lenses. The effects of small changes in lens position are most marked with very strong lenses and can cause considerable problems for patients with aphakic spectacles.

Reading segment defects

If bifocal reading segments are set too low, the patient has difficulty in looking down far enough to make use of them and is disturbed by the sudden refractive change at the top edge of the reading segment. Such a patient tends to adopt a compensatory head posture of chin elevation. If the segments are set too high, the patient has problems in looking through the distance correction and so tends to adopt an uncomfortable chin-down compensatory head posture.

Twisting of a lens within the frame

This is likely to occur only with circular lenses not fitted with a lens lock. It causes incorrect alignment of a cylinder axis, with consequent loss of visual acuity, eyestrain or pseudocyclophoria.

The optical effects of ill-fitting spectacles are more serious in children as binocular single vision is more easily decompensated and visual acuity can be adversely affected, causing or perpetuating amblyopia.

Cosmetic effects

Too wide or too narrow frames can give rise to a pseudostrabismus or increase or decrease the apparent size of a true strabismus.

Contact lenses

Contact lenses used for optical correction are of two main types, hard and soft.

Hard contact lenses

The diameter of most hard contact lenses is slightly less than that of the cornea. These lenses cannot be worn for more than 16 out of 24 h without causing corneal oedema and risking the development of peripheral corneal vascularization (pannus) in the long term. The advantages of hard lenses are:
• the optical effect of the anterior corneal surface is fully abolished, so that the lenses can be used to eliminate high degrees of regular and irregular astigmatism;
• ease of sterilization;
• durability.

The principal disadvantage is poor tolerance. Many patients never develop a wear period exceeding 8 h per day. Tolerance is rapidly lost if the lenses are not worn daily. Wear time may be improved if gaseous exchange through the lenses is increased. Lens fenestration and the use of newer gas-permeable lens materials both help in this way.

Soft contact lenses

If these are of fairly low water content (30–40%) they must be removed daily, but if the water content is high (80%) they can be used for extended wear and left *in situ* for periods of days or weeks. The principal advantages are ease of handling and very good tolerance. The disadvantages are:
• inability to correct more than approximately 1 D of astigmatism without special modifications;
• difficulties with sterilization;

- lack of durability;
- corneal vascularization;
- papillary changes in the upper palpebral conjunctiva.

Optical correction using contact lenses

The principal advantages of optical correction using contact lenses rather than spectacles are:
- The small degrees of change in image size, even for high refractive errors (e.g. a contact lens to correct aphakia increases magnification by some 8%, compared with a 20–25% increase using a spectacle lens) (Mills 1979).
- The correction of irregular corneal astigmatism, which cannot be achieved with spectacles.
- The increased field of clear vision obtained through a contact lens compared with a spectacle lens, particularly one of high power, which increases the potential for peripheral fusion.
- Most of the defects of ill-fitting spectacles are avoided.
- The increased safety factor, particularly for sportsmen.
- The cosmetic advantage of contact lenses.

Contact lenses for infants and children under 6 years of age

Contact lenses are used to correct aphakia and high degrees of myopia; they are particularly successful in the correction of unilateral and bilateral aphakia in infancy (Hoyt et al. 1982). They are rarely used for other purposes in this age group.

Principal uses of contact lenses in ocular motility disorders

Aniseikonia

The aniseikonia induced by anisometropia exceeding 6 DS usually prevents the fusion of images when wearing a spectacle correction. Contact lenses are therefore essential if binocular single vision is to be developed and maintained in patients with unilateral high myopia. The use of contact lenses in childhood to correct unilateral hypermetropic astigmatism, the common cause of anisometropic amblyopia, is more problematic but is worth considering in selected cases,

for example if spectacles are not tolerated or if there is failure to improve vision. A significant degree of astigmatism requires a hard contact lens for adequate correction.

Accommodative esotropia

Adults and older children are strongly motivated to avoid continued spectacle wear. The use of contact lenses for full correction of hypermetropia should therefore be encouraged (Calcutt 1984), especially if the patient is not wearing his spectacles all the time, thus affecting his visual acuity and risking decompensation of a fully accommodative esotropia. An accommodative esotropia often requires an increased hypermetropic correction in contact lenses compared with spectacles to control the deviation, at least when the contact lenses are first worn. High-powered convex contact lenses are less well tolerated than similarly powered concave lenses because the central thickness of the convex lens prevents free gaseous exchange.

If the esotropia is only partially accommodative, the strabismus may become more apparent when wearing contact lenses, mainly through loss of the masking effect of spectacles, although the angle of deviation does increase in some cases.

If strabismus surgery is undertaken, a conjunctival fornix incision should be considered, as a limbal excision can impair contact lens wear for a considerable period postoperatively.

Nystagmus

When a contact lens is fitted in a patient with congenital nystagmus the lens moves with the oscillations of the eye, which may result in significant visual improvement. Spectacle lenses are less effective because the optic axis is constantly changing in relation to the plane of the spectacles, resulting in optical aberrations, especially astigmatism of oblique pencils. This factor is more marked if the patient has an obvious compensatory head posture to make use of an eccentric null zone.

Occlusion

Contact lenses providing occlusion have three uses:
- In the treatment of amblyopia: total occlusion can be achieved by using an opaque black contact lens on the normal eye. There is as yet insufficient experience

of this method to permit any critical evaluation of its effectiveness.

• To overcome diplopia: a high-powered contact lens can be used to fog the unwanted image in cases of insuperable diplopia which the patient can neither fuse nor suppress.

• To mask a strabismus associated with a blind and unsightly eye: a painted contact lens may be used to cover a useless eye which has deviated and is cosmetically embarrassing to the patient.

Refractive keratoplasty

The development of computer-controlled laser surgery, photorefractive keratoplasty (PRK), has increased the accuracy of refractive surgery. PRK was first introduced to treat myopia, then later developed for hypermetropia.

Radial keratotomy is a technique used to reduce myopia. The technique involves making multiple radial partial thickness incisions in the corneas which result in a flattening of the corneal curve and reduction in its refractive power. The technique is only suitable for low degrees of myopia and uneven surgery can result in considerable astigmatism.

Epikeratophakia may be used to decrease or increase the refractive power of the patient's cornea to treat myopia or hypermetropia (including aphakia). A donor cornea is shaped to the desired curve using a lathe. The donor button is then sutured to the de-epithelialized surface of the patient's cornea.

References

Atkinson, J., Braddick, O.J. & Atkinson, S. (1984) Photorefractive vision screening of infants. In: *Transactions of the Fifth International Orthoptic Congress, Cannes* (eds A.P. Ravault & M. Lenk), pp. 53–59. LIPS, Lyon.

Bagshaw, J. (1968) Vertical deviations of anisometropia. In: *Transactions of the First International Congress of Orthoptics*, pp. 277–286. Kimpton, London.

Calcutt, C. (1984) The use of contact lenses in the treatment of accommodative esotropia. In: *Transactions of the Fifth International Orthoptic Congress, Cannes* (eds A.P. Ravault & M. Lenk), pp. 311–315. LIPS, Lyon.

Cook, R.C. & Glasscock, R.E. (1951) Refractive and ocular findings in the newborn. *American Journal of Ophthalmology* 34, 1407–1413.

Day, S.H. & Norcia, A.M. (1988) Photographic screening for factors leading to amblyopia. *American Orthoptic Journal* 38, 51–55.

Howland, H.C. & Howland, B. (1974) Photorefraction: a technique for study of refractive state at a distance. *Journal of Optometric Society of America* 64, 240–249.

Howland, H.C., Atkinson, J., Braddick, O. & French, J. (1978) Infant astigmatism measured by photorefraction. *Science* 202, 331–333.

Howland, H.C., Atkinson, J. & Braddick, O. (1979) New method of photographic refraction of the eye. *Journal of the Optical Society of America* 69, 1486.

Hoyt, C.S., Stone, R.D., Fromer, C. & Billson, F.A. (1981) Monocular axial myopia associated with neonatal lid closure in human infants. *American Journal of Ophthalmology* 91, 197–200.

Hoyt, C.S., Jastrebski, G. & Marg, E. (1982) Long-term visual results in bilateral congenital cataracts. *American Journal of Ophthalmology* 93, 615–621.

Hsu-Winges, C., Hamer, R.D., Norcia, A.N., Wessermann, H. & Chan, C. (1989) Polaroid photorefractive screening in infants. *Journal of Pediatric Ophthalmology and Strabismus* 26, 254–260.

Ingram, R.M. (1977) Refraction as a basis for screening children for squint and amblyopia. *British Journal of Ophthalmology* 61, 8–15.

Ingram, R.M., Traynar, M.J., Walker, C. & Wilson, J.M. (1979) Screening for refractive errors at age 1 year: a pilot study. *British Journal of Ophthalmology* 63, 243–250.

Ingram, R.M., Holland, W.W., Walker, C., Wilson, J.M., Arnold, P.E. & Dally, S. (1986) Screening of visual defects in pre-school children. *British Journal of Ophthalmology* 70, 16–21.

Kaakinen, K. (1979) A simple method for screening of children with strabismus, anisometropia or ametropia by simultaneous photography of the corneal and fundus reflexes. *Acta Ophthalmologica* 57, 161–171.

Kaakinen, K.A., Kaseva, H.O. & Teir, H.H. (1987) Two-flash photorefraction in screening of amblyogenic refractive errors. *Ophthalmology* 94, 1031–1042.

Mills, P.V. (1979) Aniseikonia in corrected anisometropia. *British Orthoptic Journal* 36, 36–44.

Noorden, G.K. von & Lewis, R.A. (1987) Axial length in unilateral congenital cataracts and blepharoptosis. *Investigative Ophthalmology and Visual Science* 28, 750–752.

Pratt-Johnson, J.A. & Tillson, G. (1989) Intractable diplopia after vision restoration in unilateral cataract. *American Journal of Ophthalmology* 107, 23–26.

Raviola, E. & Wiesel, T.N. (1978) Effect of dark-rearing on experimental myopia in monkeys. *Investigative Ophthalmology and Visual Science* 17, 485–488.

Sorsby, A., Sheridan, M. & Leary, G.A. (1962) *Refraction and its Components in Twins*. Medical Research Council Special Reports Series, No. 303. HM Stationery Office, London.

Wallman, J., Turkel, J. & Trachtman, J. (1978) Extreme myopia produced by modest change in early visual experience. *Science* **201**, 1249–1251.

Wood, I.C.J. (1987) A review of autorefractors. *Eye* **1**, 529–535.

4
Visual Function

The assessment and measurement of visual function is a fundamental part of the investigation of ocular motility disorders. Further examination and patient management depend to a large extent on the results obtained, particularly on the level of visual acuity and on the state of fixation.

Visual function comprises three parts.

• The *light sense*: the most primitive of the three senses, which is the ability to distinguish between light and dark. It is mediated by the transduction of light into electrical energy in the retinal receptors, and is most acute in the rods of the dark-adapted eye when the rhodopsin has been fully resynthesized. It is maximum in the range 3–8° away from the fovea.

• The *form sense*: the ability to distinguish between spatially separate visual stimuli and to discern the size and shape of objects from the position and orientation of their edges. The form sense is mediated by both the rods and cones but principally by the cones. It is most acute at the fovea, decreasing rapidly in all meridia with distance from the fovea.

• The *colour sense*: the ability to distinguish between light of different wavelengths, mediated by the cones.

Light sense

The light sense is usually recorded as a separate entity only when it is impossible to demonstrate any form vision. It can be assessed in several ways.

• Objectively by observation of the patient's reactions. A baby with light perception will turn his head towards the light source, for example a window, and look towards the source when a fairly bright light is introduced into his visual field. Great care must be taken to avoid auditory clues which may induce a confusing primitive reflex eye movement in the direction of the noise.

• Subjectively in cooperative patients by use of an on-off light stimulus, asking the patient to indicate when he sees the light.

• Electrodiagnostic tests can be used and are discussed at the end of the chapter.

The absolute threshold of light falls by a factor of approximately 10 000 during the 20 min period required for dark adaptation. The adaptation curve can be plotted using a dark adaptometer.

Form sense

The form sense comprises:

• Visual acuity, which consists of:
   1 central vision: the ability to discriminate fine high-contrast detail;
   2 peripheral vision (field of vision).
• Contrast sensitivity: the ability to perceive a less sharply delineated pattern.

Development of the form sense in the normal eye

The development of vision depends to a large extent on normal anatomical and physiological development. Other factors are adequate stimulus, continued use and intelligence.

State of the eye at birth and its subsequent development

The eyes of a full-term infant are relatively well developed compared with its other organs. All ocular tissues are differentiated but the axial length is less than that of the adult eye. The anterior chamber is shallow and the crystalline lens more spherical than it becomes in its adult form. However, these factors have relatively little effect on vision in the neonate; the blur resulting from refractive error and imprecise accommodation only becomes significant when spatial frequency increases. The retina is fully developed except for the fovea centralis. During the first 4 months of life there is an increase in the density of foveal cones and the anterior segment of each cone becomes longer (Yuodelis & Hendrickson 1986).

Postnatal foveal development is believed to contribute substantially to the rapid rise in visual acuity from birth to 6 months of age. Foveal differentiation is complete at 4 months: at this age myelination of the visual pathways and maturation of the cortical synapses are probably also complete. Mohindra *et al.* (1983) have shown that cortical maturation contributes to the early development of visual acuity; they reported that as the vision in one eye decreased, for example due to cataract or occlusion for any purpose, visual acuity in the other eye increased and became abnormally high for the age of the child.

Experimental evidence indicates that completion of anatomical differentiation is paralleled by physiological development. Accommodation reaches adult level at 2–3 months: it is accurate for targets nearer than 75 cm in 50% of newborn infants, reaching 90% accuracy at 20 months of age. The anterior segment continues growth until 16 years.

Visual acuity

Measurement of visual acuity is now possible in children under 1 year of age, using visually evoked potentials (VEP), optokinetic nystagmus (OKN) and, particularly, preferential looking techniques. The results have shown that visual acuity at birth is approximately 6/240 (20/900). The level rises rapidly in the first 6 months, followed by a somewhat slower rate of improvement from 6 to 12 months (Table 4.1). The rate of improvement is consistent whichever

Table 4.1 The development of visual acuity from birth to 3 years.

Age	Visual acuity
Newborn	6/240
1 month	6/180–6/90
4–6 months	6/18–6/6
3 years	6/6*

* Tested with single optotypes.

method of measurement is used but the visual acuity attained varies, VEP recording significantly higher levels than OKN or preferential looking methods (Atkinson & Braddick 1981; Fulton *et al.* 1981). Although VEP recording has suggested that 6/6 visual acuity is reached at 6 months it is generally accepted that this level is not attained until 2 years (Held 1988). Both central and peripheral acuities are poor at 1 month of age but the acuity decreases with increasing eccentricity. By 3 months of age acuity achieved in the temporal field is significantly higher than it is in the nasal field—this has been attributed to the corresponding anatomical asymmetries within the visual system, whereby cone density is higher in nasal retina and the cone to ganglion cell ratio is lower (Courage & Adams 1996).

Visual field

Simple tests of an infant's refixation on visually interesting targets introduced into the peripheral visual field suggest that peripheral vision is restricted in all quadrants. However, this is more likely to be due to functional and perceptual factors than to an anatomical or physiological defect.

Contrast sensitivity

At birth contrast sensitivity is approximately 1/30th of its eventual level (Held 1988). Like visual acuity, it develops rapidly during the first 6 months of life and is believed to achieve adult level at 3 months of age, at least for low spatial frequencies. The sensitive period for visual acuity and contrast sensitivity extends to 8 years of age, correlating with a 25-month period in monkeys (Harwerth *et al.* 1986). Visual depriva-

tion during this period results in loss of visual acuity and in defective contrast sensitivity for high spatial frequencies.

Assessment and measurement of form vision

Visual acuity assessment

In the context of ocular motility disorders, defective visual acuity is most likely to be due to a combination of amblyopia and refractive error, affecting one or both eyes. However, symptomatic (secondary) strabismus is not uncommon and the examiner must be aware of the pathological conditions which may present with an overt ocular deviation. As a preliminary to visual assessment, a history should be taken and the patient examined to detect the presence and type of a manifest strabismus or other features likely to affect vision, such as nystagmus. The preliminary findings, including the patient's refraction and any abnormalities of the media or fundi, give the examiner an indication of the probable visual acuity and influence the approach to visual assessment.

Guidelines for the assessment of visual acuity in young children

• Because cooperation is essential it can be beneficial if one examiner gets to know the child and tests him at each visit.

• Gaining the child's confidence by first performing less intrusive tests, such as the cover test, improves cooperation.

• Tests of resolution rather than visibility should be used whenever possible.

• Linear visual acuity should be tested as soon as possible to provide a more accurate measurement than is obtained with single-letter testing.

• The examiner must ensure that the child understands the test, first teaching him how to do it at a near distance. If necessary, the mother can teach the child at home.

• When testing for the first time it is advisable to start with both eyes open, then to test the fixing or less ametropic eye first to give the child confidence. On subsequent visits the more defective eye should be tested first.

- Uncomfortable occlusion should be avoided. Occlusive glasses such as those provided with the Cambridge crowding card test can be used if occlusion is not tolerated.
- A careful watch should be kept up to guard against peeping round the occluder or looking over spectacles, and to note screwing up of the eyes.
- The mother should be asked the best time to test an infant, when he is not hungry and is likely to be alert.
- A 6 m test distance is preferable to 3 m viewed through a mirror. A 3 m test can give a valid comparison between the two eyes but is not directly comparable to a 6 m test.
- Children tend to 'give up' when the symbols become harder to see; persuasion can lead to a significantly better level. If a symbol is seen easily the child can be encouraged to see the next smaller size by changing the letter or the chart and hinting that the new letter is easier to see.
- The examiner should note the child's mistakes. He may repeatedly get the same letter or symbol wrong, implying that he does not know it, or he may consistently miss or confuse letters in the centre or to one side of a line, suggesting a possible field defect, although a similar finding occurs in some patients with microtropia (see Chapter 15).
- If unexplained low vision is found on uniocular testing, the acuity should be retested with both eyes open.
- The examiner should note an abnormal head posture and if possible should test the visual acuity with and without the head posture.
- Near vision should be tested whenever possible. An accurate comparison with distance vision can be obtained only by testing at 33 cm, but from an educational viewpoint it is important to find out what the child sees at his optimum reading distance. He should be allowed to hold the test material in the position and at the distance at which he sees best.

Visual acuity can be assessed objectively and subjectively. Objective assessment is used when the patient is too young or too uncooperative for subjective testing. Vision may be assessed qualitatively and quantitatively.
- Qualitatively: by estimating the visual acuity from the patient's reactions and from comparison of the behaviour of the two eyes. Most tests used in qualitative assessment record the *minimal visible*, based on the target subtending the smallest angle which elicits a positive visual response; this requires less resolution than the *minimal separable* and this factor must be considered when evaluating the results.
- Quantitatively: giving a more or less precise measurement of visual acuity by assessing the *minimal separable*, requiring the identification of two sharp black edges separated by a white interval of known dimension. Normal Snellen notation vision infers a resolving power of the visual system able to distinguish as separate two edges separated by a visual angle of one minute of arc. In the universally adopted Snellen system used for optotypes, each part of each letter or shape subtends one minute of arc while the whole symbol subtends five minutes of arc at a given distance, ranging from 4 to 60 m.

Whatever the method used, good illumination of all test material is essential.

Qualitative tests of visual acuity

Visual acuity is first estimated objectively by assessing the fixation of each eye and, in the case of young children, by observing visually directed reaching.

Assessment of fixation

The position, steadiness and persistence of fixation is observed. A fixation light should be used initially to note the position of the corneal reflections and in case there is very low vision. The light should be held at eye level at 33 cm distance: it can be switched on and off or moved to attract attention; an older child can be asked to point to the light or to 'blow it out'. A more detailed fixation target should be used to induce accommodation. The most attractive formed target for the very young infant is the human face, especially his mother's. The infant can be held by the mother while the examiner observes his fixation over her shoulder. Brightly coloured mobile or audible targets are suitable for slightly older children. Once interest is obtained an occluder can be introduced in front of one eye, preferably an opaque 'paddle' or card rather than the observer's hand or thumb. Holding the occluder some distance away from the eye is less disturbing to the child. If there is an obvious strabismus it is better to cover the squinting eye first until the child's confidence grows.

The examiner should note the following:
- The position of the corneal reflections with both eyes open and as each eye fixates in turn. The reflection may be normal (central or slightly nasal) or displaced due to:
    1 a positive or negative angle kappa;
    2 eccentric fixation outside the parafoveal area, implying dense amblyopia (the reflection appears within normal limits if the fixation is close to the fovea);
    3 displacement of the macula.
- The presence of strabismus.
- Whether the strabismus is unilateral or alternating in the primary position. The preferred eye on latero-versions should also be observed, as crossed fixation may be present. Dickey and Scott (1987) have reported that crossed fixation does not exclude amblyopia.

It is essential that the behaviour of one eye is compared with that of the other, whether or not a strabismus is present.

Fixation preference in strabismus

The patient's fixation preference is used as a guide to the presence of amblyopia, or potential amblyopia, especially when visual acuity cannot be measured. The results have been graded by Zipf (1976) as follows:
- Alternation in the primary position, no fixation preference: vision equal.
- Fixation held with the squinting eye for at least five seconds on removal of the occluder from the other eye. Fixation maintained through a blink or on ocular movement: little or no amblyopia.
- Fixation held briefly with the squinting eye: probable amblyopia.
- Fixation held momentarily with the squinting eye: amblyopia present.
- Fixation not held: dense amblyopia.

This method of diagnosing amblyopia has been reported as having a high false positive rate in small-angle strabismus, which is virtually always unilateral, but greater reliability in those with large angles of deviation (Zipf 1976). The introduction of a 10 Δ base-up or down prism can facilitate identification of fixation preference in patients without strabismus and small-angle strabismus (Wright *et al.* 1981).

Other factors that must also be considered include:

- The speed with which the eye moves to take up fixation: if movement is slow, poor vision is likely.
- Whether the fixation appears central or eccentric.
- The steadiness of fixation: unsteady fixation denotes low vision in most cases.
- Reaction to occlusion of one eye: if there is consistent objection to having the straight eye covered but tolerance of the cover over the squinting eye, amblyopia is almost certainly present.
- The refractive error should also be considered: a moderate or high degree of anisometropia makes defective vision in the more ametropic eye very probable.

If amblyopia is diagnosed a more detailed examination of fixation is required (see below).

Visually directed reaching

A normal infant develops visually directed reaching between 2 and 5 months of age, when he will begin to reach out to touch or grasp a visually interesting object. This reflex can be used to aid in visual assessment in infants, but it develops even when visual acuity is as low as 3/60 and therefore does not imply good vision. However, careful observation of the behaviour of a poorly sighted child reveals that he moves his hand in an exploratory fashion rather than directly to the object. This test encourages the child to fixate and gives the examiner opportunity to assess the persistence of fixation.

Ability to locate small objects

Very small sweets such as those known as 'hundreds and thousands', commonly used to decorate cakes, can be used to assess near vision.

Method

The mother is first asked to persuade the child to eat some of the sweets. If several sweets are then placed on the examiner's or the mother's hand the child will usually pick them up. Each eye is then tested in turn using one, or preferably two, sweets and the child's reactions are noted.

Results

If the child can locate the sweet and attempts to pick it up, his near vision at 33 cm is 6/24 (20/80) or better. This is confirmed if he comes back for the second sweet. If the child is unable to see the sweet he will straighten his fingers and feel for it: this difference in behaviour is very obvious.

Value

The sweets vary in size and colour and the result cannot be regarded as an accurate measurement. However, the test is simple and very useful for detecting poor vision. It can be used when the child is 15–18 months old, and is invaluable for demonstrating to the parent that there is serious visual defect in one eye.

Dot visual acuity test

This test was devised by Rosenbaum and Kirschen (1984) to measure near vision in young children. It consists of black dots of nine sizes, subtending visual angles ranging from 40 to 1 minutes of arc, equivalent to 6/240–6/6 at the testing distance of 25 cm. The dots are displayed singly or in multiples on a uniform white background and the child is told to touch each dot. This test is probably less easy to use than 'hundreds and thousands', especially in very young children, but it has the advantages that it is standard and quantifies near vision.

Catford drum

Principle

The Catford drum uses oscillating black dots on a white ground, and is based on the principle that a child's attention is drawn to a moving target.

The observer can use the corresponding oscillatory eye movement as confirmation that the child sees the target. The oscillatory movement is generated by the pursuit system.

Apparatus

This consists of a white drum marked around its circumference with black dots corresponding in size to Snellen letters if viewed from a distance of 60 cm. The size of dot ranges from 2/60 to 6/6, printed on two interchangeable drums. The drum is mounted on the spindle of a hand-held reciprocal motor which causes the dot to oscillate horizontally. Each dot is displayed singly in the rectangular aperture of a screen which covers the other dots.

Method

The child is first shown a large-sized dot with both eyes open. It is sometimes easier to obtain fixation if the drum is turned round so that the child sees the dot on the exposed drum surface rather than through the aperture. Once the child's cooperation has been assessed, the drum is held at a distance of 60 cm, one eye is covered and dots of decreasing size are exposed in the aperture until the minimal visible has been estimated. The other eye is then tested.

The distance of the drum and the speed of oscillation can be varied to change the effective target size or to enhance the stimulus, as detailed in the instrument's instruction manual. Attention diminishes at distances beyond 90 cm.

Value

The test is mainly useful in comparing the behaviour of one eye with that of the other. It has been shown to overestimate visual acuity by a factor of four (Atkinson *et al.* 1981). It is likely that a smaller moving target can be seen in comparison with a stationary target of the same size requiring steady fixation. The moving target causes blurring of edges and therefore produces sine-wave rather than square-wave changes in contrast, so that it does not give an accurate measurement of visual acuity.

Hopkisson *et al.* (1991) introduced 'vernier' (offset) targets which can be fixed onto the drum. There are three strips with the offset corresponding to different sizes of Snellen letters ranging from 2/60 to 6/6, at 50 cm. They report a better correlation with Snellen's acuity than has been found using the dot acuity test.

STYCAR system

The STYCAR system was devised by Dr Mary Sheridan for use as Screening Tests for Young Children And Retardates. The system comprises:
- rolling balls test;
- matching miniature toys;
- matching selected letters (see below).

STYCAR rolling balls

PRINCIPLE

The principle of the rolling balls is similar to that of the Catford drum; the moving target attracts the child's attention and the observer notes the following eye movement.

APPARATUS

The test consists of 10 white polystyrene balls, ranging in size from 6 cm to 3.5 mm in diameter, which are used at a testing distance of 3 m. Clear, plain carpeted floor space is required with good illumination, providing a contrasting background against which the balls can be seen.

METHOD

The largest ball is first rolled across the child's field of vision with both eyes uncovered; the examiner notes the child's reaction to assess his cooperation. Each eye is then tested in turn using balls of decreasing size. The size of the smallest ball that elicits a following eye movement gives the measure of visual acuity.

VALUE

The criticisms which apply to the Catford drum also apply to this test: the peripheral stimulus and moving target overestimate visual acuity and partially assess contrast sensitivity. For these reasons, Sheridan (1969) deliberately did not give the Snellen's equivalents of the various ball sizes, but only the expected responses at different ages, based on her results from testing large groups of young, normal children. She reported positive following responses to the 7 mm-diameter ball by 6–9-month-old infants, and to the 3.5 mm-diameter ball from 10 months of age (measurements adapted to the metric system). An advantage of the test is that it enables distance vision to be tested in children too young for illiterate visual acuity tests. It is especially suitable for handicapped children as it does not require locomotor skills. It is more widely used by developmental paediatricians than by ophthalmologists.

The balls can be mounted on black sticks and produced in turn from behind a black screen which hides the observer, who can gauge the subject's fixation response through a slot in the screen. The method is most useful in the assessment of the visual fields.

STYCAR miniature toys

Small, silvered metal or plastic toys, comprising a car, aeroplane, chair, doll, knife, fork and spoon are shown singly to the child at a distance of 3 m against a dark background, after first familiarizing him with the toys at a nearer distance. The child either names the toy or matches it with one he selects from a tray. A child unable to point to or pick up the toy because of physical handicap can indicate that he can see it by looking at it ('eye pointing'), providing that the toys are well spaced out.

VALUE

The test is intended to give an indication of visual acuity. Although the toys are quite large, differentiation of the knife, fork and spoon requires a fairly high standard of visual acuity. The test is most useful with handicapped children and can be used to demonstrate the child's visual potential to the therapists involved in his treatment.

Quantitative tests of visual acuity

Grating acuity

The purest visual acuity test uses a square-wave grating comprising black and white stripes of equal width (Fig. 4.1). An acuity of 6/6 equates to a grating made up of stripes each subtending 1 minute of arc at the testing distance, so that the separation between two black or two white stripes is 1 minute; pairs of stripes must therefore be repeated 30 times to subtend a visual angle of 1 degree. This is termed spatial frequency and is measured in cycles per degree; the narrower the stripes the higher the spatial frequency. The highest frequency grating which elicits a response is the measure of the visual acuity. The correlation between Snellen values, stripe width and spatial frequency is shown in Table 4.2. Grating acuity has been shown to be better than visual acuity based on optotypes, especially when there is foveal pathology or dense amblyopia (Mayer *et al.* 1984). The stripes can be presented electronically on a television screen. The grating principle is used in preferential looking, VEP and OKN to measure visual acuity in infants, very young children, handicapped patients and others unable to cooperate with optotype vision tests.

Vernier acuity

Vernier acuity is defined as the smallest offset of a line which can be detected. It is measured in seconds of arc by presenting a square-wave grating, a section of which is offset by a known amount (Fig. 4.2). The effect is detected by cortical processing. Snellen's principle,

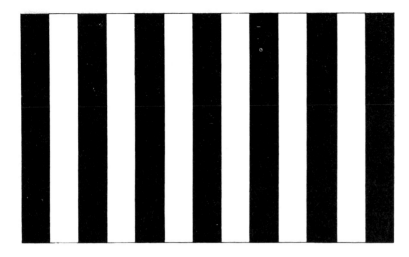

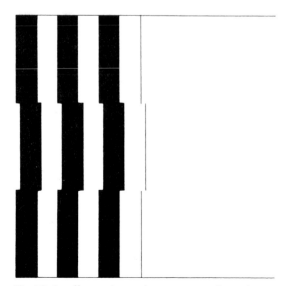

Fig. 4.1 'Square-wave' grating. There are sharp edges to the black stripes so that contrast between light and dark is 100%. This form of grating measures visual acuity thresholds.

Table 4.2 The correlation between Snellen visual acuity measurements, stripe width and spatial frequency.

Snellen		Spatial frequency (cycles per degree)	Stripe width (minutes of arc)
Metres	Feet		
6/6	20/20	30	1
6/12	20/40	15	2
6/30	20/100	6	5
6/60	20/200	3	10

Fig. 4.2 An offset grating used to measure vernier acuity.

based on the separation of foveal cones, does not apply. In consequence vernier acuity exceeds Snellen acuity, an offset measuring as little as 3–5 seconds of arc can be seen by a normal adult. For this reason vernier acuity is described as hyperacuity.

Use

The main value of vernier acuity is presently its contribution to research. It has been used to study the development of the visual system in infants. A preferential looking technique was used, the choice lying between a normal square-wave grating and a second grating of the same spatial frequency containing horizontal displacement of part of it (the vernier offset). If the offset grating was the preferred target the infant was judged to have detected the vernier effect. These studies have shown that vernier acuity is less than grating acuity in infants of 3 months or younger, but then increases until it exceeds grating acuity at 4–5 months. This increase is considered an indicator of the development of a more sophisticated cortical organization, capable of detecting the vernier effect.

Using a similar technique, obliquely orientated gratings, one with an offset section, have revealed that astigmatism in infancy can lead to meridional amblyopia, even though the astigmatism has resolved (Gwiazda et al. 1986).

Preferential looking

Preferential looking is based on the knowlege that an infant prefers to look at a patterned rather than a plain surface (Fantz 1958). When applied to the assessment of visual acuity, preferential looking is a behavioural test in which the subject is offered a choice between a black-and-white grating and a plain area of the same size and equal average luminance. If the child consistently looks at the grating rather than the plain surface he is judged to have resolved the pattern. The criterion for estimating the grating acuity threshold must be well away from chance. The minimum standard acceptable for such psychophysical procedures is 70% correct responses, and 75% correct is the standard often used.

Forced choice preferential looking (FCPL)
(Dobson *et al.* 1978)
The child is held on a parent's knee at a measured distance from a screen. A testing distance of 55 cm (57 cm from the eyes) is convenient because it allows direct conversion of cycles per centimetre to cycles per degree. However, it may be easier to test neonates and very young infants at a nearer distance, for example at 38 cm (40 cm from the eyes).

The screen contains two apertures (or uses two screens at an angle to each other, each containing an aperture); a vertical square-wave grating is displayed in one aperture and a plain surface is displayed in the other. Gratings of different spatial frequencies are changed randomly from one aperture to the other.

The test aims to eliminate observer bias: the observer should be masked as to the location of the grating and its spatial frequency. This observer is situated behind the screen and watches the child's direction of gaze and head movement through a central peephole, so that he can judge which aperture attracts the child's attention (i.e. he makes a forced choice). Another observer, who can see the screen, scores and controls the test. An average of 60 trials is needed and each examination takes a maximum of 30 min. This method has mainly been used for research purposes.

Modifications of forced choice preferential looking
The technique of forced choice preferential looking has been modified in the following ways.
• Diagnostic stripe width method: this is a screening procedure in which one grating compatible with the norm for the child's age is used (Dobson *et al.* 1978).

• Operant preferential looking: a reward system, usually comprising animated toys which appear each time a correct response is recorded, has been introduced to maintain the interest of older children. It can be used with other preferential looking techniques (Mayer & Dobson 1980).

Acuity card procedures
Teller acuity cards
Acuity cards were introduced by Teller *et al.* (1986) to provide a practical means of testing an infant's vision in a clinical situation. A set of 16 cards is available, each with a uniform grey background, containing a square on the right or left side of which is printed a square-wave grating of known spatial frequency (Fig. 4.3). The card is presented to the patient through a rectangular grating. Alternatively, it can be hand-held at a distance of 55 cm from the patient. The position of the grating can be changed by rotating the card through 180°. It is preferable to display the card through two circular apertures which mask its edges (Chandna *et al.* 1988).

Only one observer is needed. Unlike FCPL, the observer is not masked as to the location of the grating and not necessarily to its spatial frequency, since the cards are numbered on the back in ascending order. However, Pearson *et al.* (1989) recommended that a forced choice element is retained, at any rate initially, in order to avoid bias and ensure accuracy. This can be done by shuffling the cards, or having them stacked by another examiner.

Spatial frequency can be changed in octave or half-octave steps, depending on the child's response; for example, the 0.22 and 0.44 cards represent a difference of one octave and the 0.22 and 0.33 cards a difference of half an octave. The results can be expressed in octaves or converted to equivalent Snellen values, minutes of arc or cycles per degree. The testing time by an experienced operator averages 6–10 min.

METHOD OF USE
It is important to establish a routine method which is followed for all infants. A staircase or 'up and down' principle is often used. This involves sequential presentation of gratings in ascending or descending order, presenting each grating a constant number of times, moving up to the next highest frequency if there is a

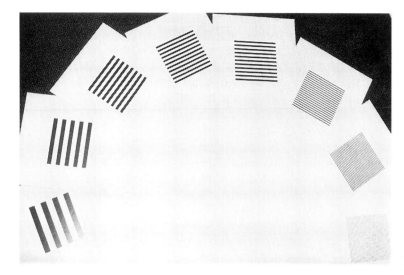

Fig. 4.3 Teller acuity cards.

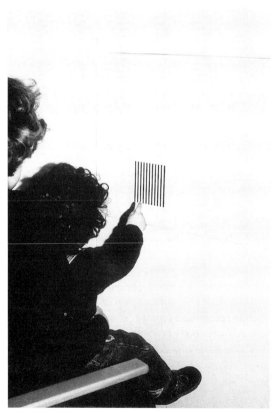

Fig. 4.4 Measurement of visual acuity using Teller acuity cards.

repeatedly correct response or down to the next lowest frequency if the response is consistently incorrect. A long or short staircase can be used; a two-step staircase (two up and one down) is practical in clinical testing.

The child's attention is first drawn to the screen, then a low-octave card is presented to gauge his understanding and response. The subsequent choice of grating is determined by the preliminary findings (history, fundi and media, refraction and the presence of strabismus), starting with a card one or two octaves lower than the expected level of vision. Initially the observer can move up or down the staircase in octave steps but as the acuity threshold is approached, half-octave steps should be used. The exposure time must remain constant. Both correct and incorrect responses for each frequency must be recorded. Two failures with a high-octave card indicate that the grating is probably not seen. If there is a correct response to all cards the acuity threshold is assumed to be an octave higher than the highest spatial frequency card. If there is an incorrect response to all cards, the acuity threshold is assumed to be an octave lower than the lowest frequency card.

If the child loses interest a toy can be introduced into the aperture to regain his interest before retesting. If it is suspected that an older child is guessing, the grating orientation can be changed from vertical to horizontal and the response compared. Older children can be asked to point to the grating (Fig. 4.4).

Vision can be tested with both eyes open or uniocularly. Obviously, it is important to obtain a uniocular response in many conditions, including strabismus, but if, for example, an infant is queried as blind, testing with both eyes open can establish whether or not he can see.

Keeler cards

These cards are printed with a circular grating patch to avoid identification of the grating by its edge (Moseley *et al*. 1988). They also have an 'empty' circle printed on the other side: this leads to a different visual response whereby the infant may look from one circle to the other before a definite fixation preference is made.

Age for using acuity card procedures

The ideal age for acuity card testing is from 8 weeks up to 12 months. The success rate is low in 4–8-week-old infants as ocular movements and head holding is not well enough developed for this method. From 12 to 24 months the infant is more restless and the response is variable. Children over 24 months can be taught to point to the grating and this may retain their interest in the test. These children usually look in the direction in which the grating last appeared and are then seen to change gaze to the new position.

Problems

Various technical problems may arise with acuity card testing.
- Inequality of luminance of the grating and the plain surface, causing the child to look towards the brighter light. Equality of luminance is essential for accuracy. Acuity cards require careful handling to preserve luminance.
- Identification of the grating by its edge, resulting in an artificially high visual acuity. Masking overcomes this difficulty.
- Variation in the speed of looking between individual patients.
- Guessing. This can be detected by retesting, changing the orientation of the grating and simply by experience of using the test.
- Observer bias.
  Clinical problems arise if there is:
- Nystagmus, which may make it difficult to assess

when the patient is looking towards the grating, especially if there is a compensatory head posture. Testing in the vertical plane can be helpful in this situation.
- Ocular motor apraxia (saccadic palsy), making it difficult for the child to look in the intended direction.
- Large visual field defects.
- Large-angle alternating esotropia with crossed fixation, when it can be difficult to know to which side the child is looking when both eyes are open.
- Loss of interest and fatigue.

Value of preferential looking techniques

RESEARCH

Preferential looking techniques have helped to establish the parameters of visual acuity and contrast sensitivity in normal infants (Dobson & Teller 1978; Atkinson *et al*. 1982) and have shown the development of grating acuity. The method has been adapted for the study of colour vision and stereopsis (Teller 1983; Birch *et al*. 1985).

CLINICAL

Preferential looking makes possible the measurement of visual acuity in infants and very young children. Teller acuity cards provide a practical means of using preferential looking which has widespread application.
- Infants with delayed visual maturation, who appear blind when seen before 10–15 weeks of age.
- Monitoring progress of children being treated for congenital cataract and associated deprivation amblyopia.
- Young children with macular disorders, when single optotype vision may overestimate what the child sees.
- Mentally retarded or severely physically handicapped patients (Jenkins *et al*. 1985).
- Early detection of gross amblyopia.

It is recognized that grating acuity overestimates vision when compared with conventional tests which assess recognition acuity. However, preferential looking techniques, particularly acuity card procedures, provide a practical method of measuring and comparing uniocular and binocular visual acuity in infants.

The Cardiff acuity test

This test was designed for the 1–3-year-olds who no longer respond well to gratings but are unable to

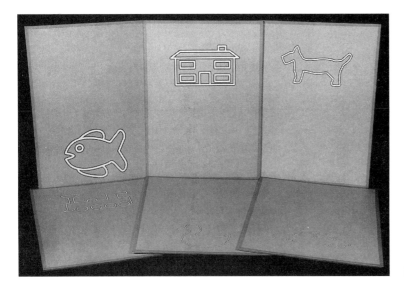

Fig. 4.5 The Cardiff acuity test.

name pictures. The principle of the test is vanishing optotypes: the targets are drawn wih a white band bordered by two black bands, each of half the width of the white band, all on a neutral grey background (Fig. 4.5). If the target lies beyond the subject's acuity limit, it merges with the grey background and becomes invisible. The acuity is given by the narrowest white band for which the target is visible. As with the acuity cards it is based on preferential looking but in this instance the separation is up or down rather than right or left.

Method

The cards are presented at eye level at a distance of 1 m. There are three cards for each acuity and two correct responses are required. The child's eye movements are observed and a judgement is made as to whether the child is fixating up or down; this response is then checked with the card. If an incorrect response is found the test is repeated with the larger target. The response is usually recorded as the Snellen equivalent, although the test is believed to produce acuities more comparable with those of grating acuity.

Value

These cards may be used to compare acuity in each eye but are known to overestimate vision in ambly-

opia (Hazell 1995). The results cannot be taken as an accurate measure of visual acuity and should, therefore, be used in conjunction with assessment of fixation and other clinical tests.

Optokinetic nystagmus (OKN)
Principle

Stripes which move across the field of vision elicit an observable eye movement, comprising a following movement as the subject fixates on one stripe and a rapid movement in the opposite direction to fixate the next stripe (Gorman *et al.* 1957).

Apparatus

The stripes are best presented as optical gratings using black-and-white stripes of equal width. To hold the infant's attention a large part of his visual field must be filled by the stripes: the vertical visual angle subtended should be ideally at least 40°. Stripes can be presented in various ways:

• rotating drum;
• moving stripes in the form of a canopy across the top of the infant's cot;
• electronically generated stripes displayed on a television screen.

An eye movement response indicates that a grating can be seen, the movement can be directly observed or, more accurately, electro-oculography can be used to trace and record eye movement (see below).

Method

The stripes should be vertically positioned and moved horizontally at both slow (3 stripes s^{-1}) and fast (30 stripes s^{-1}) speeds. The slower rate stimulates the smooth pursuit and saccadic systems, while the faster speed appears to involve a more primitive optokinetic system. Stripes of increasing spatial frequency are presented until a frequency is reached which fails to elicit an optokinetic movement. The highest spatial frequency, which produces OKN at a slow speed, is the measure of the visual acuity.

Value

The value of OKN in measuring visual acuity is limited by the problems which arise. When a large part of the visual field is filled by the stripes, peripheral as well as central vision is involved, casting doubt as to the origin of the response. There is evidence that an OKN response can be obtained in the absence of a functioning visual cortex, possibly through the primitive extrageniculostriate system (Berlyne 1958). Because the movement blurs the stripe edges, it is probable that contrast sensitivity is evaluated to some extent in addition to visual acuity. Babies will not always watch the stripes, especially when a hand-held drum is used.

Illiterate visual acuity tests

Illiterate vision tests are based on:
- Matching the letter or symbol with a replica held or indicated by the child. Tests in general use are:
  1 STYCAR letters;
  2 Sheridan–Gardiner test.
  Those less commonly used are:
  3 HOTV test;
  4 Ffook's symbols;
  5 E test;
  6 Sjögren test;
  7 Landolt's broken rings.
- Naming the picture on a chart, although several modern picture charts use a matching technique, including the Allen, Kay and Weiss charts.

Matching tests

STYCAR letters

The letters, which are based on square, circle and triangle shapes—the first to be recognized and copied by young children—are presented in three groups.
- Five letters, VTOHX, for normal children up to and including 3-year-olds.
- Seven letters, adding A and U, for 4-year-old children.
- Nine letters, adding L and C, for older children.

The letters are printed on separate cards or as a standard chart. The child is given a corresponding key card and points to the letter he sees. The test is designed for use at 6 m but can be used at 3 m, when the 6/4 letter approximates to 6/9. A near vision chart is included.

Sheridan–Gardiner test

This test uses the seven-letter STYCAR test and key card (Fig. 4.6). The letters can be viewed singly, using flip-over cards which range from 6/60 to 6/3. A linear chart is also available. Near vision can be tested with single letters, grouped letters or a standard chart.

Value

The test is easily understood by normal 3-year-olds and by some intelligent younger children. The number of letters is sufficient to eliminate guessing and the test is quick and accurate. Its advantages over other illiterate tests make it the method of choice.

HOTV test

This test, which is widely used in the USA, is similar to the Sheridan–Gardiner test but uses only four letters.

Ffook's symbols

This test uses the basic shapes of a square, circle and triangle, presented singly in sizes ranging from 6/60 to 6/6, one on each face of a cube, or as a chart. The child performs the test by picking up or pointing to a black plastic replica of the shape he sees.

E test

Capital letter Es can be presented with the short limbs directed up, down, to left or right as single letters on a

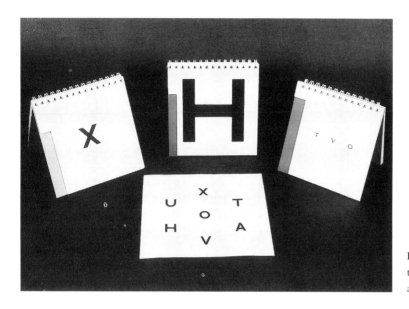

Fig. 4.6 Sheridan–Gardiner vision test: flip-over cards for use at 6 m and 33 cm.

card, on the face of a cube or as a standard chart. The child uses a replica E to copy the position of the limbs, or else indicates it by placing his fingers in the same position.

Value

The limitations of this test are:
• the lack of choice;
• the difficulty many young children have in copying right and left orientation.

Simons (1983) has stated that a three-repetition trial for each letter size reduces the chance of a correct guess to 4%, but this is a time-absorbing procedure, likely to lose the child's attention.

Sjögren hand test

This test presents a black hand with its fingers pointing up, down, to the left or right. The criticisms levelled at the E test also apply to this test, with the added disadvantage that the solid black palm of the hand can give an obvious clue to the position of the fingers.

Landolt's broken rings

This test is an extremely accurate measure of visual acuity which overcomes nearly all the disadvantages inherent in other methods (Tippings 1996), but children find it difficult to perform and the examiner

cannot be certain that a young child is indicating correctly the position of the gap in each ring.

Naming tests

The criteria for a good picture chart are:
• Each part of each picture must subtend a visual angle of one minute of arc at the stated distance.
• Each picture must depict a familiar object or animal in a form which the child can recognize.

These criteria are very difficult to meet in practice and not all picture charts are satisfactory. The Kay picture test is most widely used in orthoptic departments in the UK.

All illiterate tests should be used in their linear form as soon as possible. Using conventional charts, this can only be achieved in young children by pointing to the letters in turn, which is thought to give an artificially high level of visual acuity. Various ways to overcome this problem have been devised (see below, under visual crowding effect). Near vision should be recorded whenever possible.

Literate visual acuity tests

Literate vision tests comprise rows of letters or numbers, ranging in size from 6/60 to 6/4 or 6/3, designed for use at 6 m, and reduced in size to test near vision at 33 cm. Lower case letters are found easier by children as these letters are often taught in schools before upper case letters are introduced. Number charts can sometimes be used earlier than letters, but some numbers, for example 4, can be printed in an unfamiliar form that confuses the child. Literate tests are easier to use if only one, two or three lines are presented at one time.

Near vision can be tested using:
• Reduced distance vision charts, which provide a direct comparison between distance and near vision.
• Jaeger test types, ranging from J14 to J1.
• Faculty of Ophthalmologists N (near) test using Times Roman standard typeface sizes. Normal visual acuity at 33 cm is N5, using 5-point print letters with a height of 5/72 in.

The size range is from N48 to N4. Reading material consists of paragraphs or sentences, selected for use either with adults or children, followed by isolated single words in each size which partly avoid crowding problems and are easier to see. Special near-vision tests for children using N-sized type are:
• Maclure reading books, graded for children of different intellectual levels. The early part of this test uses script familiar to the child through his schoolwork, with a gradual transition to Times Roman typefaces.
• Moorfields bar-reading book, which also includes a useful introductory section incorporating pictures.
• Merrick reading book, which tells an entertaining, illustrated story about the treatment of amblyopia.

Recording the results of visual acuity tests

After performing visual acuity tests the examiner should record the following information:
• the test used;
• whether single-letter or linear vision was tested;
• the smallest size of type read;
• any difference in speed of reading or fluency between the two eyes;
• the optimum reading distance when testing near vision;
• any abnormal head posture adopted for distance or near vision; abnormal head movements, for example, head nodding, should also be recorded;

• any special features, such as difficulty in seeing letters at one end of a row.

Recording visual acuity in very poorly sighted patients

If visual acuity is less than 6/60 the level achieved should be recorded:
• By decreasing the distance between the patient and the chart in 1 m steps to 1 m and then to 50 cm.
• If vision is less than 1/60, by asking the patient to count the number of fingers held up by the examiner against a contrasting plain background; the result is expressed as counting fingers at the distance tested (from 1 m to 33 cm).
• If there is no measurable visual acuity, by asking the patient if he observes hand movements or to say when a bright light is shone into the eye in a darkened examination room. This would be recorded as hand movements (HM) at distance tested and perception of light (PL), respectively.

Visual crowding effect

Single optotype vs. linear testing

It is well known that a single optotype is easier to see than one of a horizontal row of the same size optotypes. The presence of contours adjacent to the letter or symbol reduces visual acuity in both normal and amblyopic subjects (Stuart & Burian 1962), but the difference in visual acuity may be as much as two or three lines when amblyopia is present. This decrease in vision is largely explained by the crowding effect, when the additional stimuli provided by the surrounding optotypes cause confusion; this factor is exaggerated in all types of amblyopia. The crowding effect does not occur when the optotypes are presented in vertical rows. Although single-optotype visual acuity is believed to show the full potential vision of an amblyopic eye (von Noorden 1980), the development of equally good linear vision indicates that the visual system has reached maturity. It is important to use linear charts as soon as possible to obtain accurate and realistic visual acuity. Pointing to the letter minimizes the crowding effect and results in a higher visual acuity. The crowding effect is greater in preschool-aged children (Atkinson *et al.* 1988).

Influence and assessment of the crowding effect

Pointing can be avoided and the influence of the crowding effect assessed if the test optotype is surrounded by similar shaped but unrelated figures or letters:
• pseudo-optotypes bearing a superficial resemblance to letters (Weiss 1973; Fig. 4.7a).
• interaction bars, forming an interrupted square of black bars each subtending one minute of arc in thickness (Parr 1981; Fig. 4.7b).
• grouped letters differing from the test letter (Cambridge crowding cards; Fig. 4.8).

Cambridge crowding cards

Cambridge crowding cards were developed to measure the crowding effect in preschool children (Atkinson *et al.* 1988). This method is a matching test in which one of five letters, H, O, T, V or X, is presented in the centre of a group of four different letters on a series of cards, graded according to size. The surrounding letters are the same size as the test letter and each inner edge is always half a letter width from the edge of the central letter. The crowding factor is therefore constant throughout the test. The patient indicates the central letter on a matching board. The arrangement of letters on the board can be changed. Visual acuity is first assessed using single letters, then retested using grouped letters: it is recorded as the

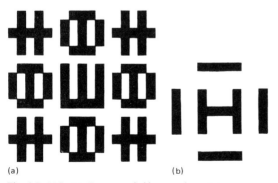

Fig. 4.7 (a) Letter E surrounded by pseudo-optotypes (after Weiss). (b) Letter H surrounded by interaction bars.

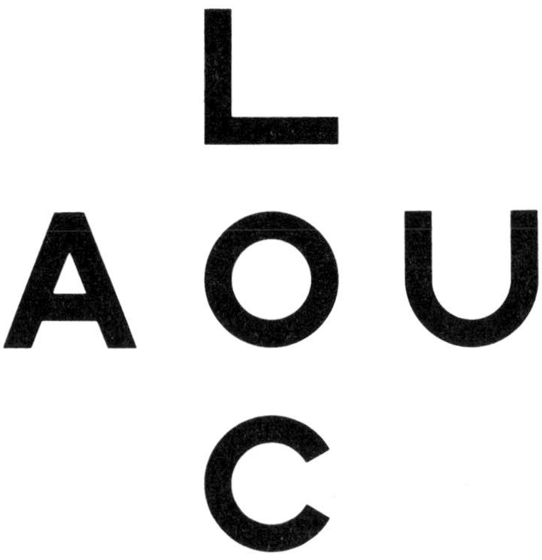

Fig. 4.8 A Cambridge crowding card used to measure the crowding effect. Only the central letter is included in the test letters (H,O,T,V,X) and is identified by the patient using a board comprising these letters.

smallest sized letter correctly identified at two out of three attempts. The crowding ratio is measured by dividing the averaged grouped-letter acuity by the single-letter acuity. If the ratio exceeds 1, crowding has occurred. Using this method, Atkinson *et al.* (1988) reported a pronounced crowding effect in children aged 3–4 years (the youngest group tested), compared with children aged 5–7 years and adults, whether vision was tested at 6 m or at 3 m. The shorter distance was easier to use and gave more reliable results.

Chart design

The design of Snellen vision charts has been criticized because of the absence of standardization. The charts lack regular progression from top to bottom, with variations in: the number of letters of each size presented; the spacing between rows and letters; and even the typeface in which the letters are printed.

logMAR charts

These charts have been developed to overcome the defects inherent in Snellen charts. The Bailey Lovie chart (Fig. 4.9) is most generally used. As the chart design is based on the LOGarithm of the Minimal Angle of Resolution (logMAR), progression in target size and lines is uniform and therefore standardized

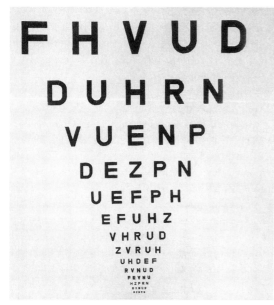

Fig. 4.9 logMAR chart for the measurement of visual acuity.

(Sloan 1959; Frank 1986). The chart can also be used at any interim distance by reading additional lines. The result can be related to vision at 6 m, which is the standard testing distance.

6/6 logMAR equals 0.00 and 6/24 equals 0.6. The scoring system gives credit for every letter read correctly. Each letter is given the value of 0.02 logMAR units, therefore each row of five letters is 0.10 logMAR units.

This method has obvious advantages over conventional Snellen charts, particularly for monitoring changes in visual acuity.

The logMAR crowded test

This test using the logMAR principle has been designed for use with preschool children, using the letters H, O, U, V, X and Y. The format is similar to that of the Sheridan–Gardiner test, comprising three flip-over books for use at 3 m, with a matching card for the child to indicate the letter seen.

It consists of one book which measures uncrowded visual acuity and two books which measure crowded acuity. The uncrowded book presents two letters, one on the right and one on the left side of each card; there are two cards of each size. The crowded test begins with three screening cards which have four letters of decreasing size surrounded by interaction bars of equally decreasing width. These are followed by cards with four letters of the same size in a line and surrounded by a crowding bar; each card decreases in size by one log unit. The range of the test is 0.7 to –0.3 logMAR.

Method

The test is performed at 3 m. Uncrowded visual acuity is assessed first: the child is asked to match the first letter from each of the 24 cards in turn until a mistake is made; the next largest letters are then re-presented; if two or more out of the possible four are correctly identified, the test continues with the next card in the series. Crowded visual acuity is first assessed using the screening cards; when an error is made the previous size letter is presented from the four letter cards. As with the uncrowded test, two or more correct responses are required to progress to the next card.

The scoring system is calculated by the lines each changing by 0.1 log unit and each letter having a value of 0.025 log unit.

Value

This test will become of greater value as more clinics change to the logMAR system. The disadvantage at present is that it is designed for use at 3 m, making it difficult to compare the response to tests using Snellen's principle.

Further investigation when defective visual acuity is recorded or estimated

Fixation

When a normal eye fixates, the image of the fixation object falls on the retinal foveola, or foveal pit, which is centrally located within the fovea and subtends a visual angle of 1.2°. The foveola can be identified by the foveal reflex, which results from the reflection of light from the pit wall. The fovea has a diameter of 5° and is characterized by the absence of retinal ganglion cells and retinal blood vessels. It is surrounded by the macula, a less well-defined area variously described as 12–18° in diameter and containing a much thickened retinal ganglion cell layer.

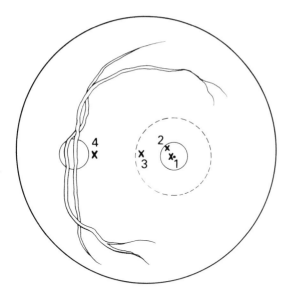

1 = **Parafoveolar**
2 = **Parafoveal**
3 and 4 = **Peripheral**

Fig. 4.10 Fundus diagram showing positions of eccentric fixation.

Classification of fixation

Fixation in an amblyopic eye may be:
• central (foveolar);
• eccentric, when the eye fixates with an area outside the foveola;
• wandering, when the eye makes quite gross random eye movements in an effort to fixate.

Eccentric fixation is classified according to the area of retina used for fixation:
• parafoveolar, when fixation is adjacent to the foveola;
• parafoveal, when it lies within the fovea but further away from the foveola;
• peripheral, when the fixation area lies outside the fovea (Fig. 4.10).

Examination of fixation

Fixation ophthalmoscope

If any level of amblyopia is present in one or both eyes the fixation should be examined in more detail using a fixation ophthalmoscope.

A fixation target is incorporated into the ophthalmoscope beam, usually in the form of a graticule which can be removed when desired. The target varies with the type of ophthalmoscope: it must be easily seen by both the subject and the examiner and must be small enough to allow identification of the foveola.

METHOD (USING THE VISUSCOPE)

The Visuscope incorporates a four-pointed star as a fixation target. The star has a clear central area, which makes it easier to identify the foveola. A green filter can be used to provide red-free light and facilitate recognition of fundus landmarks. The target is first presented to the normal eye (or the eye with the better visual acuity) so that the patient can recognize it and his cooperation can be assessed. The amblyopic eye is then examined with the other eye occluded. The patient is asked to fixate the centre of the star. The examiner should move the target and observe refixation on it. The accuracy of fixation can be confirmed by asking the patient to fixate on the points of the star.

If visual acuity is very low, fixation can be aided by reducing the illumination, increasing it once fixation is achieved. It is easier to examine the patient with the pupils dilated but with experience, dilatation is rarely necessary.

RECORDING OF RESULTS

The examiner should record:
• the position of fixation in relation to the foveola;
• whether it is steady, unsteady or wandering.

The position can be recorded verbally or on a fundus diagram. It is sometimes found that the foveola or fovea of an amblyopic eye appears less well defined than that of the fixing eye, irrespective of the refractive error. This finding should be recorded even though the fundus has been pronounced normal.

The incidence of eccentric fixation is far higher in esotropia than exotropia, although parafoveolar or parafoveal fixation is seen in microexotropia, lying temporal or, in some cases, nasal to the foveola. In esotropia fixation is nearly always nasal to the foveola. Paradoxical eccentric fixation is present if fixation falls on temporal retina in an esotropic patient; this is considered a poor prognostic sign. Fixation is quite often superior or, less often, inferior to the foveola as well as being laterally displaced, especially in those patients with parafoveal fixation.

Visual acuity in eccentric fixation

Visual acuity depends upon:

• The area of retina used for fixation: optimum vision is determined by the visual potential of that retinal area.

• The stability or instability of fixation: better vision is obtained in stable eccentric fixation.

• Superimposed amblyopia, which may reduce the visual acuity considerably. The optimum visual acuity obtainable with parafoveolar eccentric fixation is 6/9. Patients with wandering or peripheral eccentric fixation close to the optic disc will see less than 6/60. Although eccentric fixation is usually considered a uniocular condition, the occurrence of bilateral eccentric fixation has been reported (von Noorden 1963) and its presence should be suspected in cases of bilateral amblyopia due to ametropia or of unknown cause.

Fundus photography

Serial photographs of the fundus can be taken while the patient, whose pupil must be dilated, views a target incorporated in the apparatus and visible on the photograph. This method provides an accurate record and can show if fixation ranges over a retinal area, as is often the case when it lies outside the fovea. Photographs can be repeated to record changes resulting from treatment.

Pinhole test

Purpose

The pinhole test is performed to establish if defective vision is wholly or partly due to uncorrected or wrongly corrected refractive error.

Method

A black disc with a 1 mm pinhole is placed in front of the eye, the other eye being occluded. The visual acuity is tested through the pinhole, which allows the passage of only paraxial rays, so that an optically clear image is formed on the retina even in the presence of an uncorrected refractive error. It is easier to use if the patient holds the disc himself.

Results

Normal or improved pinhole vision proves that the visual defect is wholly, or partly, due to a refractive error. Correction of the error should produce a corresponding improvement in visual acuity. If pinhole vision shows no improvement the defect is due to amblyopia or an organic lesion.

Neutral density filters

Purpose

Neutral density filters are used to differentiate between defective vision due to amblyopia and that due to an organic defect.

Principle

It is known that when filters of graded neutral density are placed in front of the eye, visual acuity is reduced sooner and to a more marked extent in the normal eye, an eye with uncorrected refractive error, or an eye with an organic lesion, than it is in an amblyopic eye.

Method

The patient wears his refractive correction. The normal eye is occluded and two neutral density filters (Kodak Wratten filter 96, ND2 and ND0.50) are placed in front of the eye to be tested. Time is allowed for adaptation to the filters and the visual acuity is then recorded.

Results

If there is little difference in the level of visual acuity with and without the filters, the defect is most likely caused entirely by amblyopia. If there is a significant decrease in visual acuity, an organic lesion should be suspected.

The main indication for using this method is the presence of apparently intractable amblyopia in what appears to be an entirely normal eye.

Contrast sensitivity

Contrast sensitivity is the ability to perceive differences in contrast over the spectrum of spatial frequencies. The level of contrast at which a light and dark pattern is first discriminated is the *contrast threshold*. No consistent discrimination occurs for contrast below the subject's threshold for a particular spatial frequency. High spatial frequencies and very low spatial frequencies require higher contrast for resolution.

Fig. 4.11 'Sine-wave' grating. The contrast of the grating bars changes gradually between light and dark. This form of grating is used for assessing contrast sensitivity thresholds.

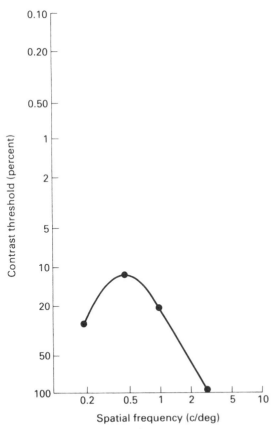

Fig. 4.12 Contrast sensitivity function curve. Contrast sensitivity thresholds as a percentage (ordinate) are plotted against various spatial frequencies of sine-wave gratings (abscissa).

Contrast sensitivity is the reciprocal of the contrast threshold. Contrast sensitivity is measured using sine-wave (sinusoidal) gratings, which show a gradual change from light to dark (Fig. 4.11). Measurement aims to record the patient's contrast threshold over a range of spatial frequencies, using gratings with different contrast levels. Because two variables are involved (spatial frequency and contrast threshold), a graph must be constructed, setting out the contrast threshold for each spatial frequency, resulting in a contrast sensitivity curve (Fig. 4.12). The normal curve has an inverted 'U' shape, with a peak at spatial frequencies of 5–6 cycles per degree (cpd). The curve shows a physiological variation according to the subject's age: children and the elderly have a higher contrast threshold for mid to high spatial frequencies. Pathological reduction in contrast sensitivity occurs in developmental and acquired visual defects, when the contrast threshold can be raised for low, high or all spatial frequencies, depending on the underlying cause.

Contrast sensitivity in amblyopia

Hess and Howell (1977), Lennerstrand and Lundh (1984), and colleagues have reported contrast sensitivity defects affecting the amblyopic eye in all types of amblyopia. Hess and Howell reported that those with strabismic amblyopia and anisometropic amblyopia showed contrast sensitivity loss affecting either all spatial frequencies or limited to high spatial frequencies. Reduction for high frequencies was found in stimulus deprivation amblyopia. Lennerstrand and Lundh found defects in contrast sensitivity for all spatial frequencies when strabismic and anisometropic amblyopia were combined. High-frequency loss was found in strabismic amblyopia without anisometropia. Contrast sensitivity measurement was used to monitor progress during treatment; improvement was reported, leaving a residual high-frequency loss.

Methods of measurement

Both preferential looking and VEP have been used to measure contrast sensitivity for research purposes. Methods which are designed for clinical use are described below.

Pelli–Robson chart
This chart presents 16 sets of letters printed in groups of three, each letter in a group having the same contrast. The contrast decreases from one triplet to the next but the letter size remains the same. Uniform illumination is important and glare must be avoided.

Method
The patient is seated at eye level to the chart at a distance of 1 m. He is asked to identify the letters, starting with the maximum contrast; provided that two out of three are named correctly, the test continues with reducing contrast. The contrast sensitivity measurement is taken as the least contrast which allows identification of at least two of the set of letters. The log contrast sensitivity is given on the score pad used for recording the results. Time must be allowed for identification of the letters, which may not be visible initially.

The test should be performed with both eyes open and each eye separately: binocular log contrast sensitivity is normally 0.15 higher than monocular.

Arden gratings (Arden 1978)
The test consists of six test plates, each of a different spatial frequency, ranging from 0.2 to 6.4 cpd (Snellen equivalent 6/900–6/28.13). Each plate presents a sine-wave grating with decreasing contrast from the top to the bottom of the plate.

Method
The test is used at 57 cm in good light. Starting with the lowest spatial frequency, the subject is first shown the area of least contrast: if this is not discriminated, areas of increasing contrast are gradually revealed until the grating is detected. The procedure is repeated for the remaining plates and a graph constructed showing the contrast threshold for each spatial frequency.

VISTECH vision contrast test system
Two models of this equipment are available, one for use at 33 cm and the other a near test used at 3 m. The test consists of 40 small circles containing sine-wave gratings randomly orientated in one of three directions: $-15°$, $0°$ and $+15°$. The gratings are arranged in five rows according to spatial frequency, 1.5, 3, 6, 12 and 18 cpd. The contrast decreases from left to right across each row.

Method
The patient is first shown circles to demonstrate the four choices available to him, i.e. the three grating orientations and a blank circle, seen when the grating cannot be identified. A high-contrast grating is situated at the beginning of each row and is used to show the patient the spatial frequency common to that row. He is then asked to 'read' the chart from left to right, starting with the lowest spatial frequency, indicating the grating orientation with his finger or a pencil. The examiner records the contrast threshold (the least contrast discriminated for each spatial frequency). This information is transferred to an evaluation chart which gives the contrast sensitivity curve. The physiological limits of the normal curve are shown on the chart for comparison.

Precautions
The test must be performed in good light, which must not fall below the recommended standard of 30–70 ft lamberts. Luminance must be constant, both during the test and on retesting. It must be consistent for all areas of the test (this applies when the larger distance test is used). A light meter is supplied.

The manufacturers warn against basing a diagnosis on the contrast sensitivity findings and stress the need for confirmatory tests, even though the curve may be typical of a specific condition.

Bailey–Lovie low-contrast visual acuity charts
The low-contrast chart is identical to the high-contrast chart, described previously under logMAR charts and shown in Fig. 4.9: the letters decrease in size in logMAR units at a constant 10% contrast. The high- and low-contrast charts should be used in conjunction to provide a simple means of identifying patients who have loss of contrast sensitivity.

Method
Once the acuity on the high-contrast chart is known, the patient should be asked to read the letters on the low-contrast chart. Normal subjects will read approximately two lines less with lower contrast. If the difference is greater than this there is a loss of contrast sensitivity, the difference in the number of letters read gives an index of the extent of the loss.

Other methods of contrast sensitivity measurement include the Regan contrast sensitivity plates (Regan & Neima 1983) and the Cambridge low-contrast gratings (Wilkins *et al.* 1988).

Value of contrast sensitivity measurement

Measurement of contrast sensitivity gives a more complete picture of the patient's visual function. It can be used in:
• the diagnosis of a number of ocular conditions;
• the early detection of visual loss;
• as a means of monitoring progress and assessing the effect of treatment.

It is stated to be more sensitive by a factor of two than visual acuity (Hess 1984). Loss of contrast sensitivity and loss of visual acuity are not necessarily correlated; it has been found, for example, that patients with 6/6 visual acuity may complain of defective vision due to reduced contrast sensitivity. Conversely, Lennerstrand and Lundh (1984) reported that patients undergoing treatment for amblyopia could show improvement in contrast sensitivity measurements without change in visual acuity. They considered this improvement an important visual gain to the patient. Contrast sensitivity measurement is therefore of value in eliciting the cause of symptoms and in regulating treatment, which would be continued as long as improvement occurred.

The tests described are relatively simple to perform for both the patient and the examiner, and take little time to use.

Precautions
The examiner must take pains to control the following parameters:
• lighting, taking care that there is no reflection from the test surface;
• distance from the test;
• patient's head position—he should look straight at the grating or letters through correctly fitted spectacles, if these are normally worn; tinted lenses invalidate the test;
• patients should not be tested immediately after gonioscopy or the use of fluorescein.

Other investigations should be used to confirm the diagnosis whenever possible.

Problems
In the past technical problems have arisen, due to fading of the gratings and discoloration of the material on which they were printed. These difficulties now appear to have been overcome.

All contrast sensitivity tests are subjective and the patient's response cannot be verified, limiting their use in children.

Visual fields

Peripheral visual function is evaluated by assessing the extent of the visual fields.

Normal visual field

The normal field, using a white target, extends approximately 100° temporally, 60° nasally, 50° upwards and 70° downwards. The fields of the two eyes overlap to give a binocular visual field 120° wide, with uniocular temporal crescents from 60° to 100° to either side. The blind spot, corresponding to the optic nerve head, is an absolute scotoma lying in the temporal half of each field between 13° and 19° from fixation, with its centre just below the horizontal meridian.

The normal peripheral visual field using a coloured target (commonly red), is considerably smaller than that with a white target of the same size, if the subject is asked to state when he first recognizes colour rather than the presence or movement of the target. This is due to a combination of the low proportion of cones in the peripheral retina and the lower luminosity of coloured targets.

Visual field defects

Uniocular field loss can be the result of damage to the retina or optic nerve. Bilateral symmetrical field loss can be caused by damage to the chiasm, tracts, radiations or cortex.

Abnormalities of the visual field are described below.

Generalized constriction
The field of one or both eyes may be constricted in advanced open angle glaucoma, and bilateral field constriction occurs in retinitis pigmentosa.

Sectoral field loss
Bilateral or hemianopic field loss results from damage to the visual pathways at, or posterior to, the chiasm. Chiasmal lesions may result in symmetrical or asymmetrical bitemporal loss. More posteriorly sited chiasmal lesions cause a homonymous defect. A field loss of this type that crosses the midline strongly suggests a chiasmal lesion.

Scotoma
A scotoma is an area of defective visual field surrounded by normal visual field. The scotoma may be absolute when the area is blind, or relative when vision is reduced. Open angle glaucoma causes loss of nerve fibres from the disc resulting in nerve fibre bundle branch defects (arcuate scotomata).

Toxic amblyopia, which may result from damage to the optic nerve from cyanide in tobacco smoke, usually causes a centro-caecal scotoma.

Principles and methods of visual field assessment

The principles and methods of assessment are described only briefly; for more detailed descriptions of methods and their uses and interpretation the reader is referred to specialist publications (Harrington 1981).

Assessment can be made using:

- stationary targets (static field);
- moving targets (kinetic field).
  The examiner can explore:
- the extent of the peripheral field (perimetry);
- details of the central field up to 25° from fixation (scotometry).

The fields are examined in many meridia radiating from the point of fixation. The positions at which targets of the same size, brightness or colour are first visible in these meridia, when joined together, form the isopter for that particular stimulus. The isopters to different targets are plotted to form the visual field chart.

Methods of testing

The subject must have sufficient visual acuity and concentration to maintain fixation on the central target. Central fields should be tested with the patient wearing any necessary near refractive correction. Good illumination is essential. Several visual field examinations over a considerable period are often required to assess both the consistency of the responses and to plot the progress of a pathological process affecting the visual system.

Confrontation tests
No apparatus is required for this simple test, which can be used at the bedside as well as in the clinic. White and red targets of some 1 cm diameter (traditionally the spherical tops of hat pins) are used at a testing distance of 50 cm. The targets should be well illuminated and should be viewed by both the patient and the examiner against a dark background. To plot the field of the right eye the patient closes his left eye and fixes on the examiner's open left eye, the right eye being closed. In this way the visual fields of the patient and the examiner should coincide and the examiner can use his own awareness of the target as a control. The target is introduced midway between the examiner and the patient:
- from the temporal mid-periphery to discover the dimensions of the blind spot;
- from the far periphery in many meridia to explore the peripheral field;
- in the central portion of the field to delineate scotomata, particularly to red targets.

If the normal blind spot can be consistently and repeatedly defined, the results should be reliable. This same criterion applies equally to other methods.

Methods of testing fields may be divided into static or kinetic and further subdivided into testing the peripheral visual field or the central visual field.

Static field testing

Static field analysers, such as the Friedmann and Henson machines, are used primarily in the assessment of the central field, mainly as a screening test for glaucoma, or to monitor field changes. Light is flashed through small apertures in prearranged parts of the vision field. The patients is asked the number of flashes he sees on each occasion (one, two, three or four). The intensity of the flash may be increased to assess the density of any scotoma found.

Computerized systems, including the Humphrey field analyser, are now available which allow the patient to test his own field with a minimum of qualified supervision. The Humphrey performs a variety of screening programmes allowing both central and peripheral fields to be tested. The intensity of the stimulus is automatically adjusted to follow the natural decrease in retinal sensitivity in the periphery. Threshold tests are then employed for monitoring the condition. The equipment is expensive but a skilled examiner is not required.

Kinetic field testing

This is based on the introduction of a moving target into the periphery of the visual field. The patient is asked to say when the target first appears and to note its disappearance and reappearance as it moves towards the fixation point. The size of the target may be increased to measure the density of any scotoma found.

Arc perimetry

This method utilizes equipment such as the Lister or Aimark perimeter. Its value was for testing peripheral fields only and is rarely employed in clinical practice today.

Bjerrum screen

This is used to test the 25° of central field; white or coloured targets of 1–30 mm may be used. Red targets are particularly useful when testing for subtle neurological field defects.

Goldmann perimetry

Here the patient sits in front of an illuminated white bowl. Moving spots of different sizes and intensity of light (white or coloured) may be projected onto the interior of the bowl. The shape of the bowl allows accurate testing of both the central and peripheral field. The light projector is coupled with a chart marker, allowing accurate recording of the field. The patient's eye is viewed by the examiner throughout the test to ensure that central fixation is maintained. The Goldmann is superior to both the arc perimeter and the Bjerrum screen.

Amsler charts

The innermost 10° of the central field can be explored in greater detail using a series of small charts comprising grids of white or red lines on a dark background at 33 cm. The patient draws the extent of variation in or absence of the pattern on a similarly sized blank grid. Distortions in the orientation of lines (metamorphopsia, which is typical of macular pathology) and scotomata can both be explored by this simple but highly subjective method.

Assessment of visual fields in children

Subjective assessment is impossible during the first three years of life and is much less reliable than visual acuity tests in children of 3–6 years because of the exteme difficulty in persuading the child to maintain fixation on a central point: he will inevitably look in the expected direction of the peripheral target display. The central fields cannot be analysed until steady central fixation can be maintained for a considerable period despite distractions. Scotometry is rarely possible before the age of 8 years. However, objective assessment can be achieved at an earlier age.

Objective assessment of peripheral fields
Peripherally introduced target

When mounted on black sticks the polystyrene balls used in the STYCAR rolling balls test can be used for objective perimetry. The observer faces the infant, who should sit on his mother's lap, the mounted balls are introduced in turn from behind the child by an assistant so as to enter the peripheral field from different directions. The child's fixation response to the new stimulus is assessed. Alternatively, and more simply, the unaided examiner can observe the infant's responses when the mother's moving fingers are introduced into various meridia.

THE TWO-TOY TEST

This method is useful when the child's attention on the central target cannot be sustained. The examiner, using two visually interesting small toys, attracts the child's attention with one of them, placed in a chosen normal part of the visual field. The second toy is then moved from a sightless into a sighted area of the field; the boundary between sighted and nonsighted areas is considered to be crossed when the infant changes fixation to the new target.

OPTOKINETIC NYSTAGMUS

Some children with homonymous field defects demonstrate asymmetrical horizontal optokinetic responses, but only if there is an extensive space-occupying parieto-occipital lesion.

Subjective assessment of the peripheral fields

Simple subjective tests are described below.

Confrontation tests

These employ the same method as for adult testing and cannot usually be carried out on patients under 8 years old.

FINGER COUNTING

Most children of 8 years upwards will cooperate with this test. A preliminary finger counting game using central fixation will evaluate numeracy and cooperation. Using the confrontation method, the examiner holds up one, two or three fingers in each quadrant of the field of one eye, the other eye being covered. If the child looks towards the fingers they can be quickly withdrawn. If a hemianopic defect is suspected, two fingers can be introduced, one each side of the vertical line separating the temporal and nasal hemifields, noting whether both appear to be seen simultaneously.

RESULTS AND VALUE

Only gross visual field defects can be diagnosed using these methods with young children. The most common visual field defect seen in childhood is homonymous hemianopia, usually occurring in association with cerebral palsy, and this can be detected fairly easily with both eyes open. Bitemporal hemianopia does not usually present difficulty but other smaller and less complete field defects cannot be assessed accurately before at least 8 years of age.

Interpretation of visual field defects

The following rules generally apply in interpreting visual field defects (though there are exceptions).
- A segmental defect centred at the blind spot is caused by optic nerve fibre pathology.
- A scotoma may have a local retinal cause or be due to an optic nerve fibre defect.
- A quadrantic or hemianopic defect, centred on the point of fixation, is due to pathology in the optic chiasm, tracts, radiations or visual cortex.
- Homonymous defects, affecting corresponding quadrants (nasal in one field, temporal in the other) are caused by pathology in the retrochiasmal portions of the visual system.
- Bitemporal defects are caused by lesions in the chiasm which affect the crossing optic nerve fibres originating in the nasal halves of the retinae.
- Generalized peripheral field constriction can be caused by widespread pathology in the retina or optic nerves.

Relationship between visual field defects and ocular motility disorders

Visual field defects may be associated with ocular motility disorders as:
- *coincident factors*, as separate aspects of neurological disease and injury;
- *causative factors*, when they reduce the stimulus for binocular single vision.

In either case, the visual field defect is an additional handicap which must be taken into consideration when determining strabismus treatment.

Effects of visual field defects on binocular single vision

The stimulus for binocular single vision is diminished when:
- the extent of the potential field of binocular single vision is reduced by visual field loss;
- central visual acuity is substantially reduced in one or both eyes by a central scotoma.

These factors may occur in combination, making maintenance of binocular single vision impossible, leading to a nonparalytic strabismus. The most likely causes are considered below.

Bitemporal hemianopia

When this is complete there is no part of the visual fields common to both eyes and diplopia results through the lack of stimulus to maintain bifoveal fixation. The strabismus is usually small but with a variable horizontal and vertical angle. This 'hemianopic slide' is associated with postfixational blindness on near fixation: the only remaining sighted area lies nasally to the converged visual axes, between the subject's face and the intersection of the visual axes at the point of fixation.

Gross restriction of both peripheral fields

Even if good central visual acuity is maintained, the total extent of the binocular field may be insufficient to provide a strong enough fusion stimulus.

Severely defective central vision in one or both eyes

If this has been present from early childhood it will have impaired the development of binocular single vision. Once binocular single vision has become established the stimulus to maintain peripheral fusion is usually sufficient to inhibit the development of acquired sensory strabismus, providing that the vision of both eyes is equally affected.

Ocular motility disorders and associated visual field defects

Certain aetiologies of strabismus may be associated with visual field defects; if these aetiologies are suspected then testing is indicated. Examples of disorders which commonly cause both incomitant strabismus and visual field defects are:
• multiple sclerosis: nystagmus, internuclear ophthalmoplegia and optic atrophy are common features;
• head injuries: third, fourth and sixth cranial nerve palsies and optic nerve or optic chiasmal lesions commonly coexist;
• cerebral tumours: bilateral sixth cranial nerve palsies may be associated with homonymous or quadrantic

field defects from direct infiltration of the optic radiations or visual cortex by the neoplasm;
• pituitary tumours: bitemporal hemianopia is caused by upward growth which compresses the chiasm, while lateral expansion into the cavernous sinuses can precipitate third, fourth and sixth cranial nerve palsies;
• suprasellar and parasellar tumours: these can similarly affect both the afferent visual pathways and the ocular motor nerves.

Visual fields should be tested in the following situations:
• All patients with acquired nonparalytic diplopia, nystagmus or gaze palsies.
• All patients with orbital pathology. For instance, ischaemic optic nerve defects caused by elevated intraorbital pressure are a sight-threatening complication of dysthyroid ophthalmopathy (see Chapter 21), calling for very urgent treatment. Lesions at the orbital apex involve the structures passing through the superior orbital fissure and also the optic nerve.
• Handicapped children whenever possible, as part of their multisystem assessment.
• Children with poor vision of unknown origin affecting one or both eyes, seeking a possible neurological cause, especially when amblyopia therapy has failed to produce improvement.

Colour sense

The ability to distinguish between light of different wavelengths within the visible spectrum—ranging from violet (400 nm) to red (760 nm) in a light-adapted eye—depends on the integrity of the retinal cones and the afferent visual pathways. Three types of cone have been identified, each containing a different visual pigment, sensitive to stimulation by a wavelength of light peaking at the same level as that of each of the three spectral primary colours: red, green and blue.

Colour vision defects

A normal subject can match any unknown colour with a mixture of the three primary colours (desaturated with added white light if necessary). Subjects

with colour vision defects have anomalous matching values as follows:
• trichromats, requiring additional amounts of one primary colour;
• dichromats, able to match all colours using only two primary colours;
• monochromats, able to match colour simply by varying the intensity of one primary colour.

Defective colour vision can be hereditary or acquired.
• Hereditary defects are caused by insufficiency or absence of one or more of the three cone types. Hereditary colour blindness predominantly affects the red (protanopic) or green (deuteranopic) parts of the spectrum. Blue blindness (tritanopia) is extremely rare.
• Acquired defects are due to disease processes affecting the retina or optic nerve, frequently affecting the yellow/blue part of the spectrum.

The varieties of colour vision defect most likely to be seen in clinical practice are considered below.

Hereditary defects
Protanopia and deuteranopia
Moderate defects in the red and green parts of the spectrum are inherited as X-linked disorders and affect some 8% of Caucasian males.

Rod achromatopsia
Rod achromatopsia is complete colour blindness associated with a marked reduction in visual acuity, severe photophobia and roving eye movement. It is caused by an autosomal recessive hereditary disorder in which there is congenital absence of all functioning cones.

Dominant hereditary optic atrophy
This is a moderate defect of colour discrimination, mainly in the yellow/blue region, associated with defective visual acuity. It is a rare but specific cause of progressive visual defect in young school-age children of either sex. Correct diagnosis relies heavily on exact identification of the colour vision defect.

Hereditary cone deficiency syndromes
In such syndromes the colour vision defect is acquired in early childhood and is associated with photophobia, progressive central visual loss and macular pigmentary degeneration.

Acquired defects
Optic nerve lesions, particularly optic neuritis, cause rather nonspecific colour vision defects which may be strictly uniocular or markedly asymmetrical, whereas hereditary defects affect both eyes equally.

Colour vision tests

Only tests in current use are considered. Tests which assess colour vision are based on the subject's ability to:
• match colours;
• arrange coloured targets in an orderly spectral sequence;
• identify numbers, letters or shapes which differ in colour from their surround.

Colour vision should be tested with each eye separately.

Matching colours
This is done using a Nagel's anomaloscope. This is the most scientifically accurate method of assessment but since the apparatus is costly and very good cooperation is required, it is little used in clinical practice.

Spectral colour sequences
The ability to arrange colours in spectral sequence is the basis of the Farnsworth–Munsell 100 hue test and of the simpler D-15 test. These tests are valuable in distinguishing different types of hereditary and acquired colour vision defects, since each type produces characteristic errors. They are difficult for children to understand and are rarely used as screening tests. They can provide a more detailed study of subjects whose colour vision deficit has been detected by simpler means.

Identification of figures
Most routine colour vision tests are based on this principle. All tests use pseudo-isochromatic plates comprising multiple coloured dots among which is a pattern made up of dots of superimposed colours. Patients with specific colour vision defects will fail to recognize the pattern, or interpret it incorrectly, for example a number 8 can be seen as a 3.

Tests using this principle are:
• Ishihara
• Gardiner test for children
• Hardy–Rand–Rittler (HRR).

All are designed to be used at near and need good illumination to enhance the colour contrasts.

Ishihara test

All patients should be shown the first plate, which presents an orange-coloured number 12 with a grey dot surround, visible even to those with total colour blindness. Children may be shown half the number (1 or 2) or shown how to trace the outline with a finger. Once cooperation has been assessed each plate is presented in turn.

Gardiner test

This test uses a matching technique in which the child picks up or points to a replica of the letter which he sees. The Ishihara test, which is more comprehensive, can generally be used successfully with the same-age-group children by modifying the testing technique.

Hardy–Rand–Rittler (HRR) test

This test is easier for young children since it uses only three symbols: a circle, a triangle and a cross. It also has the big advantage that it includes plates for evaluating the yellow/blue part of the spectrum and is therefore invaluable, for example, in the diagnosis of hereditary and acquired optic atrophy. However, the test is unfortunately not widely available.

Indications for testing colour vision

Visual screening of children

Evaluation of colour vision should be included in visual screening programmes at the start of a child's school career. Colour is increasingly used in education, for example in teaching basic arithmetic in primary schools. Certain careers are barred to people with colour vision defects, for example the electrical trades and some branches of the armed services, so that early detection of hereditary defects is important both during the child's education and for career guidance.

Diagnosis of causes of defective vision

As stated above, diagnosis of the presence and the nature of a colour deficit can be confirmatory of the cause of the visual defect.

Intractable dense amblyopia

Colour vision should be tested when there is failure to improve visual acuity in spite of adequate treatment, since the visual loss may be due to an undiagnosed organic defect. Amblyopia alone does not cause specific colour vision defects.

Electrodiagnostic tests for visual function

The electrical energy which is generated by the activity of excitable cells (nerve and muscle cells) may be recorded in a number of ways. The direct current (DC) which is generated by such activity is very small. Usually the recording electrode is sited some distance from the cells generating the potential changes so the electrical impulses recorded by the electrode are minute. The interpretation of the recording is further complicated by interference generated by other neighbouring cells.

Equipment

Averaging

The difficulties described above may be reduced by the use of computer averaging. This is a system that permits the signal from the recording electrode to be evaluated only at certain specified moments of time which are synchronized with the stimulus. Sequential recordings of random potentials will vary in their degree of either negative or positive potential and when these random potentials are summated after a sufficient number of recordings the potential change is zero. However, if a nonrandom change occurs at precisely the same point in time on repeated recordings, this potential will always be of a similar size and deflection (positive or negative). The result will be an enhanced total response as each epoch is recorded and summated.

Electrodes

The usual electrodes used for skin contact are silver–silver chloride. Good contact is essential. The skin is cleaned with alcohol and the electrode contact is improved by application of a salt-containing jelly that conducts electricity. The adequacy of the contact can be checked by measuring the resistance between paired electrodes. When the search electrode is used to record directly from the surface of the eye, a gold foil electrode is used in the lower fornix. This technique has largely replaced the older contact lens electrode and is more comfortable for the patient, so the test can be carried out on cooperative children. An earth electrode is necessary as well as recording and reference electrodes.

Amplifiers

These are an essential part of the recording and are used to increase the strength of the signal received from the electrode.

Filters

Filters are employed to screen out electrical interference.

Clinical applications

The principal electrodiagnostic tests used in testing visual function are:
- electro-oculogram
- electroretinogram
- visually evoked potential.

The electro-oculogram (EOG)

This test compares the resulting potential under scotopic and photopic conditions. Two pairs of electrodes are placed at the inner and outer canthi of each eye and an earth electrode is attached to the scalp. Two targets, usually red light-emitting diodes (LED), are sited 20° to either side of central fixation and the patient is asked to look from one to the other. The movement is carried out on command at different intervals throughout the test. The eye is a dipole with the cornea relatively more positive to the posterior pole by approximately 6 mV. When the eye moves towards the recording electrode it will cause a positive deflection. Conversely as the gaze direction is changed away from the recording electrode, there is a negative deflection.

The test is first carried out with the eye in the dark-adapted state then repeated under photopic conditions. When the eye is exposed to light there is a steady rise in the EOG potential until the eye is fully light adapted. The maximum potential in the light-adapted state is compared with the minimum potential in the dark-adapted state and expressed as a ratio, the Arden index:

$$\frac{\text{Light-adapted potential}}{\text{Dark-adapted potential}} = \text{Arden index}$$

The normal range varies in different laboratories; because of difficulties encountered in totally excluding light in the dark phase, each laboratory must establish its own normal values. Most centres expect the photopic potential to be slightly more than that of the scotopic potential, resulting in a ratio of at least 2. The potential difference between the cornea and the posterior pole is generated at a level of the retinal receptors and the pigment epithelium. Any disease affecting these tissues will reduce the potential and will be shown by a reduction in the light rise.

When measuring the EOG to assess retinal function it is the change in the potential difference recorded from the receiving electrode on right and left gaze in the dark-adapted state compared with the light-adapted state which is important.

The EOG potential may be utilized to measure saccadic velocity by measuring the rate of change of potential as the eye moves towards and away from the recording electrode as described in Chapter 6.

Value

The EOG tests the integrity of the receptors and pigment epithelium and is used to detect subclinical choroidal and retinal dystrophies, for example retinitis pigmentosa.

The electroretinogram
Principle

When a flash of bright light is shone into the eye a series of electrical changes takes place in the retina which can be recorded by electrodes placed on or around the eye.

Method

An active electrode is placed in the conjunctival sac, in a corneal contact lens or on the skin near the eye, with indifferent and earth electrodes attached to the surrounding skin. Potential changes can be measured accurately between these electrodes and displayed

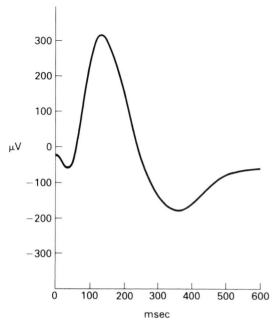

Fig. 4.13 Electroretinogram (ERG). Tracing of the fully dark-adapted response in a normal patient with a fully dilated pupil. A small negative a-wave is followed by a much larger positive b-wave.

on a visual display unit (VDU). When only corneal electrodes were available, a general anaesthetic was often necessary for young children. With more modern goldleaf electrodes and computerized summation techniques this is no longer required.

Results

The normal electroretinogram (ERG) (Fig. 4.13) consists of two major deflections; a negative a-wave followed by a larger positive b-wave. These deflections occur within the first 200 ms after the light stimulus. The b-wave is largest in the fully dark-adapted eye and with a dilated pupil, when it measures some 200 μV. If flickering light stimuli are used, the ERG responses remain separately identifiable up to some 20 stimuli s⁻¹, provided the retinal cones are functioning normally. If only the rods are active, the flicker fusion frequency of the response is much lower, at approximately 4 flashes s⁻¹. The cones are relatively more sensitive than the rods to the red end of the visible light spectrum: the ERG responses of the cones

and rods can therefore be distinguished by contrasting the amplitude of electrical responses to pink and blue light.

It is now possible to obtain a pattern ERG. The retina appears to be sensitive to a chequer-board stimulus, and by the use of averaging and summation, a response may be achieved to a chequer-board target. The role of this relatively new technique is still to be assessed.

Value

The examination is of critical importance in the early and exact diagnosis of widespread pigmentary retinal degenerations, enabling the diagnosis to be made before abnormal fundus changes are seen ophthalmoscopically. Disorders of the retinal cones alone can be distinguished by flicker and colour ERG responses, allowing early diagnosis of rod monochromatism. In congenital retinal blindness the ERG response is extinguished from early infancy.

The visually evoked potential (VEP) (visually evoked response, VER)
Principle

When a normal subject views a patterned stimulus (grating or chequer-board), small electrical potential changes occur in the occipital cortex. These can be recorded by overlying scalp electrodes and summated to give a significant wave-form response (Sokol 1978).

Method

A black-and-white grating or chequer-board of 100% contrast and known spatial frequency is presented to the subject on an oscilloscope screen subtending a visual angle of some 20°. This pattern is reversed (e.g. black changed to white) at intervals of 0.25–1 s, the mean luminance remaining constant. (Alternatively the same pattern can be displayed intermittently.) The stimulus is presented from 50 to 200 times, and repeated using gratings of decreasing size (and therefore of higher spatial frequency) until there is no observable change in electrical potential on pattern reversal. The electrical changes recorded are summated and processed using a computation of average transients which eliminates random unrelated electrical activity (Fig. 4.14). The highest spatial frequency

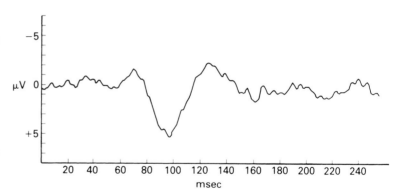

Fig. 4.14 Visually evoked potentials (VEP). This tracing is the averaged response to 128 reversing chequerboard patterned stimuli recorded from a normal subject. Positive polarity is displayed as a downward deflection. The important P_{100} wave peak is the largest positive deflection occurring some 100 ms after each change in visual stimulus.

pattern which elicits an electrical potential change is the measure of the visual acuity.

Value

Provided that the scalp electrodes are correctly positioned and that the subject is looking directly at the target, any significant potential changes will be recorded. Little cooperation is needed, and neither sedation nor anaesthesia must be used as they invalidate the result. Maintaining the child's attention is a major problem: the amplitude of the VEP decreases markedly when fixation is not maintained. Most apparatus incorporates a built-in device which suspends averaging until fixation is resumed. Bumgartner and Epstein (1982) have shown that the results can be altered by accommodation or by defocusing on the pattern. Neither of these factors can be controlled in young patients. Further doubts about this method have been raised by reports of normal VEP recordings in cortically blind children and in monkeys lacking a visual cortex (references in Hoyt 1984). There is no doubt that visual acuity is overestimated (Sokol & Moskowitz 1985). A delayed P_{100} strongly suggests optic nerve disease, for example optic neuritis.

References

Arden, G.B. (1978) The importance of measuring contrast sensitivity in cases of visual disturbance. *British Journal of Ophthalmology* **62**, 198–209.

Atkinson, J. & Braddick, O. (1981) The development of visual function. In: *Scientific Foundations of Paediatrics* (eds J.A. Davis & J. Dobbing), pp. 865–877. Heinemann Medical Books, London.

Atkinson, J., Braddick, O., Pimm-Smith, E., Ayling, L. & Sawyer, R. (1981) Does the Catford drum give an accurate estimate of visual acuity? *British Journal of Ophthalmology* **65**, 652–656.

Atkinson, J., Braddick, O. & Pimm-Smith, E. (1982) 'Preferential looking' for monocular and binocular acuity testing of infants. *British Journal of Ophthalmology* **66**, 264–268.

Atkinson, J., Anker, S., Evans, C., Hall, R. & Pimm-Smith, E. (1988) Visual acuity testing of young children with the Cambridge crowding cards at 3 and 6 years. *Acta Ophthalmologica* **66**, 505–508.

Berlyne, D.E. (1958) The influence of the albedo and complexity of stimuli on visual fixation in the human infant. *British Journal of Psychology* **49**, 315–318.

Birch, E.E., Shimojo, S. & Held, R. (1985) Preferential-looking assessment of fusion and stereopsis in infants aged 1–6 months. *Investigative Ophthalmology and Visual Sciences* **26**, 366–370.

Bumgartner, J. & Epstein, C. (1982) Voluntary alterations of visual evoked potentials. *Annals of Neurology* **12**, 475–478.

Chandna, A., Pearson, C.M. & Doran, R.M.L. (1988) Preferential looking in clinical practice: a year's experience. *Eye* **2**, 488–495.

Courage, M.L. & Adams, R.J. (1996) Infant peripheral vision: the development of monocular visual acuity in the first 3 months of postnatal life. *Vision Research* **36** (8), 1207–1215.

Dickey, C.F. & Scott, W.E. (1987) Amblyopia – the prevalence in congenital esotropia versus partially accommodative esotropia: diagnosis and results of treatment. In: *Transactions of the Sixth International Orthoptic Congress* (eds M. Lenk-Schafer, D. Calcutt, M. Doyle & S. Moore), pp. 106–112. British Orthoptic Society, London.

Dobson, V. & Teller, D.Y. (1978) Visual acuity in human infants: a review and comparison of behavioural and electrical-physiological studies. *Vision Research* **18**, 1469–1483.

Dobson, V., Teller, D.Y., Ping Lee, C. & Wade, B. (1978) A behavioural method for efficient screening of visual acuity in young infants. *Investigative Ophthalmology and Visual Science* **17**, 1142–1150.

Fantz, R.L. (1958) Pattern vision in young infants. *Psychological Research* **8**, 43–47.

Frank, J.W. (1986) Scaling of visual acuity: applying a logarithmic scale. *American Orthoptic Journal* **36**, 11–13.

Fulton, A.B., Hansen, R.M. & Manning, A.B. (1981) Measuring visual acuity in infants. *Survey of Ophthalmology* **25**, 325–332.

Gorman, T.J., Cogan, D.G. & Gellis, S.S. (1957) Apparatus for grading visual acuity of infants on basis of optokinetic nystagmus. *Paediatrics* **19**, 1088–1092.

Gwiazda, J., Bauer, J., Thorn, F. & Held, R. (1986) Meridional amblyopia does result from astigmatism in early childhood. *Clinical Visual Science* **I**, 145–152.

Harrington, D.O. (1981) *The Visual Field. A Text Book and Atlas of Clinical Perimetry*. Mosby, St Louis.

Harwerth, R.S., Smith, E.L., Duncan, G.C., Crawford, M.L.J. & von Noorden, G.K. (1986) Multiple sensitive periods in the development of the primate visual system. *Science* **232**, 235–238.

Hazell, C.D. (1995) Evaluation of the Cardiff Acuity Test in uniocular amblyopia. *British Orthoptic Journal* **52**, 8–15.

Held, R. (1988) Normal visual development and its deviations. In: *Strabismus and Amblyopia: Wenner Gren International Symposium Series*. (eds G. Lennerstrand, G.K. von Noorden & E.C. Campos), pp. 247–258. Macmillan, London.

Hess, R.F. (1984) On the assessment of contrast threshold functions for anomalous vision. *British Orthoptic Journal* **41**, 1–15.

Hess, R.F. & Howell, E.R. (1977) The threshold contrast sensitivity function in strabismic amblyopia: evidence for a two type classification. *Vision Research* **17**, 1049–1055.

Hopkisson, B., Arnold, P., Billingham, B., McGarrigle, M. & Entwistle, P. (1991) Visual assessment of infants: vernier targets for the Catford drum. *British Journal of Ophthalmology* **75** (5), 280–283.

Hoyt (1984) The clinical usefulness of the VER response. *American Journal of Ophthalmology* **93**, 704–708.

Jenkins, P.L., Simons, J.W., Kandel, G.L. & Forster, T. (1985) A simple grating visual acuity test for impaired children. *American Journal of Ophthalmology* **99**, 652–658.

Lennerstrand, G. & Lundh, B.L. (1984) Contrast sensitivity in amblyopia. In: *Transactions of the Fifth International Orthoptic Congress, Cannes* (eds A. Ravault & M. Lenk), pp. 77–84. LIPS, Lyon.

Mayer, D.L. & Dobson, V.L. (1980) Assessment of vision in young children: a new operant approach yields estimates of acuity. *Investigative Ophthalmology and Visual Sciences* **19**, 566–570.

Mayer, D.L., Fulton, A.B. & Rodier, C.O. (1984) Grating and recognition acuities of pediatric patients. *Ophthalmology* **91**, 947–953.

Mohindra, L., Jacobson, S., Zwaan, J. & Held, R. (1983) Psychophysical assessment of visual acuity in infants with visual disorders. *Behavioural Brain Research* **10**, 51–58.

Moseley, M.J., Fielder, A.R., Thompson, J.R., Minshull, C. & Price, D. (1988) Grating and recognition acuity of young amblyopes. *British Journal of Ophthalmology* **72**, 50–54.

von Noorden, G.K. (1963) Bilateral eccentric fixation. *Archives of Ophthalmology* **69**, 25–31.

von Noorden, G.K. (1980) *Burian and von Noorden's Binocular Vision and Ocular Motility*, 2nd edn, pp. 228–229. Mosby, St Louis.

Parr, J.C. (1981) Clinical assessment of visual acuity. *Transactions of the Ophthalmological Society of New Zealand* **33**, 157–167.

Pearson, C.M., Chandna, A. & Doran, R.M.L. (1989) Preferential looking: the state of the art. *British Orthoptic Journal* **46**, 66–72.

Regan, D. & Neima, D. (1983) Low-contrast letter charts as a test of visual function. *Ophthalmology* **90**, 1192–1200.

Rosenbaum, A.L. & Kirschen, D.G. (1984) A survey of visual acuity testing in the infant and preverbal child. *American Orthoptic Journal* **34**, 13–21.

Sheridan, M.D. (1969) Visual screening procedures for very young or handicapped children. In: *Aspects of Developmental and Pediatric Ophthalmology* (eds P. Gardiner, R. MacKeith, & V. Smith), pp. 39–47. Heinemann Medical Books, London.

Simons, K. (1983) Visual acuity norms in young children. *Survey of Ophthalmology* **28**, 84–92.

Sloan, L.L. (1959) New test charts for the measurement of visual acuity at far and near. *American Journal of Ophthalmology* **48**, 807–813.

Sokol, S. (1978) Measurements of infant visual acuity from pattern reversal evoked potentials. *Vision Research* **18**, 33–39.

Sokol, S. & Moskowitz, A. (1985) Comparison of pattern VEPs and preferential-looking behaviour in 3-month-old infants. *Ophthalmology and Visual Science* **26**, 350–365.

Stuart, J. & Burian, H. (1962) A study of separation difficulty. Its relationship to visual acuity in normal and amblyopic eyes. *American Journal of Ophthalmology* **53**, 471–477.

Teller, D.Y. (1983) Scotopic vision, color vision and stereopsis in infants. *Current Eye Research* **2**, 199–207.

Teller, D.Y., McDonald, M., Preston, K., Sebris, S. & Dobson, V. (1986) Assessment of visual acuity in infants and children: the acuity card procedure. *Infant Behavioural Development* **2**, 135–153.

Tippings, E.K. (1996) Measurements of visual acuity using the Snellen test, in situations of blur. *British Orthoptic Journal* **53**, 10–16.

Weiss, J.B. (1973) Measure de l'acuité visuelle du jeune enfant. *Vision Research* **13**, 1139–1149.

Wilkins, A.J., Della Sala, S., Somazzi, L. & Nimmo-Smith, I. (1988) Age-related norms for the Cambridge Low Contrast Gratings, including details concerning their design and use. *Clinical Vision* **2**, 201–212.

Wright, K.W., Walonker, F. & Fedelman, P. (1981) 10 dioptre fixation test for amblyopia. *Archives of Ophthalmology* **99**, 1242–1246.

Yuodelis, C. & Hendrickson, A. (1986) A qualitative and quantitative analysis of the human fovea during development. *Vision Research* **26**, 847–855.

Zipf, R.F. (1976) Binocular fixation pattern. *Archives of Ophthalmology* **94**, 401–404.

5
Ocular Deviation

Strabismus is a condition in which the visual axes deviate from parallelism. The strabismus can be manifest (heterotropia), in which one visual axis deviates either constantly or intermittently, or latent (heterophoria), in which the deviation is normally controlled by fusion and only becomes apparent when the eyes are dissociated. A necessary part of assessment is first to detect the strabismus then to *estimate* and if possible *measure* the deviation.

Detection of strabismus

The history may give an indication of the presence and the type of strabismus but the main methods of detection are:
• observation of the patient's appearance;
• observation of the position of the corneal reflections;
• the cover test.

Appearance

The observer should note any deviation of the visual axes and other signs which can indicate a possible ocular motor defect, such as an abnormal head position or a craniofacial abnormality.

Pseudostrabismus

A significant number of children and a few adults who are referred to an ophthalmologist or orthoptist have a pseudostrabismus rather than a true deviation of the visual axes. Apparent esotropia, exotropia, hypertropia or hypotropia can result.

Various causal factors may be involved in pseudostrabismus.
• Epicanthus affecting the inner canthi, which is the most common cause of pseudoesotropia. Epicanthus

can affect the outer canthi and cause pseudoexotropia but this is rarely seen. Most epicanthus resolves spontaneously with the development of the facial skeleton. It persists in a few children and can be treated surgically if severe.

• Asymmetry or other abnormality of the palpebral fissures can simulate a squint but can also be a characteristic of certain ocular motility disorders, for example the narrowing of the fissure seen on adduction in Duane's retraction syndrome.

• Unilateral ptosis and unilateral upper eyelid retraction can result in pseudohypertropia or hypotropia, respectively, or may mask or accentuate a true vertical strabismus.

• Asymmetry of the face, either congenital or acquired, is a possible cause of pseudohypertropia or hypotropia. Asymmetry also occurs when there is a congenital head tilt, which can be associated with a vertical muscle palsy.

• A narrow interpupillary distance (IPD) simulates and accentuates esotropia. A wide IPD gives an impression of exotropia but is also a common feature of this type of deviation.

• Deep-set eyes may result in pseudoesotropia, whereas subjects with prominent eyes are more likely to appear exotropic.

• Displacement of the orbits, either as a result of a congenital condition such as hypertelorism, or acquired following trauma, can occur without disruption of binocular single vision and can give rise to a pseudostrabismus of any type, depending on the nature of the displacement.

• A positive or negative angle kappa can result in a pseudoexotropia or pseudoesotropia, respectively (see below). Usually both eyes are affected, but the angle kappa may be asymmetrical, increasing the possibility of pseudostrabismus. Occasionally displacement of the macula can occur (heterotopia), which leads to quite marked displacement of the corneal reflection. Heterotopia can be the result of pathology, for example the temporal displacement seen in some cases of retinopathy of prematurity. If only one eye is affected the squinting appearance is accentuated.

Differential diagnosis

Pseudostrabismus and true strabismus are differentiated by tests to prove whether bifoveal binocular single vision is present. This is accomplished principally by the use of the cover test, as described below, and by proof of motor fusion, which can be demonstrated in children aged from 4 to 6 months onwards with a 15 Δ prism held base-out in front of each eye in turn. If binocular single vision is present the eye under the prism will adduct whilst the other eye first abducts and then adducts to regain fusion. A routine ophthalmic examination is of course required.

Factors causing pseudostrabismus can be present when there is a true squint and may mask or accentuate its presence. If there is any doubt about the diagnosis observation should be continued until it is resolved. Certain findings are strong indications that a child should be kept under observation even though no convincing evidence of strabismus has been found. These include:

• a family history of refractive error or strabismus;
• a significant heterophoria (even a small esophoria is significant);
• a tendency to close one eye in sunlight, indicating a possible intermittent exotropia.

Once a pseudostrabismus has been proved, the parents should be reassured and the reason for the apparent deviation explained to them.

Confirmation and measurement of strabismus

Cover test

The cover test is a simple, mainly objective test which is the cornerstone of investigation of strabismus; it is therefore described in detail. To perform it accurately and to obtain the maximum information, the test requires the correct fixation targets for use at 33 cm, 6 m and in the far distance, and an adequate cover, preferably a matt black 'paddle'. Spielmann (1986) has developed a translucent occluder made of rigid nonreflective plastic, which allows the examiner to assess the eye position behind the occluder. One or both eyes may be covered by this means. The patient's view is reduced to an indistinct blur, sufficient to minimize accommodation but less dissociating than an opaque occluder. This method could be useful in conditions such as dissociated vertical deviation (DVD) or variable deviations and when observing nystagmus.

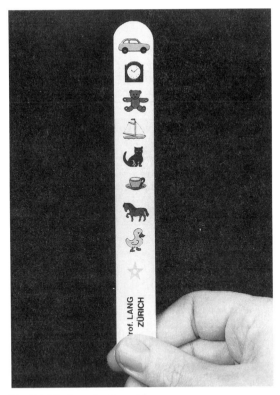

Fig. 5.1 The Lang fixation stick.

Fixation targets

Targets for 33 cm

• A spotlight, which should be used initially to observe the corneal reflections and to aid the assessment of fixation, noting whether it is central, steady and maintained, which is particularly relevant in patients with amblyopia.

• A detailed target to stimulate accommodation and assess fixation: very small pictures can be used for young children and the Lang fixation stick is excellent for this purpose (Fig. 5.1). Reduced Snellen letters or numbers are best for adults and older children.

Targets for 6 m

• A spotlight at the patient's eye level, especially when amblyopia is present.

• A Snellen's test type. If it is difficult to obtain fixation in the distance in young children, a fixed toy with an added auditory stimulus helps, and the remote-controlled mobile toys and videos are usually successful.

Target for far distance

• An easily seen landmark as close to eye level as possible, visible through a window.

It is important that the target should be held in the primary position, otherwise a false impression of the deviation may result, for example in A- and V-patterns (see Chapter 17), or when incomitance is present. When an accommodative target is used the examiner must ensure that the patient continues to see it clearly so that accommodation is controlled. If a patient wears bifocal spectacles a cover test should be performed through the appropriate bifocal segment in the position the patient uses it.

Method (Figs 5.2 & 5.3)

The cover test can be used in two ways:

1 The *cover/uncover test* in which one eye is covered and the observer notes:

(a) the movement of the uncovered eye to take up fixation;

(b) the position and movement of the covered eye, as the cover is removed.

The test is repeated, making the same observations whilst covering the other eye.

2 *The alternate cover test* in which one eye or the other is covered throughout the test; the movement of the covered eye is noted as the cover is changed from one eye to the other.

The cover/uncover test is less dissociating than the alternate cover test. Dissociation can be kept to a minimum or increased, depending on the length of time one or other eye is covered. The alternate cover test fully dissociates the eyes and cannot differentiate latent and manifest deviations.

Practical application

Stages in the detection of a manifest deviation

If the strabismus is manifest the uncovered eye will move to fixate when the fixing eye is covered. Detection involves the following stages.

1 The cover/uncover test is performed for near fixation using a spotlight, covering the straight eye if a strabismus is apparent, or the eye with the better visual acuity or least refractive error if this information is available, observing the behaviour of the uncovered eye.

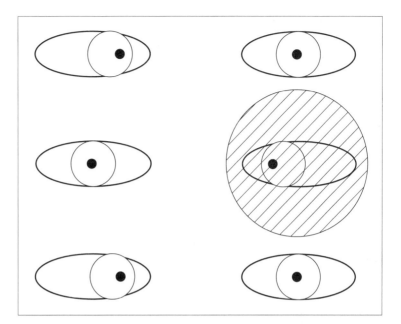

Fig. 5.2 The cover/uncover test in a right esotropia.

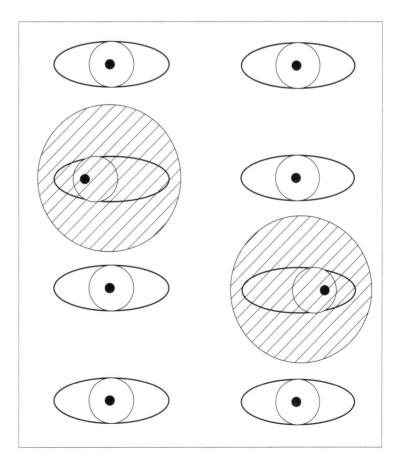

Fig. 5.3 The alternate cover test in an exophoria.

2 The spotlight is replaced by an accommodative target at 33 cm, which may be a Snellen's letter or small picture. The procedure is then repeated at 6 m.

3 An alternate cover test is performed to ensure full dissociation, noting any change in the amount or type of movement.

4 Finally the cover/uncover test is repeated to observe if the deviation returns to its original position or remains at the dissociated angle.

Stages in the detection of a latent deviation

If a latent strabismus is present the uncovered eye will not move but the eye behind the cover will deviate and should recover to a straight position on removal of the cover. Detection involves the following stages.

1 The cover/uncover test is performed at 33 cm and at 6 m, using a detailed target, first ensuring that there is no movement of the uncovered eye to exclude a small manifest strabismus, then concentrating on the behaviour of the covered eye. The speed of the recovery movement as the cover is removed is particularly important.

2 An alternate cover test is used for both near and distance fixation to dissociate the eyes and elicit the maximum deviation. The speed of the recovery movement as the cover is finally removed is noted, and can indicate the patient's ability to control the deviation. The faster the recovery the better the control.

3 This must be followed by a further cover/uncover test to ensure that the deviation has remained latent and that there is no deterioration in the speed of recovery.

Precautions

• Unnecessary dissociation should be avoided until a provisional diagnosis has been made. For this reason it is advisable to perform a cover test, keeping dissociation to a minimum by covering the eyes for the shortest possible period, before testing visual acuity; occlusion of one eye during the vision test may dissociate a precariously controlled deviation. If it appears that there is a latent or intermittent strabismus, or if the angle of deviation appears very small, tests for binocular function, particularly stereotests, should be used before the eyes are further dissociated, otherwise a misdiagnosis can be made.

• Time must be allowed for the patient to fixate when the other eye is covered and for recovery to take place when the cover is removed. A common fault is for the cover test to be performed too quickly. Slowing down the speed with which the cover is changed from eye to eye will usually overcome the tendency of the eyes to 'overshoot', for example if the eye moves out then in before finally fixating, making it difficult to estimate the amount of deviation.

• A spotlight should be used to assess the position and steadiness of fixation in the squinting eye but a detailed target must always be used to note the effect of accommodation on the deviation. To ensure that accommodation is exerted the patient should be asked to name each fixated letter or describe a picture. The pupils should be observed for constriction on accommodation.

• The squinting eye should be covered and uncovered and an alternate cover test performed even if there is a constant unilateral strabismus, otherwise a consistent increase in angle on dissociation or the presence of DVD may be missed.

• If there is a significant increase or decrease in the size of the deviation from 33 cm to 6 m a cover test should be performed using a far distance fixation target.

• It is unusual for orthophoria to be present for near and distance fixation. If no deviation is seen on cover test the visual acuity should be considered; an amblyopic eye may not move to fixate, either because it fixes eccentrically or because the visual acuity is too low for the target to be seen clearly. If the visual acuity is even slightly unequal a microtropia (a small-angle strabismus measuring no more than 10 Δ, with binocular single vision) should be considered.

Information provided by the cover test

The cover test is the main method of differentiating manifest and latent strabismus. The information which can be obtained is summarized here, and is referred to again in later sections. It comprises:

• The direction of the deviation (horizontal, vertical and torsional).

• The difference in angle from near to distance fixation.

• The effect of accommodation and of the patient's refractive error.

• Comitance or incomitance in the primary position by comparison of the deviation fixing with either eye, and in all gaze positions by means of an alternate cover test.

- Other characteristics of manifest strabismus: constant or intermittent; unilateral or alternating.
- Estimation of the visual acuity in a constantly squinting eye by a study of fixation (Dickey & Scott 1987; Calcutt 1995).
- The speed of recovery in latent strabismus.
- The presence of latent or manifest latent nystagmus. The cover test will reveal if there is a latent component in manifest nystagmus.

Recording the results of the cover test

The results of the cover test should be recorded clearly and concisely; examples are shown in Table 5.1. The information recorded should include:

- The type of deviation: whether manifest or latent.
- The direction of the deviation: horizontal, vertical or combination of the two.
- Which eye deviates.
- An estimation of size: this is assessed by observing the position of corneal reflections and by the amount of movement elicited to take up fixation.
- The speed of recovery in latent deviations: this is usually described as rapid, moderate, delayed or blink (when a blink allows fusion to be regained). Diplopia may be appreciated prior to recovery and should be noted.
- There may be no recovery in a poorly controlled heterophoria and the deviation remains manifest.

Table 5.1 Example of cover test recorded findings.

An accommodative esotropia
With glasses:

Nr.	Moderate LCS	or	Moderate LET
D.	Slight LCS	or	Slight LET

Without glasses:

Nr.	Marked LCS	or	Marked LET
D.	Moderate LCS	or	Moderate LET

A distance exotropia

Nr.	Slight exophoria with rapid recovery	or	Slight X with rapid recovery
D.	Moderate LDS	or	Moderate LXT
F.D.	Moderate LDS	or	Moderate LXT

LCS, left convergent squint; LDS, left divergent squint; LET, left esotropia; LXT, left exotropia; D., 6 m distance; F.D., distance beyond 6 m.

- Any special features, for example incomitance, nystagmus, torsion or DVD.

Estimation of size

The estimated angle of deviation is customarily classified as shown below according to size, expressed in degrees or prism dioptres.

- fractional/minimal: <5° (<10 Δ);
- slight/small: 5–10° (10–20 Δ);
- moderate: 10–20° (25–35 Δ);
- marked: ≥20° (≥40 Δ).

Standardization of description is helpful for improved interobserver reliability.

Corneal reflections

The corneal reflections should be observed with both eyes open and with each eye separately whilst the patient fixates a spotlight at 33 cm distance.

The position of the corneal reflections is measured by the angle kappa (the angle between the visual axis and the central pupillary line). If the fovea coincides with the posterior pole of the eye, the angle kappa is zero and the corneal reflection is central; more usually the fovea lies slightly temporal to the posterior pole and the reflection is nasal, giving a positive angle kappa of around 3° in an emmetropic eye. A larger positive angle kappa results in a pseudoexotropia. More rarely the fovea lies nasal to the posterior pole, resulting in a temporal corneal reflection and a negative angle kappa, simulating an esotropia. The positive angle kappa is larger in hypermetropia and smaller in myopia, when it may even be negative.

If there is a sufficiently large-angle strabismus, the corneal reflection in the squinting eye will be temporal in esotropia and nasal in exotropia when both eyes are open. When the fixing eye is covered the reflection assumes a normal position, provided that central or near central fixation is present. If there is eccentric fixation outside the macular area the reflection will remain displaced when the fixing eye is covered; this usually occurs only in esotropia. The corneal reflection will be so little displaced in a small-angle strabismus that it will appear normal.

Hirschberg's test

A spotlight is held at 33 cm and the position of the corneal reflection in the fixing eye is noted and compared with the reflection in the deviating eye: this will be displaced temporally in esotropia and nasally in exotropia. Each millimetre of displacement from the centre of the cornea equals approximately 7° of deviation, although Brodie (1987) revised this to 21° using photographic measurements. von Noorden (1977) stated that a reflection on the temporal edge of pupil indicates 15° esotropia.

Brüchner test

The Brüchner test is performed by illuminating both eyes with a direct ophthalmoscope. The position of the corneal reflections is noted and the fundus reflexes are compared; strabismus and anisometropia can produce asymmetry of the reflexes, the brighter reflex being that of the abnormal eye. This can be very useful in the uncooperative child or when the examiner is more adept at ophthalmoscopy than the cover test. It is, however, unreliable in infants under 8 months of age (Archer 1988). This principle is also used in photorefraction screening techniques.

Prism reflection test (Krimsky's test)

The patient fixes on a spotlight at 33 cm and a prism bar or loose prism is placed in front of the *fixing eye* with the apex of the prism in the direction of the deviation. The eye behind the prism moves to maintain fixation and due to Hering's law, the squinting eye makes a conjugate movement. The prism strength is increased until the reflection matches that previously noted in the fixing eye. Alternatively the prism can be placed in front of the *squinting eye*; however, the corneal reflection is more difficult to assess behind the prism and the first method is usually preferable. This test can be adapted for use at 6 m using the method of Wisnicki and Guyton (1986) described for use with Hirschberg's test. The interpupillary distance is measured and the patient is asked to fixate a distance target. A horizontally held ruler is positioned at 33 cm so that the zero mark is opposite the centre of the pupil of the fixing eye. A pen torch is held above the ruler in front of the squinting eye at the patient's exact interpupillary distance. The position of the corneal reflection is noted and the deviation calculated as it is in Hirschberg's test. Alternatively a prism can be used to centre the reflection in the squinting eye as in the prism reflection test.

Prism cover test

The prism cover test is mainly used objectively and is the method of choice in the measurement of horizontal and vertical manifest and latent deviations in the majority of suitable cases. Cyclotropia cannot be measured by this method.

The test requires horizontal and vertical prism bars and/or loose square prisms, suitable fixation targets for use at 33 cm, 6 m and in the far distance, and an adequate means of covering the eye. An accommodative target is preferable in most cases, for example a Snellen letter.

A cover test is first performed to assess the approximate size of the strabismus and to note the preferred eye in a manifest deviation. A prism of a strength approximating to the estimated angle of deviation is placed in front of the squinting eye if the deviation is manifest, or in front of either eye if it is latent and comitant, with the apex in the direction of the deviation (e.g. base-out in esotropia, base-down in hypertropia). An alternate cover test is performed, adjusting the prism strength until there is no movement of the eye under the prism when the other eye is covered. The strength of prism is increased until a reversal movement is seen to confirm the maximum angle has been elicited. The strength is then reduced until no movement is seen; this may be referred to as the null point. The angle of deviation is recorded in prism dioptres.

The test should be used in the primary position at 33 cm and 6 m and in the far distance if necessary.

If the deviation is incomitant in the primary position, the angle can be measured fixating with either eye in turn. The fixing eye is the eye without the prism; movement of the eye behind the prism is neutralized.

Measurement can be made in all or selected positions of gaze in one of two ways:

1 The fixation target can be moved into the required gaze position. Ideally, a deviometer should be used, in which fixation targets, usually small spotlights, are presented in the diagnostic positions of gaze, allowing consistent and repeatable measurements.

2 The fixation target can remain in the primary position whilst the patient's head is moved to place the eyes in the required position.

This can be repeated in the same conditions more easily if the head is turned so that the fixation target is only just visible to both eyes, thus testing at the extreme limits of gaze. This method can be used for both near and distance measurement and can be recorded on an adequately labelled chart. The same eye should be used for fixation throughout each set of measurements.

Thompson and Guyton (1983) have pointed out that ophthalmic prisms may be calibrated for use in three possible ways. These are:

• With the posterior face perpendicular to the line of sight of the deviating eye. This is termed the Prentice position, for which traditional prism bars are calibrated.

• In the position of minimum deviation with the prism power divided between the two faces of the prism.

• With the posterior face in the patient's frontal plane.

The traditional prism bar is frequently held in the frontal position rather than the correct Prentice position (Kaye *et al.* 1989). If a prism bar is used in a position for which it is not calibrated, or if two prisms are placed in apposition in front of one eye, measurement errors occur (Thompson & Guyton 1983). The error is usually slight but becomes significant when high-powered prisms are used; for example, if two 30 Δ prisms are placed together in front of one eye the combined power is 94 Δ. The inaccuracy is reduced to 6 Δ if one prism is placed in front of each eye, giving a combined power of 66 Δ. Overestimation should be taken into account when very large angles of deviation are measured.

A horizontal prism bar calibrated for use in the frontal plane position is now available (Fig. 5.4): it can be stacked with a vertical prism bar calibrated for the Prentice position (Flüeler *et al.* 1995). The bars are easy to hold correctly and the measurement of combined horizontal and vertical deviations is more accurate. The authors recommend their use.

Precautions

• It is essential:

1 to prevent fusion by the continued use of the alternate cover test. The cover should be alternated slowly enough to give the patient time to fixate accurately;

2 to control accommodation by the use of a detailed target, ensuring that accommodation is maintained by changing the letter or picture and asking the patient to identify it.

• A high-powered prism reduces the clarity of vision and makes it difficult for an amblyopic patient to fixate. Therefore it may be necessary to place the prism in front of the better eye. In very large angles the prism strength may need to be divided between the two eyes, but this should be noted or correction of the inaccuracy made using the table devised by Thompson and Guyton (1983) (see Table 5.2).

• Children can concentrate for only a short time so it is important to start the measurement with approximately the correct prism rather than to work up from a much lower strength prism.

• It is difficult to measure combined horizontal and vertical deviations using two conventional prism bars, one held with the base horizontal and the other held

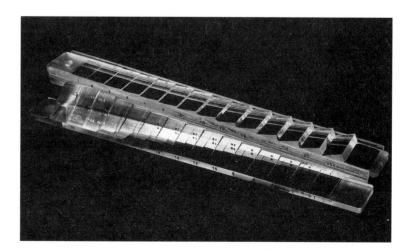

Fig. 5.4 The Gulden combination horizontal and vertical prism bars.

Table 5.2 Deviation in prism dioptres for the addition of two prisms (glass or plastic) with one prism held in front of each eye. (From Thompson & Guyton 1983.)

Left eye prism (labelled value)	Right eye prism (labelled value)											
	10	12	14	16	18	20	25	30	35	40	45	50
10	20	22	24	26	29	31	36	41	47	52	58	63
12	22	24	26	29	31	33	38	44	49	55	60	66
14	24	26	29	31	33	35	40	46	52	57	63	69
16	26	29	31	33	35	37	43	48	54	60	66	72
18	29	31	33	35	37	39	45	51	57	63	69	75
20	31	33	35	37	39	42	47	53	59	65	71	78
25	36	38	40	43	45	47	53	59	66	72	79	86
30	41	44	46	48	51	53	59	66	73	80	87	94
35	47	49	52	54	57	59	66	73	80	87	95	103
40	52	55	57	60	63	65	72	80	87	95	104	113
45	58	60	63	66	69	71	79	87	95	104	113	123
50	63	66	69	72	75	78	86	94	103	113	123	133

with it vertical. It is much easier if square prisms are used, when they can be placed in apposition and held together between the finger and thumb. The larger component of the deviation should be measured first and a prism to measure the smaller component added to the first prism. It is more satisfactory if both prisms are placed in front of the same eye rather than using a horizontal prism bar in front of one eye and a vertical bar in front of the other eye because incomitance is common in this type of strabismus and cannot be measured in this way. These difficulties are overcome using the prism bars described above.

Advantages of the prism cover test over other methods of measurement

The prism cover test is accurate to within 2 Δ; it provides complete dissociation and therefore measures the maximum angle of deviation. It gives a comparison of the angle at different distances, including the far distance.

Indications for use

Use of the prism cover test is indicated in all patients with manifest and latent deviations who meet the criteria of good fixation and sufficient cooperation.

Variants of the prism cover test

Simultaneous prism cover test

This test is used to measure the manifest deviation in manifest strabismus with a latent component, as seen in some cases of microtropia. It can also be used to measure the manifest deviation in the presence of DVD.

The prism is placed in front of the deviating eye and a cover simultaneously introduced in front of the fixing eye (Pratt-Johnson & Tillson 1994). The aim is to neutralize the movement of the squinting eye as the fixing eye is covered. Prism and cover are removed and the test is repeated with larger prisms until this is achieved. An alternate cover test is then used to measure the total deviation, comprising the manifest and latent components.

Subjective prism cover test

The principle of this test is to find the prism strength which neutralizes the movement of the images observed by the patient as the cover changes from one eye to the other. Unlike the objective prism cover test, it requires the patient to have normal retinal correspondence. This method is difficult to perform correctly and has no advantages over the conventional method but it can be combined with it when measuring small vertical deviations; the patient's observation that vertical movement has ceased through the prisms is confirmation that the measurement is correct.

Diagnostic occlusion

Diagnostic occlusion can be used to induce full dissociation when it is thought that the maximum angle of deviation has not been revealed.

Method

One eye is totally occluded for a period of 45 min to 48 h, depending on circumstances and the views of the examiner. It is most common to measure the deviation pre- and post-occlusion by the prism cover test. Occlusion must not be removed until an eye is covered by the occluder to be used in the measurement, ensuring fusion cannot occur prior to measurement.

Indications for use

Occlusion is mainly used before surgery when it is important to elicit the maximum angle of deviation in order to plan the operation. It is particularly useful in:
• intermittent exotropia (distance or nonspecific types);
• esophoria, especially of the divergence weakness type;
• congenital or long-standing vertical deviations.

Other uses for diagnostic occlusion

• To diagnose whether symptoms are due to heterophoria.

• To differentiate between real or apparent limitation of abduction in infants and young children.
• To distinguish real or apparent eccentric fixation in infants and young children.

Major amblyoscope

The major amblyoscope is a reflecting and refracting stereoscope, the basic principle of which is shown in Fig. 5.5. There are a number of different models available. Measurement requires a range of foveal, macular and paramacular simultaneous perception slides (i.e. presenting dissimilar images), subtending angles of 1°, 3° and 5° (or more), respectively, at the nodal point of the eye.

The IPD should first be corrected. The angle of deviation can be measured objectively and subjectively. It is best to use the smallest size slides compatible with the patient's visual acuity to ensure accurate measurement, but in exotropia the maximum angle is sometimes better obtained using paramacular-sized slides, which should be marked with a central fixation point to aid accurate fixation.

To obtain an *objective measurement* the tube containing the fixation slide, for example a lion, is placed at zero on the scale at the base of the instrument; the other tube containing the surround, for example a cage, is moved to the estimated angle of deviation; an alternate cover test is performed by extinguishing the light in front of each eye in turn and the angle is adjusted until there is no movement as the eye fixates. As with the prism cover test, continuing dissociation until there is a reversal of movement can confirm

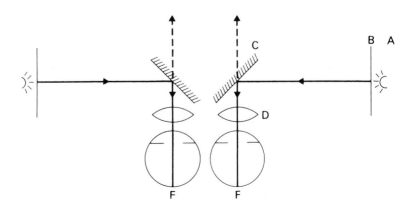

Fig. 5.5 The principle of the major amblyoscope. A = light source; B = slide at focal distance of lens; C = plane mirror; D = +6.5 lens; F = fovea.

accuracy. The test is repeated with the other eye fixating in the primary position with the instrument arm at zero on the scale. The angle is registered on the instrument's scale and should be recorded in degrees, as it is an arcuate measurement. Vertical deviations can also be measured in degrees and this is preferable to using the dioptre scale, which is limited in size and does not use prisms to displace the image: since torsion is also measured in degrees, this aids comparison and standardization.

The instrument measures the deviation at infinity but it can be used with −3.0 DS in the instrument's lens holders to induce 3 DS of accommodation, provided it is ensured that the patient can see the pictures clearly, giving a measurement with accommodation for comparison.

If a near measurement is required the tube should be set at 3×1 in prism dioptres to account for a subject's required convergence at 33 cm; this point should be taken as zero when calculating the measurement. As this is still not a true near measurement −3.00 DS lenses alone are more commonly used.

To obtain a *subjective measurement* the patient is asked to superimpose the images; provided that retinal correspondence is normal they will be superimposed at the angle of deviation and the subjective angle will therefore be the same as the objective angle. If suppression prevents superimposition larger sized slides can be used to place the images outside the suppression scotoma. Objective measurement is more accurate and should always be used to check the patient's observations.

A difference in subjective and objective measurements may indicate the presence of abnormal retinal correspondence.

Measurement using corneal reflections

A foveal-sized slide is placed in front of the fixing eye and the position of the corneal reflections is noted whilst the amblyoscope tubes are both at zero. The tube in front of the fixing eye is moved along the arc in such a way that the reflection in the squinting eye moves into a normal position (comparable with the position of the reflection noted in the fixing eye); the patient must maintain steady fixation on the foveal picture. Alternatively the tube in front of the squinting eye can be moved as in the Krimsky test. If the

angle is large the observer will need to position himself in line with the deviation to assess the reflection accurately. The angle is recorded in degrees.

Indications for use of the major amblyoscope

Horizontal, vertical and torsional deviations can be measured in the nine positions of gaze. The major amblyoscope is not the first choice method in the majority of cases because its accuracy is affected by artefacts, mainly the lack of normal seeing conditions and the patient's awareness of the proximity of the instrument, inducing proximal convergence which results in an increase in the angle in esotropia and a decrease in exotropia. However, this has not been substantiated by recent findings (Georgievski 1995a), which showed that underconvergence was just as likely to occur as overconvergence and that 'instrument convergence' is not a relevant clinical entity. It is sometimes possible to obtain measurements in children unable to cooperate with a prism cover test.

The major amblyoscope is particularly useful in the following circumstances:
• in measuring paralytic strabismus in all gaze positions, when the test conditions are better controlled than with a prism cover test and are therefore more repeatable;
• when there is complicated torsion, as in bilateral superior oblique palsies (see below).

Cyclodeviation can be measured subjectively using slides designed by Maddox for the purpose (Fig. 5.6). The patient is asked to superimpose a red cross in a white cross within the surround so that all the lines are parallel. Torsion is adjusted by rotating the slide with the tilted image and the amount of adjustment is recorded in degrees. The measurement can be made fixing with either eye and in all positions of gaze.

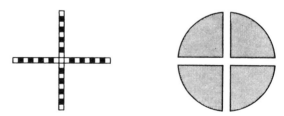

Fig. 5.6 Maddox synoptophore slides for detecting and measuring torsion.

The main value of this method is that it provides a repeatable record of cyclotropia in positions of gaze up to 20° away from the primary position. The accuracy of this method outweighs the artefacts produced by the instrument.

Maddox rod

Use of the Maddox rod provides an entirely subjective method of measuring horizontal, vertical and torsional deviations. Dissociation of the eyes is achieved by presenting a spotlight to one eye and a line image to the other eye.

The rod comprises a series of parallel ridges which have a cylindrical effect on light passing through them, converting a point source of light into a line image at 90° to the cylinder axes. The rod is traditionally coloured red and is made to fit into a trial frame. Variations are a large hand-held rod and a rod which incorporates a 10 Δ rotating prism to simplify measurement. The rod can be used in conjunction with the Maddox tangent scale (Maddox cross), which is marked in degrees along its horizontal and vertical arms for measurement at 5 m; there is also a scale for measurement at 1 m. More usually the deviation is measured using prisms. The spotlight should be viewed at eye level.

Horizontal deviations
The Maddox rod is placed in front of the nonfixing eye with the cylinder axes horizontal, the patient fixates the spotlight with the other eye and is asked on which side he sees the vertical red line. A prism is held in front of the rod with its apex in the direct direction of the deviation (e.g. base-out in esodeviations), and the strength of prism is adjusted until the line passes through the light. The measurement is repeated fixing with the other eye.

Vertical deviations
The cylinder axes are placed vertically, giving a horizontal red line. The same procedure is followed, using vertical prisms.

Torsional deviations
Torsion can be detected by asking the patient if the line image is exactly vertical (or horizontal); this information must be sought by questioning as few patients volunteer it. Measurement of cyclodeviation using the Maddox rod is described below (Maddox double rod test).

Precautions
• Other light sources should be extinguished.
• The deviation should always be measured fixing with either eye, and the patient should be asked routinely if the line appears straight or tilted. If he is unsure of this, or if the examiner expects torsion to be present, the line can be tilted deliberately and then straightened through the patient's observations.
• Time must be allowed for dissociation in latent strabismus. If the deviation measures significantly more with the second eye fixing, the measurement should be repeated fixing with the eye first tested, as the difference may be due to increased dissociation rather than incomitance.
• If the line image is intermittently suppressed it can sometimes be restored by quickly covering and uncovering the fixing eye several times.

Indications for use
The Maddox rod is useful for measuring some small deviations, especially vertical deviations which are sometimes difficult to see on a prism cover test. It is an excellent way of detecting and measuring torsion in an observant patient. Although it can be used to measure small-angle horizontal manifest strabismus, many patients with this condition have abnormal retinal correspondence, which invalidates the test. It is not suitable for the measurement of larger deviations, nor for accommodative deviations as accommodation cannot be controlled with this test.

Maddox double rod test

Two Maddox rods are placed in trial frames, one before each eye, with the cylinder axes vertical, resulting in horizontal line images when a spotlight is viewed at 6 m. If the patient has a vertical strabismus, as is usually the case, the lines will be seen one above the other. If there is little or no vertical separation, a vertical prism can be used to separate the lines. The patient is questioned about the direction of the tilt and whether it affects one or both line images. Alternatively the rods can be placed so that the lines are seen at 90° to each other, or different coloured rods can be used. The patient then adjusts the position of the lines by rotating the rods in the trial frame until they appear parallel and straight or the examiner does this for him if necessary. The amount of cyclodeviation is measured in degrees from the scale on the trial frame. The test can be used at near as well as distance and in different gaze positions.

This test is in general use in the measurement of cyclotropia. It is effective when used in the primary position providing that the vertical deviation does not exceed 20 Δ. Accuracy is reduced for larger amounts: Johnson *et al.* (1987) have reported that this method is unsuccessful more than 10–12° from the primary position, which limits its usefulness.

Maddox wing

The Maddox wing dissociates the eyes by means of two septa, arranged so that the horizontal and vertical measurement scales are visible to the left eye and the right eye sees the two arrows, one vertical to indicate the horizontal measurement and the other horizontal, indicating the vertical measurement. Horizontal and vertical measurement is recorded in dioptres at 33 cm.

The apparatus should be held in a reading position in good illumination, and reading corrections should be worn; if it proves difficult for those wearing bifocal glasses to see through the eye-pieces, appropriate lenses can be placed into the eye-piece lens holders. The patient is asked to indicate the position of the vertical arrow on the horizontal scale to record the horizontal deviation, and the position of the horizontal arrow on the vertical scale to measure the vertical deviation. Torsion is indicated if the horizontal arrow on the right-hand side is not parallel with the horizontal measurement scale; this arrow can be moved until the patient sees it parallel, when the amount of torsion is indicated on a scale on the right-hand edge of the baseplate; each division on the scale equals 2°. It is easier if the patient adjusts the position of the arrow himself.

Precautions
• The septa bend easily, allowing one eye to see both the arrows and the numbers. The examiner should check that the apparatus is functioning correctly before use.
• Time must be allowed for dissociation to take place.
• The numbers and the arrows should be seen clearly; relaxation of accommodation results in an increase in exophoria and a decrease in esophoria, giving an erroneous measurement.

Indications for use
Although the measurements may sometimes be misleading, the Maddox wing provides a quick method of checking the heterophoria for near, provided that the precautions outlined above are taken. It is particularly useful in patients complaining of symptoms for close work for which there is no obvious cause: use of the instrument may reveal a small amount of vertical imbalance or possibly an unsuspected torsional deviation which could account for the symptoms.

Hess screen

Principle
The screen is based on:
• foveal projection;
• Hering's and Sherrington's laws of innervation;
• dissociation of the eyes by means of complementary colours or a mirror.

Since the development of the original screen by Hess, several modifications and refinements have been made and new screens introduced. These include:
• Replacement of the counterweighted indicator by a pointer with a green ring which the patient places on the red dot.
• A Hess screen with a grey background used with projected red and green lights giving a linear image (Foster torches).
• An illuminated Hess screen on which each target can be lit up in turn and its position indicated by the patient using a green linear light.
• The Hess/Weiss screen, which allows the plotting of dissociated and nondissociated charts.
• The Lees screen, which uses mirror dissociation in place of complementary colours.

Modern refinements include electronic control. The Lancaster screen, more widely used in the USA, and the modification of it developed by Foster *et al.* (1953), can be used for the same purposes.

Lees screen

The Lees screen is used by the authors and it is preferred because it has certain advantages Suppression occurs less frequently because of the stronger stimulus provided by the black-and-white contrast. The patient's eyes are more visible to the observer because goggles are not required, and full dissociation is more easily achieved by the mirror than it is by red/green dissociation. It is found that children can understand and perform the test at an earlier age than they can with colour dissociation methods, so that despite its large size and greater costs its use is justified.

The plotted Hess chart aids in the diagnosis of ocular motility defects, measures the deviation and provides a reliable and repeatable record of the condition.

Apparatus

The Lees screen consists of two opalescent glass screens at right angles to each other, bisected by a two-sided plane mirror. Each screen has marked on its back surface a tangent grid (Fig. 5.7), intersected by dots at 15° and 30° intervals, giving an inner and outer square of dots (or an inner and outer field). Each small square subtends an angle of 5°. Two pointers are used, one by the examiner to indicate each dot in turn and the other held by the patient, who places the ring on the end of his pointer round the indicated dot.

Method

The test is performed with each eye fixating in turn. The patient sits facing the nonilluminated screen and fixates the dots through the mirror. The screen viewed in this way by the fixing eye is illuminated throughout the test. When the patient has placed his pointer on the dot which he projects onto a blank screen, that screen is briefly illuminated by means of a foot switch operated by the examiner. The position of the dot is then recorded on the chart, which is a facsimile of the grid on the screen and is common to all adaptations of the Hess screen. When the position of all the dots has been recorded the patient is rotated through 90° to face the other screen, the illumination is changed to the opposite side and the procedure repeated with the other eye.

Precautions when using the Lees screen

• The mirror must have a true plane surface and must exactly bisect the two screens; if it does not do so, the chart plotted with one eye fixating will be artificially larger than that plotted with the other eye fixating, implying greater incomitance than is present.

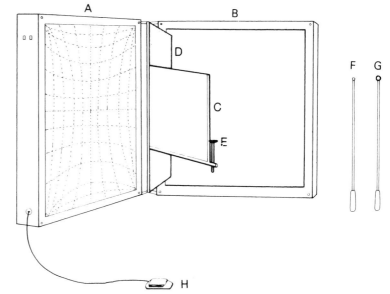

Fig. 5.7 Lees' adaptation of the Hess screen: to plot the field of the right eye the patient sits facing the nonilluminated screen B and fixates a dot on the grid on the illuminated screen A with his left eye, through the plane mirror C. The patient projects the fixated dot on to screen B and indicates its position by encircling it with his pointer G. The examiner then illuminates screen B to note and record the position of the dot. The patient's position is reversed to record the field of the left eye. D = septum; E = chin rest; F = examiner's pointer; H = foot switch used to illuminate screen B.

• The patient must be positioned so that the mirror is at 45° to the plane of his face; he should be as close to the mirror as possible otherwise it is difficult to plot the outer field.

• The patient's head must remain straight throughout the test; it may be necessary to hold it in the correct position.

• If there is a manifest deviation and no diplopia, the presence of normal retinal correspondence must first be established, i.e. the foveae must have a common visual direction, otherwise the field plotted will not be a true representation of the eye position. However, even in the presence of abnormal retinal correspondence, recent-onset incomitance will be depicted. Marked suppression may prevent the use of the Lees screen.

• The patient must fix centrally on each dot; this is not always possible when there is gross restriction of ocular movement.

• The test should be performed without spectacles if possible because the spectacle frames prevent proximity to the mirror and the lenses can induce a prismatic effect when fixating the peripheral dots.

Indications for use

A Hess chart should be plotted:

• On all patients with incomitant strabismus, provided that they have normal retinal correspondence and do not suppress the targets.

• On patients with esophoria or intermittent esotropia of the divergence weakness type to exclude a mild sixth cranial nerve palsy.

• To differentiate apparent divergence palsy from a sixth nerve palsy.

• To provide a baseline in conditions likely to develop defective ocular movement in the course of the disease, for example in dysthyroid eye disease.

Problems associated with use of the Lees screen

• Suppression, which is less of a problem when using the Lees screen than other adaptations, can be overcome temporarily by moving the pointer backwards and forwards across the dot or by using a spotlight as a fixation target instead of the pointer.

• Gross limitation of movement may prevent the patient from fixing on the dots. If both eyes are affected

the chart is of little value and other methods of recording must be used. If part of the field cannot be plotted the reason should be recorded rather than leaving the chart blank.

• Hemiretinal suppression and a variable angle prevent the plotting of a satisfactory chart in most cases of intermittent distance exotropia, when a chart might be useful in analysis of any V-pattern.

Measurement

Each small square on the grid subtends 5°, allowing the deviation in the primary position to be calculated, fixing with either eye and compared with the deviation recorded in other gaze positions.

Lees screen used to measure cyclotropia

A linear pointer for use with the Lees adaptation of the Hess screen was first devised by Dulley and Harden (1974) to measure cyclotropia in any position of gaze. This technique was modified by Johnson *et al.* (1987) as follows: the fixation dot on the screen is replaced by a horizontal blue line printed on a clear, plastic, weighted triangle, which is attached to each dot in turn by a suction cup. A screw head in the plastic corresponds to the position of the fixation dot on the screen. The patient uses a clear plastic pointer printed with a horizontal red line with a central red spot and a measurement scale, marked off at 1° intervals. He is instructed to align the red and blue lines and to place the red spot on the screw head. In this way a conventional Hess chart can be plotted and cyclodeviation measured up to 30° from the primary position.

VALUE

This method is simple and is more reliable in peripheral gaze positions than any other method of measuring cyclotropia. By recording extraocular muscle underaction and overaction, it relates the cyclodeviation to the muscle function.

Specific tests for the assessment of cyclotropia

Cyclotropia can be assessed subjectively and objectively.

Subjective tests

Double Maddox prism

This test detects but does not measure torsion. The apparatus consists of two prisms placed base to base. It is held with the bases horizontal in front of one eye so that the patient looks through the join; a horizontal line is viewed with both eyes open, resulting in three lines—the higher and lower lines are seen through the prisms and the central line is seen by the other eye. The patient is asked if the three lines are parallel to each other or if the upper and lower lines or the central line appear tilted, denoting torsion of the eye which sees the tilted images or image. The direction of the tilt indicates whether there is intorsion or extorsion.

Major amblyoscope

This has already been described (see above). The method has the advantage of being able to test accurately in all nine position of gaze and is repeatable on subsequent visits.

Maddox double rod test

This has already been described (see above). For accurate results a well-fitting trial frame is essential. Large rods aid testing in nine positions of gaze but standardization of degrees from the primary position can be difficult.

Bagolini glasses

Bagolini striated glasses were devised to assess binocular vision but have been adapted to measure cyclotropia by Ruttum and von Noorden (1984). The apparatus comprises a pair of trial frames, a spotlight and two plano glasses, each marked with fine striations which produce a line image of a spotlight, perpendicular to the direction of the striations.

The principle of the test is similar to that of the Maddox double rod test. The glasses are placed in the trial frames with the striations vertical, giving rise to two horizontal line images when viewing a spotlight. If the patient has a vertical strabismus, as is usually the case, the lines will be seen one above the other. If there is little or no vertical separation, a vertical prism can be used to separate the lines. The patient is asked

if one or both lines are tilted. The lines can be straightened subjectively by rotating the glasses in the trial frame and the degree of cyclotropia recorded, as in the Maddox double rod test.

The test is performed in almost normal conditions of seeing, which is an advantage. Suppression of one line easily occurs if there is a large vertical deviation. Johnson *et al.* (1987) reported similar problems to those found with the Maddox double rod test when measuring cyclotropia away from the primary position.

Lees screen with linear pointer

As described above, this is accurate and repeatable but can be time consuming. It relates well to ocular muscle function.

Awaya cyclo test

The test is presented in book form, showing 13 pairs of half-moons, one of each pair printed in red and the other in green, separated by a gap of 10 mm. In the first figure the half-moons are parallel to each other; in the following figures the green half-moon is tilted in steps of 1°, giving a maximum tilt of 12° for the 12th pair; the red half-moon is upright on all the figures (Fig. 5.8). Each pair is viewed through reversible

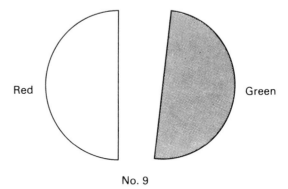

No. 9

Fig. 5.8 Awaya cyclo test: one of a series of paired red and green semicircles viewed through complementary red and green reversible spectacles. If the inner edges of the illustrated pair appear parallel to a patient wearing the red glass in front of the right eye he has 9° excyclodeviation in the right eye (assuming there is no left excyclodeviation), or a total amount of 9° excyclodeviation in both eyes. The colours are reversed to measure incyclodeviation.

complementary red and green glasses. The test is used at reading distance.

The patient wears the red glass in front of the right eye; he is shown the first pair of half-moons and is asked if they are parallel to each other, in which case there is no torsion. If the green half-moon is tilted clockwise there is intorsion and if it is tilted anti-clockwise there is extorsion. If extorsion is present the patient then views each succeeding pair until he assesses that the half-moons have become parallel; this plate records the amount of torsion in degrees. If intorsion is diagnosed on the first pair of half-moons the glasses are reversed so that the green glass is in front of the right eye and the procedure is repeated. (Awaya *et al*. 1986).

Precautions

• The red and green glasses provided with the test should be used, so that the colours are exactly complementary.

• The book must be kept upright, parallel to the plane of the patient's face, otherwise erroneous torsion is introduced by tilting it backwards or forwards.

This test is useful in assessing the problems caused by cyclotropia for close work.

Torsionometer

The test is based on complementary colour dissoci-ation; red and green goggles are worn, and red and green vertical lines are viewed. The red line is printed onto the front surface of a plastic square and a cutout in the square reveals the green line, which is printed on a separate sheet of plastic, allowing it to be rotated to the right or left. The red filter is placed in front of the right eye and the patient is asked to move the green line until it is parallel with the red line.

The test is held at 40 cm, and the amount of torsion is read off the scale printed on the back of the test. It can measure up to 25° of excyclotorsion and 10° of incyclotorsion. It can be used in all positions of gaze provided it is presented perpendicular to the visual axis. The test is quickly performed and has been shown to be comparable with the major amblyo-scope, Maddox double rod and Maddox wing (Georgievski 1995b).

Objective test

Fundus photography

This provides an objective assessment of torsion in which the relative positions of the fovea and the optic disc are noted. Normally the fovea is 0.3 disc diameters below the centre of the optic disc. There are individual variations, but these lie within 0.25 disc diameters between the two eyes. If a greater displacement is seen this should be regarded as abnormal and a cyclodeviation is present. The fovea will appear relatively high in incyclotropia and low in excyclotropia.

Indications

The main indication for measuring cyclotropia is in patients with acquired paralytic strabismus, par-ticularly in unilateral or bilateral fourth cranial nerve palsies when the presence and extent of cyclotropia is a crucial factor in the choice of ocular muscle surgery (see Chapter 9). In such cases it is not sufficient to measure cyclotropia only in the pri-mary position; it must also be recorded in other gaze positions, particularly in the lower field, in order to plan treatment. It is only rarely possible to measure torsion subjectively in other conditions in which it is known to occur, partly because the patient is unaware of it and also because binocular function is too poor. Objective measurement may be possible in such cases.

Supplementary tests

Bielschowsky head tilt test

The main purpose of the Bielschowsky head tilt test is to differentiate a palsy of the superior oblique from one affecting the contralateral superior rectus. Other possible uses are:

• differentiation of an inferior rectus and contralat-eral inferior oblique palsy, both rare conditions;

• differentiation of DVD from other vertical strabismus.

In some centres, particularly those in the USA, the head tilt forms part of the routine examination of all patients with a vertical deviation.

Method

The method is described taking as an example a right superior oblique or left superior rectus palsy. The compensatory head posture in either case involves a head tilt to the shoulder, adopted to compensate a right hyper or left hypo deviation, and in the case of a superior oblique weakness extorsion of the right eye. The patient fixates a mid-distance target on eye level and the examiner notes the eye position with the head tilted maximally (30°) to the left shoulder; the head is then tilted maximally to the right shoulder, observing the behaviour of the right eye. A cover test should be performed to compare the amount of hyperdeviation with the head tilted to either shoulder; a more accurate assessment of the deviation can be obtained by a prism cover test measurement in the two positions.

Precaution

• The examiner must use the cover test to ensure that the patient fixates with either eye. If he fixates only with the paretic eye (when a superior oblique palsy is present) the elevation of that eye can be missed.

Results

If there is a right superior oblique palsy, the right eye will probably be seen to elevate when the head is tilted to the right and there will be a significant increase in the amount of right hyperdeviation. If the left superior rectus is affected, there will be very little difference in the amount of vertical deviation on tilting to either side.

The widely accepted criterion for a positive result is an increase in hyperdeviation of at least 5 prism dioptres on tilting the head from the hypotropic side to the hypertropic side.

Explanation

When the head is tilted to the right the right eye is normally intorted by the superior oblique and the superior rectus; the depressing action of the superior oblique is balanced by the elevating action of the superior rectus and the eye remains level. If there is a superior oblique palsy the elevating action of the superior rectus is unopposed and the hyperdeviation increases. This is described as a positive result.

Jampolsky (1986) maintained that a positive head tilt test can result from superior rectus contracture rather than from this muscle's unopposed action. Levine (1969) believed that overaction of the inferior oblique, arising as part of the muscle sequelae of a superior oblique palsy, contributed to the elevation of the eye on head tilt to the affected side. This view was confirmed by Goodier (1981), whose clinical study showed that only patients with superior oblique palsy and overaction of the ipsilateral inferior oblique demonstrated a positive head tilt. Kushner *et al.* (1984) studied cyclodeviation during forced head tilt to either side in patients with unilateral superior oblique palsy, filming the eye movements with a corneal marker to show torsion. They found that both the superior and inferior vertically acting muscles were active on ipsilateral head tilt, rapid extorsion of the eye occurring due mainly to the inferior oblique action. Recession of the inferior oblique resulted in a normal head tilt test. They concluded that ipsilateral inferior oblique overaction could be in part responsible for elevation of the eye on tilting to the affected side.

Value

The Bielschowsky head tilt test provides useful confirmatory evidence of superior oblique palsy but is not infallible. It may also help in the detection of bilateral fourth nerve palsy, when a positive result is obtained when the head is tilted to either shoulder. A positive result may influence the choice of muscle surgery, since it has been found that weakening of the inferior oblique produced a negative response to this test (Goodier 1981; Kushner *et al.* 1984). Jampolsky (1986) reported that when DVD was present in both eyes, the head tilt test resulted in right hypertropia on tilting the head to the left and left hypertropia on tilting it to the right, the opposite of the findings in a superior oblique palsy, thus aiding the diagnosis in DVD.

The head tilt test in horizontal strabismus

Moore and Cohen (1987) studied the effect of head tilting in horizontal strabismus. They reported that 98% of exotropic patients showed right hypertropia on tilting to the right side and left hypertropia on tilting to the left side, averaging 8 Δ hypertropia. The converse was found in esotropia, with left hypertropia on tilting to the right and right hypertropia on tilting to the left. The hypertropia was not explained by vertical muscle dysfunction and the authors suggested that these findings might be considered normal.

Parks–Helveston 3-step test

The Parks–Helveston 3-step test can simplify the diagnosis of vertical muscle palsies.

Method

The test consists of three steps.
1   A cover test is performed in the primary position, noting which eye is hypertropic.
2   An alternate cover test is performed on dextroversion and on laevoversion, to assess the direction of greater vertical deviation.
3   The Bielschowsky head tilt test is performed, tilting the head to either shoulder and noting the difference in degree of hypertropia.

Application

If the cover test reveals a right hypertropia in the primary position which increases on laevoversion, there is either a right superior oblique palsy or a left superior rectus palsy. These two conditions can be differentiated by the Bielschowsky head tilt test, which will show an increase in right hypertropia if the superior oblique is affected. A prism cover test can be used to measure and compare the degree of hypertropia. The test can be modified by using the alternate cover test in, for example, laevoelevation and laevodepression to find the position of maximum hypertropia, rather than relying on the head tilt test. We prefer this method.

Guidelines for measuring a deviation

Assessment of the deviation can be qualitative or quantitative. Qualitative assessment includes the cover test, but it is preferable to obtain a quantitative measurement. The important aspects of each test to note are:
- is the test performed in free space?
- what is the level of dissociation incurred?
- is proximal convergence induced?
- are the distance and the amount of accommodation controlled?
- does the test require simultaneous perception (SP) and normal retinal correspondence to give an accurate subjective response?
- is central or near central fixation necessary.

In general measurements are most accurate if they are performed in free space with maximum dissociation and controlled distance and accommodation. Table 5.3 gives a brief summary of situations which may affect the choice of test.

Measurement of AC/A ratio

The AC/A ratio represents the amount of accommodative convergence exerted in response to one unit of accommodation. An individual's AC/A ratio, which may be genetically determined, has been shown to remain virtually unchanged from childhood to at least presbyopic age, providing the stimulus to accommodation is kept within narrow limits. Patients approaching presbyopic age show an increase in the

Table 5.3 Comparison of tests used to measure strabismus.

Test	Reduced VA	Limited cooperation	SP required	Nine positions	Torsion
Corneal reflections	Yes	Yes	No	No	No
Maddox rod	No	No	Yes	Yes	Yes
Maddox wing	No	No	Yes	No	Yes
Prism cover test	No	No	No	Yes	No
Prism reflection test	Yes	Yes	No	No	No
Major amblyoscope	Yes	No	Yes/No	Yes	Yes
Lees screen	No	No	Yes	Yes	Yes*

* Yes with adaptation (see text). VA, visual acuity; SP, simultaneous perception.

AC/A ratio when these limits are extended (Breinin & Chin 1973). It follows that it is the stimulus to accommodate which induces accommodative convergence rather than the physical accommodation exerted.

Two AC/A ratio measurements are defined by Alpern *et al.* (1959).
• Stimulus AC/A, in which the magnitude of vergence is measured with a unit change in accommodative stimulus.
• Response AC/A, in which the magnitude of vergence is measured with a unit change in accommodation. This method requires an objective measurement of accommodation, which can be obtained by using an optometer, an instrument able to determine the refractive state of the eye.

The two are interrelated, the latter being slightly higher.

Historically the normal AC/A ratio has been accepted as 3–5 : 1, i.e. for every 1 dioptre sphere of accommodation, between 3 and 5 prism dioptres of vergence occurs. However, much of the early data used the fixation disparity method of measurement (Martens & Ogle 1959), whereas most clinicians now prefer the gradient method. Using this method Plenty (1988) reported a ratio of less than 3 : 1 in normal subjects, with a mean of 2.13 in children and 3.03 in adults. No ratio was as high as 5 : 1. Firth *et al.* (1996) reported a mean of 2.88. Clinically it is assumed that the ratio is linear. However, this was not confirmed by Firth *et al.* Nonlinearity may be due in part to inaccuracy of accommodation, which could only be assured if the response AC/A was measured. Note should therefore be taken of the lens power used to calculate the ratio.

Methods of measurement

Clinical measurement is based on changing the stimulus to accommodation and assessing the amount of accommodative convergence which results from this change. This can be achieved in one of two ways:
• By changing the distance of the fixation target from infinity to 33 cm, as in the heterophoria method.
• By using spherical lenses to increase or decrease the amount of accommodation, as in the gradient method.

Heterophoria method
Measurement is carried out as follows:
• The IPD is measured in centimetres, as it influences the amount of convergence needed as fixation changes between distance and near and thus must be taken into account when calculating the ratio.
• The patient should wear his refractive correction.
• The deviation is measured by prism cover test at 6 m and at 33 cm, using a detailed target, preferably a Snellen letter or optotype corresponding to the patient's optimum visual acuity. If the target is seen clearly at 33 cm it is assumed that 3 DS of accommodation is exerted.

Calculation of the ratio
The ratio is calculated as follows:

$$AC/A = IPD + \frac{n-d}{D}$$

where AC = accommodative convergence; A = accommodation; IPD = interpupillary distance in centimetres; n = prism cover test measurement at 33 cm; d = prism cover test measurement at 6 m; D = accommodation in dioptres, based on the reciprocal of the focal distance (3 DS at 33 cm). A positive sign denotes an esodeviation, a negative sign denotes an exotropia or exophoria. An example of the calculation is:

$$AC/A = 6 + \frac{-20 - (-5)}{3} = 1:1$$

In this example the patient is assumed to have an intermittent exotropia of the convergence insufficiency type (near exotropia). The AC/A ratio is low.

Gradient method
The gradient method can be used with concave lenses at 6 m or with convex lenses at 33 cm. This is regarded as the most accurate method of measuring the AC/A ratio. The gradient method is the method of choice in our view because it excludes both tonic and proximal convergence, measuring only accommodative convergence.

Using concave lenses
• The patient wears his refractive correction.
• The deviation is measured by prism cover test at 6 m, using a detailed fixation target.

• Concave lenses are inserted in trial frames in strengths of up to 3.00 DS. Time is allowed for accommodation to take place: as soon as the target is seen clearly the prism cover test is repeated.

Calculation of the ratio

The ratio is calculated by the equation:

$$AC/A = \frac{+L-(-L)}{D}$$

where +L = prism cover test measurement with concave lenses (on accommodation); –L = prism cover test without lenses; D = strength of lens used. An example of this calculation is:

$$AC/A = \frac{+30-(+6)}{3} = 8:1$$

In this example the AC/A ratio is high.

The gradient method can be used by measuring the angles with a major amblyoscope instead of the prism cover test. The deviation is first measured using simultaneous perception slides and then re-measured with the addition of concave lenses. The results must then be converted into prism dioptres. This method is useful with younger patients.

Using convex lenses

• The deviation is measured using an accommodative target at 33 cm.
• Convex lenses are inserted in trial frames in strengths up to 3.0 DS. The patient must relax his accommodation to see the target clearly. The prism cover test is then repeated. This method is particularly applicable in differentiating true and simulated distance exotropia (see Chapter 13).

Indications for measuring the AC/A ratio

Measurement of the AC/A ratio is essential in the following conditions:
• accommodative esotropia with convergence excess;
• intermittent distance exotropia to differentiate true and simulated distance exotropia.

Measurement can be useful in all deviations in which there is a significant difference between the near and distance deviations.

Precautions

• Accommodation must be maintained at a constant level throughout the test. If the patient can read he can be asked to name different letters, but if he is too young the fixation picture should be changed and the child asked about details on it.
• When using the gradient method it may be better to start with a 1 DS lens, particularly with plus lenses, which many people find difficult to overcome.
• When using the heterophoria method the near fixation target must be kept at exactly 33 cm.

Problems

It is sometimes difficult for the patient to exert accommodation to clear the letters or picture at 6 m through concave lenses. It is not always possible to increase the lens strength to 3.00 DS even in children, and the ratio must be measured using –1.00 or –2.00 DS lenses instead.

Other methods of measurement

Graphic method

This method is designed for use with the major amblyoscope. Considerable cooperation is required and the method is unsuitable for young children.
• The IPD must be measured accurately. The angle of deviation is first measured subjectively using a reduced Snellen test-type slide in front of one eye and a vertical line in front of the other eye. The patient bisects the smallest line of letters visible to him with the black line.
• The measurement is repeated with the addition of concave lenses, starting with –1.0 DS, increasing the strength in 1 DS steps to –4.0 DS if possible. The patient is asked to name the letters to ensure that he is accommodating.

To calculate the ratio, the measurements are compared with the normal convergence requirements for the distance which corresponds to the accommodative stimulus for each lens strength. These are 6, 12, 18 and 24 DS for lenses of 1.0, 2.0, 3.0 and 4.0 DS, respectively, if the IPD is 6 cm. The results show whether the response is slow or fast (Duke-Elder & Wybar 1973). If slow, the amount of convergence induced will be less than the normal convergence requirement, and if fast it will be greater than the normal requirement. The results can be plotted graphically, showing the difference in change induced in angle from the convergence requirement for each dioptre of accommodation.

Fixation disparity method

The principle of this method is that the amount of fixation disparity is altered when positive or negative convergence is induced by base-out or base-in prisms and when the accommodative stimulus is changed by concave or convex lenses.

Method

The subject's fixation disparity is first measured using two centrally placed vertical lines seen against a background which is common to both eyes. The upper line, which can be moved, is seen by one eye and the lower fixed line is seen by the other eye. The subject adjusts the upper line until the two are seen one directly above the other. The amount of adjustment gives a measurement of the disparity.

Measurements are repeated as positive and negative convergence are induced by prisms. The patient's eyes are not dissociated and he maintains binocular single vision with a fusional background until convergence fails. The results can be plotted as a curve. Measurements are repeated using concave and convex lenses to change the accommodative stimulus, providing a second curve.

Calculation of the ratio

The ratio is derived by finding the stimuli for accommodation and for convergence which result in the same amount of fixation disparity. For a detailed description of this method and of fixation disparity curves the reader is referred to Ogle *et al.* (1967).

Value of these other methods of measurement

The graphic method provides information on the speed of the response as well as giving a measurement. The fixation disparity method has the advantage that the eyes are not dissociated. Both methods are time-consuming and require considerable cooperation.

Convergence accommodation/convergence ratio (CA/C ratio)

The synkinesis between accommodation and convergence is such that when convergence is initiated by disparate near images, accommodation also occurs.

Accommodation resulting directly from convergence is termed convergence accommodation (or vergence accommodation). Just as the AC/A ratio is measured to discover whether a known amount of accommodation results in excessive or, less usually, defective accommodative convergence, the CA/C ratio can be measured to assess whether a known amount of convergence results in excessive or defective convergence accommodation. It has been reported that there is a reciprocal relationship between the AC/A and CA/C ratios, so that when one ratio is very high the other ratio is likely to be very low (Schor 1988).

The CA/C ratio can be calculated by comparing the refraction of the eyes before and after convergence is initiated by a base-out prism. The ratio is expressed as the amount of convergence accommodation per metre angle of convergence. The normal CA/C ratio is in the region of 0.5 DS to 1 metre angle. For details of the methods of measurement the reader is referred to Schor and Ciuffreda (1983). In practice it is not always possible to ensure that only convergence accommodation is exerted, making it difficult to assess the significance of the ratio in conditions in which it might be abnormal, for example in intermittent esotropia and exotropia. Objective assessment of accommodation is necessary to assess this response with any degree of accuracy.

References

Alpern, M., Kincaid, W.M. & Lubeck, M.J. (1959) Vergence and accommodation III: proposed definitions of the AC/A ratios. *American Journal of Ophthalmology* 48, 141–148.

Archer, S.M. (1988) Developmental aspects of the Brüchner test. *Ophthalmology* 95, 1098–1101.

Awaya, S., Iwata, M., Miura, M. & Mizukami, Y. (1986) The 'New Cyclo Tests' and its clinical application. In: *Proceedings of the Fifth Meeting of the International Strabismological Association, Rome* (ed. E.C. Campos). ETA, Italy, pp. 225–231.

Breinin, G.M. & Chin, N.B. (1973) Accommodation, convergence and ageing. *Documenta Ophthalmologica* 34, 109–121.

Brodie, S.E. (1987) Photographical calibration of the Hirschberg test. *Investigative Ophthalmology and Visual Science* 28, 736–742.

Calcutt, C. (1995) Is fixation preference assessment an effective method of detecting strabismic amblyopia? *British Orthoptic Journal* 52, 29–31.

Dickey, C.F. & Scott, W.E. (1987) Amblyopia – the prevalence in congenital esotropia versus partially accommodative esotropia: diagnosis and results of treatment. In: *Transactions of the Sixth International Orthoptic Congress, Harrogate* (eds M. Lenk-Schafer, D. Calcutt, M. Doyle & S. Moore), pp. 106–112. British Orthoptic Society, London.

Duke-Elder, S. & Wybar, K. (1973) *Ocular Motility and Strabismus*, Vol. 6, pp. 204–206. Kimpton, London.

Dulley, B. & Harden, A. (1974) Cyclo-torsion: a new method of measurement. *British Orthoptic Journal* **31**, 70–77.

Firth, A.Y., Leach, C.M., Griffiths, H.J. & Rennie, I.G. (1996) Patterns of nonlinearity in the ratio of stimulus accommodative convergence to accommodation. *Middle East Journal of Ophthalmology* **14** (2), 123–127.

Flüeler, U.R., Elhatton, K.M. & Guyton, D.C. (1995) A combination horizontal/vertical prism bar. *Strabismus* **3**, 27–32.

Foster, J.F., Pemberton, E.C. & Bagshaw, J. (1953) Modified combination of the Lancaster and Hess tests. *British Orthoptic Journal* **10**, 32–36.

Georgievski, Z. (1995a) Synoptophore versus prism and cover test measurements in strabismus. A question of instrument convergence? *Strabismus* **3**, 71–77.

Georgievski, Z. (1995b) Comparison of 3 standard clinical tests and a new test for the measurement of torsional diplopia. Update on Strabismus and Pediatric Ophthalmology. In: *Proceedings of the Joint ISA and AAPOS and S Meeting, Vancouver*, pp. 171–174.

Goodier, H.M. (1981) The evaluation of the Bielschowsky's head tilt test. In: *Orthoptics, Research and Practice. Transactions of the Fourth International Orthoptic Congress, Berne* (eds J. Mein & S. Moore), pp. 189–197. Kimpton, London.

Jampolsky, A. (1986) Management of vertical strabismus. In: *Pediatric Ophthalmology and Strabismus: Transactions of the New Orleans Academy of Ophthalmology* (ed. J.H. Allen), pp. 141–171. Raven Press, New York.

Johnson, F., Harcourt, B. & Fox, A. (1987) The clinical assessment of cyclodeviation. In: *Orthoptic Horizons. Transactions of the Sixth International Orthoptic Congress* (eds M. Lenk-Schafer, C. Calcutt, M. Doyle & S. Moore), pp. 179–183. British Orthoptic Society, London.

Kaye, S.B., Ansons, A.M., Green, J.R. & Wylie, J. (1989) The prism bar – Prentice and frontal positions. *Eye* **3** (4), 404–408.

Kushner, B.J., Kraft, S.E. & Vrabec, D.P. (1984) Ocular torsional movements in humans with normal and abnormal ocular motility. Part 1: objective measurements. *Journal of Pediatric Ophthalmology and Strabismus* **21**, 172–177.

Levine, M.H. (1969) Evaluation in Bielschowsky's head tilt test. *Archives of Ophthalmology* **82**, 433–439.

Martens, T.G. & Ogle, K.N. (1959) Observations on accommodative convergence, especially on its non-linear relationships. *American Journal of Ophthalmology* **47**, 455–462.

Moore, S. & Cohen, R.L. (1987) The head tilt test in horizontal strabismus. *American Orthoptic Journal* **37**, 105–108.

von Noorden, G.K. (1977) *von Noorden and Maumenee's Atlas of Strabismus*, pp. 44–45. C.V. Mosby, St Louis.

Ogle, K.N., Martens, T.C. & Dyer, J.A. (1967) *Ocular Motor Imbalance in Binocular Vision and Fixation Disparity*. Lea & Febiger, Philadelphia.

Plenty, J. (1988) A new classification for intermittent exotropia. *British Orthoptic Journal* **45**, 19–22.

Pratt-Johnson, J.A. & Tillson, G. (1994) *Management of Strabismus and Amblyopia. A Practical Guide*. Thieme Medical Publishers, New York.

Ruttum, M. & von Noorden, G.K. (1984) The Bagolini striated lens test for cyclotropia. *Documenta Ophthalmologica* **58**, 131–139.

Schor, C.M. (1988) Phasic-tonic organisation of accommodation and vergence. In: *Strabismus and Amblyopia. Wenner-Gren International Symposium* (eds G. Lennerstrand, G.K. von Noorden & E. Campos), pp. 111–120. Macmillan Press, London.

Schor, C.M. & Ciuffreda, K. (eds) (1983) *Vergence Eye Movements: Basic and Clinical Aspects*. Butterworths, Boston.

Spielmann, A. (1986) A translucent occluder for studying eye position under unilateral or bilateral cover test. *American Orthoptic Journal* **36**, 65–74.

Thompson, J.T. & Guyton, D.L. (1983) Ophthalmic prisms: measurement errors and how to minimise them. *Ophthalmology* **90**, 204–210.

Wisnicki, H.J. & Guyton, D.L. (1986) A modified corneal light reflex test with distance fixation. *American Journal of Ophthalmology* **102**, 661–662.

6
Ocular Movements

Ocular motor function

The ocular motor system functions to maintain viewing in a variety of situations. There are five main types of movement:

- saccades
- smooth pursuit
- vergence
- optokinetic
- vestibular.

Normal full ocular movement is dependent on the integrity of the the ocular motor nuclei, the internuclear and infranuclear pathways and the extraocular muscles and their check ligaments. There must be integration of the different control systems, originating in the supranuclear centres. The structures involved in eye movement control are shown in Figs 6.1 and 6.2. Lesions affecting these pathways are discussed in Chapter 22.

Assessment of ocular movement establishes:
- the extent and quality of movement in all directions of gaze;
- the integrity of the movement systems and the neural pathways involved.

Ocular movement takes place around the three axes of Fick (x, y and z axes), which pass through the centre of rotation of the globe:

x = vertical eye movement, which takes place around the horizontal x-axis.

y = torsional eye movement, which takes place around the anteroposterior y-axis.

z = horizontal movement, which takes place around the vertical z axis.

Conjugate movement is movement of both eyes in the same direction (version). *Disjugate movement* is movement of the eyes in opposite directions (vergence). *Ductions* are uniocular movements from the primary position.

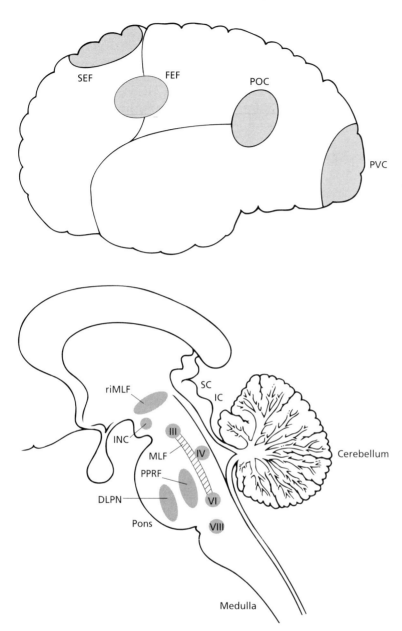

Fig. 6.1 Cortical structures involved in eye movement control. The primary visual cortex (PVC), parieto-occipital cortex (POC) and the frontal eye fields (FEF) have important roles in the generation of saccadic and pursuit movements. The supplementary eye fields (SEF) in the dorsomedial frontal lobe is involved with saccades.

Fig. 6.2 Subcortical structures involved in eye movement control. Structures involved in the generation of saccadic eye movements include the superior colliculus (SC), pontine paramedian reticular formation (PPRF) and rostral interstitial nucleus of the medial longitudinal fasciculus (riMLF). Subcortical pursuit eye commands are thought to arise from the dorsolateral pontine nuclei (DLPN) and cerebellum. The neural integrators responsible for stable gaze-holding are located in the cerebellum, medulla (vestibular nuclei (VIII)) and the interstitial nucleus of Cajal (INC). Binocular horizontal eye movement coordination involves projections along the medial longitudinal fasciculus (MLF). (IC, inferior colliculus; III, 3rd nerve nucleus; IV, 4th nerve nucleus; VI, 6th nerve nucleus.)

Laws relating to ocular movement

Donder's law

This states that a definite and invariable amount of torsion occurs for a given position of gaze, irrespective of how that position was reached.

Sherrington's law of reciprocal innervation

This states that when increased innervation is sent to a muscle to cause it to contract, decreased innervation goes to its direct antagonist, which is therefore relatively relaxed. This finely tuned interplay ensures smooth, accurate movement to take up or maintain fixation. It is a uniocular law.

Hering's law of equal innervation

This states that when an impulse goes to a muscle, causing it to contract, a simultaneous and equal impulse is sent to its contralateral synergist. For example, when looking to the right, the right lateral rectus and left medial rectus receive equal innervation to contract and the right medial rectus and left lateral rectus relax. This is a binocular law which aids the maintenance of binocular single vision (BSV).

Ocular movement systems

There are five ocular movement systems which ensure accurate fixation tracking of objects.

Saccadic system

A saccade is a fast eye movement of 400–700° s⁻¹. The purpose of a saccade is to place the image on the fovea. Saccades occur to refixate an object, to change fixation voluntarily on command, as an involuntary response to sound and as the fast phase of optokinetic nystagmus.

Control

The command for voluntary horizontal saccades originates in the frontal eyefields (FEF) (Brodmann area 8); the pathway descends via the anterior limb of the internal capsule to the superior colliculus then passes to the brainstem reticular formation in the pons. It decussates at the ponto-mesencephalic junction, hence stimulation of the FEF leads to contralaterally directed saccades. Vertical saccades are generated by signals from both FEF, with the pathway connecting with control centres in the midbrain.

The saccadic latency is the interval elapsing between the appearance of the stimulus and the start of the saccadic movement. This interval represents the time it takes the ocular motor system to process the signal before it reaches the extraocular muscles, and is normally about 200 ms.

A saccade comprises an accelerating and decelerating phase, with the peak velocity occurring a third of the way into the movement. The amplitude of the saccade has a close relationship with the peak saccadic velocity: large-amplitude saccades are associated with high veloc-ities (Bahill *et al.* 1975). Peak velocities range from 60° s⁻¹ to 600° s⁻¹ for movements of 1–30° in amplitude.

The desired position is reached by a 'pulse', which is a burst of electrical activity in the motor nerves, and is maintained by the 'step', which is an increase in electrical activity or energy to maintain eye position and counter the activity of antagonistic muscles. This sequence is coordinated by the neural integrator.

Development of saccades

Saccades can be initiated in the neonate but are inaccurate, consisting of jerky movements until the target is reached. Accuracy increases rapidly from 2 months of age. Infants use coordinated head and eye movements to change gaze to a greater extent than adults. The ability to change fixation with a single saccade has developed by 1 year of age (Fielder 1985).

Testing saccadic movement

Saccades are tested by asking the patient to look quickly from one target to another. For example, when testing horizontal saccades one target is held in the primary position and another to one side—often two pens of different colours. The patient is then instructed to look rapidly from one to the other. This is then repeated to the opposite side. The task should be repeated several times.

The saccades are observed both away from the midline and to the midline. Asymmetry between the two eyes and/or directions can sometimes be more easily detected if the left and right gaze is tested consecutively. This is achieved by holding the two pens, one to each side, within the limit of gaze; the patient is instructed to look from one pen to the observer's nose and then to the pen on the opposite side and back to the nose. Large excursions can be tested by asking the patient to look straight from the pen on right gaze to the pen held in left gaze and back. If ocular movement is significantly limited it may be necessary to hold the targets at the two extremes of the patient's gaze, asking him to look from right to left and back. Vertical saccades are tested in the same way, holding the targets above and below the patient's eye level.

Initially the head should not be restrained, so that abnormal or exaggerated head movements can be seen, for example the head thrusts seen in ocular motor apraxia, but the test should then be repeated with the head held if these occur. Small mobile or auditory toys can be used as targets for young children. The speed, accuracy and symmetry of movement in each direction should be observed and noted. Repeated testing may demonstrate fatigue or reveal inconsistencies.

Indications for testing

Saccadic movement is tested when limited ocular movement is seen or suspected. Saccadic testing is particularly important in the differential diagnosis between neurogenic and mechanical limitations: the saccadic velocity is reduced in a neurogenic palsy.

A slow peak saccadic velocity is most easily identified when there is a difference in the movement of the two eyes as in a unilateral sixth nerve palsy, resulting in slower movement of the affected eye on abduction. Global reductions in saccadic velocity, as seen, for example, in chronic progressive external ophthalmoplegia, can be harder to detect. Large-amplitude saccades accentuate small differences and may make identification easier. An optokinetic nystagmus (OKN) drum initiating multiple saccades may also accentuate differences in peak saccadic velocity and will demonstrate fatigue in conditions such as myasthenia gravis.

Saccadic velocities can be measured by electrodiagnostic techniques described later in this chapter.

Smooth pursuit system

A pursuit movement is a slow following movement which does not usually exceed 40° s⁻¹.

The pursuit system maintains stable eye tracking or combined eye-head tracking of slow-moving objects. The normal stimulus for pursuit movement is image movement in the parafoveal region (retinal slip).

Control

The higher control centres for pursuit movement lie in the parieto-occipital cortex; the fibres descend from the brainstem paramedial pontine reticular formation for horizontal pursuit commands. The cerebellum is closely associated with normal pursuit movements. Signals are generated during pursuit with the head stationary and during combined eye-head tracking.

Pursuit movements, like saccades, have a latency between the stimulus and start of movement; this is in the order of 100 ms. For target velocities up to 30–40° s⁻¹ most eyes are able accurately to track the object, with eye velocity equalling target velocity, hence the gain = 1 (gain is the ratio of eye velocity to head velocity). For higher target speeds the eyes have increasing difficulties in matching target velocity (gain < 1), either lagging behind the target or requiring a catch-up saccade to maintain fixation. Pursuit movements are influenced by the nature of the stimulus, how it behaves, the subject's attention and by certain drugs. The vestibular ocular reflex (VOR), which initiates eye movement equal and opposite to head movements, must be suppressed by the pursuit system in order to maintain stable eye tracking of objects.

Development of smooth pursuit movement

Roucoux *et al.* (1983) reported that following movements could be demonstrated in neonates when the target speed was very slow, but most 'following' movement in very early infancy is accomplished by a series of saccades. From 6 weeks of age, tracking a moving target becomes a mix of fast and slow movements, the latter gradually predominating until the smooth pursuit system is better developed at 3–4 months of age. Even at 3 months, Timms *et al.* (1987) reported a maximum pursuit velocity of 22° s⁻¹ and found that pursuit movement lagged in development compared with the vestibular system.

Testing smooth pursuit movements

Smooth pursuit movement is observed as the subject tracks a slow-moving (< 40° s⁻¹) target to the limit of gaze with the head stationary. Note is taken of the smoothness of movement, the extent of movement and if gaze position can be maintained. If regular catch-up saccades are observed then low pursuit gain may be present.

The ability of the pursuit system to cancel the VOR during combined eye-head tracking provides a sensitive measure of pursuit performance. This can be demonstrated by using a wooden tongue depressor with a small fixation target attached to one end. The subject holds the other end between his teeth, then slowly rotates his head from side to side then up and down whilst maintaining fixation on the target, which indicates a normal response. Failure of the pursuit system to cancel the VOR results in breaks in fixation, which occur as the VOR drives the eyes in the opposite direction to the head rotation. Multiple saccades are observed in the direction of the head movement as the subject attempts to regain fixation on the target.

Indications for testing

Smooth pursuit movements are tested routinely in all patients attending for orthoptic investigation in order to determine the extent and quality of movement. If an abnormality is noted or suspected during this procedure or the patient complains of symptoms of difficulty following objects, then the integrity of the system is tested as described.

Vergence system

Vergence is a disjugate eye movement generated to obtain and maintain binocular alignment. In this respect it functions entirely differently from the saccadic and smooth pursuit systems, which generate conjugate eye movement.

Vergence movement is mainly horizontal, comprising convergence and divergence, and serves to maintain binocular single vision when the fixation object approaches the eyes or recedes from them, allowing the appreciation of a single stereoscopic image. Vertical vergence and cyclovergence can also be demonstrated.

Convergence is principally brought about by:
• fusional vergence, which is generated in response to diplopia (retinal slip);
• accommodative vergence: accommodation takes place in response to a blurred image and generates convergence to maintain a clear single image.

Contributing to a much lesser extent are:
• proximal vergence, in which convergence is generated in response to the subject's awareness of the proximity of the fixation object;
• tonic vergence, in which a small amount of convergence is brought about by the tonus of the medial rectus muscles.

Convergence is normally associated with accommodation and pupillary miosis, the near triad.

Control

The higher centre control for vergence movements is poorly understood. Striate cortex neurones responding to retinal image disparity have been identified in monkeys (Poggio & Fischer 1977). Pre-motor signals are thought to originate in the mesencephalic reticular formation with separate populations of convergence cells. Three subnuclei, a, b and c, have been identified at the level of the medial rectus nucleus, with subnucleus c thought to be involved principally with vergence movements (Buttner-Ennever & Akert 1981).

Pure vergence movements have a maximum velocity of approximately $20°$ s^{-1}. However, vergence movements are more often associated with versional saccades, when the velocity of vergence is much increased (Leigh & Zee 1991). The dynamic properties of vergence movements (the relationship between peak vergence velocity and vergence amplitude) are more variable than those of saccades, being influenced by the type of stimulus, either retinal disparity or blur, its size and by whether the object is viewed monocularly or binocularly.

Development of convergence

Convergence can be demonstrated in full-term neonates but it is uncoordinated. Accurate and maintained convergence is well developed by 2–3 months of age.

Testing vergence movements

Convergence to the near point is tested routinely and can be measured using a near point rule. The horizontal and vertical vergence systems can also be tested by assessing motor fusion responses to prisms. Clinically the end-point of convergence is tested rather than the nature of the movement itself. Note should be taken of how well the convergence is maintained and if fatigue occurs on repeated testing.

Cyclovergence is best assessed using the major amblyoscope, although a sensory as well as motor response is then involved. Further detailed description of these tests can be found in Chapters 5 and 7.

The vergence mechanism may affect strabismus and its control, for example in intermittent exotropia. In these cases it may be necessary to disrupt the mechanism in order to reveal the maximum angle of deviation; prism adaptation or occlusion can be used for this purpose.

Indications for testing
Convergence should be tested in all patients.

Vestibular and optokinetic system

These systems are considered together because of their common purpose, which is to maintain a stable retinal image during head movements. A variety of sensory signals originating from the labyrinthine semicircular canals, the otoliths, the visual system and peripheral receptors are used to generate compensatory eye movements to counteract the effect of head movement. The movements comprise a slow following movement and a rapid refixation movement. During whole body rotation the vestibular ocular reflex (VOR) generates compensatory eye movements after a 16 ms latency; the slow phase is opposite to the direction of rotation and the fast phase is in the direction of rotation. This occurs due to stimulation of the semicircular canals. As a constant rotational velocity is approached the VOR declines, causing retinal image slip across the retina; this in turn stimulates the optokinetic and smooth pursuit systems, which eventually take over the generation of compensatory eye movements to stabilize the retinal image.

The semicircular canals respond only to angular acceleration, which is produced by head rotation. Translatory head movements cause linear acceleration, which occurs during head movement without rotation, for example movement of the head up and down whilst running. Static head tilts stimulate the otoliths, which are sensitive to linear acceleration.

The optokinetic system combines with the pursuit system to provide stable tracking during head rotations and during full-field moving stimulation (the optokinetic response). In the clinical situation it is difficult to isolate the optokinetic response from the more dominant pursuit response.

Control
The vestibular system comprises a peripheral component located in the middle ear and a central component situated in the medullary region of the brainstem. The peripheral vestibular apparatus consists of the three semicircular canals and the otolith organs, the saccule and utricle. Each semicircular canal connects centrally via a three neurone arc to paired extraocular muscles. The orientation of the horizontal canal is only truly horizontal with the head held at 30° in extension; in this position the lateral canal is vertical and provides a maximal response during caloric testing.

The otoliths connect centrally only to the cyclovertical muscles. The vestibular nuclei play a key role in coding information for gaze maintenance and have important connections to the cerebellum.

It is probable that there are two pathways for the neural control of optokinetic movement: one passing to the occipital cortex and mediating nasal to temporal target movement; the other a more primitive extrageniculate striate pathway, mediating temporal to nasal target movement. This subcortical pathway may function before the more sophisticated cortical pathway has fully developed, accounting for the early asymmetry seen in infants.

Development of the vestibular system
Phylogenetically this is the oldest slow eye-movement system. The horizontal VOR is well developed at birth, whereas the vertical VOR develops slightly later.

Development of the optokinetic system
Optokinetic nystagmus (OKN) can be elicited in very young infants provided that both eyes are open and that the targets are moved fairly briskly. Asymmetry of OKN is found when the infant is tested uniocularly. OKN can be demonstrated by temporal to nasal movement of the targets but there is little or no response when the movement is reversed to a nasal to temporal direction. Symmetry develops at about 4–6 months of age.

Testing the vestibular system
Vestibular dysfunction can lead to spontaneous slow eye movements which break fixation. Visual fixation must be disrupted to elicit the full extent of these movements and this can be achieved by using an opaque lens, a high convex Fresnel lens or by testing in the dark. The nystagmus produced can then be observed.

Visual acuity during head movement
The subject is asked to read down the Snellen chart: the head is then rotated from side to side at between 2 and 3 cycles per second and the subject is asked

to read the chart again. Vestibular imbalance reflected in abnormal gain will result in failure to maintain fixation, the eyes will repeatedly drift off target, using small saccades to recover fixation. The procedure is repeated moving the head vertically. The acuity will be reduced by one or two lines if abnormal gain is present. If the VOR is intact there will be no reduction in visual acuity.

Caloric testing

Caloric testing uses warm and cold water to set up temperature gradients across the semicircular canals, the resulting convection currents in the endolymph bend the cupula, so stimulating the hair cells. The subject's head is positioned 30° from supine, which places the lateral canal in the vertical plane, maximizing the effects from the convection currents. Cold water (30°C) is irrigated into the auditory meatus of first one side and then the other; this is then repeated using warm water (44°C). The normal response is nystagmus, with the fast phase to the opposite side for cold water and to the same side for warm water.

Dolls's head test

The subject fixates an object whilst his head is rotated briskly by the examiner, first in the horizontal plane and then in the vertical plane. A normally functioning VOR will result in eye movements equal and opposite to head movements. The extent of eye movement will be seen to increase in a supranuclear lesion whereas it will remain unchanged if the lesion is at a lower level.

Cooperation from the patient is not required and the response will occur even if the patient is unconscious.

This test can also be very useful in infants with childhood esotropia where there is suspected lateral rectus weakness. A normal response will indicate that the muscle function is not impaired.

Spinning baby test

This test is based on observation of the conjugate deviation of the infant's eyes in response to head movement induced by rotation. The infant is held in an upright position under the axillae, facing the examiner and on a level with his face; the neck should be supported. The examiner rotates the baby and himself through 360°, observing the infant's eyes.

Stimulation of the semicircular canals should cause a conjugate deviation in the direction opposite to that of the rotation, demonstrating that the VOR is intact. Postrotational nystagmus persists for a few seconds but is rapidly suppressed by the visual system in a sighted infant. In practice a good response is obtained by swinging through 180° instead of 360°.

Because the test must be performed in the light, the normal response is due to interaction between the vestibular and optokinetic systems. Smooth pursuit movement is unlikely to contribute in a young infant but an older infant may succeed in maintaining fixation on the examiner's face during rotation, in which case the more developed pursuit system has suppressed the vestibular and optokinetic systems and the test is invalidated.

Indications for testing the VOR

• When the patient is too ill, too uncooperative or too young for ocular movement to be tested by other means.
• To prove whether or not the VOR is functioning in an apparent gaze palsy
• When there is apparent lack of abduction in an infant.

Testing the optokinetic system

A large-field moving stimulus is required to test the optokinetic response, or alternatively the patient is rotated at a constant velocity in static surroundings. The former is preferable as it allows eye movements to be recorded and quantified. Infrared techniques have allowed very detailed analysis of these movements. A modified technique using a striped curtain and rotating chair has been used successfully to test infants.

Small hand-held striped drums or tapes are still in clinical use but these primarily test the pursuit system, particularly if the subject is instructed to look at the drum.

Indications for testing OKN

OKN should be tested in suspected gaze palsies or internuclear ophthalmoplegia. Convergence retraction nystagmus can be seen when the stripes of an OKN drum are rotated vertically from up to down, thus helping to establish the diagnosis of the dorsal midbrain (Parinaud's) syndrome (see Chapter 22).

Clinical assessment of ocular movement range

Testing the smooth pursuit system in each direction of gaze first assesses the extent of ocular movement. The subject is instructed to follow a spotlight from the primary position to the limits of each position of gaze in turn. The head must be kept stationary. Versions are tested first, comparing the angle of deviation in each position with that seen in the primary position by means of an alternate cover test, noting if there is an increase, decrease or a change in the nature of the deviation on cover test; for example, the presence of a vertical component in some gaze positions would indicate an abnormality of vertical movement.

Ductions are tested by occluding one eye and assessing the uniocular excursion. Ductions should be tested with each eye whenever limitation of movement is seen or suspected, moving the target to the limit of gaze. It is normal for ductions to be slightly greater than versions, especially on lateral gaze. In neurogenic palsies, movement will improve on ductions but no significant improvement occurs if a mechanical restriction is present. Saccades should be tested when the differential diagnosis is not clear or when fatigue is seen on testing smooth pursuit movement. OKN testing can be helpful if the integrity of either the smooth pursuit or saccadic systems is in doubt or if both up and down movement is limited.

Details which should be observed when testing ocular movements are:
- the extent of ocular movement in each eye;
- the quality of the movement, if it is steadily maintained or if catch-up saccades occur;
- whether fixation can be maintained when the limit of movement is reached or if there is end-point nystagmus or even gaze-evoked nystagmus;
- the effect of repeated testing of both smooth pursuit and saccadic movement—this is especially important in patients with a history suggestive of myasthenia gravis;
- any discomfort on movement, which can occur with mechanical restriction or an inflammatory condition;
- whether the movement ceases gradually or suddenly;
- a difference between version and duction;

- change in the position of the eyelids, for example lid-lag seen in thyroid eye disease;
- change in the position of the globe, for example globe retraction sometimes accompanies mechanical restriction;
- a change in palpebral fissure size, which can be seen, for example, in Duane's retraction syndrome;
- the presence of nystagmus and its direction—in Parinaud's syndrome this may be more obvious when testing vertical OKN.

In general a patient with limited ocular movement will fix with the unaffected or more mobile eye. Therefore control of fixation by means of the cover test is necessary in order that incomitance and contralateral movements are assessed accurately. The alternate cover test should be performed in all positions of gaze comparing the size of movement seen.

Recording of ocular movement

The information recorded must include:
- Whether movement is full, limited or excessive.
- The grade of abnormality, usually −4 to +4.
- Direction of the abnormality (this may be related to the muscle affected, if known, e.g. underaction of right superior oblique).
- Any associated signs, for example globe, fissure or lid changes, or the presence of nystagmus (methods of recording and measuring nystagmus are described in Chapter 23).

Grading of limitation and overaction
Limitation of movement is usually graded on a scale of −1 to −4; −4 indicates that there is no movement beyond the midline; −3 indicates that 25% movement remains, −2, 50% and −1, 75%. If the eye cannot reach the midline, the extent of limitation should be recorded as −5 or higher if necessary. Duction should be compared with version and any difference between them should be recorded.

Overaction is graded from +1 to +4. These movements can be more difficult to gauge, but using the inferior oblique as an example, +1 would indicate excessive elevation only in the field of main action and +4 would mean the maximum amount of elevation anatomically possible. Grades +3 and +4 of overaction usually indicate an updrift is present on horizontal movement, whereas +2 overaction indicates that the eye has to be in an elevated position before excessive movement occurs.

Examples of grading

Right superior oblique palsy:

−2 underaction (u/a) of the right superior oblique (RSO) with +2 overaction (o/a) of the left inferior rectus (LIR)

−1 u/a of left superior rectus (LSR) +3 o/a of right inferior oblique (RIO)

  Left blow-out fracture:

−3 restriction of left eye in all elevated positions with +3 overaction of right eye.

−1 restriction of left eye in all depressed positions with +2 overaction of right eye.

  Limitation and overaction can also be represented diagrammatically (O'Flynn 1994). A hatched area indicates a restriction and a minus number without hatching indicates an underaction (Fig. 6.3a,b).

  This method of recording is generally also combined with a template that includes prism and cover test measurements in nine positions of gaze (Fig. 6.4). Measurement in each gaze position should be taken and recorded on the chart. It is important to note that the two may not equate, as ocular movements are tested for near, and the prism and cover test are most commonly performed for distance. It may be necessary to measure gaze positions for near in certain circumstances—superior oblique palsies, for example—as the extent of the vertical deviation and

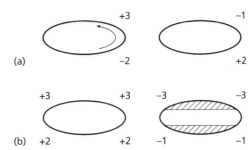

Fig. 6.3 (a) Diagrammatic representation of a superior oblique palsy. (b) A blow-out fracture.

presence of a V-pattern may only be demonstrable at near. The measurement may not reflect ocular movements in bilateral palsies or in mechanical limitation of movement. Prism cover test measurements with the head tilted to each shoulder can also be recorded on the diagram and although this can be helpful it may also be misleading (see 'Bielschowsky head tilt test' and 'Park's 3-step test' in Supplementary tests, Chapter 5).

  For those not using a template, ocular movements can be represented as a line diagram (Fig. 6.5).

Photographic/video recording

A photographic record of oculomotor disorders has the advantage that it shows relevant associated features, such as anomalies of head, lid or globe position as well as the limitation of movement. Video recording is particularly useful in subjects with nystagmus.

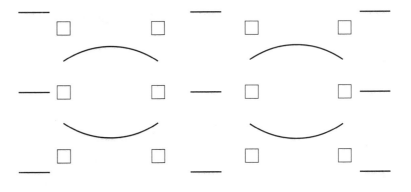

Fig. 6.4 Template for nine positions of gaze measurements.

———— Position of distance prism cover test results

☐ Position of numerical gradings of ocular movements

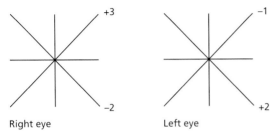

Right eye   Left eye

Fig. 6.5 Graphic representation of a right superior oblique palsy.

Diplopia chart

The diplopia chart provides a record of the separation of diplopic images in the nine positions of gaze. The patient wears red and green goggles, which must be carefully fitted so that he looks through them in all positions of gaze. He views a linear light source, usually presented vertically at 50 cm, and is questioned about the relative positions of the two images. He must be asked if the images are parallel or tilted; if torsion is present he should be asked to demonstrate it if possible by holding a pencil at the same angle.

The patient's head must be kept straight throughout the test, preferably by using a fixed head and chin rest. The distance of the light must remain constant and it must be kept upright. Once diplopia has been analysed in the primary position, the light is moved as far as possible in each gaze position in turn. If the limits of gaze are used it is easier to repeat the test under the same conditions.

If the patient sees a single image, the examiner must establish whether it is a fused image, if suppression is present, or if one image is obscured, for example by the patient's nose.

The diplopia chart is recorded as shown in Fig. 6.6. It must indicate the patient's right and left sides, and which eye sees the red image. The estimated separation of the two images should be recorded in each position, in centimetres.

The diplopia chart is not usually plotted routinely but it is useful if the patient is bedridden or handicapped and cannot plot a Hess chart and field of BSV. It can also be useful in acquired fourth nerve palsies, especially those due to head injury; this may result in a very asymmetrical bilateral palsy which can easily be misdiagnosed as unilateral: a small amount of reversed torsion recorded on the diplopia chart can indicate that both superior obliques are involved.

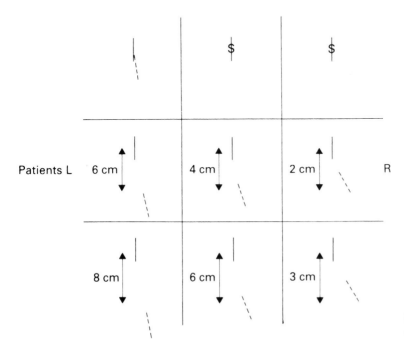

Patients L

Fig. 6.6 Diplopia chart of a patient with a right fourth nerve palsy.

Hess chart

As described in Chapter 5, the Hess chart gives a measurement in the nine positions of gaze which, provided the limitation is unilateral, will measure the amount of overaction and underaction of the extraocular muscles and provide a reliable and repeatable diagrammatic representation of the condition.

Interpretation of Hess charts

The charts of the two eyes are compared for position, size and shape.

Because the test is based on foveal projection, the position of the fields reflects the position of the eyes; for example, the higher field belongs to the higher eye, in contradistinction to diplopia, when the higher image belongs to the lower eye. The position of the central dot in each field indicates the deviation in the primary position, fixing with the right eye on the left chart and with the left eye on the right chart.

Due to Hering's law of equal innervation, the smaller field, plotted with the normal or more mobile eye fixating, belongs to the eye with primary limita-tion of movement. Underaction can be seen by noting the inward displacement of the dots; maximum displacement occurs in the direction of main action of the affected muscle. Overaction can be seen by noting the outward displacement of the dots; maximum displacement occurs in the direction of main action of the overacting contralateral synergist in the larger field (Fig. 6.7). If there is less marked inward and outward displacement in other directions, secondary underactions and overactions are present as a result of the development of muscle sequelae (Fig. 6.8). The outer fields should be examined carefully for small underactions and overactions, which may not be apparent on the inner fields.

A narrow field restricted in opposing directions of movement denotes a mechanical restriction of ocular movement (Fig. 6.9).

Equal-sized fields denote either symmetrical limitation of movement in both eyes, a nonparalytic strabismus or, sometimes, a very longstanding paralytic strabismus in which the development of muscle sequelae has led to concomitance.

Sloping fields denote A- and V-patterns. It is erroneous to interpret sloping fields as an indication of torsion.

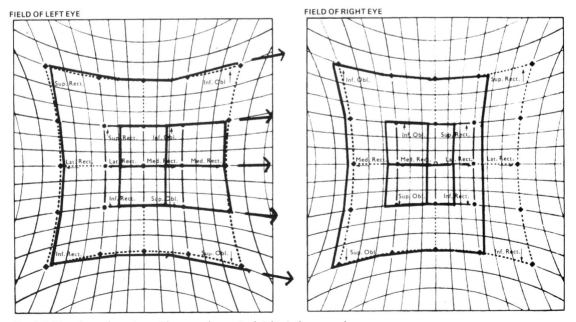

Fig. 6.7 Hess chart of a patient with a recently acquired right sixth nerve palsy.

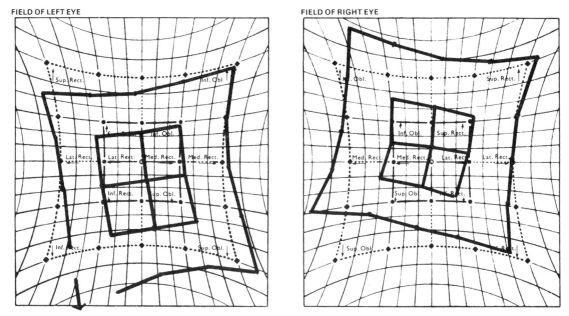

Fig. 6.8 Hess chart of a patient with a right fourth nerve palsy of several months' duration, showing the development of muscle sequelae—overaction of the left inferior rectus, overaction (contracture) of the right inferior oblique and underaction of the left superior rectus.

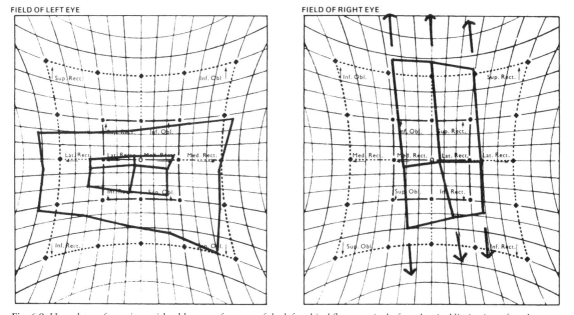

Fig. 6.9 Hess chart of a patient with a blow-out fracture of the left orbital floor, typical of mechanical limitation of ocular movement.

Each small square on the grid subtends 5° at the working distance of 50 cm, therefore the amount of deviation can be calculated by the displacement of the plotted point. It is important that care is taken in plotting as even very small inaccuracies result in significant measurement errors.

• In the primary position fixating with either eye, by the displacement of the plotted point from the centre dot.

• In the positions of maximum underaction and overaction of the affected muscles.

• Cyclotropia can be measured in degrees in the primary position and in the desired positions of gaze, using the linear pointer described by Dulley and Harden (1974) or by Johnson *et al.* (1987) (see Chapter 5).

Provided that the outer fields are plotted in every case, the charts are of diagnostic value, revealing even small limitations of movement at 30°. The accuracy of measurement in the periphery of gaze has been questioned. The main use of Hess charts is to provide a permanent record which can be used in assessing progress, planning treatment and evaluating its results, and in this they are invaluable. Hess charts should not be viewed in isolation but should be considered with the field of binocular single vision and other measurements of the deviation to give an overall picture.

Field of binocular single vision (binocular fixation)

The field of binocular single vision is plotted on a perimeter to depict the areas of the binocular field in which binocular single vision is maintained and those in which there is diplopia. The results are recorded on the appropriate binocular perimeter chart.

A field of binocular single vision should be plotted when a patient with diplopia is able to fuse the images in some part of the binocular field.

The patient is seated at the perimeter on eye level with its centre. A 2° white target or letter is used for fixation if using a Lister perimeter; a light is used in the Aimark model. If the target cannot be fused in the primary position it is moved along each meridian in turn until an area of binocular single vision is found. Usually the examiner knows where this area will be situated and can position the target accordingly. The area of binocular single vision is then plotted by moving from within it into the area of diplopia, recording the point at which diplopia first occurs. If the patient cannot see the target well or it is suppressed, a spotlight can be used instead. It may be necessary for presbyopic patients to wear their reading corrections but this should be avoided if possible.

The patient's head must remain straight. The fixation target should be moved slowly, otherwise he cannot report when it is seen as two. The target must be kept within the binocular field so that it is visible to both eyes and is not obscured by the nose; a cover test can be used to check visibility.

The patient must recognize diplopia when it occurs; although this is easier if red and green goggles are used, dissociation reduces the size of the field of binocular fixation and their use should be avoided. If there is some suppression present, an alternative method is to use Bagolini glasses and a spotlight as a means of ensuring that both images are seen.

The position, size and shape of the field of binocular fixation are examined.

The field of binocular single vision can be measured in degrees from the perimeter chart and these measurements compared with those of the normal field.

The field is displaced away from the direction of maximum limitation of movement; for example, it will be situated on dextro-elevation in a right superior oblique palsy, with diplopia on laevodepression (Fig. 6.10). The patient's comfort depends more on the position of the field of binocular fixation than it does on its size; a small field centrally placed and extending downwards will be more comfortable than a larger field displaced upwards.

The greater the limitation of ocular movement, the smaller the field of binocular single vision. However, the size is influenced by the patient's fusion amplitude; if this is good the field will be enlarged, at least in congenital vertical muscle palsies and in patients with thyroid eye disease involving vertically acting muscles.

A narrow field of binocular single vision, often relatively centrally placed, is characteristic of mechanically caused limitation of movement in opposing directions: a blow-out fracture of the orbital floor with entrapment of tissue provides a good example of this type of field (Fig. 6.11).

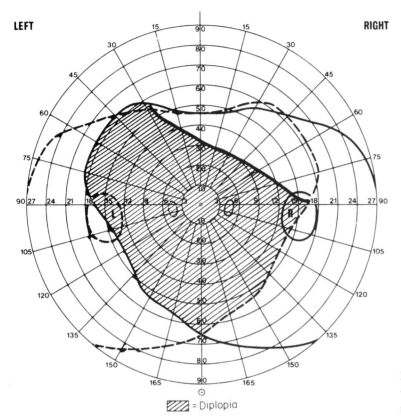

LEFT　　　　　　　　　　　　　　　**RIGHT**

⊙
▨ = Diplopia

Fig. 6.10 Field of binocular single vision of a patient with a right fourth nerve palsy.

The field of binocular single vision has some diagnostic value and, like the Hess chart, it provides a permanent and repeatable record. Its main value is that it covers a much larger area than the 30° which is the limit on the Hess screen in each direction, so that a near-normal Hess chart can be plotted in a patient who has troublesome diplopia or, conversely, a patient with a good fusion amplitude, enabling him to control his diplopia, will have a relatively large and comfortable field of binocular single vision in spite of a considerable angle of deviation and obviously displaced Hess chart fields.

Measurement of ductions

Field of uniocular fixation

The field is plotted on a perimeter and is recorded on a perimeter chart. The patient is seated at the instrument with the eye to be tested opposite the centre of the perimeter; the other eye is occluded. A 2° white target or letter is used for fixation. It must first be established that the patient can appreciate when he is fixing with the fovea rather than using peripheral retina; optimum vision is needed for this discrimination so patients should wear any spectacles necessary for the working distance of 33 cm. The target is moved from a point where foveal fixation is possible into the direction of limitation of movement, recording the position at which restricted movement prevents foveal fixation and causes the target to blur, repeating this procedure in all meridia (Fig. 6.12).

A field of uniocular fixation can be plotted if there is no binocular vision or if gross restriction of ocular movement is present, preventing the use of the Hess screen. The test is difficult to perform accurately but is particularly useful in plotting any change from visit to visit when both eyes show limitation of movement on ductions. The Hess is of limited value in these cases.

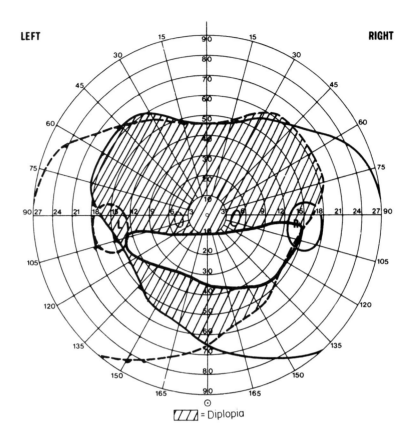

Fig. 6.11 Field of binocular single vision of a patient with a blow-out fracture of the left orbital floor (Hess chart shown in Fig. 6.9).

⊙
[///] = Diplopia

Major amblyoscope

Ductions can be assessed using the major ambly-oscope. A slide which equates to the patient's visual acuity is used and he is asked to fixate the target at zero. The arm of the synoptophore is then moved into the position of defective movement, while asking the patient to maintain fixation. When he is unable to do this, or the eye is seen to cease following the target, the instrument arm is moved back until foveal fixation is regained (Roper-Hall 1975). The result is recorded in degrees. Patients with Duane's syndrome are ideal candidates for this type of assessment.

Methods used to assess mechanical factors

Forced duction test (traction test)

The purpose of the forced duction test is to assess pas-sive movement of the globe in cases in which active ocular movement is limited. Limitation of passive movement, as demonstrated by this test, denotes that a mechanical factor is involved in the limitation, either wholly or in part. The test can be performed as an out-patient procedure or it can be integrated into the surgical procedure for strabismus.

Method
Anaesthesia

The test requires local or general anaesthesia. Topical local anaesthesia is successful in making application of the forceps painless, but attempted rotation of the globe against mechanical resistance may still be very uncomfortable. Injection of local anaesthetic around the muscles, while overcoming this difficulty, may modify the result of the test by itself introducing a mechanical factor. Small to moderate amounts of mechanical resistance can be difficult to assess using local anaesthesia. General anaesthesia is preferable and is generally used when the test is performed during

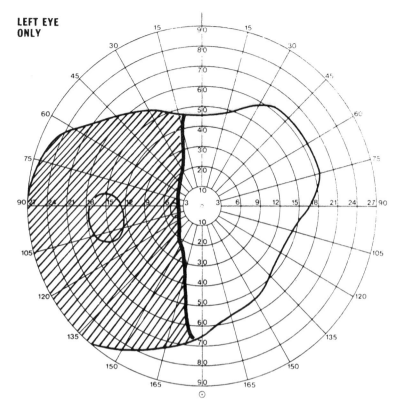

Fig. 6.12 Field of uniocular fixation of a patient with a left sixth nerve palsy.

surgery. However, it should be noted that the effect of succinylcholine, which is in general use as a short-acting depolarizing muscle relaxant, produces a sustained muscle contraction which can persist for up to 20 min, preventing the correct interpretation of the forced duction test (France *et al.* 1980). Propofol infusion anaesthesia is associated with reduced postoperative recovery time and lower levels of nausea and vomiting, and is frequently used for day-case strabismus surgery: the patient breathes spontaneously and muscle relaxation is frequently incomplete making interpretation of the forced duction test difficult.

Technique

The test can be performed using two pairs of fixation forceps or a cotton-tipped bud. Both eyes are usually examined, especially when the test is performed under general anaesthesia.

FIXATION FORCEPS

Two pairs of fine fixation forceps are applied to dia-metrically opposite limbal points. The globe is then rotated horizontally, vertically and obliquely, being careful to lift as well as rotate the eye. The examiner notes:

- limitations of movement;
- the nature of the limitations;
- resistance to rotation—considerable experience is required before a sense of normal resistance is developed;
- stretching of tight conjunctiva which can be seen indenting the globe.

COTTON BUD METHOD

This method is useful in patients who find the fixation forceps too uncomfortable under local anaesthesia. The patient is instructed to look in the direction of the limited movement and the examiner applies a sterile cotton-tip bud adjacent to the limbus diametrically opposite to the direction of rotation, and attempts to increase the range of movement of the eye. In the absence of any mechanical restriction the passive movement achieved by the examiner will be greater than the active movement achieved by the patient: mechanical restriction will result in both the passive and active movements being equal.

Precautions

• If the globe is pushed back into the orbit instead of being moved around the normal centre of rotation, a mechanical restriction can be missed because shortened muscle or tissue is better able to wrap itself around the globe in a retroposed position. Retropulsion and anteropulsion of globe can be usefully employed to differentiate mechanical restriction of rectus from oblique muscles (see Chapter 9).
• Two pairs of forceps should always be used; if only one pair is applied to the limbus diametrically opposite to the direction of rotation, retropulsion of the globe is likely to occur.
• Interpretation of forced duction under local anaesthesia can be inaccurate because of muscle tone.

Indications for use

The forced duction test should be used routinely whenever extraocular muscle surgery is performed:
• at the start of the operation (after insertion of the lid speculum);
• when each stage of surgery is completed, to monitor success in increasing passive movement;
• on completion of the operation.

It is an essential test in known or suspected mechanical restriction of ocular movement, first to establish the diagnosis and secondly to assess the degree and nature of the restriction.

Value

The forced duction test plays a very important part in the differential diagnosis and surgical management of ocular motility disorders. Although there is no standard method of quantifying the result we recommend using the same system (0–4 scale) that has already been described for grading duction eye movement. This allows the examiner to compare the patient's active duction movement with the passive rotation of the forced duction test. It should be remembered that restriction can be caused by direct and reverse leashes and can affect connective tissue and bulbar conjunc-

tiva as well as extraocular muscles. Neurogenic and mechanical conditions can coexist and this possibility should also be considered.

Measurement of intraocular pressure

The intraocular pressure can be measured in the primary position and when the eyes are turned in the direction of limited excursion. A rise in pressure of 6 mmHg is significant and is indicative of compression of the globe due to mechanical restriction. However, it should be remembered that mechanical restriction and a neurogenic muscle palsy can coexist. There is then insufficient compression of the globe to cause intraocular pressure to rise, giving a false negative result.

Spring-back balance test

This test was described by Jampolsky (1978). The purpose is to assess whether surgical adjustment of muscles has disturbed the balanced of passive muscle forces. Marked imbalance might make restoration of binocular single vision difficult or cause further incomitance.

Method

The test is used during the course of surgery, so that the patient is already anaesthetized.
• The eye is passively rotated in the chosen direction using forceps placed at the limbus.
• The forceps are then removed and the observer notes whether the eye springs back to the primary position or remains deviated in an eccentric position.
• The eye is then rotated in the opposite direction, released and the same observations made.

These procedures are repeated several times and a comparison is made between the reaction of the eye to movement in opposite directions on repetition of the test.

The eye should spring back with equal force on each occasion and whichever way it is moved. If it does not do so and remains in an eccentric position, surgical adjustment is made and the test repeated.

The spring-back balance test is also useful when grading the amount of superior oblique tuck performed (see Chapter 9).

Value

This is a rather elementary mechanical test, but taken in conjunction with the findings of the forced duction test carried out at the same time, it does give some fairly accurate and useful information about the total passive forces influencing eye position and restraining eye movement. It should be more widely used.

Muscle stretch test

A further simple test of the normal elasticity of rectus muscles can be carried out during surgery under deep general anaesthesia with full muscle relaxation. The muscle to be operated on is detached from its insertion and drawn forwards. If the muscle has no abnormal stiffness due to contracture and fibrosis, it should be possible to advance its insertion as far forwards as the centre of the cornea with eye in the straight ahead position.

Active muscle force generation test

The force generation test assesses the active muscle force which enables eye movement to take place. This force arises from the increase in tone of healthy muscle fibres which occurs when they are activated but are prevented from reducing their length. The aim of the test is to calculate the isometric contraction force in an apparently palsied muscle to indicate the muscle's potential function.

Methods

Three different techniques have been described, all requiring topical anaesthesia.

1 In the simplest and most primitive of the three, the eye is held firmly at the limbus with a pair of toothed forceps. The patient is then asked to try as hard as possible to move the eye into the field of action of the muscle under investigation, either by following a moving target or by making a voluntary saccade. For example, to assess the active contraction force in an apparently limited right lateral rectus, the right temporal limbus is grasped with the forceps and the eye is held in a slightly adducted position; as the patient tries to abduct the eye the examiner can sense muscle contraction through the tug on the forceps tip. Although this method is entirely qualitative and assessment of contraction requires considerable experience, it can readily differentiate between and total and partial horizontal rectus muscle palsy.

2 A scale with a moving pointer is attached to a pair of toothed forceps with a slightly flexible tip. The same procedure is followed and the amount of force applied to the teeth of the forceps as the muscle contracts causes the pointer to move on the scale, thus providing a quantitative assessment of active muscle contraction (Scott *et al*. 1972).

3 A suction cup with a strain gauge attached is fitted to a contact lens which is applied to the eye. Forceps are not required because the eye is held still by a handle attached to the suction cup. The same procedure is followed and the isometric force registered on the strain gauge is recorded and stored (Strachan *et al*. 1976).

Precautions

• The toothed forceps must be applied sufficiently firmly to resist any rotational force.
• The suction cup must be designed so that it will not slip.

Indications for use

The principal use of this test is to measure potential muscle force when there is known mechanical restriction of ocular movement. If, for example, there is complete loss of abduction with contracture of the medial rectus, a positive result would indicate that there is potential lateral rectus muscle force and surgery would be planned accordingly.

Value

This test is uncomfortable for the patient and it is not possible to quantify the degree of muscle activity accurately. For these reasons it is not widely used, although the results can help in the correct choice of muscle surgery.

Electrodiagnostic methods

Recording equipment may be used to measure the electrical activity within muscles (muscle potential) or to measure gaze movement.

Measurement of muscle potential

Electromyography (EMG)

Principle

When the group of muscle fibres supplied by a motor nerve axon contract due to a nerve stimulation, a change of electrical potential is produced in the area immediately surrounding this motor unit, which can be detected by a fine electrode introduced into the muscle. Whereas many large muscles have motor units in which one nerve axon supplies up to 100 muscle fibres, the extrinsic ocular muscles are unique in having very refined motor units in which one nerve axon supplies as few as four muscle fibres. Therefore, when EMG is used to investigate electrical activity in the ocular muscles, the pattern of activity closely follows that occurring in individual nerve axons.

Method

Unipolar or bipolar electrodes can be used: indifferent and earth electrodes are first attached to the skin around the eye. Using topical anaesthesia, a fine electrode, which must be fully sterilized to avoid infection, is introduced into the muscle through the conjunctiva and its position adjusted until a satisfactory pattern of electrical activity is recorded. The electrical activity within a muscle is normally maximum when the patient makes a voluntary movement into the field of action of the muscle, and is absent when gaze is directed away from its field of action. Therefore, the patient is first asked to look in the direction of main action of the muscle being tested, and then in the opposite direction. Sophisticated recording apparatus allows sampling, analysis and storage of the responses. An audio-frequency reproduction of the electrical activity gives the investigator a simple check of recording.

The investigation requires good cooperation and some fortitude on the part of the patient, and considerable skill from the examiner. It is unsuitable for most children and apprehensive adults, and requires careful selection of patients.

Indications for use

RESEARCH USES

EMG has been used in the following investigations:

• The electrical basis of Hering's and Sherrington's law governing ocular movement.
• Vergence movements, particularly to confirm the presence of active divergence through simultaneous innervation of the lateral rectus muscles, at least as a motor fusion response.
• Duane's retraction syndrome. Using this method, Breinin (1957) was the first to demonstrate paradoxical innervation of the lateral rectus muscle in this condition, with little or no electrical activity on attempting abduction of the affected eye. Simultaneous firing of vertically acting muscles with the medial rectus was found in some cases and has been cited as a cause of the anomalous up-shoots, down-shoots and retraction seen in this syndrome.
• Aberrant regeneration. EMG recordings have confirmed that the physical signs indicate a misdirection of the third cranial nerve fibres during regrowth, so that they supply inappropriate muscles (see Chapter 19).

CLINICAL USES

EMG is of value in differentiating limitation of ocular movement due to neurogenic, myogenic and mechanical causes.

Neurogenic palsies

There is partial or complete loss of motor unit activity even when the patient makes a maximum voluntary effort to look in the field of action of the defective muscle.

Myogenic disorders

• *Myopathies.* There may be decreased or abnormal electrical activity during contraction of the affected muscles.
• *Myasthenia gravis.* This disorder, sited at the neuromuscular junction, causes decreased amplitude and frequency of muscle potentials, especially after sustained voluntary action. A dramatic temporary increase in the electrical responses, which occurs within 1 min of intravenous injection of edrophonium chloride (Tensilon), is characteristic. These changes occur even when the clinical examination after injection has failed to reveal any significant improvement in ocular movement, stressing the sensitive nature of the test in these cases (see Chapter 20).

- *Lambert–Eaton–Rooke syndrome (myasthenic syndrome)*. There is an increased electrical response after sustained muscle action (see Chapter 20).

Mechanical restriction

There is increased recruitment of motor units when a muscle attempts to rotate the tethered eye in the direction of restricted movement.

Monitoring needle tip position for botulinum toxin A injection

EMG is used as an essential part of the technique of botulinum toxin A therapy (see Chapter 8). An active electrode is incorporated in the tip of the needle used to inject a minute quantity of toxin directly into the muscle belly. Observation of the potentials recorded indicates to the therapist the position of the needle tip: injection is not begun until a satisfactory level of electrical activity results when the eye is moved into the field of action of the muscle to be injected.

Problems

The main limitations of EMG as a clinical tool are:
- The invasive and, to some patients, distressing nature of the procedure. Introduction of the electrode may cause minor haemorrhage in the subconjunctival tissues or in the muscle.
- The difficulty in judging the function of a whole muscle by sampling only a fraction of it.
- Small amounts of weakness in muscle function may not be detected.

Value

EMG has undoubtedly been a very important research method in elucidating the true nature of the various types of paralytic strabismus. Its main value in clinical practice is in the differentiation of neurogenic and mechanical palsies and in the confirmation of the presence of myasthenia gravis when this is in doubt. It is essential in ensuring the accuracy of botulinum toxin A injection.

Measurement of gaze movement

The use of recording equipment for accurate measurement of eye movement has the advantage of:

- allowing a detailed study of the quality of the movement;
- producing a permanent record of the nature of the movement so that it can be compared with later measurements.

The techniques currently available are: the electro-oculogram, infrared systems, magnetic search coil and the Purkinje image tracker.

Electro-oculogram

The principles of electro-oculography for detecting changes in the potential of the eye from the dark-adapted to the light-adapted state are described in Chapter 4. The same potential may be used to measure eye movement. Recording electrodes are placed at the inner and outer canthi to record horizontal eye movement. Recording electrodes are placed above and below the eye to record vertical gaze movement. As the eye moves towards one pair of electrodes, the positive potential at the cornea will cause a rise in potential at this electrode and a corresponding decline in potential of the other. The rate of change in potential is proportional to the speed of eye movement. When measuring saccadic velocity, two targets, usually red light-emitting diodes (LEDs), are placed in front of the patient. The distance between the two targets is known, as is the distance of the patient from the targets. The patient is then asked to look from one target to the other. The distance between the targets and the distance from the patient governs the size of the saccade. The average velocity of the saccade may be calculated by the size of the saccade divided by the time taken to complete it. The result is expressed in degrees of arc per second. The saccade may be seen as a curved line on a visual display unit. More modern systems are capable of evaluating the shape of the curve and can measure the maximum peak velocity, acceleration profile and latency of saccade.

Infrared scleral reflection technique

An infrared light source on spectacle frames illuminates the eye; reflected light from the anterior surface of the globe is intercepted by two infrared-sensitive photoelectric cells adjacent to the nasal and temporal limbus (to record horizontal eye movement). As the eye moves nasally, for example, the temporal cell receives increased illumination as more light is reflected from the sclera, while the nasal cell receives less illumination. The amplitude of potential change from the two cells is recorded and is proportional to the eye movement.

Scleral search coil technique

The patient is fitted with a large-diameter soft contact lens which contains a fine wire coil (the search coil). The eye under examination is centred between pairs of large horizontal and vertical coils which generate a magnetic field. Movement of the eye within this field generates a small electrical current in the search coil, which is proportional to the amount of arc movement.

Purkinje image tracker

Purkinje images are formed by reflection from the optical surfaces; Image I by reflection at the anterior corneal surface and is erect, II by reflection at the posterior corneal surface and is also erect, III by reflection at the anterior lens capsule and is erect, image IV is from the posterior lens surface and is inverted. When the eye moves there is a proportional movement of Purkinje's images, which is tracked electronically using this method.

Value of methods of measurement

EOG is the most widely available technique. It is an accurate method of measuring large-amplitude horizontal saccades but is less effective for those of small amplitude. The infrared scleral reflection technique is an excellent method of recording horizontal eye movements, especially nystagmus, although it is less accurate than EOG for large-amplitude saccades. Both methods have limitations in measuring vertical saccades, when blink artefacts and electrode position reduce accuracy.

The scleral search coil records horizontal and vertical eye movements of quite large amplitude with a high degree of accuracy but is available in only a few laboratories. The Purkinje image tracker is the most sensitive of all the methods used but, like the scleral search coil, it is not readily available in clinical practice.

Indications for measuring gaze movements

Most static tests of ocular movement compare the position of one eye relative to the other and are more reliable than electrodiagnostic tests when defective movement is strictly unilateral. When limitation of movement is bilateral, abnormal is compared with abnormal, making the results of static tests less reliable. Eye-movement recording systems record the movement of one eye independently of the other and can provide a useful record for diagnosis and subsequent comparison, particularly in the following conditions.

Neurogenic palsies

• Differential diagnosis of neurogenic palsy and mechanical restriction of ocular movement: both amplitude and velocity of a saccade are reduced in neurogenic palsy. This is especially obvious when the tracing of a paresed muscle is compared with that of its overacting contralateral synergist. The amplitude of a saccade is also reduced when there is mechanical restriction but the velocity is normal up to the point at which the tether intervenes. Velocity is an indicator of muscle strength and is important in assessing the residual power of the paresed muscle when neurogenic palsy and tethering are present in the same patient.

• Serial recordings plot the rate and degree of recovery of a paresed muscle.

Myogenic disorders

Measurement can reveal subtle transient increases in saccadic velocity after Tensilon injection in suspected

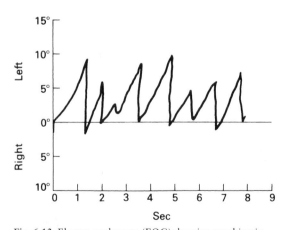

Fig. 6.13 Electro-oculogram (EOG) showing optokinetic responses elicited by stripes moving from left to right. The tracing shows slow pursuit movement to the right (upward deflection of the tracing) and fast refixation movement. The speed of movement is indicated by the steepness of the slope.

myasthenia, although the variable types of saccades in myasthenia need careful interpretation. Saccades are very slow in myopathy.

Supranuclear gaze disorders and internuclear ophthalmoplegia

Tracings are useful in differentiating asymmetrical bilateral internuclear ophthalmoplegia (INO) from strictly unilateral cases.

Nystagmus

Gaze measurements can show the typical wave form of the different types of nystagmus (Fig. 6.13). This information can be crucial in the differential diagnosis.

References

Bahill, A.T., Clark, M.R. & Stark, L. (1975) The main sequence: a tool for studying human eye movements. *Mathematical Biosciences* **24**, 191–204.

Breinin, G.M. (1957) Electromyography: a tool in ocular and neurologic diagnosis. II muscle palsies. *Archives of Ophthalmology* **57**, 165–175.

Buttner-Ennever, J.A. & Akert, K. (1981) Medial rectus subgroups of the oculomotor nucleus and their abducens internucleur input in the monkey. *Journal of Comparative Neurology* **197**, 17–27.

Dulley, B. & Harden, A. (1974) Cyclo-torsion: a new method of measurement. *British Orthoptic Journal* **31**, 70–77.

Fielder, A. (1985) Neonatal eye movement: normal and abnormal. *British Orthoptic Journal* **42**, 10–15.

France, N.K., France, T.D., Woodburn, J.D. Jr & Burbank, D.P. (1980) Succinylcholine alteration of the forced duction test. *Ophthalmology* **87**, 1282–1287.

Jampolsky, A. (1978) Spring back-balance test in strabismus surgery. In: *Transactions of the New Orleans Academy of Ophthalmology* (ed. J.H. Allen), pp. 104–111. Mosby, St Louis.

Johnson, F., Harcourt, B. & Fox, A. (1987) The clinical assessment of cyclodeviation. In: *Orthoptic Horizons. Transactions of the Sixth International Orthoptic Congress, Harrogate* (eds M. Lenk-Schafer, C. Calcutt, M. Doyle & S. Moore), pp. 179–183. British Orthoptic Society, London.

Leigh, R.J. & Zee, D.S. (1991) *The Neurology of Eye Movements*, 2nd edn. F.A. Davis, Philadelphia.

O'Flynn, E.A. (1994) Strabismus documentation: an alternative approach. *British Orthoptic Journal* **51**, 10–14.

Poggio, G.F. & Fischer, B. (1977) Binocular interaction and depth sensitivity in striate and prestriate cortex of behaving rhesus monkey. *Journal of Neurophysiology* **40**, 1392–1405.

Roper-Hall, G. (1975) Duction measurements in limited ocular rotations. *British Orthoptic Journal* **32**, 70–76.

Roucoux, A., Culée, C. & Roucoux, M. (1983) Development of fixation and pursuit eye movements in human infants. *Behavioural Brain Research* **10**, 133–139.

Scott, A.B., Collins, C.C. & O'Meara, D.M. (1972) A forceps to measure strabismus forces. *Archives of Ophthalmology* **88**, 330–333.

Strachan, I.M., Brown, B.H., Johnson, S.G. & Robinson, P. (1976) An apparatus for measuring forces in strabimus. In: *Orthoptics Past, Present and Future. Transactions of the Third International Orthoptic Congress, Boston* (eds J. Moore & L. Stockbridge), pp. 123–128. Symposia Specialists, Miami.

Timms, C., Barratt, H., Taylor, D. & Gresty, M. (1987) The development of slow phase eye movements: their relationship to the spinning test. In: *Orthoptic Horizons. Transactions of the Sixth International Orthoptic Congress, Harrogate* (eds M. Lenk-Schafer, C. Calcutt, M. Doyle & S. Moore), pp. 16–20. British Orthoptic Society, London.

7
Binocular Function

Terminology

There is sometimes confusion between the terms 'binocular single vision' and 'binocular vision'. In this book they are defined as follows:
• *Binocular single vision* is the simultaneous use of the two eyes to give a single mental impression in normal conditions of seeing. Normal binocular single vision is bifoveal and there is no manifest deviation. Anomalous binocular single vision is present when the images of the fixated object are projected from the fovea of one eye and an extrafoveal area of the other eye; a small manifest strabismus is present.
• *Binocular vision* is the simultaneous perception of two images, one from each eye. This may be demonstrable spontaneously if there is appreciation of diplopia, or apparatus such as the major amblyoscope may be needed before the patient is aware of the two images. Binocular vision can be normal when the foveae have a common visual direction, or anomalous when the visual direction of retinal elements has changed.

WORTH'S GRADES OF BINOCULAR VISION
Worth's classification of binocular vision into three grades is still useful in identifying the degree of binocular vision present:
• simultaneous perception
• fusion
• stereoscopic vision.

Aims of investigation

The main purpose of the investigation of binocular function is to determine if the aim of treatment should be to restore binocular single vision or to improve the patient's appearance and ensure that he has the best possible visual acuity. The presence of sensory and motor fusion should lead to a functional result and a good prognosis for long-term alignment of the visual axes. If fusion is absent, treatment is aimed at improving the appearance.

Investigation should include tests to determine:
• Grade of binocular vision, with emphasis on the potential for fusion.
• Presence of binocular single vision or the patient's potential for achieving it.
• Strength of existing binocular single vision.
• State of retinal correspondence either normal or abnormal.
• Presence of suppression, including its area and density.

Retinal correspondence

Definition

Retinal elements of one eye correspond with retinal areas in the other eye and have a common visual direction. Panum's fusional area allows fusion to occur despite slight disparity of fixation; the area measures at least 2° at the central retinal area and increases towards the periphery, allowing correspondence between retinal areas (Fender & Julesz 1967; Crone et al. 1978).

If binocular potential is present this may be normal or abnormal. Abnormal binocular single vision can occur when there is a constant manifest strabismus and may be associated with abnormal retinal correspondence. This is more common in esotropia measuring less than 20 Δ.

The grade of binocular single vision demonstrable may vary with the angle of deviation in that the larger the angle the poorer the binocular function.

Normal retinal correspondence
Normal retinal correspondence has the following features:
• the foveae have a common visual direction;
• nasal elements of one eye correspond with temporal elements of the other eye.

Normal retinal correspondence is expected in:
• intermittent strabismus;
• acquired strabismus, especially if onset is after the age for the normal development of binocular single vision.

Abnormal retinal correspondence
Abnormal retinal correspondence is a sensory adaptation to manifest strabismus which facilitates binocular single vision, albeit to a lesser quality than normal bifoveal binocular single vision.
• The fovea of one eye has a common visual direction with an extrafoveal area of the other eye (sometimes referred to as the pseudofovea).
• Elements nasal to the fovea correspond to elements temporal to the extrafoveal area.
• In esotropia the anatomical fovea of the deviating eye will project as temporal retina in binocular viewing.
• The objective angle of deviation will be greater than the subjective angle.

Fusion

Fusion has two components:
• *Sensory fusion:* the ability to appreciate two similar images, one with each eye, and to interpret them as one.
• *Motor fusion:* the ability to maintain a single fused image during vergence movements. The strength of motor fusion is represented by the fusion amplitude, made up of horizontal vergence (convergence forming the positive component of the amplitude and divergence the negative component), vertical vergence and cyclovergence.

Importance of fusion

The presence or absence of fusion is crucial to the prognosis and management of strabismus. If sensory and motor fusion are present the prognosis is good. Conservative and surgical management are directed to obtaining a functional result. Treatment to eliminate suppression and promote recognition of diplopia can safely be given if indicated. Surgical treatment is planned to place the visual axes parallel or to overcorrect the deviation in certain cases.

If fusion is absent, binocular single vision cannot be restored. Patients are occasionally seen with evidence of only sensory fusion but this is insufficient to maintain a stable eye position and the prognosis is poor. Orthoptic treatment of any type is contraindicated in the absence of sensory and motor fusion, and surgery is planned to leave the visual axes slightly convergent to prevent redivergence in exotropia and consecutive exotropia in esotropia.

Loss of fusion

Loss of fusion can occur later in childhood and in adult life, usually following severe head injury or brain damage due to other causes. It can apparently occur in patients with unilateral aphakia following lens extraction for acquired cataract. Loss of fusion may be relatively transitory or can be permanent.

Signs and symptoms

Diplopia is present for near and distance fixation and in all positions of gaze. The images cannot be fused with the aid of prisms or when using a major amblyoscope. The image seen by the nonfixing eye may show nonrhythmical vertical movement (bobbing).

Investigation

True loss of fusion must be differentiated from apparent loss due to other factors. These include insuperable excyclotropia in bilateral fourth nerve palsies and bitemporal hemianopia, which if complete, rules out binocular fixation. Patients who have been deprived of binocular single vision for several months or years may at first be unable to fuse the diplopic images, for example after surgery for a longstanding paralytic strabismus. In such cases it is worth using compensating prisms for a short period as fusion may result with time.

Management

There is no known treatment for patients with true loss of fusion. Symptoms may be alleviated by modifying the refractive correction before one eye or by removing a contact lens in unilateral aphakia to make the diplopia less obvious. Occlusion on spectacles or by means of a contact lens can be used if the diplopia is very troublesome.

It is very difficult to explain the loss of fusion seen in association with unilateral aphakia. Pratt-Johnson and Tillson (1989) reported on these rare cases, and we have seen others which exactly fitted their description. Characteristically, there was exotropia, hypotropia and excyclotropia. Fusion could not be achieved when the hypotropia and cyclotropia were corrected on the major amblyoscope. Aniseikonia was insignificant when a contact lens was worn. Patients observed constant vertical movement of one image and fusion was impossible. There was no evidence to suggest that defective binocular vision was present before the onset of the cataract. We have not seen this occur with intraocular lens correction.

Stereopsis

The perception of the relative depth of objects is based on the ability to fuse images stimulating disparate retinal elements within Panum's fusional areas. These disparities may be crossed or uncrossed: crossed disparity gives the effect of the image being perceived in front of the background and uncrossed behind the background.

Development of stereopsis

Stereopsis is not present at birth but has been demonstrated at 3–4 months of age. It appears to have an abrupt onset with rapid subsequent development to adult levels within weeks (Held 1988), and occurs significantly earlier in females than males. The development of segregated cortical ocular dominance columns is thought to play a major role in the onset of stereopsis. Stereopsis has been studied experimentally in normal and squinting infants using preferential looking techniques to compare the infant's response to stereoscopic and nonstereoscopic targets (Teller 1983; Stager & Birch 1986). Archer *et al.* (1986) used EOG monitoring of infants' eye movements in response to a dynamic random dot stereogram, confirming that stereopsis has developed in the normal infant at 4 months of age. Worth (1901) postulated a progression from one grade of binocular vision to the next, with stereopsis as the highest grade. However, it is possible to have sensory and motor fusion with no stereopsis or, much more rarely, stereopsis without motor fusion. It is probable that fusion of images and disparity detection are separate cortical functions.

Suppression

Suppression is the inhibition of unwanted stimuli; it can be either physiological or pathological.

Physiological suppression occurs in normal binocular single vision. It is demonstrable, for example, by the lack of awareness of physiological diplopia and by retinal rivalry, when there is alternating and fluctuating suppression of conflicting stimuli.

Pathological suppression occurs in constant and intermittent strabismus, in some latent deviations and in patients with anisometropic amblyopia. Although suppression is a cortical function descriptions are referred to in relation to the retina.

Purpose

Suppression develops in order to overcome symptoms of:
• Binocular diplopia, occurring in a manifest strabismus when the image of the fixated object stimulates a noncorresponding peripheral area in the deviating eye.
• Confusion, which occurs in manifest strabismus because the image received by the fovea of the fixing eye is different from the image falling on the fovea of the deviating eye. As the foveae have a common visual direction, the images are seen superimposed, providing that retinal correspondence is normal. However, confusion is rarely a symptom even in strabismus acquired in adult life. Pratt-Johnson and Tillson (1984) have stated that confusion is not recognized because the brain is unable to appreciate simultaneously two different images falling on corresponding points.
• Incompatible images, which can occur when there is a significant degree of anisometropia. The foveae are stimulated by images of the same object but are sufficiently different in size and/or shape to prevent fusion. Peripheral fusion is maintained but central suppression develops in the more ametropic eye.

Development

Suppression develops rapidly in early childhood before the neurophysiological processes involved become fixed. It develops more slowly in older children up to around 10 years of age, although it is impossible to state a definitive upper age limit. Some children with strabismus do not suppress and appear to tolerate diplopia well.

Suppression rarely develops in adults but it is not uncommon for elderly patients to be able to ignore an unwanted image.

Suppression developed in childhood can occasionally be lost in adult life following brain damage, usually due to head injury.

Characteristics

Suppression can affect one or both eyes and can be constant or intermittent; these factors depend largely on the type of strabismus and on the size of the angle of deviation. Most patients with constant manifest strabismus show constant suppression, affecting one eye in unilateral strabismus and affecting either eye if the deviation is alternating. Patients with intermittent or latent strabismus may suppress when binocular single vision cannot be maintained.

Suppression varies in area and in density, depending on the characteristics of the strabismus.

Area of suppression

Initially suppression in manifest strabismus involves two areas:
• the fovea;
• the peripheral retinal area stimulated by the fixation object.

In esotropia these two areas merge to form an elliptical shaped scotoma with its long axis horizontal; its size is proportional to the size of the deviation. In exotropia suppression is more widespread; in intermittent distance exotropia in particular it may involve the whole temporal retina (Jampolsky 1955). However, Awaya et al. (1976) and Pratt-Johnson et al. (1981) demonstrated that patients with this type of exotropia have very similar-shaped scotomata to those found in esotropia. A few individuals with intermittent distance exotropia can recognize diplopia, and it is evident that by no means all patients with this condition have hemiretinal suppression.

Pratt-Johnson and Tillson (1984), using an Aimark perimeter with fusion targets, showed that there is suppression of images falling on both nasal and temporal retina in all types of strabismus, with the exception of the monocular temporal crescent, which has no correspondence with the other eye. Only patients with microtropia show a circumscribed fovealparafoveal suppression scotoma.

Even so, suppression usually occurs when the vertical mid-line is crossed. Sudden reversal of esotropia or exotropia by surgery or overcorrecting prisms often results in diplopia.

Density of suppression

Suppression affecting the fovea is very dense and obdurate. As the suppression scotoma extends into the periphery it generally becomes progressively less dense, with the exception of large-angle infantile strabismus in which there is marked suppression involving a large scotoma, often alternating in character.

Investigation of binocular vision

General factors to be considered

History

It should be possible to infer the state of binocular function from the age at onset, duration and characteristics of the strabismus. The younger the age of onset and longer the duration of a constant manifest strabismus the less likely normal binocular function will exist. Obviously these factors must be taken into account, but the history is often inaccurate, particularly if the deviation is small or if it is variable, when it may be described as intermittent.

Refractive error

The presence of anisometropia may indicate the presence of central suppression and possible microtropia. Other refractive errors may indicate the nature of the deviation rather than the binocular potential; for example, a moderate degree of hypermetropia can indicate an accommodative element.

Visual acuity/fixation

The level of visual acuity has little bearing on the patient's binocular function; equal visual acuity is often present in infantile esotropia without binocular vision, while some patients with amblyopia have useful binocular vision. The appreciation of finer disparities may be prevented by amblyopia, resulting in poor stereopsis: improvement may follow occlusion therapy.

If fixation is eccentric, normal binocular single vision is not present but there may be abnormal binocular single vision.

Abnormal head posture

An abnormal head posture is most often adopted to overcome diplopia, mainly in congenital and acquired ocular muscle palsies. A few patients with long-standing palsies retain the head posture but lose binocular single vision: in these cases it may be possible to restore binocular single vision with the appropriate therapy. However, other ocular causes for the head posture must be excluded, for example improvement in visual acuity and facilitation of foveal fixation.

Cover test

A recovery movement on removal of the cover can indicate both the presence of binocular single vision and its strength. If a latent or intermittent deviation is present the rate of recovery will be a useful indication of control. If a manifest deviation increases on dissociation and is seen to make a recovery movement when the cover is removed, it is indicative of normal or abnormal binocular single vision.

Appreciation of diplopia

If diplopia is appreciated spontaneously and the patient can consciously control it, by adopting an abnormal head posture for example, binocular single vision is present. Failure to control the diplopia may be due to wide separation of the images, insuperable hypertropia or cyclotorsion, a poor fusion amplitude, or lack of fusion.

General guidelines for selecting binocular vision tests

The selection of tests for binocular vision may be assisted by the following guidelines:
• Visual acuity and particularly fixation influence the selection and interpretation of tests and should therefore be known.
• Age and cooperation of the patient will influence the choice; e.g. the patient must be able to count to perform Worth lights (see below).
• Tests using normal seeing conditions are preferable; those giving monocular clues should be avoided if possible.
• Cover test indicates normal binocular single vision, as in heterophoria, stereoacuity may be measured without the need to prove that fusion is present first as this

has already been demonstrated by the response to the cover test.

Tests for binocular vision

Bagolini glasses

The apparatus consists of a pair of plano glasses marked with fine parallel striations at 45° on one glass and 135° on the other. When a spotlight is viewed through the glasses each produces a line image at 90° to the axis of the striation. A patient with the peripheral suppression scotoma typical of a unilateral horizontal manifest strabismus more easily sees an oblique image.

The glasses can be used in trial frames or are obtainable mounted in a reversible lorgnette for convenience. The test can be used at 6 m, 33 cm or in any desired gaze position, for example on up- and down-gaze in A- and V-patterns.

The test should be performed in good illumination but with extraneous light sources extinguished. The glasses must be clean, otherwise more than one image can be seen: the test uses normal conditions of seeing and is minimally dissociating and therefore more likely to elicit a correct and true response.

Method of use

This method entails the following steps.
• The patient fixes on a spotlight on eye level at 6 m with his refractive correction in place. The glasses are placed in front of his eyes and he is questioned about the number of lights seen and the number and position of the lines. If two lines are seen he should be asked if they cross or are seen separated.
• It is advisable first to show a child the line image with each eye separately. All patients are asked to describe or draw the exact position of the lines. Difficulties arise if the lines are reported as crossing: the examiner must establish if they cross through the light or above or below it (Fig. 7.1). It is easier, especially for children, if the possible responses are drawn for the child; alternatively the light and line seen by the fixing eye can be drawn by the examiner and the child asked to add the second line.
• The patient should be asked if he sees two lines all the time or if one or other of them disappears. If both lines are seen to cross on the light he should be ques-

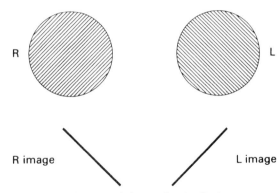

Fig. 7.1 Bagolini striated glasses, showing line images perpendicular to the striations.

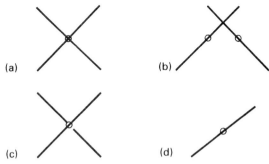

Fig. 7.2 Results of the Bagolini striated glasses test. (a) Bifoveal or anomalous binocular single vision. (b) Two lines, signifying a manifest strabismus with normal retinal correspondence (or inharmonious abnormal retinal correspondence). (c) Central or paracentral suppression scotoma in one eye. (d) Suppression of one line image.

tioned about a possible gap in one line resulting from a central or paracentral scotoma. This is to be expected in microtropia but in practice it is rarely reported. It is advisable to repeat the test at 33 cm.

Results

See Fig. 7.2.

Indications for use

Bagolini glasses are used in the following circumstances.
• To diagnose or confirm the presence of normal or abnormal binocular single vision in the primary position or in an eccentric position of gaze.
• To assess if a patient with a manifest strabismus is suppressing or if binocular vision is present.

• To assess if a patient able to appreciate two lights and lines can obtain and maintain a symmetrical cross when the deviation is corrected with prisms, implying the presence of at least sensory fusion.

• As a means of checking or controlling the accuracy of other tests, for example the field of binocular single vision.

Worth lights

These consist of four circular lights, two green one red and one white, which are viewed through complementary red and green goggles. The red light is seen through the red filter and the green lights through the green filter; the white light is common to both eyes.

There are three sizes of Worth lights:

• Distance (usually located on the base of a vision chart) for use at 6 m, subtending an angle of 1.25°.

• Macular, presented as a sleeve which fits over a pen torch for use at 33 cm, subtending an angle of 1.25°.

• Near, a large stimulus in the form of a bicycle lamp for use at 33 cm or at any intermediate distance, subtending an angle of 6° at 33 cm.

Method of use

• The patient is seated at 6 m and the goggles are placed in front of his eyes so that the red filter is over the right eye. The Worth lights are switched on and the patient is questioned about the number and colour of the lights seen. If five lights are present he should be asked to indicate whether the red lights are to the right or left of the green lights.

• Occluding one eye then the other to familiarize the patient with the lights can help his understanding.

• Patients with binocular single vision often report the white light as pale red or green; it is important to establish how many lights are seen.

• If the patient sees five lights, prisms should be used to correct the angle of deviation and assess whether or not the lights can be fused: the presence of fusion is confirmed if four lights are maintained when the prism strength is increased or decreased by a small amount.

• If central suppression is suspected, it is advisable to repeat the test for near using the macular Worth lights.

Results

• Four lights indicate binocular single vision, either normal or, less usually, abnormal.

• Two lights are seen if left suppression is present.

• Three lights are seen if right suppression is present. The lights may change from one colour to another if alternating suppression is present.

• Five lights are appreciated when there is a manifest strabismus without suppression. Homonymous diplopia is present if the red lights are seen to the right of the green lights, and heteronymous diplopia if they are seen to the left.

Indications for use

• To diagnose or confirm the presence of normal or abnormal binocular single vision.

• To assess if a patient with a manifest strabismus is suppressing or can appreciate diplopia, and if so, the type seen.

• To determine the presence or absence of fusion; if four lights can be maintained with a prism, fusion is present.

• To detect a central suppression scotoma, although it should be noted that the macular lights subtend an angle greater than 1° and therefore a small number of patients with central suppression may appreciate four lights on this test.

Polaroid 4-dot test

This test uses polarization as a means of dissociation. Polarizing glasses are worn to view four polarized lights which are illuminated by a flashlight. Two are seen with the left eye and three with the right eye.

The test is designed to be used at 6 m, where the four dots subtend an angle of 0.26°, and is therefore a test for bifoveal fusion.

Method of use

• The glasses are placed in front of the patient's eyes and the flashlight is viewed at eye level at 6 m. If suppression is found at 6 m, peripheral fusion can be tested by moving the test nearer the patient to increase the angle subtended: at 33 cm this is 5.25°.

Results

• Four lights at 6 m indicate normal bifoveal fusion.

• Five lights indicate diplopia. If fusion occurs when the flashlight is moved nearer to the patient, this distance is also recorded. Two lights indicate right suppression; three lights left suppression.

- If prisms are used to assess the patient's response, they must be placed between the glasses and the patient's eyes to avoid degradation of the polarization.

Indications for use
- To detect or confirm the presence of bifoveal fusion or central suppression.
- To estimate the size of the suppression scotoma in those patients appreciating four lights at distances less than 6 m.

Prism reflex test
This test is used to determine the presence of motor fusion and to prove the presence of binocular single vision (BSV). A 20 Δ or 15 Δ base-out prism is generally used. A response should be obtained in infants aged 6 months and upwards.

Method of use
- A prism is placed base out in front of one eye whilst the patient fixates a near target. The prism shifts the image of the fixation object onto temporal retina which elicits an inward movement to regain foveal fixation. Due to Herings' law the other eye will make a conjugate outward movement resulting in diplopia, which stimulates convergence to regain fusion. If all three components are seen the patient is said to 'overcome' the prism, demonstrating both sensory and motor fusion.
- When the prism is removed the compensatory movements to resume binocular single vision can be seen. It is advisable to repeat the test with the base-out prism in front of the other eye in order to confirm the findings.

Results
- If all three movements are seen, motor fusion is present. However, asymmetry of movement may occur and should be noted; for example, one eye may be slower to respond than the other.
- If the eye behind the prism fails to adduct or the other eye fails to converge, motor fusion is either absent or insufficient to overcome the strength of prism used.
- Lack of recovery may indicate that suppression is preventing fusion or that there is poor motor fusion.

Indications for use
- This test is particularly useful in infants and when

the fusion amplitude cannot be measured. It is commonly used to confirm pseudostrabismus in the very young.

4 Δ prism test
The main purpose of this test is to prove the presence or absence of normal binocular single vision. A central or paracentral scotoma is revealed in the absence of bifoveal binocular single vision.

Method of use
- The principle of the test is the same as for the prism reflex test but a 4 Δ prism is used. Therefore the eye under the prism will be seen to move in, and the other eye will make a conjugate movement out, followed by a movement in to regain fusion. This size of prism keeps the image within the central retinal area and elicits the smallest movement reliably detected by experienced observers.
- It is preferable if the patient fixates a small Snellen target. The test can be performed for any distance although it is often easier to observe the response for distance. Although most often used base out, the prism may also be used base in or vertically.
- The test is repeated placing the prism in front of the other eye.

Results (Fig. 7.3)
- The movements seen will be extremely small but if all three movements are seen with the prism placed in front of either eye, bifoveal fusion is present.
- If there is central suppression the affected eye will not move behind the prism nor will it make a corrective fusional movement when the prism is placed over the contralateral eye.
- A base-out prism is used in suspected microesotropia and a base-in prism in microexotropia. In practice the affected eye may move and not recover with the prism placed both base-in and base-out in front of the suppressed eye, indicating a larger suppression scotoma, irrespective of the type of horizontal microtropia.
- Four atypical responses found in subjects with bifoveal binocular single vision were described by Romano and von Noorden (1969). These patients had either an esophoria not exceeding 5 Δ or poor fusional convergence.

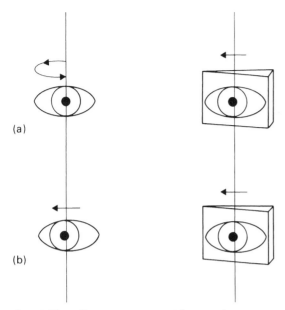

Fig. 7.3 The 4-dioptre prism test. (a) The normal response: the right eye moves out as the prism is placed in front of the left eye but rapidly moves in to regain foveal fixation. (b) The response if bifoveal binocular single vision is absent: the right eye moves out and remains in that position.

- The suppressed eye will make a motor response and is seen to move out when a base-out prism is placed in front of the contralateral eye. However, Bagolini (1985), using Bagolini striated glasses, has demonstrated that a cross can be maintained after interposition of the prism, suggesting that sensory adaptation rather than suppression has taken place. This may be accounted for by the patient's difficulty in appreciating a small gap in the line seen by the affected eye, which results from a central or paracentral suppression scotoma.

Indications for use
- The test is of most use in patients with slight inequality of vision who show no manifest deviation on cover test (this aspect is further discussed in Chapter 15).

Prism fusion amplitude
Horizontal vergence movements occur to maintain binocular single vision when base-out and base-in prisms are introduced. Vertical vergence occurs in response to base-up and base-down prisms. The prism fusion amplitude is recorded as the maximum strength of prism which can be fused: the positive amplitude is assessed using base-out prisms and the negative amplitude with base-in prisms.

The full motor fusion amplitude can be measured irrespective of whether the fixation target is clear or blurred, or prisms can be used to measure positive and negative relative convergence. Positive relative convergence occurs when convergence is exerted in excess of accommodation, and is measured by the maximum strength prism which can be fused whilst maintaining a clear image. Convergence is relaxed in relation to accommodation in negative relative convergence, and is measured by the strength of base-in prism which can be fused whilst accommodating to see clearly.

Before measuring the prism fusion amplitude the patients near point of convergence and the type and extent of any heterophoria should be investigated. There is evidence that once a vergence has been initiated the tonus for the response persists after removal of the stimulus. Therefore, testing the negative amplitude immediately after measuring the positive amplitude, for example, can result in an apparently lower negative amplitude than is the case. For this reason it is advisable to measure the positive amplitude first in exophoria and the negative amplitude first in esophoria.

Method of use
- The patient fixates an accommodative target for near. The prisms are introduced in front of one eye and gradually increased in strength, while asking the patient to keep the image single as long as possible and report when it becomes double. The observer watches the patient's eyes, concentrating on the non-dominant eye if known, to note when binocular single vision is lost.
- It is important that the distance of the target remains static so that the only variable is the disparity caused by the prism.
- The test should be carried out in normal illumination. The amplitude is believed to be larger if the peripheral background contains objects which also stimulate fusion.
- The break point is recorded when diplopia occurs. The strength of prism should then be reduced until

fusion is regained: this is recorded as the recovery point.

• The test can also be used to assess positive and negative relative convergence by asking the patient to report when the image blurs prior to the break point.

• The test is repeated for distance and then the same procedure used with the prisms in the opposite direction.

• The vertical fusion amplitude is mainly measured in patients with thyroid eye disease and those with long-standing vertical muscle palsies, who often have an increased fusion amplitude. The measurement is useful in determining prism strength and can influence the amount of surgery performed.

Normal reported fusion amplitudes are as follows (BO = base-out; BI = base-in; BU = base-up; BD = base-down):

• Distance   15 Δ BO, to 5/7 Δ BI;
• Near   35/40 Δ BO, to 15 Δ BI;
• Vertical   3 Δ BU, to 3 Δ BD;
• Cyclo   3° excyclo, to 3° incyclo (motor): there is also a large sensory amplitude.

Any heterophoria present may bias the amplitude as the deviation is not corrected first; for example, a 10 Δ exophoria may give an amplitude of 10 Δ BO, to 20 Δ BI for distance and still have a 'normal' amplitude. This is important when determining management options.

Major amblyoscope
All grades of binocular vision can be assessed using the major amblyoscope.

Method of use
• Firstly, simultaneous perception slides are inserted into the slide-holders, the image size relating to the patient's visual acuity. If the patient can appreciate both pictures at once simultaneous perception is present. If he can put the lion in the cage, for example, superimposition is present. When suppression prevents superimposition, larger images may be used until simultaneous perception occurs or suppression is found even with the largest sizes.

• If superimposition is obtained, fusion slides of comparable size should be used. The images are the same except for the controls, for example one rabbit without a tail holding a bunch of flowers, the other with a tail and no flowers. When the patient reports only one image, he should be questioned to ensure both controls are present, indicating sensory fusion. This may be confirmed by locking the tubes and moving them on versions to determine if the fused image is maintained, providing that the deviation is concomitant.

• The tubes are then locked and first converged and then diverged. If the patient is able to maintain fusion over a range of 6° then motor fusion is present. The amplitude is measured in degrees. Unlike the prism fusion amplitude method, this method accounts for the angle of deviation present.

• If fusion is absent the images will break and join without movement of the tubes, or one image will appear in front of the other, indicating superimposition rather than fusion.

• The major amblyoscope provides the only way of measuring cyclovergence: a combination of the motor and sensory components recorded 10° in either direction is usually achieved.

• Gross stereopsis is also assessed on the major amblyoscope: more detailed assessment is possible using the Braddick slides (see below).

Indications for use
• Although a very artificial method of assessing binocular vision, the major amblyoscope is extremely useful in patients with a constant manifest deviation and possible potential binocular function, for example those with a history of late-onset strabismus.

Binocular visual acuity (BVA)
BVA is a measure of the level of visual acuity obtained whilst binocular single vision is maintained.

Method of use
• The test is performed by asking the patient to read down a Snellen chart at 6 m whilst the eyes are observed to note any manifest deviation. It is occasionally necessary to perform a quick cover/uncover test to check the response, mainly in small deviations. The patient may report diplopia or blurred vision at the threshold.

• The test is repeated for near and without glasses if binocular single vision can be maintained.

Indications for use
• To elicit whether the patient's positive and negative relative vergences are sufficient for his needs.

- To assess the control of the deviation under accommodative duress.

It is useful to monitor the BVA in all intermittent deviations and in latent deviations where control is uncertain. It is essential in accommodative esotopia, when it should be recorded for near and distance with and without the patient's hypermetropic correction if BSV can be maintained. It is also invaluable in ensuring that control of a distance exotropia is not dependent on excessive accommodation.

Bar reading

This test is similar to the BVA test for near except that the presence of crossed physiological diplopia of the bar is used as a control to ensure binocular single vision is maintained. A subject with binocular single vision can see the print behind the bar on the left side of the page with the left eye and print on the right side with the right eye, allowing him to read without the bar obscuring the print. Several types of bars have been described, but the thumb bar is most universally used (Fig. 7.4). It is necessary that accommodation and convergence are in the correct relationship to achieve a normal response on this test. Bar reading is quite difficult; if small print can be read with the bar in position it indicates that binocular single vision is well established at 33 cm.

Method of use

- Crossed physiological diplopia should first be taught if necessary.
- Print which is a size larger than the near binocular visual acuity is selected and the bar is held by the examiner in the centre of the page. The book is held at 33 cm. The patient's head should be kept stationary, and it is advisable to hold the head during testing.
- The patient is asked to read the print. If this is achieved the size of print is reduced until he is no longer able to read the text or BSV is lost.
- The text should be sufficiently wide for the two images of the bar to fall on it. The bar should be far enough away from the page to allow complete separation of the diplopic images.
- Well-known text such as nursery rhymes should be avoided as the patient could guess words obscured by the bar. The patient can be asked to spell more difficult words to reduce the reading speed, making observation easier.

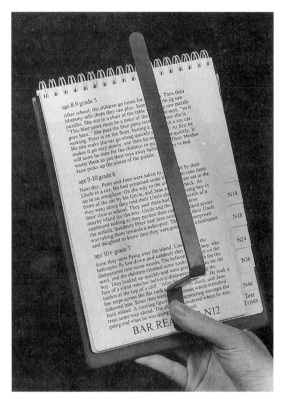

Fig. 7.4 Bar-reading, showing a short-thumb bar in position on a book.

Results

- If the patient reads well with the bar in position, binocular single vision is present. Not all patients recognize diplopia of the bar, and responses can be checked by occluding each eye to ensure that reading is not being achieved by moving the head or alternating fixation.
- If the bar covers the print, either suppression or a manifest strabismus is indicated. If suppression is monocular the bar will remain on one side of the page but if there is alternation it will jump from one side to the other.
- The print may become blurred or double either because the patient cannot accommodate sufficiently whilst controlling the deviation, or because he fails to control it.

Indications for use

- Bar reading gives a further measure of binocular visual acuity for near.

• It can be used as an exercise to improve negative or positive relative convergence (see Chapter 8) and is most commonly used in the treatment of accommodative esotropia.

Sbisa bar

The Sbisa bar consists of 17 filters ranging from palest pink to very dark red. Its purpose is to assess either the density of suppression or the strength of normal or abnormal binocular single vision. In order to interpret the results correctly the examiner must first establish whether the patient is suppressing in free space or is maintaining normal or anomalous binocular single vision.

Method of use

• The test is usually performed for near. The patient fixates a spotlight and the bar is placed with the palest filter in front of the fixing eye, or in the case of heterophoria, the eye least likely to deviate on dissociation, as revealed on the cover test.
• The filters are then increased in density until diplopia is appreciated or a manifest deviation is observed. The filter prior to this is recorded.

Results

• Diplopia is reported by the patient indicating that either fusion or suppression has been disrupted. The density of the filter eliciting diplopia is a measure of the depth of suppression or the strength of normal or abnormal binocular single vision.
• The spotlight is seen to change from red to white without appreciation of diplopia, indicating that fixation has changed and that the eye behind the filter is suppressed.

Indications for use

• To determine how well abnormal retinal correspondence is established.
• To determine the density of suppression. This is most important in gauging the risk of intractable diplopia when considering occlusion in an older child, or before treatment is given to eliminate suppression.
• This test can be especially helpful in patients whose deviation readily becomes manifest on dissociation but not necessarily on accommodation.

Tests for stereopsis

Stereopsis is the perception of the relative depth of objects on the basis of binocular disparity; stereoacuity is an angular measurement of the minimum resolvable binocular disparity necessary for the appreciation of stereopsis. Qualitative tests reveal the presence or absence of stereopsis, whilst quantitative tests provide a measure of the stereoacuity recorded in seconds of arc. The disparity is the measure of lateral displacement produced, but actual acuity will vary depending on interpupillary distance, distance from the target, and whether the object is seen in front of or behind the background.

Qualitative test

Lang two pencil test

This is a rudimentary test for the presence of stereopsis which compares the patient's responses with both eyes open and with one eye covered, both in manifest strabismus, to assess if abnormal binocular single vision is present, and in apparently straight eyes when it can confirm the presence of binocular single vision. It is a very simple test requiring only two pencils and a cover.

Method of use

• The patient is given a pencil to hold vertically and is asked to place this on top of the examiner's vertically held pencil, so using horizontal disparity detectors to locate the correct position.
• The test is then repeated with one eye occluded (the deviated or amblyopic eye, if present).
• It is important that the subject is not given too long to perform the test so that he does not use any monocular or motion clues to depth.
• The test should be repeated several times and the responses compared.

Results

• If accuracy in locating the examiner's pencil is repeatedly better with both eyes open then stereopsis is present thus confirming normal or abnormal binocular single vision.
• If the response is comparable with both eyes open and with the squinting eye covered, the squinting eye is suppressed and binocular vision is absent (Fig. 7.5).

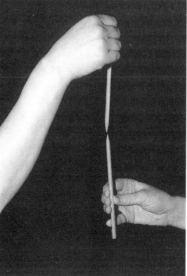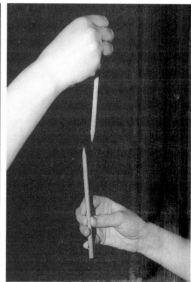

Fig. 7.5 The Lang two-pencil test. (a) The response with both eyes open in the presence of BSV. (b) The response with one eye covered in the same subject.

Quantitative tests

TNO test

The TNO is based on random dot stereograms and complementary red and green glasses. The red and green anaglyphs are computer-generated random dots, the image disparities ranging from 1980 to 15 seconds of arc. The first plate contains two butterflies, the second plate contains four circles, and the third five different shapes; each plate has at least one image which can be appreciated monocularly. There is a suppression test plate with three circles. The decreasing stereoacuities from 480 to 15 seconds of arc are incomplete circles.

Method of use

• The red and green glasses are worn and the apparatus is held at 40 cm perpendicular to the patient.
• The screening plates subtending 1980 seconds of arc are shown first, and if these are successfully completed the graded plates from 480 to 15 seconds of arc are presented until the patient is unable to locate the three-dimensional shape correctly.
• If the screening plates are not appreciated the response can be checked with the suppression plate, which consists of three circles, the middle one being common to both eyes.

Indications for use

• This test is often the method of choice as there are no monocular clues or contours, making it a useful tool in the diagnosis of bifoveal BSV. It can be difficult for children under 3 years to understand the test.

Wirt test (also referred to as Titmus test)

The targets are presented as vectographs. The image seen by one eye is polarized at 90° to that seen by the other eye when viewed through the polarized spectacles. The disparities range from 3000 to 40 seconds of arc. The targets comprise a housefly, animals and sets of circles, one of which is disparate in each set. The test gives monocular clues, especially when viewing the first three sets of circles, when it is easy to see monocularly that one circle is displaced and therefore different from the others.

Method of use

• The test is performed at 40 cm with the patient wearing the polarizing spectacles.
• The fly is shown first, although the effect of this can frighten some young children, in itself an indication that stereopsis is present, while others are fascinated by it. The patient is asked to 'pick up' the wings of the fly. The animals and circles should then be presented until the stereoscopic image cannot be identified.

• If only gross stereopsis is demonstrated the apparatus should be turned through 90°, when there is no depth effect, or one eye occluded and the response compared.

Indications for use

Gross stereopsis is tested, making this a useful method for patients with abnormal binocular single vision, when this may be the optimum of stereoacuity obtained. It has been shown that patients with abnormal retinal correspondence (ARC) recognize stereopsis more readily when contours are present. (Lang 1987).

Randot test

This test also uses polaroid vectographs but in conjunction with random dots. Geometric shapes easily recognized by children are seen in three of each of two sets of four boxes. As with the Wirt test there are also rows of animals and sets of circles; in this case one in each row is disparate. The level of stereoacuity measured ranges from 500 to 20 seconds of arc. Unlike Wirt there are no monocular clues.

Method of use

• The polarizing glasses are worn and the apparatus presented at a distance of 40 cm. The patient identifies the objects in the boxes and then indicates the circles and animals seen stereoscopically.

Indications for use

• In young children, who can understand this test more easily than the TNO.

Randot preschool stereoacuity test

This test also uses random dots and polarized glasses, using the four boxes containing three stereoscopic shapes, as in the Randot test. The range of stereoacuity is 800–40 seconds of arc. The targets are presented in three booklets.

Method of use

• Booklet one is presented at 40 cm: the infant either names the shape or matches it to that printed on the opposite page. Two out of three correct answers are required to proceed to the next set of shapes. If the patient responds correctly to book 1 he can proceed to book 2, which contains stereoacuities of 60 and 40 seconds of arc. If he fails to respond to book 1 he

should proceed to book 3, which contains shapes of 800 and 400 seconds of arc.
• If his understanding is in doubt, his familiarity with the shapes can be checked by asking him to name those printed on the opposite side.

Indications for use

• The test can be used successfully in children as young as 2 years of age and provides a fairly quick screening tool in this age group.

The Frisby stereotest

This is the only test based on actual depth. Random shapes are printed on three clear plastic plates of different thickness. Each plate comprises four squares of curved random shapes; one square contains a 'hidden' circle, which is printed on the opposite surface of the plate. The thickness of the plates provides different disparities, or the test can be moved further away or closer to the subject to change disparity. The range is from 600 to 15 seconds of arc. This test has the advantages of not requiring glasses and the facility to repeat the test an infinite number of times without the correct response being learnt.

Method of use

• The 3 mm plate is held in front of a plain white background ensuring that the plate is not touching the surface and that the patient does not use gross head movements, either of which will provide monocular clues to the test. The patient is questioned as to the position of the hidden circle; the plate is then turned around and the patient questioned again. The target can be presented in either the crossed or uncrossed position by reversing the plate as many times as necessary to be certain of the result. If this plate is recognized successfully the 2 mm and, if successful, the 1 mm plate is presented. The plate can be moved further away from the patient to reach the threshold, when the tape measure provided is used to measure the distance from the patient.
• If there is difficulty interpreting the response, the child can be trained to see the target by twisting the plate, to demonstrate the depth effect, or placing it flat against a surface when binocular vision is not required to perceive the circle; this helps to assess his understanding of the test. Further modification has included a flashlight reward to help in testing

in the under-24-month age group (Frisby *et al.* 1996).

Indications for use
• Very young infants often perform this test quite well, and responses have been found in subjects as young as 9 months, especially when training is undertaken and a reward given.
• It is useful for patients who will not tolerate glasses or for those in whom dissociating spectacles may cause a deviation to become manifest.

Reinecke E test
This method employs polarized spectacles and random dots, with two plates. An E is depicted on one plate but not the other. The range of stereoacuity is 504–50 seconds of arc.

Method of use
• The test is first performed at 50 cm. The two plates are viewed and the patient chooses the one which displays the E. The examiner then moves back one metre at a time up to five metres, repeating the test.

Indications for use
The test can give an indication of stereopsis for distance, but a disadvantage is the 50% chance of guessing correctly.

Lang stereotest
This test combines panography with random dots. The targets are fine vertical sections that are seen alternately by each eye as they are viewed through the built-in cylindrical lens elements. Displacement of the random dots creates the disparity. The test comes in two versions: Lang I, with a disparity range of 1200–550 seconds of arc; and Lang II, with a disparity range of 600–200 seconds of arc.

Method of use
• The card is held at normal reading distance and the child is asked to name or point to the pictures. On the Lang II test a star can be seen monocularly.
• Preverbal children may be seen to look at the pictures shown.

Indications for use
• The Lang test is often used for screening pur-

poses as it is interesting to young children. There are, however, only three pictures, which can easily be remembered.

Randot stereo smile test
This test combines the use of random dots and polaroid spectacles with preferential looking. It consists of three cards: a training card printed with a face without a depth effect displaced to one side of the card, and two cards printed with a smiling face of disparate random dots either to right or left of the card. Each card has a central peephole so that the examiner can obscure the child's response: identical targets are printed on both sides of the card, so that the position of the face can be changed by turning the card round. The disparity range is 480 and 120 seconds of arc at the testing distance of 55 cm (Fig. 7.6).

Method of use
• The child wears polaroid spectacles and his response to the training card is assessed by the examiner through the peephole. Very young children should be seen to look to the side of the face: older children can be taught to point to it. The card should be reversed several times to ensure that the response is consistent.
• The test cards are then introduced, starting with the maximum disparity, changing the face position several times. Four consecutive correct answers are required to record a positive response.
• The test can be repeated at 110 cm distance, where the disparities will range from 240 to 60 seconds of arc.

Indications for use
• The test is designed to be used with preverbal children. The test's similarity to Teller acuity cards, for example, makes it suitable for preverbal children able to cooperate with preferential looking or pointing tasks (Ciner *et al.* 1996).
• The full value of this relatively new test has yet to be determined.

Major amblyoscope
Both gross and detailed targets can be used to establish whether or not stereoscopic vision is present in patients with manifest strabismus. The Braddick random dot slides provide a means of measuring stereoacuity, using disparities ranging from 720 to 90 seconds of arc.

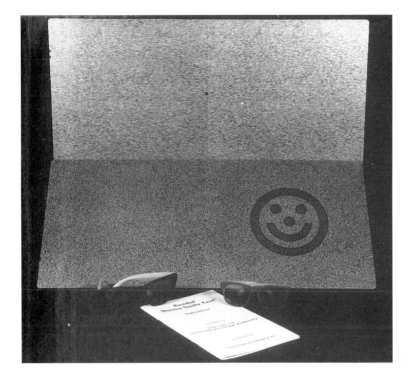

Fig. 7.6 Randot stereo smile test.

Method of use
• Stereopsis slides are used and the patient is questioned as to the direction of the object, which should be seen stereoscopically, or in the case of the more detailed slides, the order in which the objects are seen from front to back.
• The Braddick slides seen stereoscopically will produce a C, H or +; a key card is provided to help younger children identify the shape.

Indications for use
• In manifest strabismus with deviations exceeding 40 Δ when testing by other methods is not possible.

Tests specifically used to assess retinal correspondence

Comparison of the subjective and objective measurements
If the objective and subjective measurements of the deviation are the same, normal retinal correspondence is present. If the difference exceeds 3°, abnormal retinal correspondence is implied. However, testing should be repeated in case this difference is due to a variable angle. These observations are usually made using the major amblyoscope.

Tests for foveal projection
The presence of binocular single vision in patients with a manifest deviation on cover test implies the possible presence of abnormal retinal correspondence. Tests for projection will indicate whether or not the foveae are projecting straight ahead.

After-image test
The principle of the test is to produce after images by presenting a bright light to each eye in turn. The images can be obtained by using special slides in the major amblyoscope or with a hand-held flash apparatus, which is the author's preference and is described.

The apparatus consists of a linear light with a central black band within a circular black background, mounted on the flash apparatus. The line can be presented horizontally or vertically. The apparatus is flashed while the patient fixates the black band.

Method of use

The patient must have steady foveal fixation:

• The deviating eye is covered and the line is presented horizontally at a distance of approximately 50 cm. The fixing eye is then covered and the process repeated with the line presented vertically. A vertical line is more likely to fall outside the suppression scotoma.

• The patient looks at a blank wall in normal illumination and should see two negative linear afterimages, each with a central gap corresponding to the fixation and, therefore, representing the visual direction of the fovea. He is asked to draw or describe the position of the lines. Blinking may aid appreciation of the images. Alternatively the position of positive after-images can be assessed in a dark room.

Results (Fig. 7.7)

• A symmetrical cross with coincident gaps indicates normal retinal correspondence.

• Displacement of the lines indicates abnormal retinal correspondence; the separation between the gaps is determined by the size of the angle of anomaly. There will be crossed projection in esotropia.

• If eccentric fixation is present the results will need to be assessed accordingly; a symmetrical cross would then indicate ARC.

Indications for use

• The test is difficult for the patient to perform and to interpret, which limits its application. Testing conditions are entirely artificial and abnormal retinal correspondence is only diagnosed if it well established, in contrast to the results of tests using more normal seeing conditions, which have largely superseded this test in routine clinical examination.

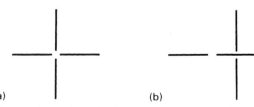

(a)   **(b)**

Fig. 7.7 The results of the after-image test. (a) Normal retinal correspondence. (b) Abnormal retinal correspondence.

Binocular Visuscopy (Cüppers test; fovea-foveolar test)

This test was devised by Cüppers and is sometimes referred to simply as Cüppers test. It can be performed if the patient has central fixation or steady eccentric fixation: the state of fixation must be known in order to interpret the results. Good cooperation and understanding are required from the patient and he should be given a careful explanation of the procedure before starting the test.

Apparatus

The test requires:

• A spotlight: the patient sits at 6 m distance at right angles to the light, which he views at eye level through a plane mirror held at 45° to the plane of his face (Fig. 7.8).

• A Visuscope, which is used by the examiner, who sits facing the patient.

• A Maddox tangent scale, which is not essential but which allows the findings to be recorded in degrees from the scale.

Method (using a plane mirror)

The patient views the light with his normally fixing eye:

• the Viscuscope star is projected onto the fovea of the squinting eye by the examiner and the patient is asked to state its position on the tangent scale in relation to the spotlight;

• if the star and the spotlight are not coincident, the patient adjusts the Visuscope until the two are

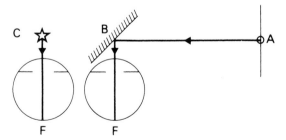

Fig. 7.8 Binocular visuscopy: the right eye fixates on a spotlight through a plane mirror, the left eye fixates on the Visuscope star. A = spotlight viewed by the fixing eye through the mirror; B = plane mirror; C = Visuscope star projected onto the fovea of the squinting eye; F = fovea.

superimposed. The examiner then notes the position of the star on the retina.

Results
• If the star is seen superimposed on the light whilst projected onto the fovea, retinal correspondence is normal.
• If the star consistently appears to one side of the light, abnormal retinal correspondence is present. When the patient claims they are superimposed, the Visuscope star will appear eccentric to the fovea, confirming the presence of abnormal retinal correspondence.

An alternative method of performing this test is for the patient to sit facing the spotlight, using a Lang periscope instead of a mirror.

In practice this test is very difficult to perform. Suppression of the star image is frequently found and it is hard to maintain the star on the fovea when the patient is asked to interpret its position, as fixation reverts to eccentric as he looks at the star in many cases.

Prism adaptation test
The principle of the test is to completely correct or slightly overcorrect the angle of deviation with Fresnel prisms and to observe the patient's motor response over a period of time. The patient must have:
• equal or nearly equal visual acuity;
• an angle of deviation not exceeding 40 Δ.

It is easier if glasses are worn, but if not, plano lenses in frames can be used. The test is most commonly used in acquired esotropias as reported by the Prism Adaptation Study Research Group (1990) and Ohtsuki *et al.* (1993). The prisms should be divided between the two lenses. The patient should be reassessed before leaving the clinic and if the visual axes have reconverged, producing a manifest deviation greater than 8 Δ, the prism strength is increased. The patient is reviewed one week later.

There are four possible responses to overcorrecting prisms:
• The visual axes become straight and binocular single vision can be confirmed, for example with Bagolini glasses.
• There is a residual microtropia with demonstrable binocular single vision.

• The visual axes reconverge to the original angle, referred to as 'eating up' the prism, which Bagolini (1982) suggested was indicative of abnormal retinal correspondence.
• The visual axes remain convergent, indicating a lack of binocular cooperation. Suppression or, more rarely, diplopia occurs.

If the esotropia measures more than 8 Δ and no binocular single vision is demonstrable after one week of prism use, the prism strength is increased to correct the total deviation. The patient is seen at weekly intervals until a stable angle measuring less than 8 Δ is achieved or the esotropia exceeds the limits correctable with prisms, usually over 50–60 Δ. Binocular single vision may be demonstrable in some who maintain a small stable angle, but is assumed to be absent in those who continue to 'eat up' the prisms.

The test is useful in determining the presence of binocular vision and in planning surgery:
• If there is demonstrable binocular single vision, either bifoveal or with a microtropia, the patient is classed as a prism responder and the prism strength is gradually increased to assess the maximum angle of deviation, seeing the patient at weekly intervals until a stable angle measuring less than 8 Δ is achieved. Surgery is then performed to correct the maximum angle measured.
• If binocular potential cannot be demonstrated the patient is classed as a nonresponder and any surgery performed is based on the angle of deviation first measured (or measured at the commencement of the test).

Botulinum toxin
Ketley *et al.* (1987) suggested that botulinum toxin A could be used to investigate potential binocular function in patients with manifest strabismus. They reported a small series of patients requesting surgery to improve their appearance who underwent botulinum toxin injection preoperatively. The results showed that 20 out of a total of 113 patients unexpectedly demonstrated binocular function following injection, and 7 of the 13 patients who were thought to have potential binocular function failed to demonstrate it postinjection. Shah *et al.* (1996) suggested the use of botulinum injection in patients who had apparently lost motor fusion whilst main-

taining sensory fusion. If no improvement in motor fusion occurred following injection, surgery was considered inadvisable.

Tests for suppression

Presence

The presence of suppression can be diagnosed by using the tests for binocular vision (BV) described above, mainly Worth lights and Bagolini glasses. Central suppression is diagnosed by the 4 Δ prism test and the polarized four dot test.

Area

A defined area of suppression is referred to as a suppression scotoma. It is useful to measure the area of suppression preoperatively to elicit whether diplopia would follow a change in the angle of deviation, either as a result of strabismus surgery or due to the passage of time. The scotoma can be measured with prisms.

Method

• A prism bar is introduced in front of the deviating eye or a bar can be placed in front of each eye to minimize blur, reduce the steps between prisms and avoid the inaccuracies resulting from the need for stacked prisms in large deviations.
• The prism strength is gradually increased until the patient reports diplopia.
• The prisms should be used base-out, base-in and vertically to measure the scotoma in all directions. The prism strength prior to appreciation of diplopia is recorded.

Postoperative diplopia test

Testing for postoperative diplopia is performed in a similar way. A base-out prism is introduced in esotropia, usually by means of one or two prism bars, and the strength slowly increased until the patient notices diplopia of the fixation target. It is suggested that both illuminated and nonilluminated targets are used (Gray *et al.* 1996). Exotropic patients are tested with base-in prisms. The results can be recorded as for the suppression scotoma or graphically with the corrected angle at the mid-point, showing undercorrection to the left and overcorrection to the right, as shown in Fig. 7.9.

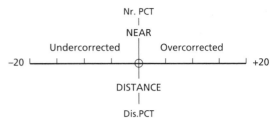

Fig. 7.9 Recording the postoperative diplopia test.

Major amblyoscope

As described earlier, suppression is diagnosed by the patient's inability to superimpose images and by the total or partial disappearance of the target presented to the squinting eye.

Method of use
• The tube in front of the suppressing eye is rotated by the patient in a convergent, divergent or vertical direction until both pictures are perceived at the same time. The angle in each direction is recorded in degrees.
• The density of suppression can be estimated by reducing the illumination on the side of the fixing eye until simultaneous perception is achieved.

Binocular perimetry

The apparatus must be arranged so that the fixation target is common to both eyes but the test object is seen only by the eye under examination. This can be achieved using one of the following methods or types of apparatus:
• two Bjerrum screens at 90° to each other (Travers 1938);
• the Lees (Hess) screen (Pratt-Johnson *et al.* 1981);
• polarization or colour dissociation (Parks 1971);
• the Aimark or other modern perimeter (Pratt-Johnson & Tillson 1984).

Retinal rivalry must be avoided by using fusional targets.

Parks method of binocular perimetry
The patient fixates a central 5 mm black target on an illuminated screen, which appears a diffuse red to him when wearing complementary red and green glasses. A 1 mm green light is projected onto the screen, which the patient moves along an isopter to within the

fixation target. If there is a suppression scotoma the green light will disappear as it approaches the target; the scotoma can be plotted by moving the light from the periphery inwards along each isopter, recording when it disappears and reappears.

Amsler grid

Lang (1984) has described how the Amsler grid can be used to plot a central or paracentral suppression scotoma in observant patients, either monocularly, using a conventional red-and-black or white-and-black grid, or binocularly, using specially designed slides for use in a major amblyoscope. One slide presents the full grid and the other slide shows only a central fixation point within a linear border (see Chapter 15).

Density

The density of suppression is tested using the Sbisa bar, as described above.

Quality of binocular single vision

The quality of binocular single vision can be assessed by:
- the speed of recovery on cover test;
- the size of the fusion amplitude;
- stereoacuity;
- binocular visual acuity;
- the size of print which can be bar-read.

All of these provide a measure of the patient's ability to control a latent or intermittent strabismus.

References

Archer, S.M., Helveston, E.M., Miller, K.K. & Ellis, F.D. (1986) Stereopsis in normal infants and infants with congenital esotropia. *American Journal of Ophthalmology* **101**, 591–596.

Awaya, S., Nozaki, H., Itoh, T. & Harada, K. (1976) Studies of suppression in alternating constant exotropia and intermittent exotropia: with reference to the effects of fusional background. In: *Orthoptics: Past, Present and Future. Transactions of the Third International Orthoptics Congress, Boston* (eds S. Moore, J. Mein & L. Stockbridge), pp. 531–546. Symposia Specialists, Miami.

Bagolini, B. (1982) Anomalous fusion. In: *Documenta Ophthalmologica Proceedings Series No. 32* (eds A.Th.M. van Balen & W. Houtman), pp. 41–51. Junk, The Hague.

Bagolini, B. (1985) Objective evaluation of sensorial and sensorimotor status in esotropia: their importance in surgical prognosis. *British Journal of Ophthalmology* **69**, 725–728.

Ciner, E.B., Schanel-Klitsch, E. & Herzberg, C. (1996) Stereoacuity development: 6 months to 5 years. A new tool for testing and screening. *Optometry and Vision Science* **73** (1), 43–48.

Crone, R.A., Vrooland, J.L. & Hardjowito, S. (1978) Proportionregelung der Fusion. Integralregelung der willkurlichen konvergenz. In: *Disorders of Ocular Motility* (ed. G. Kommerell), pp. 323–327. Bergmann, Munich.

Fender, D.H. & Julesz, B. (1967) Extension of Panum's fusional area in binocularly stabilised vision. *Journal of the Optical Society of America* **57**, 819–825.

Frisby, J.P., Davis, H. & McMorrow, K. (1996) An improved training procedure as a precursor to testing young children with the Frisby stereotest. *Eye* **10** (2), 286–290.

Gray, C., Ansons, A. & Spencer, A. (1996) A study of the method of testing and recording of the post-operative diplopia test. In: *Transactions of the 22nd Meeting of the European Strabismological Association, Cambridge* (ed. M. Spiritus), pp. 79–84. Aeolus Press, Cambridge.

Held, R. (1988) Normal visual development and its deviations. In: *Strabismus and Amblyopia: Wenner Gren International Symposium Series* (eds G. Lennerstrand, G.K. von Noorden & E. Campos), pp. 247–258. Macmillan Press, London.

Jampolsky, A. (1955) Characteristics of suppression in strabismus. *Archives of Ophthalmology* **54**, 683–696.

Ketley, M.J., Powell, C.M., Lee, J.P. & Elston, J. (1987) Botulinum toxin adaptation test: the use of botulinum toxin in the investigation of the sensory state in strabismus. In: *Orthoptic Horizons. Transactions of the Sixth International Orthoptic Congress, Harrogate* (eds M. Lenk-Schafer, C. Calcutt, M. Doyle & S. Moore), pp. 289–293. British Orthoptics Society, London.

Lang, J. [trans. Cibis, C.W.] (1984) *Strabismus*, pp. 90–97. Slack, Thorofare, New Jersey.

Lang, J. (1987) Anomalous retinal correspondence update. In: *Orthoptic Horizons. Transactions of the 6th International Orthoptics Congress, Harrogate*, pp. 124–126. British Orthoptic Society, London.

Ohtsuki, H., Hasebe, S., Tadokoro, Y., Kobashi, R., Watanabe, S. & Okano, M. (1993) Preoperative prism correction in patients with acquired esotropia. *Graefe's Archives in Clinical and Experimental Ophthalmology* **231**, 71–75.

Parks, M.M. (1971) The monofixation syndrome. In: *Symposium on Strabismus. Transactions of the New Orleans Academy of Ophthalmology* (ed. J.H. Allen), pp. 121–153. Mosby, St Louis.

Pratt-Johnson, J.A. & Tillson, G. (1984) Suppression in strabismus, an update. *British Journal of Ophthalmology* 68, 174–178.

Pratt-Johnson, J.A. & Tillson, G. (1989) Intractable diplopia after vision restoration in unilateral cataract. *American Journal of Ophthalmology* 107, 23–26.

Pratt-Johnson, J.A., Pop, A. & Tillson, G. (1981) The complexities of suppression in intermittent exotropia. In: *Orthoptics, Research and Practice. Transactions of the Fourth International Orthoptic Congress, Berne* (eds J. Mein & S. Moore), pp. 172–173. Kimpton, London.

Prism Adaptation Study Research Group (1990) Efficacy of prism adaptation in the surgical management of acquired esotropia. *Archives of Ophthalmology* 108, 1248–1256.

Romano, P.E. & von Noorden, G.K. (1969) Atypical responses to the four-diopter prism test. *American Journal of Ophthalmology* 67 (6), 935–941.

Shah, S., Spencer, A.L. & Ansons, A.M. (1996) Intractable diplopia due to non-traumatic loss of motor fusion. In: *Transactions of the 22nd Meeting of the European Strabismological Association, Cambridge* (ed. M. Spiritus), pp. 73–78. Aeolus Press, The Netherlands.

Stager, D.R. & Birch, E.E. (1986) Preferential looking and stereopsis in infantile esotropia. *Journal of Pediatric Ophthalmology and Strabismus* 23, 160–165.

Teller, D.Y. (1983) Scotopic vision, color vision and stereopsis in infants. *Current Eye Research* 2, 199–207.

Travers, T.àB. (1938) Suppression of vision in squint and its association with retinal correspondence and amblyopia. *British Journal of Ophthalmology* 22, 577–604.

Worth, C. (1901) The orthoptic treatment of convergent squint in young children. *Transactions of the Ophthalmological Society of the United Kingdom* 21, 245–258.

II
PRINCIPLES OF MANAGEMENT

8
Nonsurgical Management

Optical management
Use of spherical lenses
Use of prisms

Orthoptic exercises
Criteria for selection
Dangers of orthoptic exercises
Purpose of exercises
Exercises to aid control of the deviation
Improving the near point of convergence

Pharmacological management
Miotic drugs
Cycloplegic drugs

Botulinum toxin
Mechanism of action
Ophthalmological use of botulinum toxin

References

The goals of the management of strabismus are the restoration of visual acuity and of comfortable binocular single vision. Obviously these goals cannot be achieved in all cases but, generally, correct management can go some way towards them and at worst it should result in good ocular alignment, with its attendant social advantages. The restoration of visual acuity is discussed in Chapter 10.

Nonsurgical management of the ocular deviation comprises:
• optical treatment;
• orthoptic exercises;
• pharmacological management.

Although the principles of each are discussed separately, in practice they overlap and are frequently integrated with surgical management. Any deviation measuring greater than 20 Δ will almost certainly require surgery in addition to other forms of treatment.

Optical management

Optical management comprises:
• the use of lenses;
• the use of prisms.

Use of spherical lenses

In addition to spectacles or contact lenses to correct the refractive error, spherical lenses can be used, usually as a temporary measure, to aid in the management of strabismus. Temporary lenses can be used as:
• Fresnel lenses attached to the patient's spectacles or to plano glasses.
• Clip-on lenses on the patient's spectacles (although these are no longer commercially available).
• In spectacle frames prescribed for the purpose.

Fresnel lenses have the advantages that they are lightweight, are certain to fit (provided that the spectacles are well fitted) and are generally more acceptable to the patient than clip-on lenses. The slight reduction in visual acuity is usually tolerated. Spherical lenses up to 3 DS can be used. However, ordering the lenses as a temporary spectacle correction is often more satisfactory.

Principle

Spherical lenses induce relaxation or exertion of accommodation in order to obtain clear vision through the lenses and thereby influence the amount of convergence which is exerted. In addition, convex lenses may be used to supplement defective accommodation in accommodative fatigue or insufficiency (see Chapter 16).

Following a successful trial of lenses in the clinic, a temporary presciption may be useful to determine if lens therapy is indicated.

Diagnostic uses
- Low-power convex lenses (up to +2 DS) can be worn for 2–4 weeks to assess if the prescription of such a low hypermetropic correction is justified, in that a patient with an esotropia will obtain binocular single vision with the lenses.
- To assess if binocular single vision with a satisfactory near binocular visual acuity can be achieved in accommodative esotropia with convergence excess. It is better to start with the lowest strength convex lenses which appear to result in binocular single vision for near, increasing the strength in stages if necessary. The lenses should be worn for approximately two weeks and the patient reassessed using:
- the cover test;
- assessment of the near binocular visual acuity with the lenses.

If the distance visual acuity is reduced by an unacceptable amount with an extra plus correction, Fresnel lenses can be applied to the lower half of the spectacle lenses, bisecting the pupil. The strength of the near addition required in bifocal spectacles can be assessed in this way. It also helps the examiner to judge if the patient will use bifocal spectacles correctly should they be prescribed.

Low concave lenses up to −3.00 DS may be used in patients with intermittent distance exotropia. Assessment of their control for distance will help determine if they are a suitable form of therapy and indicate the strength of lens required.

Therapeutic uses

Spherical lenses are used in the treatment of strabismus only when there is a good potential for binocular single vision. Convex lenses are used to relax accommodation, and convergence and concave lenses are used to stimulate accommodation and convergence, using the lowest strength lens which achieves the desired result.

The success of therapeutic lenses is in part dependent on the AC/A (accommodative convergence : accommodation) ratio. A good response to lens therapy is often found when the ratio is high, provided that the initial angle is less than 20 Δ.

The main objectives of therapeutic lenses are:
- to achieve binocular single vision in intermittent or residual deviations;
- to improve the binocular visual acuity.

To achieve binocular single vision

Lenses can be of value in the following types of strabismus.

ACCOMMODATIVE ESOTROPIA OF THE CONVERGENCE EXCESS TYPE

Convex lenses up to +3.00 DS can be used to control the esotropia at near and provide the patient with a binocular visual acuity sufficient for his needs.

INTERMITTENT DISTANCE EXOTROPIA

Concave lenses up to −3.00 DS are used to stimulate accommodation and convergence in order to control the exotropia for distance fixation.

POSTOPERATIVE ESOTROPIA

Residual esotropia

Every effort should be made to obtain binocular single vision in patients with sensory and motor fusion as soon as possible.

The patient should be prescribed his maximum hypermetropic correction. If this is insufficient, additional plus lenses may be tried to ascertain if binocular single vision can be achieved.

Consecutive esotropia after surgery for an intermittent exotropia

The patient should be observed for at least 2–3 weeks after the operation to allow time for spontaneous relaxation. If esotropia persists, convex lenses can be used, either for near and distance if any hypermetropia present has not been corrected, or in bifocal form if esotropic only at near.

Convex lenses are more likely to succeed in either residual or consecutive esotropia measuring 15 Δ or less. Success is limited in larger deviations.

Once stable binocular single vision is maintained with lenses, steps should be taken to reduce the lens strength in 1 DS or 0.5 DS stages over several weeks, the time depending on each patient's progress. This is easier to achieve if exercises to improve the fusional reserves are combined with the use of lenses.

Improvement of binocular visual acuity

FULLY ACCOMMODATIVE ESOTROPIA

Once the esotropia can be controlled without the patient's hypermetropic correction, efforts should be made to improve the binocular visual acuity without spectacles in suitable cases, mainly those wearing corrections of +3.00 DS or less without significant astigmatism.

To achieve this, concave lenses can be applied to the patient's spectacles, starting with –0.50 DS or –1.00 DS. The patient must accommodate to see clearly, and use negative relative convergence to maintain binocular single vision. The lens strength can be slowly increased in stages, up to –3.00 DS if necessary. When there is already good control of the esotropia without glasses, it may be possible to commence treatment to improve the binocular visual acuity (BVA) without glasses, dispensing with the need for the initial use of concave lenses.

Details of the treatment outlined above can be found in Chapters 12 and 13.

Use of prisms

Prisms are used in several forms, as outlined below.

• Fresnel prisms, which are the method of choice for temporary use. Up to 30° can be applied to either eye but high-powered prisms may not be tolerated because of their adverse effect on visual acuity; usually up to 20° can be worn comfortably, at least by children.

• In spectacle frames: if the patient has a high refractive error the spectacle lenses can be decentred to give the desired effect, providing that the prism strength is not too great. Patients with lower refractive errors and those who are emmetropic can be prescribed additional prisms. These methods are used when permanent or long-term use of prisms is envisaged.

• Clip-on prisms: generally used only when the patient cannot tolerate Fresnel prisms. The strength is limited to $10–12 \Delta$ in front of each eye because of the weight involved. These are no longer commercially available.

Application of Fresnel prisms

• Care must be taken to ensure that the spectacle lens is clean and that the prism is cut so that it is marginally smaller than the spectacle lens, otherwise it is very difficult to prevent the formation of air bubbles.

• The prism can be placed horizontally, vertically or obliquely to correct horizontal, vertical or combined horizontal and vertical deviations, respectively. It is important not to tilt the prism when fitting it in purely horizontal or purely vertical deviations, otherwise an added and unwanted vertical or horizontal component is introduced. In combined horizontal and vertical deviations the prism is deliberately tilted to compensate for both components. If, for example, a base-out prism is tilted down it acts as a base-down vertical prism, the amount depending on the degree of tilt, decreasing the base-out effect by the amount of vertical prismatic effect produced.

• The prism is normally fitted to the back surface of the spectacle lens. Problems can arise with some high-powered lenses because of the amount of curvature; occasionally it is easier to fit the prism onto the front surface of the lens.

• In children it is preferable to place the prism in front of the eye with better acuity to help prevent suppression and amblyopia.

• Most patients with incomitant deviations are more comfortable if the prism is placed over the affected eye unless the visual acuity is unequal, when it is preferable to confine the prism to the side of the weaker eye in an adult patient.

• The patient should be instructed on the care of the prism.

Not all patients accept the reduction in vision and the slight distortion which is caused by the prisms, but some become more accustomed to this with long-term wear. A Fresnel prism bar is useful to demonstrate the effect, or the prisms can be held in front of the patient's eyes before they are prescribed.

Temporary prisms can be used diagnostically and therapeutically.

Diagnostic uses

• Prism adaptation is used to investigate the potential for BSV by initially overcorrecting the deviation to induce diplopia, dividing the prism strength between the two eyes and assessing the presence or absence of BSV after a trial wearing period. If the angle of deviation increases after wearing prisms, higher strength prisms are used until there is no further increase and the maximum angle of deviation is reached. Correction of this angle has been shown to improve the surgical outcome (Prism Adaptation Study Research Group 1990).

• When there is a combined horizontal and vertical deviation one element, usually the vertical component, can be corrected with prisms and the patient reassessed to ascertain if he can then control the horizontal component, indicating that vertical muscle surgery alone should be successful. Alternatively, or if the horizontal element is much the larger, this component can be corrected with prisms and the effect on the vertical component assessed before deciding on the choice of surgery.

• Base-up or base-down prisms can be used to correct the vertical deviation in a patient who also has cyclotorsion, to assess if the torsion is then superable or if it prevents fusion and will require surgical correction. This situation most commonly occurs in unilateral fourth nerve palsy.

• Prisms can be used to help in planning the amount of vertical muscle surgery required in congenital or long-standing vertical muscle palsies with a large vertical fusion amplitude. These patients are usually more comfortable if surgically undercorrected. The lowest strength of prism which results in comfortable BSV is then used as a guide to the amount of surgery to perform.

• Prisms can help to determine if a patient's symptoms are due to his heterophoria, especially when there is a small esophoria which can give rise to severe symptoms, or when the symptoms are atypical. If the symptoms are relieved when the deviation is corrected with prisms, the heterophoria can be treated, but if they persist, further investigation is indicated.

Therapeutic uses

• Prisms can be used to restore and maintain BSV in children with late-onset strabismus, usually esotropia, who are waiting for surgical treatment. Maintenance of BSV will prevent the development of suppression and amblyopia and thus improve the prognosis.

• Prisms can be used to obtain BSV if there is a small surgical undercorrection or overcorrection in a patient with a good prognosis for a functional result. Once BSV is established, efforts should be made to reduce the prism strength in stages until BSV can be obtained unaided. This is more easily achieved if diplopia is present as the patient will have some conscious control over the deviation. Diplopia is more likely if the strabismus is overcorrected.

Relieving prisms

• Prisms are used in patients with ocular motility defects, such as neurogenic palsies, to relieve symptom-producing diplopia. The aim is to give the patient comfortable binocular single vision and possibly allow him to return to work. The strength of prism can be adapted to any change which occurs while waiting for spontaneous recovery or treatment. Patients with diplopia due to thyroid eye disease respond well to relieving prisms.

Assessment of prism strength

• The angle of deviation for near and distance fixation is first measured using the prism cover test.

• To fuse diplopia: starting at the distance at which the diplopia is maximum, a prism bar is placed in front of one eye and the prism is gradually increased until the images join and fusion can be maintained without undue effort. The effect of the prism is then assessed at other distances, adjusting the strength if necessary. It is simpler and more comfortable for the patient if the same strength of prism can be tolerated for near and distance fixation. If this is impossible, Fresnel prisms can be fitted as 'bifocals', using different powers on the upper and lower halves of the spectacle lens or on plano glass if there is no refractive error. The prism may be required only on one half of the lens; for example, a patient with a sixth nerve palsy may read binocularly without a prism.

A useful way of confirming that the prism strength is correct is to ask the patient to read the smallest line he can see on a Snellen's vision chart for distance and near, asking him to note any difference in the clarity of the letters as the prism strength is changed by 1 or 2 Δ. The prism which gives the clearest vision is likely to result in comfortable binocular single vision. The Bagolini glasses test can also be used as confirmation, prescribing the minimum power which results in a BSV response.

General guidelines

In principle the patient should be given the lowest-powered prism which makes him comfortable. The guideline generally applied is to correct two-thirds of the deviation, but the variation found in different conditions and among patients with the same condition make this rule of little value. Useful guidelines are:

• Patients with acquired vertical muscle palsies usually require a prism equal or nearly equal to the angle of deviation, whereas those with congenital or long-standing palsies and most patients with dysthyroid eye disease involving vertical eye movement, may require as little as half the amount measured. There is some indication that patients with long-standing vertical strabismus caused by retinal detachment surgery behave in a similar way, needing only a small prism correction.

• Patients with esodeviations, especially those which increase in the distance (divergence weakness type), are harder to control and therefore require a larger prism in relation to the angle of deviation than do those with exodeviations.

• Patients with paralytic strabismus who have been deprived of binocular single vision for many months may not be able to fuse the images immediately prisms are introduced. Although it may not be possible to demonstrate fusion in the clinic, it is worthwhile fitting trial prisms for a period to see whether binocular single vision can be obtained with more time.

• Patients with very incomitant deviations are thought to be unsuitable for prism therapy because the area of binocular single vision achieved will be too small; however, even a very small field of binocular fixation is welcomed by some patients, while others find the intermittent diplopia too distracting. It is often worth a short period of trial prisms in these cases.

Long-term use of prisms

The prescription of prisms incorporated into the patient's spectacle lenses or in plano glass in spectacle frames may be considered after successful wear of Fresnel prisms. The circumstances in which prisms might be preferred to muscle surgery are:

• When there is a small symptom-producing vertical deviation which could easily be overcorrected by surgery.

• When patients refuse surgery or are unfit for it.

• Patients with dysthyroid eye disease whose condition may change and who may have to wait a long time until it is sufficiently stable for surgical correction.

• Symptom-producing heterophoria which has failed to respond to other forms of treatment. Small degrees

of esophoria, especially of the divergence weakness type, may be unresponsive to orthoptic treatment and can be compensated with base-out prisms (see Chapter 16).

Orthoptic exercises

Orthoptic work has become increasingly diagnostic and less therapeutic over the years. In our experience, exercises can undoubtedly prove beneficial in certain conditions, providing that the patients are carefully selected and sufficiently motivated. Some types of latent and intermittent strabismus can be improved solely by this means; in others, exercises can augment optical, pharmacological or surgical treatment and can enhance the success of these methods (see Chapters 12 and 13). The authors' aim is to describe the exercises in sufficient detail and clarity to enable the ophthalmologist either to prescribe and carry them out himself if he so wishes or to take a more informed interest in this aspect of the patient's management.

Orthoptic exercises may be given:
• to compensate a latent strabismus;
• to improve control of an intermittent strabismus;
• as a pre- or postoperative measure in constant strabismus.

Treament necessitates regular attendance and follow-up with exercises carried out at home.

Criteria for selection

Exercises are only given to patients who have or have had binocular single vision. Suitable patients must fulfil the following criteria.

• The examiner must be certain that normal sensory and motor fusion can be achieved.

• The visual acuity must be equal or nearly equal. The refractive error must be corrected (with certain exceptions already discussed) and spectacles worn as directed.

• The patient must be able to attend regularly.

• A pathological cause for the strabismus must have been excluded.

• The patient must be fit for surgery if it is indicated. The patient, or the parents if the subject is a child, must be willing for it to be carried out.

• The patient must be sufficiently cooperative to

understand and perform the exercises; the parent's cooperation is equally important in children.
• Symptoms must be attributable to the deviation and not to other causes.

Not all patients who fulfil these criteria are suitable for exercises. Controversy exists as to their benefit in certain conditions, for example in intermittent distance exotropia. These aspects will be discussed in the relevant chapters.

Dangers of orthoptic exercises

The main risk of ill-judged treatment is that it can give rise to insuperable diplopia if given to patients lacking adequate motor fusion. More rarely, a convergence or accommodative spasm can be caused by over-enthusiastic convergence exercises or by promoting control of a large exodeviation.

Purpose of exercises

The aims of orthoptic exercises can be divided into the following categories:
• elimination of suppression;
• control of a deviation;
• extension of the fusion amplitude;
• improvement of relative (fusional) convergence;
• improvement of the near point of convergence.

Elimination of suppression

In the past exercises to eradicate suppression were given extensively using a major amblyoscope and other apparatus, such as the Maddox cheiroscope; this treatment is now rarely given and probably has little value. The methods in current use are less artificial and are directed at promoting diplopia in order to provide a stimulus for fusion.

Indications

The use of orthoptic exercises to eliminate suppression is indicated in the following circumstances:
• Convergence insufficiency or exophoria of the convergence insufficiency type, when diplopia is not recognized on failure of convergence.
• Selected cases of intermittent strabismus as a preliminary to teaching control of the deviation. Diplopia recognition is rarely possible in intermittent distance

exotropia, but can usually be achieved in other types of strabismus.
• Constant strabismus of late onset preoperatively, to promote control of the deviation postoperatively.

Methods

COLOURED FILTERS

These comprise either red and green glasses, a red filter or the Sbisa bar (Bagolini filter bar) used with a spotlight for near and distance fixation. The deviation must remain manifest; it may be necessary to use an accommodative target as well as a light when treating accommodative esotropia to ensure that the strabismus is not controlled. It is helpful to show the patient the likely position of the second image, starting with red and green glasses and proceeding to one filter, removing it at intervals to obtain spontaneous recognition of diplopia. The Sbisa bar is useful as the density of the filters can be reduced in stages until diplopia can be maintained without the bar. Unless suppression is very dense, these methods are usually successful. The presence of diplopia can be checked by asking the patient to look from one light to the other, taking care that he is not alternately suppressing one image. Worth's four-lights test is another method of proving that diplopia is present.

SEPTUM

A card can be used as a septum, holding it at 90° to the plane of the face, resting on the nose. This can be combined with a cover test to show both images. This method is often successful in fully accommodative esotropia.

The septum can be made smaller or a transparent septum used until diplopia is recognized without it.

PRISMS

If the above methods fail, prisms can be used to move the image out of the suppression scotoma. A 10 Δ vertical prism is usually successful in horizontal strabismus. Nearly all patients can appreciate diplopia in this way, which gives them an indication of the horizontal separation of the images and shows them that diplopia is possible. If a vertical prism bar is used, the prism strength can be reduced slowly while the patient tries to maintain the two images. Coloured filters can be used in addition if necessary.

RED FILTER DRAWING

A red filter is worn on the spectacle lens of the fixing eye and the patient is asked to draw using a red pencil or crayon; if the red of the crayon and of the filter are identical, the drawing will be seen only by the suppressed eye whilst the paper is seen by both. Children enjoy this exercise, which is very suitable for use at home. (This method should not be confused with red filter occlusion, used in the past in the treatment of eccentric fixation.)

OCCLUSION

Part-time occlusion is sometimes used to encourage the use of the squinting eye.

If there is a constant strabismus, steps should be taken to prevent resuppression. This can be achieved by:
- occlusion;
- the use of Fresnel prisms.

Prisms have the advantage that the patient fuses the images while waiting for surgery, thus improving the prognosis for binocular single vision postoperatively.

Exercises to aid control of the deviation

Methods

Essentially, the patient must appreciate when the strabismus is manifest by recognizing diplopia. Some patients can differentiate clear vision when squinting from blurred vision when accommodation is relaxed. However, diplopia recognition is a more reliable means of achieving control and it ensures that binocular single vision is present. Diplopia provides a stimulus to fusion and its recognition quite often results in spontaneous control of the strabismus. If not, this can be taught by:
- Using a prism to fuse the images, then slowly reducing the prism strength while the patient maintains binocular single vision.
- Working from the point of intersection of the visual axes, extending to distance over which binocular single vision is maintained by moving the target towards or away from the eyes.
- Using the patient's accommodation to achieve control, either by stimulating it with detailed targets in exodeviations or promoting relaxation in esodeviations, encouraging the patient to blur the image. Dif-

ficulties can occur with this method as the patient may then find it difficult to clear the image when required.

The longer term use of prisms and lenses is described under 'Optical management' above. The aim is to reduce the prism or lens strength in stages over a period of weeks or months until binocular single vision can be maintained unaided.

Extension of the fusion amplitude

Improvement of the fusion amplitude enables comfortable binocular single vision to be maintained and prevents recurrence of symptoms. Exercises are directed to improving the positive and negative horizontal amplitude: the vertical and torsional amplitudes are not usually improved by treatment.

Methods

The horizontal fusion amplitude can be improved for near and distance using:
- prism bars;
- the major amblyoscope.

The use of prisms is by far the more effective method and should be used whenever possible. A prism bar may be made using small pieces of Fresnel prisms, allowing the patient to perform the exercises at home.

Positive fusion amplitude (convergence)

This is increased by using a prism bar base-out, gradually increasing the prism strength while the patient fuses the images. When convergence fails, the patient should be encouraged to rejoin the diplopia with only a small reduction in prism strength until he can fuse the images through a $40-45\,\Delta$ base-out prism at 33 cm, and a $20-25\,\Delta$ base-out prism at 6 m.

Convergence must be smoothly maintained. In the later stages of treatment the patient should be able to fuse images when a $20-30\,\Delta$ prism is introduced, rejoining the diplopia immediately it is removed and rejoining it again when the prism is replaced. Relaxation of convergence must be emphasized at all stages. Improvement of the positive amplitude is indicated in exodeviations.

Negative fusion amplitude (divergence)

A prism bar is used base-in. Patients with esophoria of the divergence weakness type often have a very poor negative fusion amplitude at 6 m. Even a $1\,\Delta$ or $2\,\Delta$

prism is sufficient to disrupt binocular single vision, and improvement of the amplitude is difficult. These patients can be helped by lending them low-powered loose or Fresnel prisms to use at home, advising them to start by fixing on an object at an intermediate distance, gradually increasing the fixation distance once fusion is maintained. Extension of the negative amplitude is indicated in esodeviations and can be used to ensure that there is adequate relaxation after convergence exercises in exodeviations.

Improvement of relative (fusional) convergence

Improvement of relative convergence is not the same as improvement of the fusion amplitude, which utilizes all three components of convergence (accommodative, fusional and proximal). Whenever the amount of accommodation is changed, accommodative convergence is either exerted or relaxed by a predetermined amount (the AC/A ratio), but if accommodation is constant, relative convergence can be exerted or relaxed whilst maintaining a static amount of accommodation.

Positive relative convergence

Convergence is exerted in excess of accommodation. This component is improved in exodeviations so that relative convergence can be used to control the strabismus whilst the correct amount of accommodation is exerted to give clear vision at all distances.

Negative relative convergence

Convergence is relaxed in relation to the amount of accommodation exerted. The negative amplitude is improved in esodeviations so that sufficient accommodation can be used for clear vision at all distances without associated convergence.

The purpose of improving relative convergence is therefore to:
• improve the binocular visual acuity (the level of visual acuity achieved while binocular single vision is maintained);
• to allow the continued use of clear binocular single vision.

Methods

Many of the exercises used are based on physiological diplopia, so this must first be taught if it is not recognized spontaneously. Most patients can appreciate the two images using red and green filters. Those with esodeviations find crossed physiological diplopia easier and those with exodeviations have less difficulty appreciating it in the uncrossed position. The easiest position should be taught first but ideally all patients should eventually recognize both the crossed and uncrossed positions spontaneously.

If the patient has difficulty in seeing the second image, he can be helped by telling him where to look for it and by rapidly covering and uncovering the unsuppressed eye. Recognition of physiological diplopia alone is a useful method of improving control of the deviation when this is precarious. The methods described below can all be used for this purpose.

STEREOGRAM CARDS

Apparatus

The cards are printed with two figures: by looking in front of the card uncrossed diplopia is obtained, resulting in four figures. The distance of the near fixation target or the card can be adjusted until the innermost figures fuse to give a central figure common to both eyes, with two peripheral figures, each seen by either the right or left eye. The same effect is obtained by fixating on a distance target beyond the card, obtaining crossed physiological diplopia of the figures. To be called stereograms the central figure should be three-dimensional but the term is used loosely and a commonly used card presents two-dimensional drawings of cats.

Method

It is best to start with the large simple cat card, first teaching the patient the position he finds easiest, progressing to more detailed cards as he improves (Fig. 8.1). The card is held at approximately 33 cm from the patient's eyes: it is easier if the patient holds the card and the near fixation object himself. The near object should be unobtrusive, such as a pencil. The position of the target is changed until three figures can be seen; the patient is then encouraged to see them clearly, but this is easier to judge using detailed stereograms. The crossed position is best taught by telling the patient to fixate a target just visible over the top of the card, but eventually he must be able to look 'through' the card, relaxing his convergence, in order to see the figures clearly.

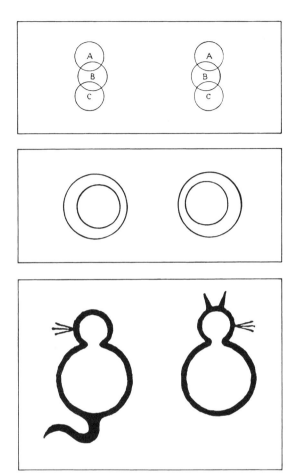

Fig. 8.1 Stereogram cards.

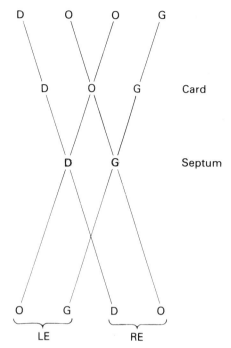

Fig. 8.2 The construction of the diploscope, showing the combination of letters seen at the different fixation distances.

To make it easier for the patient to see three figures the following measures can be taken:

• A vertical coloured stripe can be drawn down the centre of the card. The patient obtains physiological diplopia of the stripe, separating the lines sufficiently to admit the central fused figure and adjusting the position of the fixation target until this is achieved.

• The separation between the figures can be reduced (by cutting the card). In the later stages the separation can be increased to make it more difficult. The Mayou stereograms have a variable separation.

• If the patient has difficulty in looking through the card to obtain crossed physiological diplopia, holes can be cut in the two figures. Esophoric patients often have great difficulty in achieving three figures with stereogram cards and it may be necessary to use a very

simple transparent 'stereogram', in order to teach them how to obtain crossed physiological diplopia.

DIPLOSCOPE

Apparatus

The apparatus consists of a shaft 27 cm in length, having a nose rest at the proximal end and a card at the distal end. A septum with four holes is placed 7 cm in front of the card. The card is printed with the letters D,O,G signifying 'Droit ou Gauche' (Right or Left). D and O are visible to the right eye and G and O are visible to the left eye; red and green control marks are seen by the right and left eyes, respectively. The letters on the card can be seen in several combinations through the central holes in the septum (Fig. 8.2). The control marks are seen through the top and bottom holes.

Method

The diploscope can be used in four positions to exercise positive or negative relative convergence (Table 8.1). When physiological diplopia of the card

Table 8.1 Use of the diploscope to exercise positive and negative relative convergence.

Position	Fixation distance	Letters seen	Physiological diplopia	Relative convergence
1	Card	DOG	Crossed of holes	Convergence and accommodation equal
2	Septum	DG	Uncrossed of card	Positive
3	Between septum and nose	OGDO	Uncrossed of card and septum holes	Positive
4	Beyond card	DOOG	Crossed of card and septum holes	Negative

is obtained, the unwanted letters are obscured by the septum. The patient holds the instrument by a handle on the shaft.

BAR-READING
The principle of bar-reading has already been explained (see Chapter 7). The purposes of bar-reading in treatment are:
• to exercise maintenance of binocular single vision when reading;
• to improve relative positive or negative convergence with the use of lenses.

To exercise binocular single vision
The patient wears his refractive correction and reads the print using the bar as a control. Provided that two bars are seen and the print is not obscured, he is reading correctly. If he has difficulty in seeing two bars the patient can be helped by first holding the bar closer to the eyes when the wider separation of the two images makes recognition easier.

To exercise relative convergence
• Negative relative convergence: concave lenses are used to increase the amount of accommodation exerted. Large print is used initially, but the size of print is reduced as the binocular visual acuity improves. Hypermetropes may be taught to bar-read without their spectacles if the correction is +3 DS or less, without significant astigmatism; otherwise concave lenses are added in stages up to −3 DS.

• Positive relative convergence: additional convex lenses are used to relax accommodation. Convergence remains static for the distance of the page.

Bar-reading is little used to improve positive relative convergence and is mainly of value in improving the near binocular visual acuity in accommodative esotropia.

REMY SEPARATOR
This instrument is based on foveal projection rather than physiological diplopia. It consists of a septum which rests on the nose. Transparencies are placed in the holder at the opposite end of the apparatus. The transparencies present either dissimilar simultaneous perception targets or fusion targets. The patient looks through the transparency and relaxes his convergence, causing the images to fall on the foveae, when they should appear superimposed or fused. If they are seen clearly, negative convergence is exercised. The original purpose of the instrument was to treat esodeviations but it has very limited value in this condition.

Precautions when improving relative convergence
• Negative and positive relative convergence are only exercised if the targets are seen clearly, and this should be the aim of all the exercises. Detailed targets should be used as soon as possible (e.g. when using stereograms) and the patient should be questioned on what he sees.
• These exercises are very suitable for use at home but the examiner must ensure that they are clearly under-

stood by the patient and that adequate supervision can be given if the patient is a child. This is particularly important in bar-reading, when the patient's head must be kept straight and the bar maintained in the centre of the page.

Improving the near point of convergence

Many patients with symptoms of blurred vision, headaches, jumbling of print or diplopia have a primary or secondary convergence insufficiency. Improvement in the near point of convergence can often be achieved easily and should relieve the patient's symptoms.

Smooth convergence

This is exercised by asking the patient to follow an accommodative target moved slowly towards the nose. When convergence fails and diplopia is recognized the target should be withdrawn until single vision is regained. The target is again moved slowly forwards, encouraging the patient to maintain single vision. The aim of this treatment is to achieve a normal near point of 10 cm or less without effort.

Jump convergence

A number of patients are able to achieve a better near point when a target is moved slowly towards them than if a target is introduced and a 'saccadic' vergence movement is required (jump convergence).

This is improved by asking the patient to look into the distance and then at a near target. Fixation should return to the distance position whilst the target is moved towards the nose. As with smooth convergence this should be repeated with the fixation target held at a point approximating to the break point, aiming to achieve accurate vergence to the same extent as smooth convergence.

Jump convergence can also be exercised with prisms as described above, and by using the dot card.

Dot card (Fig. 8.3)

A series of small circles is spaced out along a line drawn the length of a card some 30 cm long.

Method

The patient first fixates the farthest dot and should obtain crossed physiological diplopia of the line and

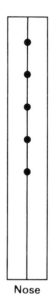

Nose

Fig. 8.3 Dot card used to improve convergence.

the closer dots. He then fixates each dot in turn, fusing the images. The more remote dots and line then appear as uncrossed diplopia. The patient can also be asked to look at one dot and then into the distance and back again to exercise jump convergence.

Voluntary convergence

Voluntary convergence is the ability to converge without the aid of a fusional stimulus. In some centres it is taught to patients with convergence insufficiency as a final stage in treatment. There is a belief that failure to achieve voluntary convergence leads to a recurrence of symptoms. It can be taught by:

• Instructing the patient to converge using a fine fixation target, for example a piece of thread. When the near point is reached, this can be removed and the patient tries to maintain convergence at the same distance.

• The first finger and thumb can be held in apposition at 8–10 cm and the patient instructed to fixate on the space between them. This space can gradually be widened and then the hand is removed while the patient continues to converge.

Eventually, the patient shoud be able to converge voluntarily and unaided. He can combine voluntary convergence with the use of stereograms in the uncrossed position.

Pharmacological management

The drugs used in the management of strabismus are miotics, cycloplegics and botulinum toxin A. The uses of drugs in refraction and in the premedication, anaesthesia and immediate postoperative care of strabismus patients are not considered here, neither is the experimental use of systemic drugs in the treatment of amblyopia.

Miotic drugs

The principle underlying the use of miotics is that accommodation is brought about by direct action on the ciliary muscle, and therefore without synkinesis with convergence, while increased depth of focus reduces the need for accommodation.

Miotics may be:
• anticholinesterases (i.e. choline esterase inactivators); or
• acetylcholine analogues (i.e. agents that directly stimulate the muscle end-plate).

They are instilled into both eyes in the form of drops.

Choice of drugs

The two drugs which have been in common use are phospholine iodide (ecothiopate iodide) and pilocarpine. Phospholine iodide (PI) has now been withdrawn from the UK market but remains available in other countries.

Pilocarpine
• Action: parasympathomimetic
• Strength: 0.5–4%
• Dosage: 6-hourly
• Duration: 4–6 h
• Side-effects: no serious side-effects at correct dosage levels.

Although the absence of side-effects makes pilocarpine a safer drug, its short action, necessitating frequent instillation, makes it less practical than PI, especially for schoolchildren. A short period of blurred vision when its action is at its peak, and discomfort when it is instilled make pilocarpine unpopular with patients. Providing its use is carefully monitored, PI is more effective and better accepted by the patient.

Care of patients during miotic therapy
General advice
Instructions must be given on storage, effect and instillation. The parents should be told to observe the pupil size in fairly poor light and to ensure that the drops are put carefully into an eye with a larger pupil.

If PI is used, a card should be issued giving the name and strength of the drug. This card must be shown to the doctor if the child is involved in an accident or is ill. The parents should inform the ophthalmologist if any side-effects develop; a slight conjunctival inflammation for the first few days is normal.

It is important to strike the right balance between making the parents aware of the risks and deterring them from using the drug.

Supervision
The patient should be seen two weeks after commencing therapy in the first instance. The following observations should be made:
• Observation of pupil size and reaction to light.
• Visual acuity—should be tested on every visit for near and distance.
• Assess.
• Measurement of the deviation, the binocular visual acuity.
• Slit-lamp examination if PI is used. The presence of iris cysts is an indication to cease treatment, whereupon the cysts spontaneously resolve. The combination of PI with a sympathetic mydriatic, phenylephrine 2.5%, is sometimes used to avoid the formation of iris cysts but the reduction in miosis makes the treatment less effective.

Uses
Miotic drugs may be used diagnostically or therapeutically. The main therapeutic uses of miotics are in the management of accommodative esotropia, particularly of the convergence excess type, and in the postoperative control of residual esotropia in patients with a good prognosis for binocular single vision.

Optimum conditions for use of miotics
The ideal conditions which will give the best chance of success are:

- equal visual acuity;
- absence of suppression;
- good cooperation.

Not all these criteria can be met in all cases.

Duration of treatment

If no improvement occurs after one month, further progress is unlikely and the drug should be discontinued. An objection to the use of miotics is that the improvement obtained with them is not maintained; in some cases regression may occur because the duration of treatment is too short. In successful cases, the drug should be continued for 2–3 months after maximum improvement has been obtained. It should then be discontinued in stages by reducing the strength of the dosage or number of instillations over several weeks. James *et al.* (1993) found success with treatment by miotics alone in 15% of primary convergence excess and in 28% of those whose deviations were reduced by surgery to less than 20 Δ at near.

Cycloplegic drugs

The principle underlying the use of cycloplegic drugs is the prevention of accommodation. This blurs near vision (and also distance vision in uncorrected hypermetropic patients). The drugs are parasympatholytic in action, preventing contraction of the ciliary and sphincter pupillae muscles by blocking acetylcholine. They therefore also act as mydriatics. Parasympatholytic agents (atropine, cyclopentolate and tropicamide) are used diagnostically in the refraction of young children (see Chapter 3). The only drug in general therapeutic use is atropine.

Atropine

- Action: parasympatholytic.
- Strength: atropine sulphate 0.5–1% eye drops or ointment.
- Dosage: usually once daily when used in strabismus treatment.

Onset and duration of actions

- Cycloplegia: within 2 h and largely reversed in 3–5 days, although some residual effect may persist for up to 10 days.

- Mydriasis: within 15 min and persisting for 10–12 days.

Side-effects

- Local hypersensitivity reaction, usually after prolonged use. This causes swelling, redness and irritation of the conjunctiva, eyelids and surrounding skin.
- Systemic poisoning due to gastrointestinal absorption of the drug following passage through the nasolacrimal duct. The principal features are restlessness, fever, rapid pulse, dry mouth and flushed skin. Infants are especially susceptible and it is advisable to use ointment in 0.5% concentration in this age group.

Uses

- In the treatment of amblyopia.
- To treat accommodative spasm.

These uses are discussed in the relevant chapters.

Botulinum toxin

Botulinum toxin is a potent neurotoxin which selectively binds to cholinergic synapses, blocking the conduction of the nerve impulse. In nature, botulinum toxin is the exotoxin of the organism *Clostridium botulinum*, which is responsible for botulism, a serious form of food poisoning. Botulism presents as an acute symmetrical descending paralysis resulting from an infection by *Clostridium botulinum*. The route of infection is usually from contaminated food, although wound botulism has been reported.

Early features are:
- dry mouth;
- nausea and vomiting;
- extraocular muscle paralysis;
- difficulty with speech and swallowing.

Late features include:
- autonomic nervous system involvement resulting in raised blood pressure;
- reduced respiratory rate.

Management may involve the use of antitoxin, antibiotics and supportive measures including respiratory assistance.

The use of botulinum toxin in clinical practice arose from an investigation into ways of identifying a suitable pharmacological agent for the treatment of strabismus. Experimental work on monkeys pioneered by

Scott *et al.* (1973) involved injecting different agents into extraocular muscles and examining their effect on the muscle and the surrounding tissue. The agents used were:
- DFP (diisopropyl fluorophosphate)
- alcohol
- cobra neurotoxin
- rattlesnake venom
- botulinum toxin.

The results of these investigations suggested that botulinum toxin was the most promising agent for creating a temporary extraocular muscle paralysis. Clinical studies were then started on patients with strabismus, confirming its usefulness (Scott 1980). Since its introduction, botulinum toxin has proved effective in the management of patients with strabismus and other disorders affecting skeletal muscles. It is available commercially in a freeze-dried crystalline form, which, when reconstituted with saline, releases the active dichain subunit consisting of heavy and light chains of combined molecular weight 150 000 Da.

Mechanism of action

Botulinum toxin binds specifically to peripheral cholinergic synapses, selectively blocking the release of evoked acetylcholine whilst leaving the mechanism responsible for spontaneous release relatively intact. Botulinum toxin achieves its effect by the following stages.
- Binding (Fig. 8.4). The heavy subunit binds to receptor sites on the unmyelinated areas of the cholinergic nerve terminal in the region of the neuromuscular junction.
- Internalization (Fig. 8.5). After the heavy chain has bound to the receptor site the light chain is internalized into the cell by the normal synaptic vesicle recycling process, thereby activating the toxin.
- Paralysis (Fig. 8.6). The mechanism by which muscle paralysis occurs is largely unknown. However, it is assumed to result from the toxin causing an alteration in the intracellular calcium levels thereby preventing the release of acetylcholine vesicles across the myoneural junction.

The paralytic effect of botulinum toxin is dose dependent; clinical paralysis occurs in around 3 days, and the maximum therapeutic effect is reached 5–7 days after injection. It takes about 3 months for

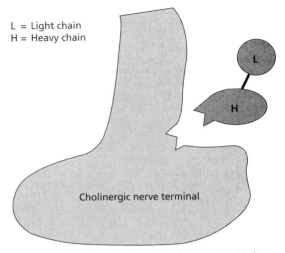

L = Light chain
H = Heavy chain

Fig. 8.4 Mechanism of action of botulinum toxin. Binding of the heavy chain subunit of the toxin to the unmyelinated portion of the cholinergic nerve terminal.

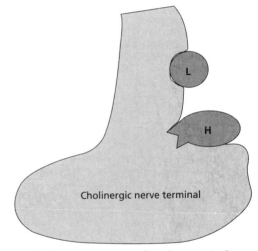

Fig. 8.5 Mechanism of action of botulinum toxin. Internalization of the light chain subunit of the toxin into the cell.

the clinical effects of the toxin to wear off, although this may be delayed in some cases. Recovery of muscle function is associated with re-sprouting of myoneural junctions at the nerve terminal. Histopathological examination of the injected muscle shows areas of muscle atrophy; however, the clinical function of the muscle appears to be unaffected once the effects of the toxin have worn off. Permanent changes in ocular alignment can occur following botulinum toxin injection,

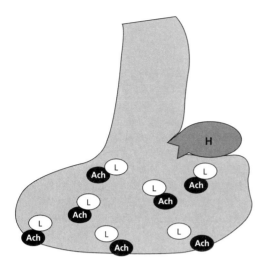

Ach = acetylcholine vesicle

Fig. 8.6 Mechanism of action of botulinum toxin. Paralysis resulting from prevention of acetylcholine release.

and the possible mechanisms responsible for this are discussed below. Repeat injection of the toxin into the extraocular muscles is not recognized by the immune system.

Mechanism of action in paralytic strabismus

In paralytic strabismus the imbalance of force between the affected muscle and its ipsilateral antagonist and yoke muscle results in altered alignment of the visual axes. Additional mechanical factors from muscle and tissue contracture may be present in some cases. For example, in sixth nerve palsy there is an imbalance between the paralysed lateral rectus and its ipsilateral antagonist, the medial rectus, resulting in an esotropia. Injecting the ipsilateral antagonist with botulinum

toxin both weakens and lengthens the muscle, restoring the balance of force between the two muscles and reducing the size of the esotropia in the short term: any long-term effect depends largely on the outcome of the lateral rectus palsy:

• If recovery of the lateral rectus palsy does not occur, there is usually a recurrence of the esotropia as the effect of the botulinum toxin wears off (Fig. 8.7). Further management involves repeat injections to maintain alignment or the use of prisms or surgery.

• If recovery of the lateral rectus palsy occurs, stable alignment may be maintained as the botulinum toxin wears off and these patients are said to be cured (Fig. 8.8). Controversy still exists as to whether the eventual chances of recovery are improved by the early use of botulinum toxin in this situation: if contracture of the medial rectus can be prevented in this way, a major obstacle to recovery of lateral rectus function is removed. Prevention of contracture also facilitates later surgical intervention in persistent lateral rectus palsy.

Mechanism of action in nonparalytic strabismus

The medial rectus in the squinting eye is injected in esotropia and the lateral rectus in exotropia. The injected muscle is weakened and lengthened following the injection.

In most cases of nonparalytic strabismus botulinum toxin is used diagnostically, in the expectation that the strabismus will recur when the effect of the toxin has completely worn off (Fig. 8.9). Histological studies of extraocular muscle after injection show that it is the orbital singly innervated fibres which selectively show long-term atrophic changes, which on their own would probably account for only minor lasting changes in alignment.

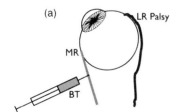
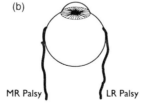
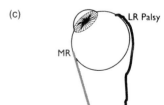

Fig. 8.7 Mode of action of botulinum toxin in paralytic strabismus (unrecovered lateral rectus palsy). (a) Ipsilateral medial rectus injected. (b) Medial rectus weakened, eye straightened. (c) Botulinum toxin no longer effective, lateral rectus palsy persists, requiring repeat injection, prisms or surgery.

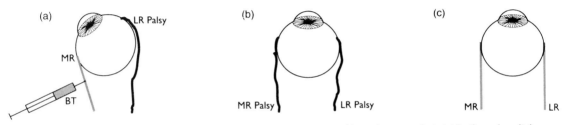

Fig. 8.8 Mode of action of botulinum toxin in paralytic strabismus (recovered lateral rectus palsy). (a) Ipsilateral medial rectus injected. (b) Medial rectus weakened, eye straightened. (c) Eye remains straight, no further treatment required.

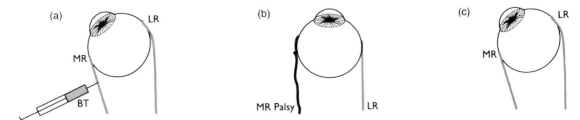

Fig. 8.9 Mode of action of botulinum toxin in nonparalytic strabismus (esotropia). (a) Ipsilateral medial rectus injected. (b) Medial rectus weakened, eye straightened. (c) Botulinum toxin no longer effective, requiring repeat injection or surgery.

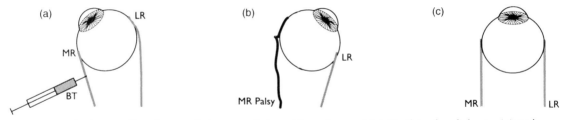

Fig. 8.10 Mode of action of botulinum toxin in nonparalytic strabismus (esotropia). (a) Ipsilateral medial rectus injected. (b) Medial rectus weakened, consecutive exotropia develops. (c) Eye remains straight, no further treatment required.

Long-term changes in alignment can result from the use of botulinum toxin. For this to occur it is probably necessary for the ipsilateral antagonist of the injected muscle to become contracted, usually secondary to a significant consecutive deviation (Fig. 8.10). Stable long-term changes in alignment are facilitated by the potential for fusion, which allows binocular single vision to develop while the toxin is effective and can enable it to be maintained after the effect has worn off.

Ophthalmological use of botulinum toxin

Botulinum toxin has been used to treat a variety of disorders; those of interest to the ophthalmologist include:
- muscle spasm involving the facial muscles;
- strabismus;
- nystagmus;
- corneal ulceration and exposure keratitis.

Its use in strabismus and nystagmus will be discussed in more detail.

Indications
The main indications for the use of botulinum toxin can be divided into diagnostic and therapeutic categories.

DIAGNOSTIC
Botulinum toxin can be used diagnostically:
- To reduce the angle of strabismus and allow sensory investigation in free space:
  1 in the investigation in patients at risk of postoperative diplopia;

2 to investigate the presence or absence of fusion before deciding on surgical treatment.
• In patients with sixth nerve palsy who cannot abduct past the mid-line. Improved abduction after injection indicates a partial palsy, failure to improve indicates a complete palsy.
• To help predict the effect of surgery on patients with incomitant deviations.
• In combination with electromyography (EMG) recording to confirm the presence of miswiring in Duane's syndrome.
• As a means of further investigation when a slipped or lost muscle is suspected.

THERAPEUTIC
Botulinum toxin can be used therapeutically:
• To restore fusion, especially in patients with decompensating strabismus and partially recovered sixth nerve palsy (Figs 8.11 & 8.12).
• In the rehabilitation of patients with cosmetic strabismus.
• As an adjunct to strabismus surgery and in the management of acute surgical undercorrections and overcorrections.

• In acquired nystagmus to dampen the amplitude of the ocular oscillation and improve visual acuity.

Method of administration
Botulinum toxin is usually administered under local anaesthesia in adults; general anaesthesia is required in children.

Local anaesthesia
For the successful administration of botulinum toxin attention needs to be directed at:
• patient preparation;
• the environment in which the toxin is administered;
• toxin dilution and patient monitoring facilities;
• the injection technique;
• postinjection management, including multidisciplinary collaboration.

PATIENT PREPARATION
It is important to exclude patients in whom either the use of botulinum toxin is contraindicated or who are not suitable candidates for its use under local anaesthesia. These include:

Field of Left Eye (fixing with right eye)

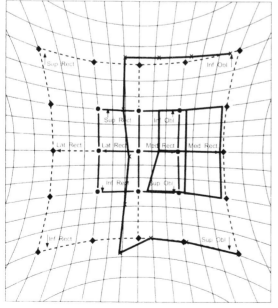

Field of Right Eye (fixing with left eye)

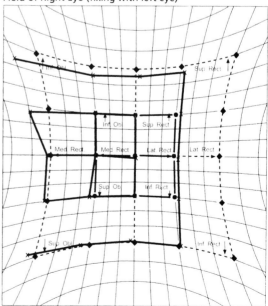

Fig. 8.11 A Hess chart of a patient with a left lateral rectus palsy. A large esodeviation is present in the primary position and no further recovery in lateral rectus function was observed.

Field of Left Eye (fixing with right eye)   Field of Right Eye (fixing with left eye)

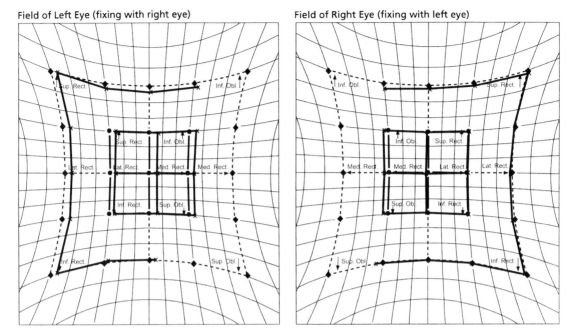

Fig. 8.12 A Hess chart of the same patient 12 months after a botulinum toxin injection into the left medial rectus showing restoration of alignment and a full range of ocular movement.

- children;
- pregnant women;
- patients with needle phobia;
- patients with mental deficiency and behaviour problems who are unlikely to cooperate with the procedure.

In our practice very few patients refuse treatment with botulinum toxin outright. We have only had to abandon an injection in two cases, one due to pain intolerance and the other because of a vasovagal episode prior to administering the injection.

All patients are given detailed instructions about what to expect prior to having treatment, and these instructions are reinforced on the day of injection. They include:

- The aim of the procedure. In most cases the toxin is used for diagnostic purposes and its effects are expected to wear off completely. Further treatment is likely to required.
- The degree of discomfort likely to be experienced during treatment. The procedure results in a degree of pain which is of a deep aching quality and poorly localized, similar to the pain with dental anaesthesia.

- The effectiveness of the procedure. In our hands the toxin injection is effective in 80% of patients; in 10% a further injection is required and in the remaining 10% a significant overcorrection results.
- Likely complications. Upper eyelid ptosis occurs in 1 in 20 patients; it is usually mild and recovers in 4–6 weeks. Local bruising around the injection site rarely occurs and usually resolves in a few days.

Local anaesthetic drops are instilled into the eye every 5 min for a period of 15 min prior to treatment.

ENVIRONMENT

A quiet, spacious and well-ventilated treatment area is important: patients are apprehensive and anxious, and vasovagal attacks during or after treatment can be reduced by providing the right environment. We prefer the patient in a semirecumbent position, with facilities available to lay him supine if necessary.

TOXIN DILUTION AND PATIENT MONITORING FACILITIES

Botulinum toxin is provided in a powdered crystalline form. There are presently two products available commercially:

- Botox (Allergan), which has 100 units of toxin in each vial;
- Dysport (Ipsen), which has 500 units of toxin in each vial.

The 100 units of Botox has a different efficacy to the 500 units of Dysport. The dilution instructions that follow relate to a vial containing 500 units of botulinum toxin (Dysport).

Dilution

Equipment for reconstituting the botulinum toxin comprises:

One vial of botulinum toxin type A (Dysport)
One 10 mL vial of 0.9% preservative-free sterile saline
Two 1 mL tuberculin syringes
Two 5 mL syringes
One 25 gauge (orange) needle.

Handling the botulinum toxin

- The toxin is stable in freeze-dried form when refrigerated at 4°C.
- Botulinum toxin requires careful reconstituting as it can be denatured by violent bubbling, agitation or repeated passage through the needle.
- Alcohol from a skin wipe can inactivate the toxin; the alcohol must be allowed to dry before proceeding with the injection.

Two and a half millilitres of saline suitable for intravenous injection is used to reconstitute the toxin, this is then further diluted as follows, depending on the volume required:

- 0.5 mL is combined with 4.5 mL saline;
- 0.3 mL is combined with 2.7 mL saline;
- 0.1 mL is combined with 0.9 mL saline.

These quantities result in 20 units of toxin per millilitre of solution: we use 2 units (0.1 mL) for each extraocular muscle. We recommend preparing a second solution of double-strength botulinum toxin using 1 mL of the solution combined with 4.0 mL of saline, or proportionately smaller quantities as required.

PATIENT MONITORING

Muscle generates an electrical signal which can be monitored using EMG even in its resting state. The EMG circuit is made of 2 electrodes, one a silver/silver chloride skin electrode and the other a unipolar electrode connected to a partially insulated 27 gauge retrobulbar needle: the insulation covers the shaft of the needle leaving the tip bare, therefore the signal obtained on the EMG reflects the location of the needle tip.

MUSCLES SUITABLE FOR INJECTION

The medial rectus, lateral rectus and inferior rectus muscles are most frequently treated with botulinum toxin. The overacting inferior oblique muscle can be injected in superior oblique palsy. Treating the superior rectus muscle results in ptosis and is therefore not recommended. The superior oblique is not treated with toxin.

INJECTION TECHNIQUE

We use 0.1 mL of the standard solution for each extraocular muscle injected unless the angle of strabismus is less than 20 Δ, when 0.05 mL is used initially; this applies particularly to decompensating exophoria and residual sixth nerve palsy with small esotropia. If the angle exceeds 30 Δ, 0.1 mL of double-strength solution is used rather than increasing the amount of standard solution, which could increase the risk of 'spillover' to other muscles.

The first step is to draw up 0.4 mL of the solution into the tuberculin syringe, and the 27 gauge unipolar needle is connected and flushed through, leaving 0.2 mL of the solution in the syringe. Although only 0.1 mL of the toxin will be injected, having 0.2 mL available ensures that the injection procedure can continue even if there is a leak around the luer lock of the needle. If a leak occurs, the luer lock is re-secured and sufficient toxin should still be available in the syringe to complete the injection.

The procedure for injection is as follows:

1 Right-handed operators should stand behind the patient when injecting the muscles used for left gaze —for example the left lateral rectus and the right medial rectus muscles—and to the patient's right when injecting muscles used for right gaze—for example the right lateral rectus and the left medial rectus muscles.

2 The patient is instructed to look in the opposite direction to the muscle being injected, for example to the left if injecting the right lateral rectus, and the conjunctiva is penetrated approximately 5 mm posterior to the limbus.

3 The needle is passed subconjunctivally along the path of the muscle for 5 mm.

4 Instruct the patient to look slowly in the direction of action of the injected muscle: the operator must take care to keep the needle in the subconjunctival position by following the movement of the globe.

5 When the eye is fully rotated the needle is slowly advanced into the muscle belly whilst monitoring the EMG signal.

6 The patient is instructed to look slightly away from the injected muscle and back again to confirm that the maximum EMG signal has been reached.

• 0.1 mL of the toxin is injected, keeping the needle in place for 30 s to reduce the risk of toxin tracking back along the needle's path

• reusable needles should be flushed out with air before sterilizing to minimize the chance of blockage.

POSTINJECTION MANAGEMENT

Whenever possible, patients are encouraged to maintain binocular viewing but if intolerable diplopia follows injection for diagnostic purposes, one eye should be occluded. Patients are usually reviewed one week after the injection. Close collaboration with the optometric service is required for contact lens provision in the sensory investigation of patients with aphakia and secondary exotropia. A second or occasionally a third injection may be necessary if the initial injection was ineffective: if the effect is excessive, the patient may need to be reviewed several weeks later.

COMPLICATIONS

Botulinum toxin is largely free of major side-effects; those which have been reported include:

• Complications arising from the injection:
  1 conjunctival haemorrhage;
  2 retrobulbar haemorrhage;
  3 globe perforation.

• Complications occurring as a result of the toxin:
  1 insufficient effect;
  2 excessive effect;
  3 ptosis;
  4 involvement of adjacent extraocular muscles;
  5 sensitivity reaction.

General anaesthesia

Children and uncooperative adults can be treated with botulinum toxin under general anaesthesia. Ketamine anaesthesia potentiates the resting muscle action potential, facilitating the recording of the EMG signal, whereas it is depressed with most other anaesthetics. If the EMG signal cannot readily be monitored, the doll's head manoeuvre can be used to induce conjugate eye movements as the vestibular pathway remains functional under ketamine anaesthesia. The indications for botulinum toxin use under general anaesthesia are similar to those with local anaesthesia, with the majority of patients having sixth nerve palsy or acute undercorrection and overcorrection. We have noted a higher incidence of ptosis after using botulinum toxin under general anaesthesia.

References

James, L. & Wood, R. (1993) Isoflurophate (Floropryl) ointment as the initial treatment of various esotropias: a survey and a review of 279 cases. *Binocular Vision* 8, 11–20.

Prism Adaptation Study Research Group (1990) Efficacy of prism adaptation in the surgical managment of acquired esotropia. *Archives of Ophthalmology* 108, 1248–1256.

Scott, A.B. (1980) Botulinum toxin injection into extraocular muscles as an alternative to strabismus surgery. *Ophthalmology* 87, 1044–1049.

Scott, A.B., Rosenbaum, A.L. & Collins, C.C. (1973) Pharmacological weakening of the extraocular muscles. *Investigative Ophthalmology and Visual Science* 2, 924–929.

9
Surgical Management

Operations on the extraocular muscles are indicated when conservative treatment cannot succeed or has failed to achieve the desired result.

Aims and objectives

The aims of surgery are:
• to straighten the eyes for functional and/or cosmetic reasons;

• to restore or maintain concomitance;
• to relieve symptoms.

These goals should be achieved with the minimal number of procedures, aiming to complete the surgery at one session whenever possible, preferably with a procedure that is reversible, for example a recession rather than a resection or posterior fixation suture.

It is rarely necessary to plan surgery in stages, except when:

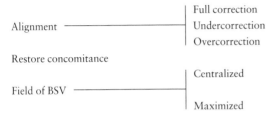

Tree 9.1 The objectives of strabismus surgery.

• there is a risk of anterior segment ischaemia, usually when surgery is required on more than two muscles in the same eye;
• the effect of surgery cannot be predicted, as in complex conditions such as fourth cranial nerve palsy.

The patient, or his parents in the case of a child, should always be informed of the likely success rate of the procedure and what further options are available if it proves unsuccessful.

Further options may include:
• spectacles
• prisms
• botulinum toxin
• further surgery.

The objectives of strabismus surgery are:
• Accurate alignment of the visual axes, indicated when, for example, there is a concomitant strabismus with normal sensory and motor fusion or an acquired paralytic strabismus.
• Undercorrection of the angle of deviation, indicated when operating on esotropia for cosmetic reasons, in many congenital cranial nerve palsies and in thyroid eye disease.
• Overcorrection of the angle of deviation, preferred by many surgeons when treating intermittent exotropia and when correcting acquired primary esotropia with potential for binocular single vision.
• Restoring concomitance, which is important in providing a stable deviation.
• Centralizing and maximizing the field of binocular single vision in situations where it is impossible to restore near normal ocular movement. One way is by weakening an overacting muscle sufficiently to restrict its movement, thus 'matching the defect' and going some way to restoring concomitance; for example, limiting adduction of the contralateral eye in lateral rectus paralysis or abduction in the ipsilateral eye in third nerve palsy.

Principles of surgery

Surgery alters the muscle balance around one or more of the axes of rotation (x, y, z axes of Fick) (Fig. 9.1a,b). Changing the position of insertion or the muscle length results in a change in the magnitude and direction of muscle force.

Operations are of three main types:
• weakening (diminishing the action);
• strengthening (augmenting the action);
• transposing (altering the direction of action).

Procedures can be combined for greater effect; for example, weakening of an agonist and strengthening of its ipsilateral antagonist is more effective when the procedures are carried out simultaneously rather than at different times.

The effectiveness of an operation is also influenced by:
• the age of the patient: more surgery is required in adults than children to obtain the same effect;
• the duration of the strabismus, which influences the state of the muscles;
• anatomical and mechanical features;
• the contractile function of the muscle;
• the size of the deviation;
• whether a muscle is overacting.

Anatomical considerations

Developmental aspects

The adult dimensions of the anterior segment of the eye are not reached until the age of approximately 18 months. Before that age the relationship of the rectus muscles to the limbus varies, therefore the measurement should be taken from the limbus and not from the point of muscle insertion in order to standardize the effect (Helveston & Ellis 1980).

Orbital connective tissue

Tenon's capsule lies beneath the conjunctiva and extends from the optic nerve to the limbus as a fascial layer that envelops the extraocular muscles and separates the orbital fat into intraconal and extraconal compartments. It forms the capsule around the muscles and the intermuscular septum connecting the

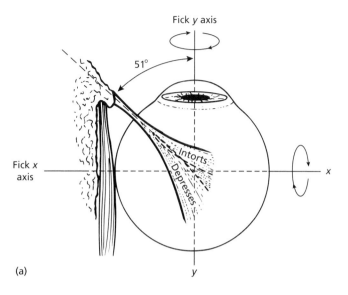

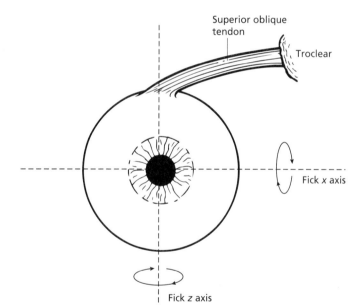

Fig. 9.1 (a) Superior oblique muscle of the right eye seen from above, demonstrating the near transverse insertion of the anterior portion of the tendon with a principal action of intorsion: the functionally distinct posterior insertion with a principal action of depression.
(b) Anteroposterior view of the right eye demonstrating the *z*-axis of Fick.

extraocular muscles. The check ligaments are condensations of connective tissue connecting the orbital surface of the muscle to the overlying Tenon's capsule and conjunctiva.

The orbit contains a complicated arrangement of connective tissue extending between extraocular muscles, Tenon's capsule, the globe and the orbit. Koornneef (1979) has described its structure. Recent studies have added to our understanding of the role

that these connective tissue septae play in normal and abnormal ocular motility. The major component of connective tissue is collagen, the fibres of which encircle and interconnect with the extraocular muscles, especially between the superior and lateral rectus muscles and the medial and inferior rectus, where there are dense concentrations. There are also dense condensations of collagen with elastin surrounding the extraocular muscles between the equator of the globe and the

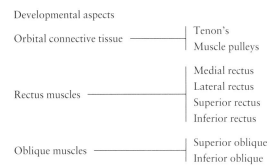

Developmental aspects

Orbital connective tissue ——— | Tenon's
| Muscle pulleys

Rectus muscles ——— | Medial rectus
| Lateral rectus
| Superior rectus
| Inferior rectus

Oblique muscles ——— | Superior oblique
| Inferior oblique

Tree 9.2 Anatomical considerations when planning strabismus surgery.

globe–optic nerve junction; these act as a sleeve that the rectus muscles and the inferior oblique muscle can slide through. These areas are known as extraocular muscle pulleys; because they are suspended from the adjacent orbital wall by means of collagen, elastin and smooth muscle bands, they make only small movements with gaze. It was once thought that the direction of pull of an extraocular muscle was determined by its line of action between the anatomical origin at the annulus of Zinn and its point of contact with the globe; it is now known that each pulley acts as the functional origin of the relevant muscle in terms of direction of pull, preventing significant sideslip. The extraocular muscle bellies have stable paths in relation to the orbit (Miller & Robinson 1987); only the anterior part of the rectus tendons move to any significant extent. It is possible to predict the three-dimensional location of extraocular muscle pulleys and observe changes with gaze by using currently

available neuro-imaging techniques (Clark *et al.* 1997). Abnormalities in pulley position have been shown to to be present in patients with A- and V-pattern strabismus (Clark *et al.* 1997), and may be important in the aetiology of some alphabet patterns as well as in other conditions.

Rectus muscles

All four rectus muscles are inserted anterior to the equator, but at different distances behind the limbus. Their common ring origin, the annulus of Zinn, around the optic foramen and the nasal end of the superior orbital fissure, is somewhat medial to the anteroposterior axis of the eye, therefore the medial rectus is significantly shorter than the lateral rectus, and the vertical recti are of intermediate length. If a muscle is resected too much a mechanical tether will be produced, limiting movement in the direction opposite to its field of action; this is most frequently seen after surgery on the medial rectus. If the muscle insertion is recessed behind its tangential point of action on the surface of the globe, restriction of movement in the direction of action of the muscle will ensue. A larger recession can be performed as a single procedure before limitation of movement occurs, compared with a combined recession and resection. The relevant measurements for the four rectus muscles are shown in Table 9.1. In addition, recession or resection of the vertical rectus muscles in excess of the measurements shown in Table 9.1 alters the vertical relationships of the globe with the upper and lower

Table 9.1 Important measurements for rectus muscle surgery. These figures are intended as a guide. Individual surgeon's techniques can result in different effects from the same amount of recession or resection.

Muscle	Distance of normal insertion behind the limbus (mm)	Maximum surgery without limiting motility	
		Recession (mm)	Resection (mm)
Superior rectus	7.5	8	8
Lateral rectus	7.0	8	8
Inferior rectus	6.5	5*	6*
Medial rectus	5.5	6	6

* Although this amount of surgery on the vertical recti should not cause limitation of movement, in practice recession or resection of the inferior rectus by more than 3.5 mm is liable to cause changes in lid position.

eyelid margins without changing the height of the palpebral aperture.

The medial and lateral recti have purely horizontal actions of adduction and abduction, respectively. The vertical recti, being inserted at an angle of 23° medial to the anteroposterior axis of the globe, have more complex actions:
• Superior rectus: elevation, adduction and intorsion. The principal action is elevation, and this is the sole action in 23° abduction.
• Inferior rectus: depression, adduction and extorsion. The principal action is depression, and this is the sole action in 23° abduction.

Both vertical recti act as weak abductors when the eye is abducted more than 23°.

Medial rectus

The medial rectus has the shortest arc of contact with the globe and is the only muscle without an intermuscular septum connecting it to an oblique muscle; therefore if it becomes inadvertently detached from the globe it can retract posteriorly within its capsule and can be difficult to relocate. Check ligaments connect the muscle to the adjacent plica and caruncle and inadequate division of these at surgery can lead to distortion and retraction of these structures.

Lateral rectus

The lateral rectus has a well-developed intermuscular septum connecting it inferiorly with the inferior oblique muscle. Incomplete dissection of this septum when operating on the lateral rectus, especially when performing a resection, will cause traction on the inferior oblique and its incarceration into the lower insertion site of the lateral rectus. Failure to divide this septum adequately can also lead to traction on the inferior oblique when the lateral rectus is transposed vertically.

Superior rectus

The nasal part of the superior rectus muscle insertion is reflected posteriorly and care is required that the tendon is not inadvertently split by the muscle hook when capturing it during surgery, leaving the temporal portion behind. Dissection carried out on the temporal side of the superior rectus requires special care to avoid damaging the anterior fibres of the super-

ior oblique tendon. An intermuscular connective tissue septum or frenulum connects the under-surface of the superior rectus muscle and the fascia surrounding the superior oblique tendon and serves to limit the amount of recession that can be performed on the muscle before exerting excessive traction on the superior oblique. When performing superior rectus recession of less than 8 mm the frenulum acts to the surgeon's advantage by moving the superior oblique tendon posteriorly, facilitating direct scleral attachment of the muscle. When carrying out larger recessions or using 'hang back' or adjustable sutures, the frenulum should be divided. Large recession of the superior rectus in the order of 10–12 mm, is not associated with significant change in upper eyelid position in our opinion.

Inferior rectus

The inferior rectus has a strong indirect attachment to the lower eyelid that can result in lower eyelid retraction after a recession of 4 mm or more, especially in patients with thyroid eye disease who may have pre-existing lid retraction. The strong intermuscular septum between the inferior rectus and inferior oblique, the ligament of Lockwood, may be responsible for the increased incidence of posterior slippage of the inferior rectus muscle reported following its surgical recession (Sprunger & Helveston 1993).

Oblique muscles

Superior oblique

The actions of the superior oblique are intorsion, depression and abduction. In full adduction, the muscle acts as a pure depressor, while in full abduction it is almost entirely an intorter. Helveston *et al.* (1982) made a number of observations following a study of the anatomy and physiology of the trochlea and intratrochlear superior oblique tendon. These included:
• A bursa-like structure separating the tendon and trochlea, the distension of which could result in an acquired Brown's syndrome, with or without a 'click'.
• The intratrochlear superior oblique tendon is normally enveloped in a vascular sheath, which may be important for maintaining the smooth passage of the tendon through the trochlea. The vascular sheath may help maintain the relatively high metabolic demands

of the region and help dissipate the heat and repair the 'wear and tear' generated through the normal movement of the tendon through the trochlea.

• The superior oblique tendon itself is made up of fibres that span the whole length of the tendon with little in the way of connections between adjacent fibres. Movement of the tendon through the trochlea is believed to be achieved by differential movement of individual fibres; those situated centrally move more extensively than the peripheral fibres during periods of contraction and relaxation of the superior oblique muscle. The tendon therefore does not move like a cord through a pulley, but rather behaves like a telescope, with the component parts of the tendon sliding over each other.

The reflected tendon turns laterally and posteriorly from the trochlea at an angle of some 51° to the sagittal plane, and penetrates Tenon's capsule 3 mm nasal to the medial border of the superior rectus muscle. The tendon fans out beneath the muscle and makes a curved insertion, convex laterally, extending forwards and laterally for some 12 mm from a point 5 mm from the optic nerve and adjacent to the scleral penetration of the superior temporal vortex vein.

The fan-shaped insertion determines that the tendon can be considered as having two functionally separate insertions (Fig. 9.1a):

• The anterior portion: this is aligned in an almost transverse direction, and so has a predominantly torsional action.

• The posterior portion: this is inserted more parallel to the globe's anteroposterior axis, well behind the equator, and so has principally depressing and abducting actions.

The intermuscular septum, often termed the 'tendon sheath', surrounds the tendon as far as its insertion and connects it to the overlying superior rectus sheath; this connection is termed the frenulum. This surrounding tissue has fine fibrillary connections with the tendon, so that complete tenectomy within the 'sheath' in the upper nasal quadrant deep to Tenon's capsule is followed by only a limited retraction of the proximal portion of the divided tendon towards the trochlea. The tendon alignment remains unchanged and some indirect postequatorial attachment to the globe is maintained via the intermuscular septum. The presence of the frenulum of the superior oblique

means that a complete tenotomy performed on the temporal side of the superior rectus results in even less retraction of the tendon towards the trochlea.

Inferior oblique

The principal actions of the muscle are extorsion, elevation and abduction. In full adduction, the inferior oblique is a pure elevator, and in full abduction it is almost entirely an extorter. The inferior oblique muscle passes posteriorly and temporally from its orbital floor origin at an angle of 51° to the sagittal plane. It penetrates Tenon's capsule beneath the inferior rectus muscle and the capsules of the two muscles are closely associated with each other in this area, forming part of Lockwood's suspensory ligament. Because the muscle tendon is only 1 mm in length the muscle hook will capture the muscle rather than the tendon when identifying the inferior oblique at surgery: careful dissection and haemostasis are required to avoid damaging it. In the lower temporal quadrant the muscle sheath is firmly attached to Tenon's capsule within the muscle cone as far as its insertion, which lies under the lateral rectus and extends as far back as the macular area, closely related to the short posterior ciliary arteries. The lower temporal vortex vein is close to the deep surface of the muscle near the lateral border of the inferior rectus. The muscle insertion can be viewed as having two distinct actions as with the superior oblique muscle. The anterior portion has a predominantly extorting action and the posterior part elevates and abducts the eye.

Preoperative assessment

A preoperative orthoptic examination should include the following information:

• Measurement of the angle of deviation for near and distance and in other directions of gaze when indicated. Measurement should be made using the up-to-date refractive correction, which should not have any incorporated prisms. Accurate measurement of torsion in paralytic and mechanical strabismus is particularly important.

• Estimation of binocular function, which will govern whether a full or partial correction of the deviation is required, or even an overcorrection is indicated.

- Whether postoperative diplopia is likely to occur in patients undergoing cosmetic surgery.
- Other relevant tests, including Hess charts and fields of binocular fixation and uniocular fixation.

Orthoptic findings may reveal an increase in esotropia or a decrease in exotropia that may be explained by preoperative anxiety. The surgeon should therefore also take account of measurements recorded at recent previous examinations. Occlusion should be discontinued a few days before the measurements are made.

Postoperative diplopia

The possibility of postoperative diplopia must be considered in adult patients and in children 5 years or older requesting strabismus surgery for cosmetic reasons. To correctly interpret the patient's responses during the test, the examiner must confirm the sensory status, using Bagolini glasses or Worth's four dots. The postoperative diplopia test investigates the presence of diplopia or suppression in patients without the potential for binocular single vision. If fusion is unexpectedly demonstrated during the procedure then in effect the measurements obtained are the prism fusion amplitude and not a measure of postoperative diplopia. The patient's visual acuity should be considered, although even deep amblyopia does not exclude postoperative diplopia. The postoperative diplopia test is summarized below.

The patient should be asked at presentation if they are already aware of diplopia. In our series of patients requesting surgery for consecutive exotropia, 38% were already aware of diplopia but did not find it troublesome, and the presence of diplopia preoperatively was the best predictor of it postoperatively (Spencer *et al.* 1995).

The patient is asked to view a fixation target appropriate to his level of acuity at near and distance through prisms. The aim of the procedure is to use the prism to simulate an alignment from 20 Δ undercorrected to 20 Δ overcorrected and assess for diplopia risk. The patient should be asked what he observes and the purpose of the test explained. If he does not recognize diplopia, the authors hold the view that no effort should be made to elicit it. If there is spontaneous recognition of diplopia, the strength of prism should be changed to map out the region where it can be elicited and this should be recorded on the postoperative diplopia chart (see Chapter 7), and should be taken into account when planning the surgery. If it is likely to occur, the patient should be informed and the diplopia demonstrated to him by means of prisms so that he can decide whether to have the operation. Botulinum toxin can also be used to temporarily correct the strabismus and provide additional information about postoperative diplopia risk and its likely tolerance (Ketley *et al.* 1987). The incomitance caused by the toxin can usefully be employed to explore a wide range of deviations in free space without the need to resort to prisms.

Normally projected diplopia is more likely to persist postoperatively, whereas anomalously projected diplopia (paradoxical or incongruous diplopia in which the projection of the images does not tally with the type of strabismus or the angle of deviation) is more likely to be transitory.

Diplopia can arise from postoperative restriction of movement following over-liberal recession or resection of a muscle and occurs when gaze is directed away from the primary position. This diplopia is also likely to persist.

Preparation for surgery

Premedication

Prophylactic topical antibiotics and trimming of the eyelashes are unnecessary and should be avoided. Adrenaline (epinephrine) 0.01% or phenylephrine 2.5% eye drops can be instilled immediately before surgery to constrict the conjunctive blood vessels and so reduce bleeding. Following the instillation of adrenaline there is an initial vasodilatory phase lasting

Premedication

Anaesthetic ——————| General
                    | Local

Eye position

Sutures / needles ——————| Temporary traction
                         | Conjunctival / muscle

Forced duction test

Tree 9.3 Factors to consider in the preparation for strabismus surgery.

1–2 min before vasoconstriction occurs. The pupillary dilation caused by both these drugs will result in blurred vision, making the subsequent use of adjustable sutures difficult. As a general principle, drugs used for preoperative sedation should decrease a patient's apprehension without delaying his total recovery from anaesthesia or altering the ocular muscle balance. This is particularly important in proposed day-case surgery and when muscle suture adjustments with the patient's full cooperation are planned, either during an operation carried out under local anaesthesia or within 24 h after general anaesthesia (see subsequent section on other surgical procedures, adjustable sutures).

Anaesthesia

General anaesthesia

This is essential for children and may be preferred by some adult patients. It also allows a thorough ophthalmoscopic examination through dilated pupils and a cycloplegic retinoscopy if this was not achieved in the clinic.

Succinylcholine should not be used as a depolarizing muscle relaxant if:
• A forced duction test is to be carried out, because extraocular muscle tone is paradoxically increased by this drug for at least 10 min after its injection.
• The patient's strabismus has been treated during the previous month by instillation of phospholine iodide eye drops—systemic absorption of the drug dangerously reduces the concentration of cholinesterases in the plasma. Phospholine iodide is no longer available in the UK.

Pancuronium is a suitable nondepolarizing alternative (France *et al*. 1980).

Propofol infusion anaesthesia is associated with reduced postoperative recovery time and lower levels of nausea and vomiting when compared with inhalational anaesthetics and is an ideal agent for day-case surgery and when adjustable sutures are used.

Operative bleeding can be reduced by:
• a slight head-up position of the patient on the operating table;
• avoidance of excessive blood carbon dioxide levels by hyperventilation if necessary.

Discharge from hospital on the day of operation is now normal practice for children and most adults.

Consideration of home conditions, distance from the hospital and the need for adequate immediate postoperative supervision may necessitate an overnight stay.

Local anaesthesia

Peribulbar or retrobulbar anaesthesia

Peribulbar anaesthesia can be used in adults when a general anaesthetic is unsuitable or when local anaesthetic is preferred. Intraoperative adjustable sutures cannot be used with peribulbar anaesthetic and we have observed cases where the effects of the anaesthetic have persisted for 18 h, complicating postoperative adjustment. Operations that do not require postoperative adjustment, for example surgery on the inferior oblique muscle, are ideal procedures to perform under this form of anaesthesia.

Topical anaesthesia

Adequate local anaesthesia can be achieved by topical anaesthesia alone. Benoxinate hydrochloride 0.5% or amethocaine (tetracaine) 1% is effective. Injections of local anaesthetic (lidocaine hydrochloride 1% with adrenaline 1 : 200 000) into the muscle sheaths and the retrobulbar spaces induce a more profound anaesthesia, but they distort the local anatomy, altering the normal action of the extraocular muscles, and must be avoided if intraoperative suture adjustment is planned. Adrenaline results in pupillary dilation and therefore should be used with caution in patients who are undergoing adjustable suture surgery.

Those suitable for topical anaesthesia include:
• cooperative adults;
• cases where the muscles to be operated on have not undergone previous surgery;
• patients who can lie flat and supine for up to one hour;
• cases in which the eye can be voluntarily rotated into a position allowing surgical access.

It is also of particular value in allowing sutures to be adjusted during surgery with the patient's full cooperation (Fells 1984).

Eye position at start of surgery

The normal eye position under deep general anaesthesia is approximately 10° exotropia. The eye position of strabismic patients varies in individuals and is not a reliable

guide to the type and amount of surgery needed as normal tone is eliminated. The position is influenced by:
• Mechanical factors: strabismus entirely due to mechanical restriction tends to be relatively unchanged from the patient's conscious state. Any degree of mechanical restriction will modify the eye position.
• The type of strabismus in the absence of mechanical restriction: many exotropic patients show an increased angle of deviation; esotropic patients may also diverge or show less esotropia.

Note should be taken of any change which has occurred.

Although the eye position under deep general anaesthesia should not be used as a guide to the type and amount of surgery to perform, the alignment shortly after an intraoperative injection of succinylcholine has been shown to correlate closely with the preoperative angle (Mindel *et al.* 1980). In man, there are two basic subtypes of extraocular muscle fibres: the slow, or tonic fibres and the fast, or twitch fibres. The slow subsystem is selectively stimulated by succinylcholine, while the fast fibres are inhibited (Bach-y-Rita & Ito 1966). If the slow system is responsible for alignment in the primary position, it would explain why the succinylcholine-induced ocular position under anaesthesia correlates with the preoperative position.

Surgical sutures and needles

Temporary traction and stay sutures
Gauge 5.0 Ethibond is appropriate.

Muscles and conjunctiva
An absorbable, synthetic, nonantigenic suture material such as vicryl is preferable to catgut because:
• the material is stronger;
• it absorbs more slowly;
• it induces much less tissue reaction.

Passage through the tissues is smoother if the sutures are coated; extra precautions must then be taken to tie the knots securely. Size 6.0 is ideal for muscles and conjunctiva, or 7.0 can be used for conjunctival closure if preferred. Permanent sutures such as Prolene 6.0 gauge or ethibond 5.0 are occasionally required, for example in superior oblique plication operations and as posterior fixation sutures or with looped recessions. We prefer to use prolene sutures

because of a significantly reduced incidence of granuloma formation.

Small, spatulated, edge-cutting 3/8-circle needles are very suitable as they neither pass too deeply nor cut out from the sclera. They are swaged on to the material to form double-ended sutures.

Fixation of the globe
The globe can be held steady in the chosen position by means of:
• A temporary 5.0 gauge stay suture attached at the limbus in the same quadrant as the conjunctival incision. This is our preferred method when operating on the cyclovertical muscles.
• A light, curved artery forceps in the same position.
• Two sutures applied at diametrically opposite sides of the limbus and at right angles to the conjunctival incision. This gives better control, the sutures do not interfere in the operative field, and it is our method of choice when operating on the horizontal recti.

The advantages of using limbal stay sutures routinely during strabismus surgery have been described by us (McElvanney & Ansons 1996) and are summarized below:
• Placement of stay sutures at the 12 and 6 o'clock positions at the limbus provides a fixed landmark and accurate reference point when determining the location and position of a muscle during surgery. This is particularly important with reoperations as well as aiding the identification of congenital anomalies of muscle insertions, thereby minimizing the risk of operating on the wrong muscle. Stay sutures can help with positioning the globe when operating on the vertical recti or the oblique muscles.
• Limbal stay sutures facilitate accurate and reproducible traction testing. Forced duction tests performed at the start of the procedure are aided by gentle anteropulsion of the globe (produced by tension on stay sutures), thus resisting retropulsion that may give rise to a false negative response.
• When recessing a horizontal muscle, selective tension on the upper stay suture facilitates the placement of the upper muscle suture by creating a space between muscle insertion and the hook, and likewise for the lower suture.

More extensive globe rotation can be achieved later in the operation using sutures passed directly through rectus muscle insertions after division of the tendon in recession procedures.

Forced duction test

A forced duction test should be performed at the start of all strabismus operations and repeated during and at the end of the procedure. The globe should be gripped firmly and rotated in all the cardinal positions of gaze: we prefer to hold the stay sutures rather than put excessive traction on the conjunctiva. Although care should be taken not to anteropulse or retropulse the globe significantly whilst performing the forced duction test, the result of such manoeuvres can help identify which structures are contributing towards any mechanical restriction of movement.

Retropulsion of the globe results in:
• a decrease in the result of the forced duction test if the conjunctiva or rectus muscles are tight;
• an increase in the response to the forced duction test if the oblique muscles are contracted.

Anteropulsion of the globe results in:
• an increase in the forced duction test if the conjunctiva and rectus muscles are tight;
• a decrease in the forced duction test if the oblique muscles are contracted.

The forced duction test is repeated once the conjunctiva has been opened to assess its contribution to any restriction. The test is repeated again after the extraocular muscle is detached. In the reverse situation, following reattachment of muscle and conjunctiva, the forced duction test can alert the surgeon to mechanical restriction caused by these structures and allow him to modify the procedure accordingly, for example by performing a conjunctival recession.

Methods to attempt to quantify the results of the forced duction test have been developed, employing some form of calibrated spring balance, but are rarely used clinically.

Conjunctival incisions

Rectus muscle surgery

Limbal incisions with radial extension give good access to the rectus muscles and are to be preferred, especially when there are circumferential conjunctival

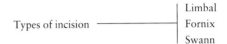

Tree 9.4 Types of conjunctival incision.

scars over the muscle insertions from previous surgery. Limbal incisions are essential if the conjunctiva is to be recessed because of tightness causing mechanical restriction of movement. Sutures can be preplaced in the corners of the conjunctival flap at this stage, serving to retract it and allow accurate reapposition. These sutures encroach slightly on the operative field during the remainder of the operation, but this is not a serious disadvantage.

Fornix incisions can be used on the medial rectus muscle; access is difficult but cosmesis is good as the result of the absence of visible conjunctival scars.

The Swann incision, which involves cutting through the conjunctiva directly over the muscle insertion, offers no real advantage over the other two approaches and can result in significant postoperative adhesions between the conjunctiva and underlying muscle.

Oblique muscle surgery

The inferior oblique muscle is best approached through a circumferential incision near the inferotemporal fornix, which will be hidden by the eyelids. Although the superior oblique can be approached through a similar incision near the superotemporal fornix, we prefer a limbal approach that facilitates identification of the superior rectus insertion before proceeding with dissection of the superior oblique.

Exposure of muscles

Exposure of rectus muscles

Adequate exposure is essential for accurate and safe surgery (Fig. 9.2). The steps by which this is achieved are:
• The conjunctiva is incised at the limbus and retracted and a radial incision made in Tenon's capsule and any overlying conjunctiva on both sides of a rectus insertion. The intermuscular septum should be

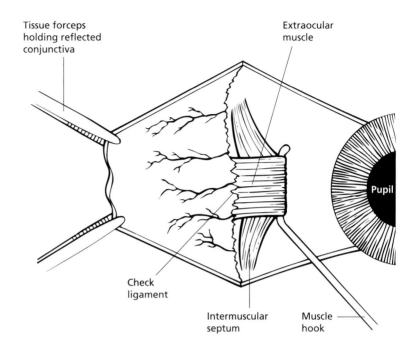

Fig. 9.2 Adequate exposure of a rectus muscle involves division of the check ligament and the intermuscular septum.

dissected along the upper and lower borders of the muscle to identify the full extent of the insertion: a greater posterior dissection is required when performing a resection compared with a recession.

• A squint hook is passed behind the muscle insertion under direct vision. The hook must at all times remain anterior to the equator and in close contact with the globe to avoid disturbing the orbital fat pad and the vortex veins. If resistance to the passage of the hook is felt further dissection should be carried out.

• The check ligaments and muscle sheaths are disturbed as little as possible to avoid bleeding and subsequent scarring, although any attachments to the lids and plica are divided. This must be done, otherwise recession of the underlying rectus muscle will cause mechanical retroposition of these structures, giving rise to:

1 retraction of the plica on adduction following medial rectus recession;

2 retraction and furrowing of the lower lid in down-gaze following inferior rectus recession.

The intermuscular connective tissue between the lower border of the lateral rectus and the inferior oblique should be divided to avoid unnecessary traction on the inferior oblique. The intermuscular connective tissue connecting the under-surface of the superior rectus to the superior oblique, commonly referred to as the frenulum, should be divided when performing a large superior rectus recession or when using adjustable or hang-back sutures. The check ligament on the orbital surface of the inferior rectus is divided when performing a recession to reduce the amount of lower eyelid retraction postoperatively.

Exposure of oblique muscles

The oblique muscles can be approached through circumferential conjunctival incisions some 10 mm behind the limbus, although we prefer to approach the superior oblique through a limbal incision.

Superior oblique
Limbal approach

A superior limbal conjunctival incision is made and the conjunctiva and overlying Tenon's capsule reflected superiorly. A radial incision of the conjunctiva and Tenon's is made temporal to the superior rectus when operating on the superior oblique insertion, and nasal to it when operating on the tendon. A muscle hook is passed behind the superior rectus insertion and the eye rotated downwards. Better exposure is achieved if a separate small tissue retractor is used to retract the upper eyelid and bulbar conjunctiva upwards and posteriorly rather than maintaining the use of a lid speculum. The check ligaments and fascia on the orbital surface of the superior rectus are divided on the temporal or nasal borders of the muscle for approximately 10–12 mm posteriorly, depending on whether the superior oblique tendon or insertion is being operated on. Care must be taken to avoid trauma to the vortex veins that emerge just medial and lateral to the superior rectus a little behind the equator of the eye; the lateral vein lies close to the posterior part of the superior oblique insertion and is a useful landmark. Passing an iris repositor between it and the underlying sclera from anterior to posterior can identify the full extent of the tendon insertion. The tendon is identified within its 'sheath' in the upper nasal quadrant and is hooked forwards for further dissection using a small muscle hook.

Fornix approach

The conjunctival incision is made in the upper fornix. The insertion is approached by an incision in the upper temporal quadrant, and the tendon aproached through an upper nasal incision. Tenon's capsule is divided separately and a muscle hook is placed beneath the superior rectus insertion to rotate the eye downwards. The rest of the procedure is identical to that described for the limbal approach.

Inferior oblique

A stay suture is placed in the limbal conjunctiva at the 6 o'clock position and the globe rotated up and nasally. The inferior oblique can usually be seen as a bulge in the inferolateral conjunctival fornix and the conjunctiva incised just anterior to it in the lower temporal quadrant. The lateral and inferior rectus muscles are identified and squint hooks placed under the muscle insertions to rotate the eye upwards and inwards. The belly of the inferior oblique muscle is identified under direct vision behind the equator between the two retracted rectus muscles, and Tenon's capsule is pulled forwards until the inferior oblique is visible at the incision site. A third squint hook is placed behind the inferior oblique from its deep to its superficial surface, making sure that no portion of the muscle remains posterior to the hook tip at any time and that the fat pad is not disturbed; the muscle is then

captured and hooked forwards into the wound. Surrounding Tenon's capsule is dissected free, being careful to avoid the inferior temporal vortex vein. Failure to ensure that the whole muscle has been identified, or when congenital anomalies result in the muscle splitting into an anterior and posterior part at the capture site, can result in leaving part of it behind. To avoid this complication we recommend:
• Reflecting the captured muscle inferiorly to reveal a 'white triangle' which represents the connective tissue between the proximal and distal parts of the muscle at the capture site. If the whole muscle is not on the hook, the uncaptured posterior fibres obscure the triangle.
• Always identifying the insertion site after capturing the muscle and performing a disinsertion or recession rather than a myectomy so as to directly visualize the full posterior extent of the insertion.

Haemostasis

Slight temporary bleeding may occur from conjunctival vessels, but dissection in the correct plane should reduce the amount of blood in the operating field.

Bleeding is most likely to occur:
• if the dissection is carried too close to the fleshy portion of a rectus muscle through the muscle sheath;
• when anterior ciliary vessels in the rectus muscle insertions are divided;
• when a muscle belly is divided or incised.
Bleeding can be controlled by:
• Application of local pressure for up to a full minute. Most bleeding will then cease spontaneously, and this is the method of choice.
• Cauterization, most accurately using bipolar cautery for localized occlusion of small persistent bleeding points. Cauterization causes scar tissue formation and should be avoided as much as possible.
• Application of topical adrenaline (epinephrine) 0.01% eye drops, with the full knowledge and agreement of the anaesthetist.

Surgical procedures, methods and indications for use

As the anatomy of the rectus and oblique muscles differs very considerably, it is convenient to consider

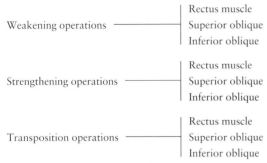

Tree 9.5 Types of surgical procedure.

these two muscle groups separately. Common muscle procedures are described in detail; others which have only occasional indications or are of particular historical significance are mentioned more briefly. The indications for each type of operation are discussed, but their applications are set out in more detail in subsequent chapters dealing with the management of specific motility disorders.

Weakening operations

Rectus muscle weakening operations

Recession
The aim of recession is to weaken the muscle without causing limitation of movement, with certain exceptions discussed below.

PRINCIPLE

The insertion of the muscle is moved closer to its point of origin in the same plane, producing a slackening of muscle fibres and weakening the muscle's action. There is a linear relationship between the weakening effect and the amount recessed until the new insertion coincides with the tangential point of the globe when the eye moves into the field of action of the recessed muscle. Recession beyond this point significantly compromises the muscle action, resulting in a restriction of movement.

When the movement is limited by mechanical contraction, recession of the contracted muscle will reduce limitation of movement by a progressive amount.

METHOD

Recession is performed in stages:

1 Sutures are placed 1 mm posterior to the tendinous insertion of the exposed muscle. Placing the suture too close to the insertion risks cutting the suture when detaching the muscle or part of it slipping. Some surgeons place whipped sutures around opposite edges of the tendon (Fig. 9.3a); others prefer to interweave a single double-ended suture across the entire width of the insertion (Fig. 9.3b).

2 The muscle is detached by transecting the tendon as close to its insertion as possible. This minimizes bleeding, makes the recession measurements more accurate and avoids an ugly muscle stump that may otherwise be visible through the bulbar conjunctiva after the operation.

3 The desired amount of recession is measured out in millimetres using callipers directed posteriorly from both ends of the original insertion; the sclera is marked at the intended reinsertion points. If there is doubt concerning the exact position of the original insertion, appropriate measurements can be made directly from the limbus immediately anterior to the muscle insertion.

4 The rectus tendon is reinserted parallel to its original attachment. The two needles of a double-ended interwoven suture are each passed transversely through the sclera to emerge adjacent to each other along the line of intended reattachment and tied. If marginal whipped sutures are used, additional sutures may need to be positioned and tied along the anterior edge of the tendon if there is any sign of posterior sagging after its corners have been sutured to the globe at the measured points (Fig. 9.4). The vertical rectus insertions are curved with the convexity forwards and should follow parallel contours when recessed.

Recession can be combined with resection of the ipsilateral antagonist so that the globe is rotated within the muscle cone. The effect of a combined procedure is greater than if recession and resection are carried out as separate procedures. The effect of simultaneous recession of both medial recti exceeds that of recession of one medial rectus followed later by recession of the other.

The effect of a specific amount of muscle recession is influenced by the type of strabismus and by the technique used by individual surgeons, which differs in

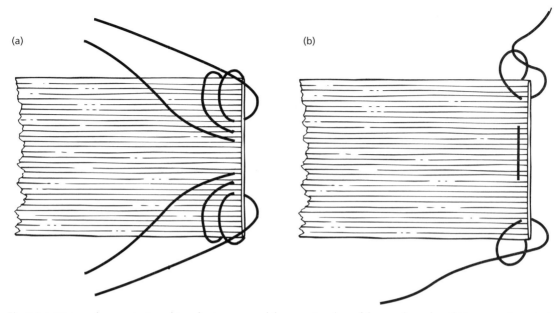

Fig. 9.3 (a) Suture placement using whipped sutures around the opposite edges of the muscle tendon. (b) Interweaving a single double-ended suture across the entire width of the tendon's insertion.

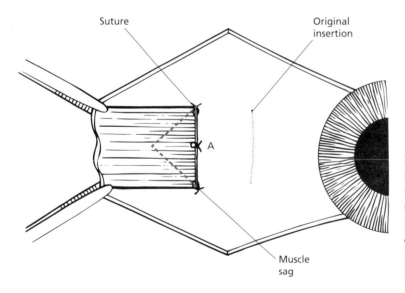

Fig. 9.4 The central portion of a rectus muscle may sag posteriorly when sutures are inserted only at the corners of the detached muscle (dotted line). A central suture (A) ensures that the recessed muscle is reattached parallel to the original insertion.

small but important ways, making it impossible to tabulate accurately the exact change in the angle of deviation per millimetre of recession.

The maximum amount of recession that can be performed without causing restriction of ocular movement varies with each muscle (Table 9.1). In some circumstances recession in excess of this amount has been proposed. The surgeon must decide whether the probable effect on the strabismus or on the patient's symptoms justifies the loss of full excursion that will result. The long-term effect should also be considered before such surgery is undertaken.

POSSIBLE INDICATIONS FOR LARGE RECESSION

Large amounts of recession have been advocated in the following conditions

• Convergence excess esotropia, as an alternative to using a posterior fixation suture.

• Dissociated vertical deviation (DVD), to prevent the up-drift by recessing the superior recti up to 13 mm.

• Congenital nystagmus with a marked face turn to use a null area, recessing the medial rectus in one eye and the lateral rectus in the other.

• Lateral rectus paralysis:

1 recession of the contracted ipsilateral medial rectus to enable the eye to abduct;

2 recession of the contralateral medial rectus to limit adduction and increase concomitance, indicated when the lateral rectus is not innervated.

• Duane's syndrome, recessing the contralateral medial rectus to enlarge the field of binocular fixation.

• Graves' disease, where large inferior and medial rectus recessions may be necessary to restore fixation in the primary position.

• Esotropia associated with a blind microphthalmic eye.

• Infantile esotropia, which may be treated by large recessions of both medial recti. von Noorden (1988) reported good alignment following this single procedure whereas conventional recession/resection procedures required at least two operations.

• Ciancia's syndrome to overcome a face turn, recessing the medial rectus on the side to which the face is turned. It may be necessary to recess both medial recti if the face is turned to either side.

VARIATIONS IN METHOD

• The amount of recession can be varied between one end of the new insertion and the other (oblique recession). For example, the inferior pole of the medial rectus insertion can be recessed more than the superior pole, thus weakening muscle action more on down-gaze. This method may be useful in some alphabet patterns (Fig. 9.5).

• The insertions of the horizontal recti can be raised or lowered up to a full muscle width after recession in order to weaken muscle action more on up-gaze or down-gaze, respectively (Fig. 9.6). See section on Rectus muscle transposition operations p. 192 for more details.

• The anterior ciliary arteries can be dissected free from the muscle before it is recessed, resected or transposed (McKeown *et al.* 1989). This vessel-sparing procedure is useful when there is a high risk of anterior segment ischaemia.

INDICATIONS

Recession is by far the commonest rectus muscle weakening procedure and is widely used in the treatment of concomitant and incomitant (paralytic) strabismus, including those patients with mechanical restriction of movement.

VALUE

The operation has great value in changing the resting

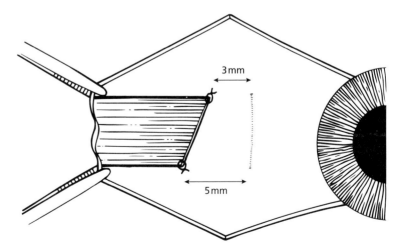

Fig. 9.5 Oblique recession where the inferior pole of the muscle insertion is recessed more than the superior pole.

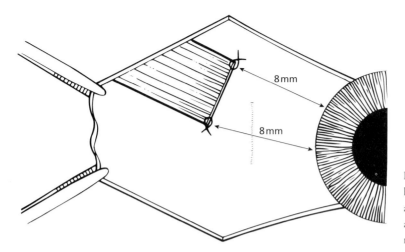

Fig. 9.6 The insertion of the horizontal rectus muscle is raised approximately half a tendon width after recession in order to weaken muscle action more on up-gaze.

position of the eye. It is the best method of reducing the mechanical limitation of movement caused by a contracted rectus muscle.

The operation can be adjusted or reversed at a later stage if necessary. A conventional amount of recession alone is not usually effective in conditions such as DVD, when the aim is to weaken markedly excessive movement in one direction of gaze without significantly changing the resting position of the eye, i.e. without altering the deviation in the primary position.

PROBLEMS

Its usefulness is limited by the amount by which each muscle can be recessed without causing a limitation of movement. For example, recession of the medial rectus by 6 mm may be insufficient to correct an accommodative esotropia with convergence excess, but a larger recession would result in significant limitation of adduction and convergence weakness.

Using standard callipers as opposed to a curved rule can result in an error larger than 0.5 mm when a recession exceeds 10 mm, because of the difference between the cord and arc measurements (Scott *et al.* 1978).

When measuring the recession the use of toothed forceps to fix the insertion site after detaching the muscle can result in splitting the sclera and displacement of the insertion site anteriorly, resulting in errors of measurement (Kushner *et al.* 1987).

Augmented recessions

These operations aim to increase the weakening effect of recession beyond the amount conventionally achieved without causing significant limitation of movement.

PRINCIPLE

Provided the insertion of a rectus muscle remains at or in front of the point tangential to the globe's surface, the muscle can be slackened without limiting movement.

METHODS

Loop sutures

The muscle is maximally recessed and is reattached to the globe by loop sutures through the corners of the disinserted tendon, so that the muscle is reinserted at this maximum recession point but can contract further back towards its origin (Fig. 9.7). The loops can be formed by tying over a metal rod; the size of the loop can be varied as required by using rods of graded diameters (Gobin 1968). A better way of fashioning the loop is to pull the muscle up to the insertion and tie the first knot, sliding it towards the insertion until the desired size of the loop is reached; the assistant grasps the suture just below the knot with nontoothed forceps and the knot is secured with two more throws. Nonabsorbable suture material is preferable. In the authors' experience, this operation has a useful place when conventional surgery has failed. Clark *et al.* (1989) reported success with this procedure and

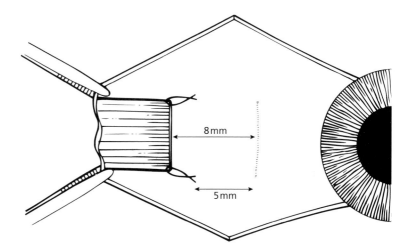

Fig. 9.7 Augmented recession using loop sutures. The medial rectus muscle has been allowed to retract posteriorly by a full 8 mm while still being indirectly reattached by the sutures to the 5 mm maximum conventional recession points.

found it particularly useful in patients with persistent esotropia. It was less effective in cases of persistent exotropia.

'Hang-loose' technique

The muscle is disinserted and reattached to its original insertion using extended absorbable or nonabsorbable sutures of predetermined length (Fig. 9.8). Not only does this allow very extensive recession, but it also avoids the problems of surgical exposure involved in direct suturing of rectus muscles far back on the globe.

INDICATIONS

The use of these operations is advocated in the management of conditions in which maximum recession gives inadequate correction, for example large-angle infantile esotropia and accommodative esotropia with convergence excess. They may also be useful when reoperation on a previously recessed muscle is indicated or on eyes with thin sclera, as the needle is placed though the thicker sclera at the insertion site and the risk of penetration is less. This is also the method commonly used in adjustable sutures.

PROBLEMS

The site at which the tendon insertion becomes reattached is largely uncontrolled. Indirect reattachment through connective tissue formation around the loops and sutures does not usually occur at the point of maximum conventional recession, as implied

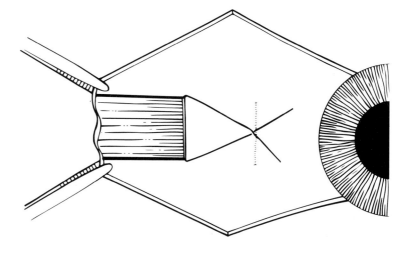

Fig. 9.8 Augmented recession using the 'hang-loose' technique. The rectus muscle has been allowed to retract far posteriorly while remaining indirectly attached to its original insertion via long absorbable or nonabsorbable sutures.

by advocates of these techniques, but the muscle acts from a new direct insertion. If this is excessively posterior, limitation of movement occurs due to loss of muscle action. We do not recommend its use on the superior rectus muscle because the muscle's attachment to the superior oblique is likely to prevent it 'hanging back' sufficiently, making its site of eventual reattachment uncertain.

Z-myotomy

This is another weakening procedure that can be used to augment the effect of recession.

PRINCIPLE

The muscle is lengthened by means of transverse incisions and thereby weakened, but continues to act from its unchanged insertion point.

METHOD

The area of muscle to be cut is first crushed with strong, straight arterial forceps. Three transverse incisions are made through two-thirds of the muscle width at 5 mm intervals behind the muscle insertion, two being placed on one side and the other between them on the opposite side.

INDICATIONS

Although Z-myotomy can be performed as a primary weakening procedure on a rectus muscle, it was more commonly used when a muscle had already been maximally recessed, when it would augment the effect of the recession. There are few indications for using a Z-myotomy in modern strabismus surgery and a recession is preferable, using looped sutures if necessary.

PROBLEMS

The muscle can become adherent to the globe if cauterization is used, therefore this should be avoided. Adhesions do not have the same effect as a posterior fixation suture procedure because lengthening slackens the muscle behind the anomalous reattachments, resulting in loss of muscle action and limitation of movement. The procedure is of limited value.

Posterior fixation suture (Faden operation, retro-equatorial myopexy)

Adelstein and Cüppers (1968) first described this re-latively new concept as a weakening procedure on the contralateral synergist of a paresed lateral rectus. It has subsequently been used in the treatment of a number of different conditions.

The aim of the posterior fixation suture is to produce progressive weakening as the eye moves into the field of action of the operated rectus muscle.

PRINCIPLE

When a rectus muscle contracts, its rotating action is the product of muscle force and the effective length of the lever arm between the centre of rotation of the eye and the muscle's tangential point of contact with the globe. When a muscle is conventionally recessed, the muscle force diminishes because the distance between the muscle's origin and insertion is decreased and the muscle becomes slack. Unless recession is greater than the accepted maximum amount, the lever arm length remains the same as the eye moves from the primary position into the position of main action, because the muscle continues to act through a point tangential to the surface of the globe. The weakening effect is therefore approximately the same in all positions of gaze in which the muscle contracts.

The posterior fixation suture attaches the muscle to the globe well posterior to its insertion, using sutures through the edges of the muscle, causing the lever arm to shorten progressively as the muscle contracts, but without appreciable muscle slackness. Therefore the weakening effect increases as the eye moves further into the field of action of the operated muscle (Scott 1977). Weakening the muscle action is less marked in the straight-ahead position than it is after a conventional recession. The difference between the effect of the posterior fixation suture and that of over-recession is that although the lever arm progressively shortens in both procedures, only over-recession results in increased muscle slackness.

The effect of the posterior fixation suture operation is similar to that of an augmented recession procedure, but limitation of movement is less because muscle slackness is largely avoided. It is very much as if the muscle had been recessed to the point of insertion of the posterior fixation sutures, but also resected by a similar amount.

Probable additional effects of the posterior fixation suture are:

• The sutures through the muscle belly may produce some ischaemia and fibrosis, thus weakening the anterior portion of the muscle.

• A reverse leash effect may be produced, so that there is some progressive mechanical restriction as the eye moves further into the field of action of the operated muscle.

• Some incomitance of movement is produced with contracture of the ipsilateral antagonist and overaction of the contralateral synergist muscles.

• The use of heavy fixation sutures produces quite a large area of scarring, which acts rather like a brake shoe in resisting rotation of the underlying globe.

• The sutures may hold back the orbital fat pad, causing resistance that damps the rotation of the eye.

METHOD

The posterior fixation sutures must be strong and permanent: 5.0 or 6.0 prolene or 3.0 or 4.0 Dacron or Supramid are suitable suture materials. The procedure may be combined with a recession of the muscle.

The principal methods used are as follows:

• The rectus muscle is detached from its insertion and one or more circumferentially placed mattress sutures are used to attach the muscle belly to the underlying sclera. The muscle is then reinserted in its original position or it can be recessed by a given amount (Fig. 9.9a).

• The muscle remains inserted. The edges of the muscle are attached to the globe, including approximately one-fifth of the marginal portion in each suture. The fixation sutures should have three interlocking turns (de Decker 1981) and should be inserted into the sclera a distance of approximately 0.5 mm from the muscle border (Fig. 9.9b).

As the four rectus muscles are attached at different distances behind the limbus and have a common origin medial as well as posterior to the eye, the tangential points of action also differ. The appropriate distances of posterior fixation sutures behind the normal muscle insertions are shown in Table 9.2.

The amount of alteration in the deviation in the primary position produced by the posterior fixation suture largely depends upon how much the muscle is stretched at the time of fashioning its new point of posterior fixation. If the eye is rotated away from the operation site the muscle will be pulled forwards so that the sutures pass from their scleral insertion through the muscle more anteriorly. The muscle behind the point of anchoring is slackening when the eye returns to the straight-ahead position, thus weakening the isometric muscle tone. This results in a significant change in the resting position of the operated eye similar to that induced by muscle recession. The opposite effect is achieved by rotating the eye towards the operation site as the sutures are passed through the muscle.

Posterior fixation may be performed alone (Fig. 9.9b) or can be combined with recession of the muscle insertion (Fig. 9.9a): the effect of recession is increased by the posterior fixation sutures because all muscle slackness is taken up by the length of muscle between the sutures and its point of origin. This combined procedure is rarely used when the marginal fixation technique is employed as it is claimed that, contrary to the original belief, the posterior fixation suture performed using this method weakens the muscle action in the primary position, making additional recession unnecessary. This effect may be the result of damage to the muscle fibres anterior to the whipped marginal sutures as well as to muscle stretching.

INDICATIONS

The procedure is used only on the medial, superior, and inferior rectus muscles. Although it is theoretically possible to perform a posterior fixation suture operation on the lateral rectus, this is rarely if ever carried out and is usually ineffective. Conditions in which the posterior fixation suture operation can be used are:

• lateral rectus palsy, when it is performed on the contralateral medial rectus, producing progressive weakness on adduction to match the existing weakness on abduction;

• accommodative strabismus with convergence excess, particularly when it persists after treatment by other means, including surgery;

• infantile esotropia with face turn to the side of the fixating eye and in the rare cases of the nystagmus blockage syndrome, usually combined with medial rectus recession;

• DVD, when a posterior fixation suture on the superior rectus can reduce elevation without producing hypotropia in the primary position.

The posterior fixation suture may be useful to augment the effect of recession in other cases of manifest strabismus.

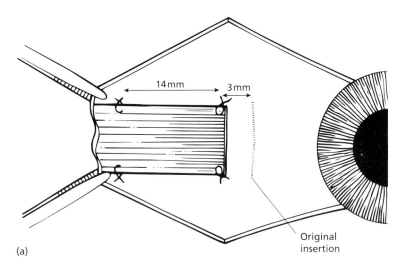

(a)

Original insertion

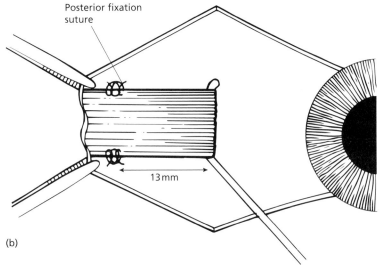

Posterior fixation suture

13 mm

(b)

Fig. 9.9 Two methods of performing a posterior fixation suture (Faden operation). (a) Nonabsorbable sutures applied to both edges of the muscle, which has also been recessed by 3 mm. (b) Strong permanent sutures whipped three times around both edges of the muscle are placed 13 mm behind its undetached insertion.

Table 9.2 Recommended distance of posterior fixation suture behind the normal muscle insertion.

Muscle	Distance
Medial rectus	11–13 mm
Superior and inferior recti	12–14 mm
Lateral rectus*	17–19 mm

* See under Indications for use.

PROBLEMS

The technique of the posterior fixation suture is considerably more difficult than that of recession because the sutures are inserted so far back on the globe. The problems created by this technique are:

• The vortex veins emerge from the sclera close to the edges of the vertical recti at approximately the same distance behind the limbus as the desired fixation sites. This is a particular problem if whipped marginal sutures are used.

- When mattress sutures are placed through the muscle belly they must be attached to the underlying sclera where it is especially thin.
- If dissection is carried out too far posteriorly the orbital fat pad may be opened and fat then prolapses forwards to produce scarring and visible subconjunctival thickening and vascularization. Such a prolapse needs to be excised subsequently, using very hot cautery dissection.
- The heavy permanent sutures may in time cut out, produce significant muscle scarring or result in granuloma formation.
- The operation is not entirely reversible in the medium or long term because of fibrosis.
- Particular problems arise if the posterior fixation suture is performed on the superior rectus (e.g. for DVD): exposure is especially difficult because of the proximity of the orbital roof; the superior oblique tendon lies in the area where the sutures are to be placed. This can be dealt with in one of three ways:

    1 the sutures may be passed through the tendon;
    2 the tendon can be deflected anterior to the sutures;
    3 the tendon can be disinserted and reinserted superficial to the superior rectus muscle after the sutures are in position.

VALUE

The popularity of this method of surgery varies considerably, even in those Western European countries where it is most widely used. The difficulties of technique make it a procedure that should be used only by ophthalmologists with considerable experience in strabismus surgery in carefully selected cases.

Superior oblique muscle weakening operations

The superior oblique muscle can be approached on the nasal or temporal side of the superior rectus muscle. Weakening the action of the muscle can be achieved by a complete or partial tenotomy or a tendon spacer or expander.

Complete tenotomy or tenectomy

Division of the tendon can be carried out nasal or temporal to the superior rectus. Division in the upper nasal quadrant is preferable; the lateral approach has a very uncertain effect as the cut tendon is likely to reattach itself to the superior rectus sheath or to the globe anterior to the equator, changing the secondary actions of the muscle to those of adduction and elevation of the eye.

METHOD

The tendon is identified just medial to the superior rectus muscle. Tenon's capsule and the intermuscular septum surrounding the superior oblique tendon in this position are disturbed as little as possible to maintain the residual indirect postoperative tendon attachments. The tendon within its 'sheath' is brought forward on a muscle hook under direct vision. The intermuscular septum is incised longitudinally and the exposed tendon is completely divided within this septal 'sheath'; the cut ends usually retract some 2–4 mm from each other without change in alignment. The effect of the surgery is more profound if the surrounding tendon 'sheath' is also divided, if a short length (3–4 mm) of the tendon is excised (tenectomy) or if the procedure is carried out closer to the trochlea.

INDICATIONS

Principal uses of the operation are described below.

Brown's syndrome

The operation eliminates or reduces the mechanical limitation of elevation-in-adduction. Overcorrection is not unknown.

A-pattern exotropia

This condition is usually associated with underaction of the inferior rectus muscle and overaction of the superior oblique muscle, often bilateral. Treatment can be directed to weakening the superior obliques or strengthening the inferior recti. Parks (1977) advised bilateral superior oblique tenotomy for large A-patterns in which the exotropia on down-gaze increased by at least 20°, but this procedure can result in insuperable excyclotropia with torsional diplopia (Parks 1986). Buckley and Flynn (1983) reported significant overcorrection. A posterior tenotomy carried out on the temporal side of the superior rectus muscle is effective in collapsing an A-pattern and does not result in significant cyclotorsion. Resection of the inferior rectus muscles is a less effective alternative, which can be augmented by medial transposition of the inferior rectus insertions. Additional horizontal muscle surgery may be required.

Complete third cranial nerve palsy
The constant marked exotropia causes contracture of the lateral rectus and also of the ipsilateral superior oblique. Tenotomy then helps to maintain the eye in the primary position when combined with an extensive recession of the lateral rectus and resection of the medial rectus: it also decreases associated hypotropia and intorsion.

PROBLEMS
The degree of residual superior oblique function is unpredictable: bilateral superior oblique tenotomy may therefore result in some vertical and torsional muscle imbalance in the primary position. Tenotomy in Brown's syndrome can cause superior oblique palsy, requiring additional surgery. In the past, surgeons hooked forwards the superior oblique tendon in the upper nasal quadrant through a small conjunctival incision without direct visual control. This potentially dangerous manoeuvre risked damage to the superior vortex veins, Tenon's capsule and the intermuscular septum, sufficient in some cases to cause extensive fibrosis and an adhesive syndrome. Proper exposure makes such complications very unlikely. Sometimes the cut tendon ends gradually reunite; this risk is less after tenectomy.

Partial tenotomy
In order to maintain the superior oblique's intorting action while reducing its actions of depression and abduction, the posterior four-fifths of the tendon can be divided at its insertion, leaving the anterior part intact.

METHOD
The tendinous insertion is approached at the lateral side of the superior rectus muscle. The eye is rotated downwards and the conjunctiva and Tenon's capsule are retracted upwards to allow tendon dissection under direct vision. An iris repositor can be placed under the insertion to aid identification, care being taken to avoid the upper temporal vortex vein, which

is usually found just posterior to the insertion site. The insertion is buttonholed just behind its most anterior fifth and the posterior tendon is disinserted and allowed to retract under the superior rectus (Fig. 9.10).

Replacing the eyelid speculum with a lid retractor creates more space and gives better posterior access to the insertion.

INDICATIONS
This operation, carried out on both eyes simultaneously, corrects a considerable degree of A-pattern associated with clinically discernible superior oblique overaction (down-drifting of each eye in adduction). It is less likely to cause symptoms from extorsion in down-gaze and a secondary vertical deviation than is complete bilateral superior oblique tenotomy. A unilateral procedure is not very effective in reducing the vertical component of an overacting superior oblique muscle.

Superior oblique tendon expander
A silicon tendon expander produces a quantifiable weakening of the superior oblique muscle and avoids the disadvantages of a complete tenotomy. The procedure was first described by Wright (1989) as a way of controlling the separation of the cut ends of the superior oblique tendon, using a length of silicon retinal detachment band.

METHOD
The superior oblique tendon is approached in an identical way to the complete tenotomy described above, taking care to keep the nasal intermuscular septum intact. The tendon within its 'sheath' is brought forwards on a muscle hook under direct vision, the intermuscular septum is incised longitudinally, and the exposed tendon captured on two small muscle hooks. Two 5.0 double-armed prolene sutures are secured to the tendon using two locking bites; the first is placed 3 mm nasal to the superior rectus muscle and the second 2 mm nasal to the first. The tendon is divided between the two sutures and a length of silicon 240 retinal detachment band (size 2.5×0.6 mm), presoaked in an antibiotic solution, is inserted into the gap and secured to the cut ends of the superior oblique tendon using the sutures (Fig. 9.11). Excess suture is removed

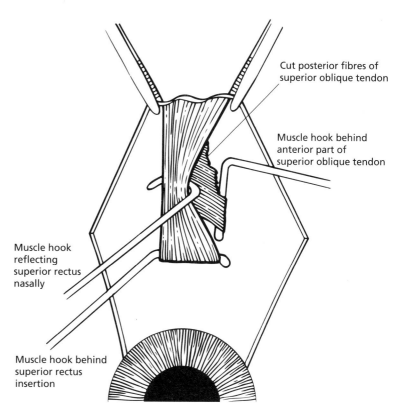

Cut posterior fibres of
superior oblique tendon

Muscle hook behind
anterior part of
superior oblique tendon

Muscle hook
reflecting
superior rectus
nasally

Fig. 9.10 Superior oblique posterior
tenotomy. The muscle hook is placed
behind the insertion of the superior
oblique and the posterior fibres
divided.

Muscle hook behind
superior rectus
insertion

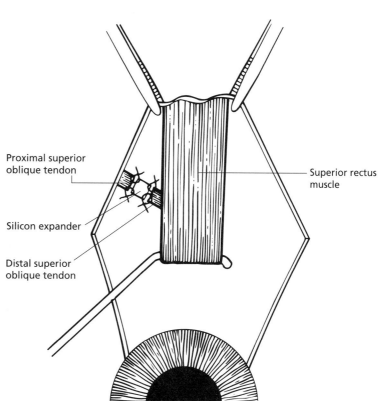

Proximal superior
oblique tendon

Superior rectus
muscle

Silicon expander

Distal superior
oblique tendon

Fig. 9.11 Superior oblique tendon
expander. The superior oblique is
divided on the nasal side of the
superior rectus muscle and the
silicon expander secured to the free
ends of the superior oblique tendon.

Table 9.3 Length of silicon expander and degree of superior oblique overaction.

Superior oblique overaction	Length of silicon expander (mm)
+1	4
+2	5
+3	6
+4	7

Note: When using the expander for Brown's syndrome a minimum length of 6 mm is recommended.

and the intermuscular septum is carefully closed using vicryl sutures to prevent extrusion of the band. Tenons's capsule and conjunctiva are then closed.

The length of silicon expander can be varied depending on the degree of superior oblique overaction or magnitude of the Brown's syndrome (Table 9.3).

INDICATIONS

The indications for use are the same as for complete tenotomy.

Superior oblique tendon expanders are not without complications, those reported include:
• extrusion of the band;
• chronic inflammation requiring the removal of the band;
• residual superior oblique muscle overaction due to missing part or all of the superior oblique tendon.

Superior oblique recession

Recession of the superior oblique tendon is rarely performed, largely because of the technical difficulties arising from its insertion behind the equator. However, the operation was described by Ciancia and Prieto-Diaz (1970) and later modified by Caldiera (1975). Buckley and Flynn (1983) compared the effectiveness of tenotomy and recession of the superior oblique and concluded that tenotomy corrected a larger amount of hypotropia but could result in overcorrection when performed bilaterally. Recession was a more predictable procedure and could be used with adjustable sutures to counter possible undercorrection.

Inferior oblique muscle weakening operations

An overacting inferior oblique can be weakened by:
• disinsertion;
• graded recession;
• myectomy, either temporal or nasal to the inferior rectus muscle;
• Z-tenotomy;
• extirpation.

Disinsertion and recession

Disinsertion

If the inferior oblique muscle belly is simply divided (myotomy) the two cut ends commonly grow together again. Division at the muscle insertion, however, leads to a permanent and effective weakening (Jones *et al.* 1984). This weakening is along the original line of muscle action and although it is uncontrolled, it is usually of only a moderate degree. The cut muscle end may reattach directly to the globe or continue to act indirectly through surrounding connective tissue. In our experience this is an effective procedure; there is less likelihood of postoperative haemorrhage than there is following myectomy, but the operation is potentially more hazardous due to the need to divide the muscle so far posteriorly in proximity to the macula and blood vessels at the posterior pole.

Recession

The aim of this operation is to produce controlled, graded and reversible weakening of all the muscle's actions.

METHOD

The muscle is disinserted, taking special care not to damage the posterior ciliary vessels. The amount of recession can be assessed by three points of reference for reattachment of the anterolateral pole of the muscle insertion:
• 6 mm posterior and 6 mm inferior to the lower pole of the lateral rectus insertion (Fink 1962) gives approximately 8 mm recession (Fig. 9.12a).
• 3 mm posterior and 2 mm temporal to the lateral pole of the inferior rectus insertion gives 10 mm recession (Apt & Call 1978; Fig. 9.12b).
• Reinsertion at the scleral exit of the inferotemporal vortex vein gives maximum 14 mm recession.

The posteromedial pole of the inferior oblique

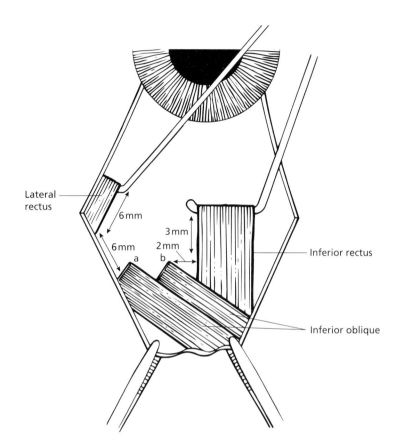

Fig. 9.12 Inferior oblique muscle recession points. The anterolateral pole of the muscle can be reattached. (a) 6 mm posterior and 6 mm inferior to the lower pole of the lateral rectus insertion (8 mm recession). (b) 3 mm posterior and 2 mm lateral to the lateral pole of the inferior rectus insertion (10 mm recession).

insertion can be reattached some 6 mm horizontally behind the anterolateral pole. These new attachment points all leave the line of action of the weakened muscle virtually unchanged.

INDICATIONS
• Primary inferior oblique overaction, often as one aspect of a V-pattern esotropia.
• Secondary inferior oblique overaction, as the ipsilateral antagonist in superior oblique palsy, or as the contralateral synergist in superior rectus palsy.

PRECAUTIONS
Good exposure is essential in order to avoid damage at the muscle insertion close to the macula and to the orbital fat, fascia and inferotemporal vortex vein.

Myectomy
The aim of the operation is to produce a predictable weakening of the inferior oblique muscle without altering its line of action, using a simpler method than recession. Although the procedure is uncontrolled, residual inferior oblique function remains on account of:
• The maintenance of an indirect attachment of the proximal portion to the globe via surrounding connective tissue.
• The attachments of the proximal part of the divided muscle to the inferior rectus sheath, which limit the amount of separation of the cut ends.

Because the normal relationships of the muscle to the inferior rectus sheath and the intermuscular septum have not been disturbed, the residual actions of the muscle are largely unchanged in direction.

METHOD
• The anterior margin of the inferior oblique is identified in the lower temporal quadrant under direct vision. Dissection is carried backwards until the posterior edge of the muscle has been identified.

• The muscle belly is hooked forwards and separated from its sheath and from Tenon's capsule for a distance of some 6 mm, midway between the inferior border of the lateral rectus and the lateral border of the inferior rectus.

• The muscle is crushed with haemostatic forceps and a portion of some 4 mm in length is excised using hot cautery.

• The inferior temporal quadrant is again carefully explored to ensure that no anomalously inserted separate portion of the muscle has been left undivided. The incisions in Tenon's capsule and conjunctiva are then closed.

PRECAUTIONS

Great care must be taken not to damage the inferotemporal vortex vein while dissecting out and hooking forwards the inferior oblique. The muscle belly is very vascular, so that thorough crushing and cauterization is essential before complete division in order to avoid a postoperative haematoma, which would be likely to result in the development of adhesions and mechanical tethering.

PROBLEMS

There is continuing controversy surrounding the efficacy and safety of this operation. Most alarming have been the reports from Parks (1974, 1975) of the common occurrence of a type of adhesive syndrome, which he found postoperatively in 13% of a large series of his own patients. It was caused by anomalous reattachment of the proximal portion of the divided muscle to Tenon's capsule with cicatrized fibrofatty tissue adhering to the temporal border of the inferior rectus or to the inferior border of the lateral rectus. This resulted in progressive hypotropia of the operated eye, with mechanical limitation of elevation. This has not been reported as a common complication by other authors. Toosi and von Noorden (1979) did not encounter this complication at all in more than 1000 patients who had undergone inferior oblique myectomy. Harcourt *et al.* (1981) found no such cases in a series of 156 inferior oblique myectomy operations followed up for a mean period of more than 4 years.

INDICATIONS

These are essentially the same as for inferior oblique recession. One exception is cases in which it is possible that the weakening procedure will need to be reversed. A recession would then certainly be preferred, although reattachment of the insertion near the posterior pole of the eye is a potentially hazardous procedure. In practice, the need for such a reversal very rarely arises.

Comparative value of inferior oblique recession and myectomy

Personal surgical preference depends both on individual experience and on the comparative weight given to the conflicting reports of long-term postoperative complications. Myectomy is certainly a simpler operation, requiring no direct suturing to the globe, which is particularly difficult at the posterior pole of the muscle insertion and close to the inferotemporal vortex vein. The less-experienced surgeon is therefore more likely to prefer myectomy. Published reports suggest that the ability to grade the amount of recession as against the uncontrolled nature of myectomy is of little practical advantage, the long-term results of the two different procedures being very similar (Dunlap 1972; Helveston & Haldi 1976). Harcourt *et al.* (1981) also demonstrated that although the effects of myectomy are variable, there is a noticeable tendency for a large preoperative inferior oblique overaction to be markedly reduced by surgery, whereas a moderate or small initial overaction is much less altered. The residual function of the muscle is therefore approximately the same regardless of the degree of preoperative overaction. We recommend that surgeons should be familiar with a recession of the inferior oblique to enable them to safely perform an anterior transposition of the muscle.

Z-tenotomy

Partial tenotomy of the inferior oblique can be performed in the lower temporal quadrant using essentially the same technique as that employed in weakening rectus muscle function. This produces a variable and uncontrolled reduction of the muscle's power and there is a tendency for the locally crushed and partially divided muscle to adhere postoperatively to the adjacent sclera and surrounding connective tissue.

Extirpation

Complete eradication of inferior oblique muscle function can be achieved by removal of the muscle after disinsertion. The muscle is traced by direct vision towards the floor of the orbit. It is divided by cautery at the point near the origin at which it pierces Tenon's capsule. The stump is oversewn and the nerve and blood supply are cauterized and divided. The stump is then pushed downwards so that it comes to lie external to Tenon's capsule, thus avoiding any risk of adhesion to the inferior rectus (Parks 1976).

This is rarely indicated but may be useful as a secondary procedure when less radical inferior oblique weakening operations have failed to produce the desired profound degree of reduction in muscle function. When the primary weakening of the inferior oblique has failed to reduce the muscle's overaction, the surgeon should always consider that the updrift in adduction may not be due to inferior oblique overaction but can be the result of mechanical or innervational factors.

Effect on the horizontal angle

A weakening procedure on the inferior oblique would be expected to have a secondary effect on the horizontal angle since the muscle is an abductor. However, there is contradictory evidence on whether or not this occurs. We do not routinely adjust the amount of horizontal surgery when combining this with weakening one or both inferior oblique muscles.

Strengthening operations

Rectus muscle strengthening operations

Resection

PRINCIPLE

The muscle is shortened and therefore strengthened, and maintains its action through the point of original insertion. Maximum amounts of resection that will avoid mechanical limitation of ocular movement in the opposite direction are shown in Table 9.1.

METHOD

There are two principal methods:

• Sutures are woven and locked transversely through the muscle belly at the required distance behind the insertion, which is mobilized. The portion of muscle in front of the sutures is excised and the shortened muscle is reattached to the original insertion.

• The muscle tendon is grasped in a muscle clamp. The tendon is divided close to the globe. Mattress sutures are passed through the tendon stump and then through the muscle belly for the required distance posteriorly. After these have been tied the anterior redundant portion of the muscle and tendon is excised.

Surgeons have their individual preferences between the two methods and there is no overwhelming superiority of one over the other.

PRECAUTIONS

If the clamp method is used, the amount of resection is greater if the sutures are passed from behind the tendon stump to exit in front of it than if they are passed in the opposite direction. This is particularly important when performing a small resection. If the central portion of the cut muscle sags behind the new insertion when using the direct suturing method, an additional suture can be inserted through the centre of the tendon stump and the muscle.

INDICATIONS

This is the principal strengthening operation used on the rectus muscles in the treatment of many types of concomitant and incomitant strabismus.

VALUE

Resection is preferable to advancement, in which the muscle insertion is moved a measured amount towards the limbus, both because it is more effective and because the muscle does not become visible through the conjunctiva postoperatively.

The disadvantages of resection are:

• It cannot be reversed, which poses particular problems if over-resection occurs.

• It produces more reaction postoperatively than most other surgical procedures for strabismus because the muscle is transected in a very vascular area, and muscle sutures are inserted not very far behind the limbus.

As already pointed out the effect of resection increases when it is combined with recession of the ipsilateral antagonist.

Advancement is now only rarely carried out except on a recessed muscle that has resulted in overcorrection.

Tucking (plication)

PRINCIPLE

Tucking strengthens the muscle's action by folding the terminal portion of the muscle and tendon, thereby decreasing the muscle length.

METHOD

The muscle is not disinserted. Mattress sutures are passed through the muscle belly at the required point and locked before being passed through the tendinous insertion, tightened and tied. The tendon then forms a tuck superficial to the plane of the muscle.

PRECAUTIONS

• The muscle should not be shortened by more than 3–4 mm, otherwise an ugly raised fold of muscle forms under the conjunctiva.
• The use of permanent sutures creates a risk of granuloma formation and of long-term suture migration and erosion through the conjunctiva.

Rectus muscle tucking is of very limited value and is rarely performed.

Superior oblique muscle strengthening operations

Tucking (plication)

PRINCIPLE

On account of the fibrillary nature of the terminal expansion of the superior oblique tendon, advancement and resection operations, both of which required mobilization and reinsertion of the tendon, are technically difficult and generally unreliable in their effects. Some form of tendon tucking is therefore most widely used as a strengthening procedure.

METHOD

Tucking should only be performed on the temporal side of the superior rectus muscle, close to the tendon insertion.

A tendon tucker is introduced with the middle prong deep to the tendon, lateral to the superior rectus muscle. The tucking screw is tightened until some resistance is felt in the tendon. The fold is then sutured together with 6.0 prolene or equivalent non-absorbable sutures. The tucker is removed and the tucked tendon is folded over laterally and fixed to the sclera by additional sutures if necessary (Fig. 9.13).

Alternatively, a muscle hook can be used to capture the superior oblique tendon and sutures placed into the folded tendon.

The maximum amount that a tendon can be tucked is determined by the degree of iatrogenic Brown's syndrome that may be induced. A normal tendon cannot usually be tucked more than 8 mm before causing an unacceptable Brown's syndrome, but Helveston and Ellis (1983) pointed out that the tendon is often lax in superior oblique palsy, allowing larger tucks of up to 20 mm, and suggested that the degree of laxity rather than the degree of hypertropia should dictate the amount tucked. It is generally accepted that superior oblique tendon tucks are graded intraoperatively and the amount of tuck performed is based on the degree of tendon laxity, on intraoperative forced duction testing and on the spring-back test.

GRADING THE TUCK

The tuck can be graded using an intraoperative forced duction test or by the spring-back test.
• Intraoperative forced duction test. After securing the tuck the limbal conjunctiva is grasped at the 6 o'clock position using toothed forceps and the eye is rotated medially then superiorly. If the tuck is adequate, firm resistance will be felt as the 6 o'clock limbus reaches an imaginary line drawn between the medial and lateral canthus. If the tuck is excessive, resistance will be felt before that point is reached and the induced iatrogenic Brown's syndrome is unlikely to be tolerated by the patient and the tuck should be revised. If the eye can be rotated above this line then the tuck is inadequate: if this is the case the tuck should be revised and the forced duction test repeated.
• Spring-back test. The eye is grasped at the 6 o'clock limbus on completion of the tuck, rotated upwards and then released, when it should spring back to a position just below an imaginary line drawn between the medial and lateral canthi. If the eye returns to a position well below this line or remains above it the tuck is taken down and modified and the spring-back test repeated.

Both tests are useful in grading the amount of superior oblique tuck performed.

This operation can be modified to achieve a moderate increase in intorsion without altering the depressing and abducting actions of the superior oblique

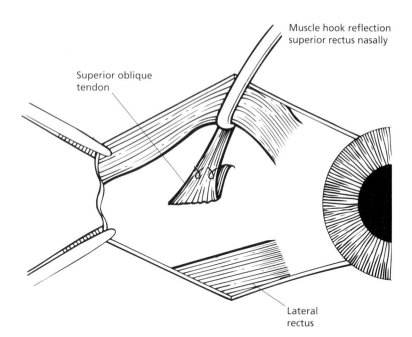

Muscle hook reflection
superior rectus nasally

Superior oblique
tendon

Lateral
rectus

Fig. 9.13 Superior oblique tuck (plication). The whole of the terminal portion of the tendon has been folded over laterally and the apposing surfaces secured together using nonabsorbable sutures.

muscle. Only the anterior portion of the tendon is folded laterally at the insertion. An iris spatula can be laid along the line of the insertion and a triangular portion of tendon folded laterally with its apex posterior. This fold is sutured to the sclera.

INDICATION

Tucking is a useful procedure when a superior oblique palsy is characterized by hypertropia that is greatest on down-gaze. It is most effective in congenital superior oblique palsy when considerable tendon laxity is often present. The risk of producing a significant iatrogenic Brown's syndrome means that this procedure should be used with caution in acquired palsies.

PROBLEMS

Mechanically induced limitation of elevation in adduction due to shortening of the tendon is common postoperatively. However, if intraoperative grading of the tuck is used it is rarely problematic. Patients should be warned that diplopia is likely to occur in up-gaze and that the aim of the procedure is to exchange diplopia on down-gaze for some diplopia in less-used up-gaze. Transient insuperable cyclotorsion is common postoperatively and usually resolves spontaneously.

VALUE

This procedure provides a practical means of strengthening the superior oblique. It is largely reversible and if a troublesome Brown's syndrome results, the tuck can be taken down. Helveston and Ellis (1983) found that this method was effective in reducing all three elements of the palsy—the head tilt, hypertropia and excyclotropia. If used appropriately it is an important procedure in the management of superior oblique palsy.

Inferior oblique muscle strengthening operations
Advancement

The inferior oblique lacks a tendinous portion and cannot be plicated. Its far posterior insertion close to important delicate structures makes surgery hazardous and strengthening is very rarely undertaken. Conrad and de Decker (1984) have described advancement of the muscle as part of their complex procedure for reduction of a head tilt associated with congenital nystagmus.

Transposition operations

Transposition refers to moving the whole or part of a muscle in order to change its primary or secondary actions.

Rectus muscle transposition operations

Whole muscle transposition

Either the horizontal or the vertical recti can be transposed. Muscles can be transposed singly, in ipsilateral pairs—for example, the right lateral and medial rectus, or the right inferior and superior rectus—or in contralateral pairs—for example, the medial recti or the lateral recti.

AIMS

Ipsilateral pairs of muscles are transposed in order to rotate the eye in the direction of the transposition. Contralateral pairs of muscles are transposed symmetrically and ipsilateral pairs asymmetrically in order to alter V- and A-patterns. Ipsilateral pairs can be transposed asymmetrically to correct cyclotropia.

METHOD

The tendon is disinserted and reattached in the indicated position. To change a V- or A-pattern or correct cyclotropia, a half to full rectus muscle width of transposition may be required. To assist the action of an adjacent rectus muscle, for example lateral transposition of the vertical recti in lateral rectus palsy, a minimum of a whole rectus muscle width transposition is needed (Fig. 9.14), and in cases of severe limitation of ocular movement the transposed muscles should be reinserted alongside the adjacent rectus insertion. Unless weakening or strengthening of the transposed muscle's main action is intended through recession or resection, respectively, the new insertion should maintain the same distance behind the limbus. The new insertion can be 'bunched up' without interfering with its function.

PRECAUTIONS

Care should be taken to transpose pairs of muscles an equal amount otherwise muscle imbalance is created which can be an obstacle to binocular single vision.

Jampolsky (1986) has reported immediate or delayed overcorrection following whole muscle transposition.

INDICATIONS

• V- and A-patterns can be treated by transposition of the horizontal recti and, more rarely, by transposition of the vertical recti. These operations are commonly associated with recession or resection, usually performed symmetrically on the medial recti and less often on the lateral recti.

• Horizontal transposition of the vertical recti can be used to correct cyclotropia or induce a cyclodeviation when managing head tilts in congenital nystagmus associated with a null zone (von Noorden & Chu

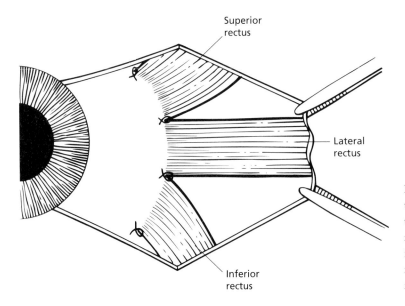

Superior rectus

Lateral rectus

Inferior rectus

Fig. 9.14 Whole muscle transposition procedure. In the treatment of a total lateral rectus muscle palsy the superior and inferior recti are detached and the muscles transposed laterally one full muscle width.

1990). This is one of the few procedures that can correct insuperable incyclotropia. Surgery to both vertical recti of one eye can correct 6–8° of cyclotropia; the amount of correction achieved can be doubled by operating on both eyes. Vertical transposition of the horizontal recti is a less effective alternative in our hands but may be indicated if previous surgery has been carried out on the horizontal muscles.

• The Knapp procedure used to correct double elevator palsy: the medial and lateral recti are reinserted alongside the medial and lateral borders of the superior rectus insertion to elevate the eye (Knapp 1969). This is also effective in correcting moderate amounts of hypotropia when operating on the horizontal recti for esotropia or exotropia.

• The inverse Knapp procedure for inferior rectus palsy: the medial and lateral recti are reinserted alongside the medial and lateral borders of the inferior rectus insertion to augment the action of the muscle. This is also effective in correcting moderate amounts of hypertropia when operating on the horizontal recti for esotropia or exotropia.

• Lateral rectus paralysis: the superior and inferior recti are transposed to the upper and lower poles of the lateral rectus insertion (Fig. 9.14). This must be combined with a medial rectus and conjunctival recession if contracture has occurred, causing a significant risk of anterior segment ischaemia in the older patient. The injection of botulinum toxin A into the medial rectus before contracture occurs and at the time of surgery will avoid the necessity of medial rectus recession and should be regarded as the management of choice for total lateral rectus palsy.

• Duane's syndrome, type A: the procedure used for lateral rectus paralysis is carried out.

• Medial rectus paralysis: the superior and inferior recti are first resected by 5 mm then transposed to the upper and lower poles of the medial rectus insertion. Resection is required to compensate for the slackening that occurs when the muscles are medially transposed.

• Lost muscle: a rectus muscle may retract to the orbital apex outside the muscle cone after accidental injury or during or after strabismus surgery. If it cannot be located and reinserted, the two adjacent rectus muscles can be transposed to its severed insertion in

order to stabilize the eye in an approximately straight position.

Part-muscle transposition

In part-muscle transposition only half the muscle is mobilized and transposed, reducing the risk of anterior segment ischaemia (see below). Usually two muscles are utilized and transposed to a third.

The main types of part-muscle transposition are outlined below.

Hummelsheim's operation

The lateral halves of the superior and inferior recti are disinserted and the medial and lateral fibres of each muscle are separated for a distance of approximately 15 mm behind their insertions. The lateral half of each muscle is reinserted alongside the upper and lower poles of the lateral rectus.

This procedure is used in lateral rectus paralysis, and in nearly all cases it is also necessary to recess the contracted ipsilateral medial rectus (see Chapter 19).

Variations on Hummelsheim's operation

• The same principle can be applied to treat limitation of adduction, although this is a very rare condition. The medial halves of the vertical recti are first resected by 5 mm and are then transposed to the borders of the medial rectus.

• The medial and lateral recti can be similarly used, for example in cases of double elevator palsy, when the upper halves of the horizontal recti are transposed to the borders of the superior rectus. This procedure is rarely used.

Jensen's operation

Jensen's operation utilizes transposition without disinserting the tendons of the muscles involved, thus maintaining the anterior segment blood supply with greater certainty. Three adjacent rectus muscles are split in half along the line of their muscle fibres from just behind the insertion to a point 15 mm posterior to it. If this procedure is used for lateral rectus paralysis, the lateral halves of the superior and inferior recti are tied fairly loosely to the upper and lower halves of the split lateral rectus, using strong nonabsorbable sutures (Jensen 1964). The ties are made some 12 mm

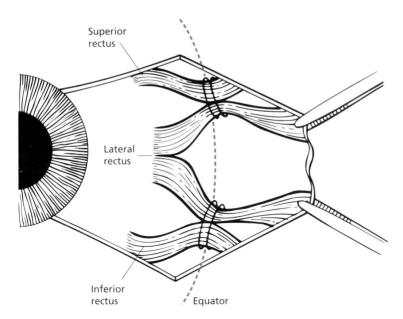

Superior
rectus

Lateral
rectus

Inferior
rectus

Equator

Fig. 9.15 Jensen's transposition operation. The lateral, superior and inferior rectus muscles have been split longitudinally. The apposing halves of the lateral and inferior recti, and the lateral and superior recti have been sutured together at the level of the equator.

behind the limbus (Fig. 9.15). Jensen's operation has been adapted for the correction of hypotropia, achieved by splitting the superior rectus muscle (Callahan 1981) and both horizontal recti and creating a posterior union between them.

PRECAUTIONS

The sutures should be tied loosely in Jensen's operation to avoid crushing the muscle fibres and causing ischaemia, but should be tight enough to prevent the suture loops gradually migrating forwards from their original positions.

INDICATIONS FOR USE

Part-muscle transpositioning is used in muscle paralysis and double elevator palsy, particularly if the patient is elderly with a poor blood circulation or when a third rectus muscle is disinserted on account of tethering or contracture. Although severe acute anterior segment ischaemia is very rare (Simon *et al.* 1984), it is more likely to occur if more than two rectus muscles are operated on, even if there is an interval between operations (see below).

PROBLEMS

Apart from the risks of anterior segment ischaemia the main problems are:

- Vertical muscle imbalance when Hummelsheim's operation is used for lateral rectus paralysis.
- Long-term changes in the position of the eye due to slippage of the permanent sutures following Jensen's operation.

Other part-muscle transposition procedures

Lateral rectus muscle stabilization

In the treatment of up-shoot and down-shoot that occurs on adduction in Duane's retraction syndrome a stabilization procedure on the lateral rectus muscle can effectively prevent the globe slipping over the ipsilateral lateral rectus muscle on attempted adduction. Jampolsky (1984) advised recession and bifurcation of the lateral rectus, suturing one half of the muscle to the globe above its original insertion and suturing the other half below the original insertion to prevent slippage of the globe (Fig. 9.16).

Anterior ciliary vessel sparing procedure

The anterior ciliary arteries can be dissected from the rectus muscle before performing the transposition to minimize the risk of anterior segment ischaemia. This is a delicate procedure requiring the cauterization of the collaterals from the main anterior ciliary vessels before separating them from the muscle. See section on Rectus muscle weakening operations p. 175 for more details.

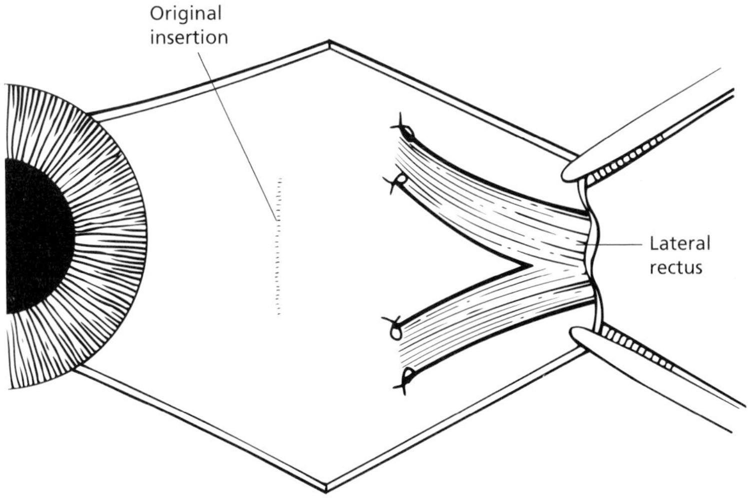

Original insertion

Lateral rectus

Fig. 9.16 Lateral rectus muscle stabilization procedure. The lateral rectus muscle has been split longitudinally 8 mm posteriorly and the muscle recessed, suturing one half of the muscle to the globe above its original insertion and suturing the other half below the original insertion to prevent slippage of the globe.

Value of rectus muscle transposition

Whole-muscle transposition of the horizontal recti is a valuable and successful method of treating V- and A-patterns (see Chapter 17). Hummelsheim's operation and the Jensen's procedure have been largely superseded in cases of muscle paralysis by whole-muscle transposition of the horizontal or vertical recti combined with botulinum toxin. This method provides a means of achieving good eye position with some degree of movement, particularly in lateral rectus paralysis in which the eye cannot move to the mid-line preoperatively. Part muscle transposition or anterior ciliary vessels sparing procedures still have a role when there is a high risk of anterior segment ischaemia.

None of these operations will be successful if there is mechanical limitation of ocular movement. Preoperative forced duction tests are therefore of critical importance. All tethers must be released as a preliminary surgical procedure, taking care to minimize the risks of acute anterior segment ischaemia by transecting no more than two whole rectus tendon insertions from the globe at a single operation.

Superior oblique muscle transposition operations
Harada–Ito procedure

The intorting action of the superior oblique muscle can be increased without significantly disturbing its depressing and abducting actions if only the anterior half of the tendon insertion is mobilized and reinserted more laterally and anteriorly. Although this procedure was first suggested by Harada and Ito (1964), the most commonly used modification was described by Fells (1976) and is outlined below.

METHOD

The anterior third of the superior oblique tendon is disinserted and split from the posterior portion along the line of its fibres for some 10 mm. The mobilized portion is then reattached 8 mm posterior to the lateral rectus insertion and just above that muscle's upper margin (Fig. 9.17). Parks (1983) has stated that bilateral reinsertion at the lateral rectus upper border corrects 15–20° of excyclodeviation, while bilateral reattachment 4 mm above the border corrects 4–8° of excyclodeviation.

Metz and Lerner (1981) have described the use of adjustable sutures in the Harada–Ito procedure.

INDICATIONS

This is the operation of choice in patients with unilateral or bilateral superior oblique palsies whose symptoms are mainly due to the excyclodeviation. It is more satisfactory in those circumstances than an inferior oblique weakening procedure, which mainly reduces extorsion on elevation of gaze. It is also preferable to superior oblique tucking, which not only increases all the muscles' actions, but also commonly causes mechanical limitation of elevation-in-adduction (acquired Brown's syndrome).

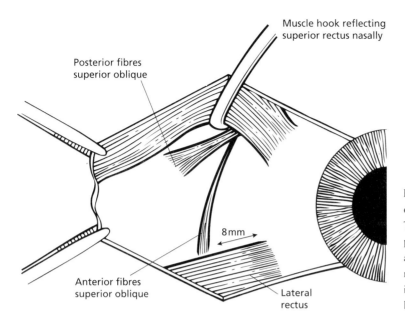

Muscle hook reflecting
superior rectus nasally

Posterior fibres
superior oblique

8 mm

Anterior fibres
superior oblique

Lateral
rectus

Fig. 9.17 Harado–Ito superior oblique transposition procedure. The anterior third of the terminal portion of the tendon has been advanced and anteroposed, being reattached 8 mm behind the insertion and just above the upper border of the lateral rectus muscle.

PROBLEMS

A vertical deviation may sometimes be revealed after operation, and overcorrection may occur, inducing intorsion in the less-used elevated positions of gaze. Neither of these complications is very serious and secondary adjustment of the transpositions can be carried out satisfactorily if required.

Inferior oblique muscle transposition operations
Desagittalization

The extorting action of the inferior oblique can be enhanced and the elevating and abducting actions decreased if the muscle is disinserted and reattached in a more transverse direction relative to the antero-posterior axis of the globe.

METHOD

Desagittalization can be achieved by total disinsertion and reattachment of the anterolateral pole of the muscle insertion at the equator of the globe midway between the lateral and inferior recti.

INDICATIONS

Gobin (1969) has claimed that one of the principal precipitating causes of strabismus in early childhood is a developmental defect in the angles at which the oblique muscles are inserted into the globe (see Chap-

ter 17). V-pattern esotropia results when the line of action of the inferior obliques is orientated in a more anteroposterior direction than normal (sagittalization). He believed that the correct treatment in such cases was bilateral medial rectus recession, often requiring augmentation with loop sutures, together with recession and desagittalization of both inferior obliques. This procedure is rarely performed today.

Inferior oblique anterior transpositioning

Transposition of the inferior oblique insertion anteriorly so that it lies alongside the inferior rectus muscle insertion is an effective treatment for DVD.

METHOD

The inferior oblique muscle is disinserted from the globe through a standard inferior-temporal conjunctival incision close to the lower fornix. Absorbable sutures are placed at the anterior and posterior extent of the insertion and the muscle transposed anteriorly and medially so that it lies adjacent to the lateral border of the inferior rectus muscle insertion (Fig. 9.18). The anterior suture is placed adjacent to the inferior rectus insertion, and the posterior suture approximately 2–3 mm lateral to this, taking care not to position it more anteriorly or laterally. The mechanism by which the inferior oblique anterior transposition

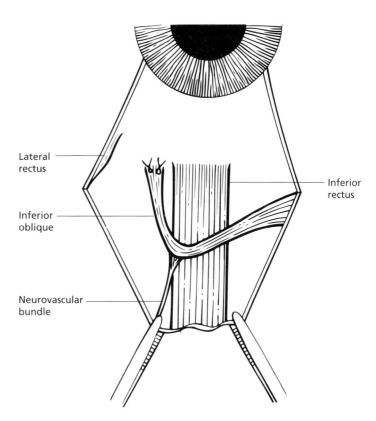

Lateral
rectus

Inferior
oblique

Neurovascular
bundle

Inferior
rectus

Fig. 9.18 Inferior oblique anterior transpositioning. Absorbable sutures are placed at the anterior and posterior extent of the inferior oblique insertion and the muscle transposed anteriorly and medially so that it lies adjacent to the lateral border of the inferior rectus muscle insertion.

works has been discussed recently (Stager 1998). The nerve and vascular supply to the inferior oblique share a common entry into the muscle, the neurofibrovascular bundle, 2 mm temporal to the lateral border of the inferior rectus or 12 mm from the inferior oblique insertion. The bundle is a taut, inelastic structure and in the normal situation does not appear to have any effect on the function of the inferior oblique. However, when the posterior fibres of the inferior oblique are transposed adjacent to the inferior rectus insertion they are put on stretch between the neurofibrovascular bundle and this new insertion; the bundle then effectively acts as the new origin for these fibres (Fig. 9.18).

This changes the function of the inferior oblique and is effective in the treatment of DVD by:
• Increasing the tonic depression force in the primary position. Most anterior transpositions are bilateral and symmetrical, minimizing the risk of inducing a hypotropia in the primary position. Performed unilaterally it has proved useful in the treatment of large angle nonrestrictive hypertropia in patients without

fusion. The anterior transposition should not move the new insertion anterior to the inferior rectus insertion nor place the posterior fibres in an excessive lateral position, as this can exaggerate the effect of the procedure and result in an elevation deficiency in the abducted position or pseudo-overaction of the contralateral eye (Stein & Ellis 1997).
• Contracture of the inferior oblique when the eye attempts to elevate. The neurofibrovascular bundle acting as the new functional origin of the muscle leads to paradoxical contraction of the inferior oblique, exerting a depressor force on the globe. Up-gaze is only mildly restricted by this procedure, but problems can occur if the posterior fibres of the inferior oblique are reattached in a more lateral position, resulting in abduction of the eye on elevation and a V-pattern on up-gaze (Kushner 1997).

INDICATIONS

Inferior oblique anterior transpositioning is indicated for the treatment of DVD and large nonrestrictive hypertropias in patients without binocular single vision.

The surgical treatment of DVD is influenced by whether or not there is associated oblique muscle dysfunction:

• DVD with inferior oblique muscle overaction, with or without a V-pattern. Bilateral inferior oblique anterior transposition is recommended.
• DVD with superior oblique muscle overaction with an A-pattern. A bilateral superior oblique posterior tenotomy combined with recession of the superior rectus muscle is the preferred option.
• DVD without an alphabet pattern. Recession of the superior rectus muscles is the procedure of choice.

Conjunctival closure

The conjunctival incisions are best closed with 6.0 or 7.0 absorbable sutures, taking care not to trap any Tenon's capsule in the incision line, which may result in granuloma formation. Bulky knots at the limbus should be avoided as they interfere with the corneal tear film and may cause 'dellen', areas of marginal corneal thinning due to dryness. Dexon and Vicryl sutures take some weeks to absorb, but if the material is tied tightly the sutures will usually cut out of the conjunctiva within a few days, which is sufficient time to allow adhesion of the incision.

Other surgical procedures

Adjustable sutures

The ability to modify the position of a newly operated muscle by the use of adjustable sutures has given the ophthalmologist control over the early postoperative surgical outcome. Adjustable sutures were reintroduced to strabismus surgery by Jampolsky in 1975 after an absence of more than 50 years (Jampolsky 1975). Previous techniques failed to gain popularity probably because the surgeon lacked the thin absorbable suture of high tensile strength and low antigenicity that is now available. Although adjustable sutures afford the modern strabismus surgeon control over the early postoperative alignment, they are not a substitute for a careful and complete strabismus examination or a poor operative technique.

Selection of patients

The use of adjustable sutures should be considered in any cooperative patient undergoing strabismus surgery. Those unlikely to tolerate the procedure can usually be identified following careful preoperative evaluation. The reasons for not proceeding with adjustable sutures include:

• Surgical procedures that do not benefit from the use of adjustable sutures. Examples include inferior and superior oblique weakening and superior oblique tuck.
• The patient is too young. Most patients below the age of 14 years do not cooperate well with adjustable sutures, although we have successfully treated some 11- and 12-year-olds.
• An uncooperative adult. Behavioural, psychological or medical handicaps obvious during the examination make it unsafe to use adjustable sutures. A few adult patients are apprehensive about the procedure and any doubts about their likely compliance can be assessed by instilling local anaesthetic drops into the conjunctival fornix and moving the globe with either nontoothed forceps or a cotton-tipped bud (Fells 1988). Patients tolerating this procedure are likely to be cooperative with adjustable sutures.

Indications

Adjustment can be applied to all the extraocular muscles but is less often used in oblique muscle surgery. Postoperative adjustment can be employed in recession, resection and transposition procedures although it is most commonly used with recession operations. The sutures allow adjustment of the amount of recession when the effects of the anaesthetic have worn off but before the healing process has commenced, or before completing an operation if carried out under topical anaesthesia.

Adjustable sutures are particularly useful when:
• it is difficult to predict the outcome of conventional surgery;
• the restoration of binocular single vision is expected;
• there is a risk of postoperative diplopia.

The following conditions respond well to postoperative or intraoperative adjustments:
• Dysthyroid eye disease, when just sufficient surgery to enable the patient to fuse his diplopia can be achieved by adjustment.

• Vertical muscle palsies: patients with congenital palsies are often more comfortable when undercorrected, whereas accurate correction is essential in acquired palsies. The patient's diplopia can be used as a guide to the amount of adjustment needed.

• Patients undergoing cosmetic surgery who are at risk of developing postoperative diplopia. Adjustment can alter the deviation to place the unwanted image in the suppression scotoma.

• Reoperations, when the amount of muscle surgery is difficult to gauge and its effect is unpredictable.

Methods

Sutures can be adjusted under local or general anaesthesia: surgery and adjustment can be performed as a one-stage procedure when local anaesthesia is used whereas adjustment is postponed until the patient is awake and alert when using general anaesthesia. In other respects the technique used is the same.

At operation

The initial recession technique must be modified to allow later adjustment. The surgical guidelines were laid down in detail by Jampolsky (1978), and many minor modifications have since been described. The important points are:

• The conjunctival incision must be left sufficiently open for the muscle sutures to be accessible.

• The recessed muscle must be sutured to the globe in such a way that the sutures can be loosened and

the muscle tendon either drawn forwards or allowed to retract posteriorly at the time of adjustment (Figs 9.19–9.21). This requires that:

1 the temporary suture knots can easily be untied but will not slip spontaneously prior to readjustment;

2 the suture material can run freely through the intrascleral channels at the time of adjustment. The material must be strong enough to allow this delayed manipulation: coated Dexon or Vicryl, gauge 5.0 or 6.0, are excellent for this purpose. The easy passage of the sutures through the sclera can be aided by widening the scleral tunnels at operation, moving the sutures backwards and forwards with sideways pressure before the temporary slip-knots are tied.

• To hold the eye steady during adjustment a temporary heavy gauge loop 'handle' suture can be placed at the lower border of a horizontal rectus insertion or at the nasal edge of a vertical rectus. This avoids the need to apply fixation forceps during adjustment and aids performing a re-recession. A 6.0 prolene suture is suitable.

• Using material differing in colour as well as gauge can simplify identification and differentiation of the sutures.

• The scleral attachments of the muscle sutures must be arranged so that the tendon insertion will maintain a stable, designated position during the healing period after the sutures have been finally tied.

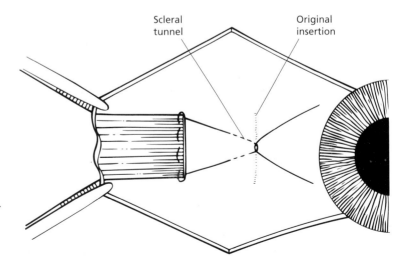

Fig. 9.19 Bow-tie type adjustable suture. The sutures are passed through scleral tunnels, which commence just posterior to the original muscle insertion and are angled forwards towards each other. A temporary knot consisting of a double throw and a half bow-tie is used to secure the suture.

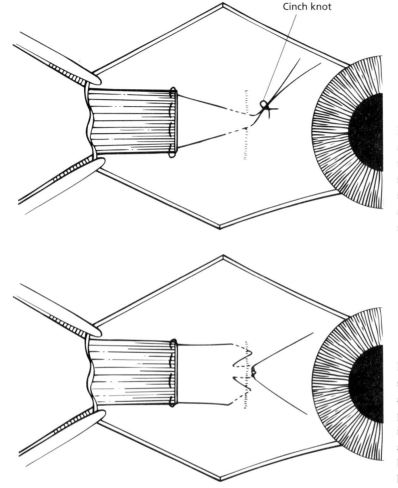

Cinch knot

Fig. 9.20 Cinch or sliding knot adjustable suture technique. The technique is similar to the crossswords except the two arms of the suture brought out close together at the insertion are lassoed with a second piece of vicryl.

Fig. 9.21 Fells type of adjustable suture technique. The two sutures are first passed forwards through the poles of the original rectus muscle insertion, and then passed forwards again a second time, more centrally, before being tied in a temporary knot.

Intraoperative adjustment

If the surgery is carried out using only topical conjunctival anaesthesia, successful adjustments can be made before the completion of the operation if the patient is fully alert and cooperative. A fixation target above the operating table can be used, otherwise an adjustable operating couch which allows the patient to be sat upright during the measurement then lain back down again for the adjustment is our preferred choice. The operating lamp is extinguished to avoid dazzle and ocular alignment is assessed by means of the cover test or prism reflection test at near and distance.

Chow (1989) compared the results of one-stage adjustable sutures, in which adjustment was made on the table, with a series of patients treated using twostage adjustable sutures. Comparable results in terms of stability were reported.

Postoperative adjustment

This is by far the more common method employed. The surgery is reviewed and any necessary adjustment is made within 24 h of the operation—either the same day, in which case the procedure can be performed as a day case, or the following morning. Postoperative adjustment can be carried out in the ophthalmic examination room; however, our preferred place is at the bedside. An ophthalmic-trained nurse familiar with adjustable sutures is an important member of the team and can relieve the patient's anxiety and apprehension. The patient must be alert and cooperative, with no residual effects of the anaesthetic that might influence the resting and active muscle tone. It has been shown that postoperative alignment can change shortly after the eye pad is removed and we therefore recommend waiting at least 30 min before starting any adjustment; during this period local anaesthetic drops are instilled in the eye being adjusted.

Sixty per cent of our patients require adjustment after surgery, and the stages in adjustment are as follows:

• The muscle balance is first assessed by observation of the corneal light reflexes and by a cover test for near and distance. The deviation is measured in the primary position using the prism cover test.

• The assistant positions the light source so that the eye is well illuminated; a light fixed to a headband allows the assistant's hands to be free to help during the procedure.

• The lid speculum is inserted and the patient instructed to move the eye into the desired position; the loop handle suture, held by the assistant, can be used if necessary.

• The temporary knot is untied and adjustment made. It is easier to reduce the slack of an over-recessed muscle than it is to augment under-recession. The sutures soften slightly overnight and great care must be taken not to break them by overstrong traction.

• The muscle balance is reassessed, both in the primary position and in the field of action of the operated muscle; further adjustment is made if necessary.

• Once a satisfactory eye position has been achieved the sutures are tied and cut. The conjunctiva is usually sutured, in a recessed position if necessary, although we did not find any difference in the cosmetic outcome when leaving the conjunctiva recessed or replacing it (Simmons *et al.* 1997).

Postoperative suture adjustment was not required in 40% of our patients. In such cases the suture can be secured and the loop handle removed before replacing the conjunctiva.

Problems

• Any delay between surgery and subsequent adjustment in the two-stage procedure leads to an increased likelihood of the muscle adhering to the sclera and surrounding tissues, making any subsequent adjustment more difficult. Tissue oedema is also likely to increase postoperatively and can further hamper adjustment.

• Traction on the extraocular muscles can slow the heart rate through the ocular cardiac reflex and result in serious problems during general anaesthesia (Apt *et al.* 1973), but may go unnoticed by patients during postoperative adjustment (Eustis *et al.* 1992).

• Access to the superior rectus is made difficult by the overhanging superior orbital margin and by a strong Bell's phenomenon, which makes it more difficult to control the adjustment procedure. Improved postoperative knot access can be obtained by placing the sutures anterior to the original insertion.

• Helveston (1987) reported slippage of the inferior rectus when adjustable sutures were used (see below), and other authors have recommended using nonabsorbable adjustable sutures when recessing this muscle. In our practice we have not found slippage of the inferior rectus muscle to be a significant problem and we continue to use absorbable sutures.

Anchoring sutures

These can be used in an attempt to prevent the recurrence of tethering due to muscle contracture and to help stabilize large angle deviations associated with muscle paralysis. Muscle contracture is a preoperative feature of long-standing large-angle strabismus with a marked mechanical element. The aim is to anchor the eye in a position opposite to that of the tether: for example, if the medial rectus is severely contracted, the eye is anchored in an abducted position.

Indications

Conditions in which anchoring sutures may be helpful include:

• Total third nerve palsy. The exotropia associated with medial rectus paralysis is managed by a large lateral rectus recession and medial rectus resection. Despite the use of an extensive amount of surgery there is still a tendency for the exotropia to recur. The combined use of horizontal rectus surgery and traction sutures to anchor the eye in adduction for a 6-week postoperative period is therefore recommended (Lee & Gregson 1993). We perform a 12–16 mm recession of the lateral rectus combined with a 8–10 mm resection of the medial rectus muscle and use anchoring sutures to fix the eye in adduction for 4–6 weeks.

• Large-angle fixed divergent or convergent strabismus.

• Lateral incomitance due to contracture of the medial rectus muscle or surrounding tissue. If there is diplopia on side-gaze without a significant deviation in the primary position, recession of the contracted tissue or botulinum toxin injection to the medial rectus can be used, augmented by anchoring the eye in abduction.

Method

When muscle surgery has been completed, ethibond traction sutures are passed under the insertion sites of both vertical recti and brought out through the medial or lateral aspect of the upper and lower lids. The sutures are tied over short lengths of rubber bolster or silastic retinal detachment explant, providing the necessary tension to keep the eye anchored in adduction or abduction for 4–6 weeks (Fig. 9.22).

Problems

Postoperative problems include:

• absence of eye movement, forcing the patient to use extensive head movement.

• overlapping diplopia, preventing the lifting of any ptosis.

• overaction of the contralateral synergic muscles, which can cause a variable and unsightly deviation if the affected eye is used for fixation;

• erosion of the anchoring sutures through the skin, requiring premature removal.

Value

The results are generally good although postoperative discomfort can necessitate premature removal of the sutures.

Conjunctival recession

Mechanical restriction of eye movement may be due to contracture not only of muscles or fascia, but also of conjunctiva. If an eye has been held habitually in an eccentric position, then the conjunctiva overlying the tight muscle will certainly have contracted and this

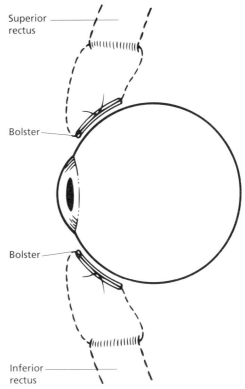

Fig. 9.22 Anchoring sutures. Ethibond traction sutures have been passed under the insertion sites of both vertical recti and brought out through the medial aspect of the upper and lower lids. The sutures are tied over short lengths of rubber bolster or silastic retinal detachment explant, providing the necessary tension to keep the eye anchored in adduction for 4–6 weeks.

must be taken into account at operation. The conjunctiva is resutured directly onto the sclera well back from the limbal incision, possibly as posterior as the underlying rectus muscle insertion. The epithelium rapidly regrows over the exposed sclera.

Surgical complications

Strabismus surgery is essentially safe, and serious complications are few, although events as catastrophic as division of the optic nerve in mistake for the inferior oblique muscle have occasionally been reported. However, various complications can arise, and these are considered below.

Infection

Prevention

Surgery must be postponed if there is clinical evidence of conjunctivitis or blepharitis in the immediate preoperative period. If there has been a recent history of either condition but with no sign of active inflammation on admission to hospital, the operation can proceed but should be covered by a systemic antibiotic. A drug with a broad spectrum of activity, especially against coagulase-positive staphylococci, is needed; ampicillin is appropriate unless the patient is allergic to penicillin, in which case erythromycin is a satisfactory alternative.

Topical antibiotics need not be given routinely during or after strabismus surgery unless there has been a suggestion of preoperative infection.

Treatment

If a postoperative infection is suspected, a conjunctival swab should be taken for Gram's stain and culture. Synthetic penicillin such as ampicillin or cloxacillin is given systemically in high dosage in the absence of allergy until the infection organism has been isolated and the antibiotic sensitivities are known.

Sterile inflammation

Excessive inflammatory response may be mechanical and chemical rather than infective, especially if catgut sutures have been used or following reoperation. A slowly reducing regimen of topical steroid eye drops should then be prescribed.

Damage to a vortex vein

If a vortex vein is torn, it bleeds profusely, and if it cannot be cauterized successfully it should be tied off using a fine absorbable suture. Occlusion of one vortex vein occasionally causes choroidal haemorrhage, but usually no complication ensues.

Penetration of the globe with a suture needle

This is uncommon and usually only occurs to a minimal and harmless extent. If the needle penetrates deeply into the eye, then the risk of complications depends on the exact site of injury.

• If the perforation is anterior to the ora serrata (7 mm behind the limbus), it passes through the pars plana of the ciliary body and complications are rare. Endophthalmitis can develop if infection is introduced, and incarceration of vitreous in the wound may eventually lead to tractional retinal detachment. The scleral wound should be carefully closed.

• If the perforation is behind the ora serrata, the pupil must immediately be fully dilated so that thorough internal examination can be made using the indirect ophthalmoscope and scleral indentation. If the penetrating needle has passed through the choroid and incised the retina there is a strong risk that a retinal detachment will develop. The area surrounding the retinal break should immediately be treated with cryotherapy in such cases. If the retina is elevated around the retinal tear, a small plomb may need to be applied to the overlying scleral surface to buckle it inwards, producing chorioretinal contact and permanent adhesion.

Anterior segment ischaemia

The blood supply of the anterior segment of the eye is distributed through the major arterial circle of the iris, formed from seven penetrating anterior ciliary arteries and two posterior ciliary arteries. The lateral rectus insertion contains one ciliary vessel, and each of the other three recti contains two, those of the vertical recti being situated in the medial halves of the muscles. Disinsertion of the recti divides these anterior ciliary arteries, and the loss of blood supply is such that simultaneous division of more than three muscles in patients under 20 years of age, and more than two muscles in older patients, risks inducing some degree of acute anterior segment ischaemia, especially following ipsilateral carotid ligation for earlier caroticocavernous fistula (Fells 1972).

Lee and Olver (1990) studied the effect of strabismus surgery on the iris circulation in the immediate postoperative period in a group of adult patients. They reported that the type of surgery performed was the most important factor in determining whether ischaemic problems occurred. All patients who had primary vertical rectus surgery showed sector filling delay on the first postoperative day, especially when the inferior rectus muscle was operated on. No delay was seen in patients who had primary horizontal rectus muscle surgery nor in those who had secondary vertical rectus muscle surgery. When surgery was performed in stages, the incidence was less, suggesting that this is a safer approach. The type of conjunctival incision used was not considered significant. These findings were not influenced by the presence of dysthyroid eye disease nor by the patient's age.

Features

Severe ischaemia produces symptoms of pain and blurred vision in the affected eye within 24 h of operation. The eyelids, conjunctiva and deep layers of the cornea all become oedematous. The pupil is dilated with a diminished light reflex and is often irregular in shape. The anterior chamber is deep with a heavy flare and circulating pigment; the vitreous is hazy and the intraocular pressure is low. Iris angiography shows very poor arterial filling, at least in the portions of the iris adjacent to the divided rectus muscles. The circulation slowly re-establishes itself, but permanent segmental iris atrophy is common, with avascularity of the pupillary margin, pupillary distortion and permanently defective pupillary reflexes. Delayed cataract formation is also common.

Lesser degrees of acute ischaemia usually resolve with no permanent sequelae apart from pupil irregularity. This may occur following division of only two adjacent rectus muscles in adult patients, especially those undergoing simultaneous medial and inferior rectus recessions for mechanical tethering caused by dysthyroid ophthalmopathy (Fells & Marsh 1978).

Treatment

In the acute stage, pain is treated with atropine 1% eye drops, which induce cycloplegia, abolishing painful smooth muscle spasm. Administration of topical and systemic steroids in high dosage for a few days reduces the ischaemic uveitis, while local circulation is improved by intravenous therapy with dextran 40 in 5–10% dextrose-saline solution. For the first two days 1 L per day is given, followed by 500 mL per day for the next three days. Blood urea and serum electrolyte concentrations must be closely monitored throughout this period.

Detached extraocular muscle

An extraocular muscle can become inadvertently detached from the globe as a result of:
• the muscle being cut free and lost during squint surgery;
• the muscle snapping whilst being held on a muscle hook during surgery;
• slippage of the muscle in the early postoperative period;
• blunt or penetrating trauma to the face or orbit (MacEwen et al. 1992).

The prognosis for the retrieval of the muscle depends on the mechanism by which it was lost; those lost during squint surgery have the poorest outcome (MacEwen et al. 1992). Other factors that affect the prognosis include:
• a long delay before reoperation to retrieve the muscle;
• which rectus muscle is involved—detachment of the medial rectus carries the poorest prognosis;
• the finding at reoperation—a lost muscle is more difficult to locate than a slipped muscle.

Lost muscles

When a rectus muscle is completely and freely detached it can retract very markedly, particularly if its check ligaments, intermuscular septum and other attachments to Tenon's capsule have also been divided, resulting in loss of both direct and indirect contact with the globe. It may come to lie in a very inaccessible position, rolled up outside the muscle cone well behind the globe.

Slipped muscle

The muscle may slip back if it is not tightly and adequately sutured to the globe at the time of operation. The muscle and tendon can slip back within the sheath or capsule, as described by Parks (1975) and Helveston (1987), and maintain attachment to the globe only through the capsule. Partial slippage of a muscle results when one pole of the insertion slips back and the other remains still attached to the globe; this is a common finding when exploring the previously operated medial rectus muscle in patients presenting with late consecutive exotropia following surgery for primary esotropia (Heaven & Ansons 1995). In these patients at reoperation there is an apparently normal muscle capsule spanning the full extent of the insertion with a reduced-width muscle within. Presumably one pole of the muscle has slipped lose from the suture leaving capsule still attached. Slippage of the muscle can produce underaction of a recessed muscle and an undercorrection when the muscle has been resected.

Helveston (1987) described progressive late slippage of the inferior rectus after the muscle had been recessed on adjustable sutures. The firm attachments between the inferior rectus and the ligament of Lockwood, and between the muscle and the inferior oblique resulted in the operated muscle moving over the globe during horizontal eye movements. Reattachment to the sclera was retarded and contraction of the inferior rectus resulted in further recession.

Features of detached muscles

Most surgeons who have lost a muscle at the time of surgery recognize the fact and make attempts to retrieve it. We have seen cases in which the inferior rectus muscle has been mistaken for the inferior oblique during a planned inferior oblique myectomy. In these cases the preoperative hypertropia in the primary position increased postoperatively and there was limitation of movement of the affected eye on down-gaze.
• A detached muscle should be suspected in the early postoperative period or after facial or orbital trauma if there is an unexpected limitation of eye movement, with widening of the palpebral fissure when the eye looks in the direction of action of the detached muscle. Movement into the muscle's field of action may still be possible because of the remaining intermuscular septum or muscle capsule attachments (Ansons *et al.* 1997).
• A detached inferior rectus muscle is associated with lower eyelid retraction and deepening of the inferior conjunctival fornix because of its intimate connections with these structures.
• Late slippage of the inferior rectus muscle is associated with a progressively increasing hypertropia. Helveston advised against the use of adjustable sutures in inferior rectus muscle surgery.

Management

A CT or MR scan can be useful in locating the site of reattachment of the detached muscle, although cases have been reported where diagnostic imaging showed the muscle to be discontinuous but a normal muscle was found at surgery (Ticho *et al.* 1993). This is because imaging cannot easily differentiate extraocular muscle from surrounding tissue oedema, haemorrhage and scar tissue. Tracing back the nearer edge of an adjacent intact rectus or oblique muscle may then sometimes relocate it. If the retracted muscle is not relocated at the time of the original operation, or is found to be very fibrosed and contracted at subsequent exploration, a transposition operation should be carried out, moving the nearer halves or the whole of the two adjacent rectus muscles to the original insertion of the lost muscle. If this operation is delayed, the ipsilateral antagonist muscle will have contracted and will also need to be extensively recessed, together with its overlying conjunctiva, until there is no residual sensation of tethering on forced duction testing. Surgery may need to be carried out in two stages to avoid anterior segment ischaemia.

The slipped muscle should be located, carefully detached from its new insertion and advanced. The results of reoperation can be disappointing and further surgery on other muscles may be required.

Adhesions

These are caused following strabismus surgery by abnormal attachments developing between structures in the orbit as the result of damage to the muscle cone, Tenon's capsule or the connective tissue amongst the orbital fat.

If the surgeon is careless and causes muscle trauma and excessive bleeding, the exposed deep muscle surface may adhere to the underlying sclera and the superficial surface may adhere to the opposing Tenon's capsule. Passing a muscle hook, or dissecting too posteriorly and without direct observation may tear Tenon's capsule behind the point of penetration of the rectus muscles, allowing part of the orbital fat to enter the anterior sub-Tenon's space. There it excites an inflammatory reaction with the development of fibrofatty scarring between sclera, muscle and the inner surface of the anterior part of Tenon's capsule. This scarring may extend posteriorly to involve the fat pad outside the muscle cone and cause additional adhesions, either to other muscles or to the orbital wall.

Management

The principles of management of adhesive complications are those which apply to any mechanical strabismus. They include extensive ipsilateral antagonist and contralateral synergist muscle weakening operations, perhaps using adjustable sutures, conjunctival recession and the division of all restricting fascial bands as far as possible, without causing additional scarring. Corticosteroid injections, plastic sheets and sleeves around muscles (not widely believed to be useful) and anchoring sutures may all have a part to play, but the results of reoperation are generally disappointing. The reduction of torsional muscle imbalance is of greatest importance, as this cannot be corrected optically, whereas residual horizontal and vertical imbalance can possibly be compensated by the use of prisms.

General problems of reoperation

Reoperation entails various problems, and the following important points should be considered.

- When previous surgery has been carried out elsewhere, the operation details may not be available.
- Inspection of the conjunctiva with the slit-lamp microscope will usually demonstrate the sites of all previous incisions, which at least helps to indicate which muscles of each eye have already been operated on.
- Forced duction tests at all stages of reoperation are essential.
- The sites of previous surgery should be fully explored, as there can be no complete certainty about the present situation merely from a second-hand written account of a previous operation.
- Accurate dissection of scar tissue and the avoidance of haemorrhage are essential to minimize the development of additional postoperative fibrosis.
- Conjunctival recession, anchoring sutures and adjustable sutures all have a possible role, together with the use of local steroid injections to reduce postoperative inflammation.
- Modifications may need to be made to the original surgical plan in the light of findings at operation; for example, a rectus muscle may be 'lost', having retracted far back outside the muscle cone.
- The patient and his family must be advised that the exact surgical measures required cannot be entirely anticipated before the operation and that yet further surgery may be necessary.

Postoperative care

Care of the eye

Antibiotic drops are best avoided during operation; the cornea should be kept moist with normal saline. Local and systemic antibiotics should be reserved for postoperative use only if there is evidence of developing infection, thus avoiding unnecessary drug reactions and reducing the likelihood of bacterial resistance. Discharge from hospital must be at a time agreed with the anaesthetist, either later on the day of operation or the next day. Padding of the operated eye is not necessary. Before discharge, the surgeon must check particularly for any evidence of a slipped muscle and for any significant infection. Correcting glasses should continue to be worn unless they include inappropriate prisms or require temporary modification to control a residual deviation. Any occlusion worn preoperatively should be removed to avoid the risk of infection and to prevent dissociation of potential binocular single vision. Children can return to school the week after surgery but should avoid swimming and sports for a further three weeks. Adults can return to office work within a few days, but those involved in dirty manual work require a longer absence.

Management

If a functional result is anticipated, every effort should be made to control any residual deviation and establish binocular single vision. The patient should be encouraged to fuse the images if diplopia is present. Control of a small esotropia can be aided by temporary use of Fresnel or clip-on convex lenses, Fresnel prisms placed base-out or miotic drugs. A small consecutive exotropia is more likely to resolve spontaneously but if it persists for two or more weeks, or if a residual exotropia is present, it can be treated by temporary concave lenses, base-in prisms and by improving the positive fusional amplitude. The patient should be closely supervised and the strength of the lenses, prisms or miotic drug should be decreased as improvement occurs.

Transitory diplopia may be present in patients operated on for cosmetic reasons. If it persists, its significance should be minimized and the patient encouraged to ignore it, at least until the deviation is more stable in 6–8 weeks time. If it is then distressing to the patient, efforts should be made to move the unwanted image back into the suppression scotoma by using Fresnel prisms. If this is unsuccessful, the image may be made less obvious by modifying the refractive correction in front of the squinting eye. An occlusive contact lens can be considered as a last resort.

References

Adelstein, F.E. & Cüppers, C. (1968) Probleme der operativen Schielbehandlung. *Bericht Deutsche Ophthalmologische Gesellschaft* **69**, 580–593.

Ansons, A.M., Denning, A., Spencer, A.L. & Kranemann, C. (1997) Pre-operative simulation of detached extraocular muscles during strabismus surgery under topical anaesthesia. In: *Transactions of the 24th Meeting of the European Strabismological Association, Vilamoura, Portugal* (ed. M. Spiritus), pp. 114–118. Aeolus Press, The Netherlands.

Apt, L. & Call, N.B. (1978) Inferior oblique muscle recession. *American Journal of Ophthalmology* **85**, 95–100.

Apt, L., Isenberg, S. & Gaffney, W.L. (1973) The oculocardiac reflex in strabismus surgery. *American Journal of Ophthalmology* **76**, 533–536.

Bach-y-Rita, P. & Ito, F. (1966) In-vivo studies on fast and slow muscles fibres in cat extraocular muscles. *Journal of General Physiology* **49**, 1177–1198.

Buckley, E.G. & Flynn, J.T. (1983) Superior oblique recession versus tenotomy. A comparison of surgical results. *Journal of Pediatric Ophthalmology and Strabismus* **20**, 112–117.

Caldiera, J.A. (1975) Graduated recession of the superior oblique. *British Journal of Ophthalmology* **59**, 553–557.

Callahan, M. (1981) Surgical mismanagement of ptosis associated with double elevator palsy. *Archives of Ophthalmology* **99**, 108–122.

Chow, P.C. (1989) Stability of 'one-stage' adjustable suture for the correction of strabismus. *British Journal of Ophthalmology* **73**, 541–546.

Ciancia, A.O. and Prieto-Diaz, J. (1970) Retrocesco del oblicui superior. Primeros resultados. *Archives Oftâlmologica (Buenos Aires)* **45**, 193–200.

Clark, D.I., Markland, S. & Trimble, R.B. (1989) A study to assess the value of Dacron slings in the management of squints which are not amenable to conventional surgery. *British Journal of Ophthalmology* **70**, 623–629.

Clark, R.A., Miller, J.M. & Demer, J.L. (1997) Location and stability of rectus muscle pulleys inferred from muscle paths. *Investigative Ophthalmology and Visual Science* **38**, 227–240.

Conrad, H.G. & de Decker, W. (1984) Torsional Kestenbaum procedure: evolution of a surgical concept. In: *Strabismus 11* (ed. R.D. Reinecke), pp. 301–314. Grune & Stratton, Orlando, Fla.

de Decker, W. (1981) The faden operation. When and how to do it. *Transactions of the Ophthalmological Society of the United Kingdom* **101**, 264–270.

Dunlap, E.A. (1972) Inferior oblique weakening. Recession, myotomy, myectomy or disinsertion? *Annals of Ophthalmology* **4**, 905–912.

Eustis, H.S., Eiswirth, C.C. & Smith, D.R. (1992) Vagal responses to adjustable sutures in strabismus correction. *American Journal of Ophthalmology* **114**, 307–310.

Fells, P. (1972) Vertical rectus muscle transplantation to restore abduction. In: *Orthoptics. Transactions of the Second International Orthoptic Congress, Amsterdam* (eds J. Mein, J.J.M. Bierlaagh & T.E. Brummelkamp-Dons), pp. 229–237. Excerpta Medica, Amsterdam.

Fells, P. (1976) Surgical management of extorsion. *International Ophthalmology Clinics* **16**, 161–170.

Fells, P. (1984) Strabismus surgery under local anaesthesia: one-stage technique using adjustable sutures. In: *Transactions of the Fifth International Orthoptic Congress, Cannes* (eds A.P. Ravault & M. Lenk), pp. 501–505. LIPS, Lyon.

Fells, P. (1988) Adjustable sutures. *Eye* **2**, 33–35.

Fells, P. & Marsh, R.J. (1978) Anterior segment ischaemia following surgery on two rectus muscles. In: *Strabismus* (ed. R.D. Reinecke), pp. 375–380. Grune & Stratton, New York.

Fink, W.H. (1962) *Surgery of the Vertical Muscles of the Eye*, p. 404. Thomas, Springfield.

France, N.K., France, T.D., Woodburn, J.D. Jr & Burbank, D.P. (1980) Succinylcholine alteration of the forced duction test. *Ophthalmology* **87**, 1282–1287.

Gobin, M.H. (1968) Recession of the medial rectus muscle with a loop. *Ophthalmologica* **156**, 25–27.

Gobin, M.H. (1969) *Cyclotropia and Squint*, p. 49. Krol & Courtin, Antwerp.

Harada, M. & Ito, Y. (1964) Surgical correction of cyclotropia. *Japanese Journal of Ophthalmology* **8**, 88–96.

Harcourt, B., Almond, S. & Freedman, H. (1981) The efficacy of inferior oblique myectomy operations. In: *Orthoptics, Research and Practice. Transactions of the Fourth International Orthoptic Congress, Berne* (eds J. Mein & S. Moore), pp. 20–23. Kimpton, London.

Heaven, C.J. & Ansons, A.M. (1995) Operative findings in patients with consecutive divergent strabismus. In: *Transactions of the 22nd Meeting of the European*

Strabismological Association, Cambridge, UK (ed. M. Spiritus), pp. 216–221. Aeolus Press, The Netherlands.

Helveston, E.M. (1987) Slipped inferior rectus after adjustable sutures. In: *Orthoptic Horizons. Transactions of the Sixth International Orthoptic Congress, Harrogate* (eds M. Lenk-Schafer, C. Calcutt, M. Doyle & S. Moore), pp. 421–426. British Orthoptic Society, London.

Helveston, E.M. & Ellis, F.D. (1980) *Pediatric Ophthalmology Practice*, pp. 34–35. Mosby, St Louis.

Helveston, E.M. & Ellis, F.D. (1983) Superior oblique tuck for superior oblique palsy. *Australian Journal of Ophthalmology* 11, 215–220.

Helveston, E.M. & Haldi, B.A. (1976) Surgical weakening of the inferior oblique. *International Clinics in Ophthalmology* 16, 113–126.

Helveston, E.M., Merriam, W.W. & Ellis, F.D. (1982) The trochlea: a study of the anatomy and physiology. *Ophthalmology* 89, 124–133.

Jampolsky, A. (1975) Strabismus reoperation techniques. *Transactions of the American Academy of Ophthalmology and Otolaryngology* 79, 704–717.

Jampolsky, A. (1978) Adjustable strabismus surgical procedures. In: *Symposium on Strabismus. Transactions of the New Orleans Academy of Ophthalmology*, pp. 321–349. Mosby, St Louis.

Jampolsky, A. (1984) Unusual eye movements in alert humans with attached and detached eye muscles. In: *Transactions of the Fifth International Orthoptic Congress, Cannes* (eds A.P. Ravault & M. Lenk), pp. 245–248. LIPS, Lyon.

Jampolsky, A. (1986) Management of vertical strabismus. In: *Pediatric Ophthalmology and Strabismus: Transactions of the New Orleans Academy of Ophthalmology* (ed. J.H. Allen), pp. 141–171. Raven Press, New York.

Jensen, C.D.F. (1964) Rectus muscle union: a new operation for paralyses of the rectus muscles. *Transactions of the Pacific Coast Ophthalmological Society* 45, 359–387.

Jones, T.W., Lee, D.A. & Dyer, J.A. (1984) Inferior oblique surgery. Experience at the Mayo Clinic from 1960 to 1981. *Archives of Ophthalmology* 102, 714–716.

Ketley, M.J., Powell, C.M., Lee, J.P. & Elston, J. (1987) Botulinum toxin adaptation test: the use of botulinum toxin in the investigation of the sensory state in strabismus. In: *Orthoptic-Horizons. Transactions of the Sixth International Orthoptic Congress, Harrogate* (eds M. Lenk-Schafer, C. Calcutt, M. Doyle & S. Moore), pp. 289–293. British Orthoptics Society, London.

Knapp, P. (1969) The surgical treatment of double elevator palsy. *Transactions of the American Ophthalmological Society* 67, 304–321.

Koornneef, L. (1979) *Sectional Anatomy of the Orbit*. Esculapius, Birmingham, USA.

Kushner, B.J. (1997) Restriction of elevation in abduction after inferior oblique anteriorization. *Journal of the American Association for Pediatric Ophthalmology and Strabismus* 1, 55–62.

Kushner, B.J., Preslan, M.W. & Vrabec, M. (1987) Artifacts of measuring during strabismus surgery. *Journal of Pediatric Ophthalmology and Strabismus* 24, 159–164.

Lee, J.P. & Gregson, R.M.C. (1993) Traction sutures in the management of fixed divergent strabismus. In: *Transactions of the 21st European Strabismological Association Meeting, Salzburg* (ed. H. Kaufmann), pp. 397–399.

Lee, J.P. & Olver, J.M. (1990) Anterior segment ischaemia. *Eye* 4, 1–6.

MacEwen, C.J., Lee, J.P. & Fells, P. (1992) Aetiology and management of the 'detached' rectus muscle. *British Journal of Ophthalmology* 76, 131–136.

McElvanney, A.M. & Ansons, A.M. (1996) Letter to the editor. *Eye* 6, 405–406.

McKeown, C.A., Lambert, H.M. & Shore, J.W. (1989) Preservation of the anterior ciliary vessels during extraocular muscle surgery. *Ophthalmology* 96, 498–506.

Metz, H.S. & Lerner, H. (1981) The adjustable Harada–Ito procedure. *Archives of Ophthalmology* 99, 624–626.

Miller, J.M. & Robinson, D. (1987) Extraocular muscle sideslip and orbital geometry in monkeys. *Visual Research* 27, 381–392.

Mindel, J.S., Raab, E.L., Eisencraft, J.B. & Teutch, G. (1980) Succinylcholine-induced return of the eyes of the basic deviation. *Ophthalmology* 87, 1288–1295.

von Noorden, G.K. (1988) Current concepts of infantile esotropia. *Eye* 2, 343–357.

von Noorden, G.K. & Chu, M.W. (1990) Surgical treatment options in cyclotropia. *Journal of Pediatric Ophthalmology and Strabismus* 27, 291–293.

Parks, M.M. (1974) The overacting inferior oblique muscle. *American Journal of Ophthalmology* 77, 787–797.

Parks, M.M. (1975) *Ocular Motility and Strabismus*, p. 145. Harper & Row, Hagerstown, Md.

Parks, M.M. (1976) Extirpation of the recurrent overacting inferior oblique muscle. In: *Orthoptics, Past, Present and Future. Transactions of the Third International Orthoptic Congress, Boston* (eds S. Moore, J. Mein & L. Stockbridge), pp. 449–451. Grune & Stratton, New York.

Parks, M.M. (1977) The superior oblique tendon. *Transactions of the Ophthalmological Society of the United Kingdom* 97, 288–304.

Parks, M.M. (1983) *Atlas of Strabismus Surgery*. Harper & Row, Hagerstown, Md.

Parks, M.M. (1986) Overacting superior obliques in pediatric ophthalmology and strabismus. In: *Transactions of* the New Orleans Academy of Ophthalmology (ed. J.H. Allen), pp. 409–418. Raven Press, New York.

Scott, A.B. (1977) The faden operation: mechanical effects. *American Orthoptic Journal* **27**, 44–47.

Scott, W.E., Martin-Casals, A. & Braverman, D.E. (1978) Curved ruler for measurement along the surface of the globe. *Archives of Ophthalmology* **96**, 1084.

Simmons, I., Ansons, A.M. & Spencer, A.L. (1997) Is there a cosmetic penalty in leaving the conjunctiva recessed following adjustable squint surgery? In: *Transactions of the 24th Meeting of the European Strabismological Association, Vilamoura, Portugal* (ed. M. Spiritus), pp. 411–414. Aeolus Press, The Netherlands.

Simon, J.W., Price, E.C., Krohel, G.B., Poulin, R.W. & Reinecke, R.D. (1984) Anterior segment ischemia following strabismus surgery. *Journal of Pediatric Ophthalmology and Strabismus* **21**, 179–184.

Spencer, A.L., Gray, C.M. & Ansons, A.M. (1995) Investigating diplopia and suppression with the post-operative diplopia test. In: *Transactions of the 22nd Meeting of the European Strabismological Association, Cambridge* (ed. M. Spiritus), pp. 362–367. Aeolus Press, The Netherlands.

Sprunger, D.T. & Helveston, E.M. (1993) Progressive overcorrection after inferior rectus recession. *Journal of Pediatric Ophthalmology and Strabismus* **30**, 145–148.

Stager, D.R. (1998) Surgery for dissociated vertical deviation: for transposition of the inferior oblique muscle. *American Orthoptic Journal* **48**, 34–37.

Stein, L.A. & Ellis, F.J. (1997) Apparent contralateral inferior oblique muscle overaction after unilateral inferior oblique muscle weakening procedures. *Journal of the American Association for Pediatric Ophthalmology and Strabismus* **1**, 2–7.

Ticho, B.H., Kaufman, L.M. & Mafee, M.F. (1993) The 'Pseudo-lost' muscle: limitations of clinical, surgical and diagnostic imaging techniques in the identification of extraocular muscles after trauma. *Journal of Pediatric Ophthalmology and Strabismus* **30**, 392–395.

Toosi, S.H. & von Noorden, G.K. (1979) Effect of isolated inferior oblique muscle myectomy in the management of superior oblique muscle palsy. *American Journal of Ophthalmology* **88**, 602–608.

Wright, K.W. (1989) Surgical procedure for lengthening the superior oblique tendon. *Investigative Ophthalmology and Visual Science* **30** (ARVO Suppl.), 377.

III
CLINICAL FEATURES, AETIOLOGY AND MANAGEMENT OF SPECIFIC DISORDERS

10
Amblyopia

Amblyopia is defined as defective visual acuity in one or both eyes which persists after correction of the refractive error and removal of any pathological obstacle to vision.

Classification

Amblyopia can be classified under the following headings.

Stimulus-deprivation amblyopia (form vision deprivation amblyopia)

Stimulus-deprivation amblyopia is characterized by the following features:

• it affects one or both eyes;

• stimulus deprivation can be virtually complete, when little or no light enters the eye and no image is formed, as in ptosis covering the pupil, or it can be partial, allowing some passage of light and the formation of a poor-quality image, as in a corneal nebula;

• other conditions which may result in this type of amblyopia are congenital cataract, hyphaema and vitreous opacity;

• von Noorden (1985a) has suggested that bilateral stimulus-deprivation amblyopia can result from congenital nystagmus, in which constant movement across the retinae prevents the formation of well-defined images.

Strabismic amblyopia

Strabismic amblyopia has the following features:
• it is the consequence of constant or near constant unilateral strabismus with onset in childhood;
• it occurs mainly in esotropia, probably because many exotropias remain intermittent, at least during childhood.

Anisometropic amblyopia

Anisometropic amblyopia is characterized as follows:
• there is a significant difference in the refraction of the two eyes such that one eye sees better for all distances;
• the refractive error can be predominantly spherical or predominantly astigmatic.

Hypermetropia

The common finding is anisometropic hypermetropia in which the difference in refraction usually amounts to at least 2 or 3 DS, although it can be as small as 1 DS.

Myopia

If the more myopic eye is used for reading and the less myopic eye is used for distance viewing, amblyopia does not develop. However, the difference in refraction is often marked and the far point of the more myopic eye may be too close for that eye to be used for near, leading to amblyopia, which may not respond well to amblyopia treatment.

Astigmatism (meridional amblyopia)

A relatively clear image is formed along the more emmetropic axis, but a blurred image is formed along the more ametropic axis, giving rise to meridional amblyopia in the more ametropic direction. Gwiazda *et al.* (1986) reported that meridional amblyopia can follow the small amount of physiological astigmatism commonly found in infancy, but clinically these patients have astigmatism of at least 1 D and often considerably more.

In all types of anisometropic amblyopia accommodation will be correct for the more emmetropic eye and there will be a blurred image in the more ametropic eye. There may be some degree of aniseikonia although it is unusual for patients to comment on this.

Ametropic amblyopia

The salient features of ametropic amblyopia are as follows:
• It is bilateral and occurs when there is a high degree of insuperable refractive error in each eye, such that a blurred image is present at all distances.
• It occurs in association with high bilateral hypermetropia in excess of 6 DS, which cannot be compensated by accommodation.
• Visual acuity is defective in severe bilateral myopia but degenerative retinal changes may account for at least part of the vision loss.
• Meridional amblyopia occurs when there is a moderate or high degree of uncorrected astigmatism in both eyes.

Idiopathic amblyopia

von Noorden (1985b) reported on amblyopic children with no refractive error and normal binocular single vision except for a foveal suppression scotoma detected with a 4 Δ base-out prism. The amblyopia responded well to occlusion but repeatedly recurred when the occlusion was removed. It was assumed that recurrence was due to the continuing effect of inhibition from the normal eye and that these patients had at one time been anisometropic, an assumption supported by Firth and Davis (1994).

More than one type of amblyopia can occur in the same patient. For example, many patients with strabismus also have anisometropia, resulting in both strabismic and anisometropic amblyopia.

Mechanisms

Two factors are involved in the production of amblyopia, namely deprivation of form vision and abnormal binocular interaction.

Deprivation of form vision

Deprivation of form vision is either complete, when no stimulus reaches the fovea or, more commonly, partial, when there is a degraded image. This factor is the passive or static element in the development of amblyopia. It is debatable whether complete stimulus deprivation exists, as some light (or 'white noise') enters the eye even in dense cataract or unilateral complete ptosis (Jampolsky 1978).

Abnormal binocular interaction or competition

Binocular competition forms an integral part of normal binocular single vision, as seen, for example, in retinal rivalry. Abnormal binocular competition is involved in all types of unilateral amblyopia but not in bilateral amblyopia, when each eye is affected to the same extent. It occurs when incompatible images are formed on the fovea. In stimulus-deprivation amblyopia, competition is between the normal image and the 'white noise' or degraded image formed in the affected eye. In strabismic amblyopia, competition results from visual confusion, in which images of different objects are projected from the fovea and are seen superimposed. In anisometropic amblyopia, competition occurs when a defocused, distorted or different-sized image of the fixation object is superimposed on the image projected from the normal fovea. Neurones from the two eyes are thought by physiologists to compete for control over cortical connections during the developmental period: those from the better eye gain control at the expense of neurones from the affected eye. This factor is active or dynamic, in contrast to the static deprivation factor. Both factors are involved in all types of unilateral amblyopia, although von Noorden (1985a) has stated that abnormal binocular competition is predominant in strabismic amblyopia. He suggested that a peripheral object lying on the visual axis of the squinting eye could form a clear image on the fovea sufficiently often to minimize deprivation.

Only form vision deprivation occurs in bilateral amblyopia.

Critical period

Amblyopia develops only in the critical period, when neural plasticity makes the visual system vulnerable to any abnormal experience such as strabismus, a blurred image or occlusion. Once this period is over amblyopia does not develop. It is now believed that there are several overlapping critical periods, each for a specific visual function (Harwerth *et al.* 1986). In monkeys these are thought to be as follows:

- scotopic vision: 0–3 months
- photopic vision: 0–6 months
- form vision: 0–25 months
- binocular summation: 0–25 months
- stereopsis: 0–25 months.

The ratio between monkey and human infants is considered to be 1 : 4. The comparable period in man in which form vision develops and amblyopia can occur is therefore 100 months, or approximately 8 years. This corresponds to the 'period of flux' described by Chavasse (1939).

The most marked improvement in vision occurs in the first 6 months of life (Dobson & Teller 1978), suggesting that this is the time when the infant is most at risk from amblyogenic factors. However, Held (1988) considered that the visual system was not at risk during the first 4 months. Awaya *et al.* (1987) studied the effect of short periods of occlusion at different ages: they concluded that occlusion during the first month of life, due to unilateral blepharoptosis or macular haemorrhage, did not cause amblyopia. Occlusion was most damaging from 2 to 18 months of age, especially towards the end of that period.

Epelbaum *et al.* (1993) reported maximum improvement in strabismic amblyopia if occlusion is started before 3 years of age, but some improvement is possible up to 12 years. Hardman Lea *et al.* (1989) demonstrated improvement in anisometropic amblyopia up until the age of 8 years. In our experience improvement is often seen beyond this age.

Research background

The causes and effects of amblyopia have been extensively studied in kittens and young monkeys, stemming from the work of Hubel and Wiesel in the 1960s. Wiesel and Hubel (1963) demonstrated the columnar arrangement of cells in the striate cortex of cats and in monkeys (Hubel & Wiesel 1972), known as ocular dominance columns. Peripheral columns responded to input from either the right or left eye but the more central columns responded to input from both eyes (binocularly driven cells). Binocularly driven cells responded to successive rather than simultaneous stimulation from each eye.

Studies of the electrophysiological and anatomical changes which take place in the cortex and lateral geniculate nucleus following disruption of the stimulus during the critical period in an animal's life have shown that:

• If binocular vision is prevented by, for example, lid suturing or an induced strabismus, there is a reduction in the number of binocularly driven cells from a norm of 80% to 10–20% (Wiesel & Hubel 1965). Loss of binocularly driven cells occurs in monkeys after unilateral or bilateral deprivation (Crawford *et al.* 1975).

• Binocularly driven cells no longer respond to stimuli from the deprived eye and undergo a change in function, becoming monocularly driven by stimuli from the sound eye. There is no change in the number of monocularly driven cells responding to stimuli from the deprived eye but the reduction in the total cell population driven by this eye provides electrophysiological evidence of cortical changes occurring in amblyopia (Wiesel & Hubel 1963).

• An alternating strabismus results in an equal number of cells driven from the right and left eyes; there are virtually no binocularly driven cells (Crawford & von Noorden 1979).

• Bilateral deprivation results in an equal reduction in the number of cells responding to stimuli from each eye (Crawford *et al.* 1975).

• Loss of stereopsis is believed to follow the loss of binocularly driven cells (Crawford *et al.* 1984).

• Cells in the visual cortex respond to line stimuli orientated in a specific direction. If an animal is subjected only to vertical black-and-white stripes, there is an increase in the number of cortical cells responding to vertical line orientation and a decrease in cells responding to other line orientations (Blakemore & Cooper 1970).

• Cells in the lateral geniculate nucleus (LGN) are arranged in layers, each layer receiving input from one eye. Cell shrinkage occurs in the layers of the LGN which are related to the eye deprived of stimulus by lid suturing (von Noorden & Middleditch 1975).

• Two types of retinal ganglion cells have been demonstrated: Y cells, which respond to transient firing and are mainly found in peripheral retina; and X cells, which respond to sustained firing and are most dense in the foveal area (Ikeda & Wright 1974). Ikeda and Tremain (1978, 1979) showed that the resolving power of retinal and LGN X cells is reduced in kittens with unilateral strabismus or a defocused image. These authors proposed that this loss of cellular activity formed the basis of at least some types of amblyopia.

Amblyopia has been produced experimentally in kittens and young monkeys by:

• unilateral or bilateral lid suturing (stimulus-deprivation amblyopia);

• unilateral strabismus (strabismic amblyopia);

• defocusing of the image, either by instillation of atropine in one eye or by placing a high-powered convex lens in front of the eye (anisometropic amblyopia);

• restricting visual stimuli to stripes orientated in one direction (meridional amblyopia).

The electrophysiological and anatomical changes outlined above have been supported by behavioural evidence of vision loss, which can include depression of contrast sensitivity function (Blakemore & Vital-Durand 1983). The most severe amblyopia results from total deprivation of stimulus following unilateral lid suturing. In general the effects of binocular deprivation on the visual system are believed to be less severe. However, von Noorden (1987) has shown that while short periods of binocular deprivation (up to 6 weeks in the monkey) have a relatively mild effect, longer periods exceeding 6 weeks can result in irreversible visual loss.

Changes in the distribution of cortical neurones and a decrease in size of the layers of the LGN referable to the deprived eye are common to all forms of unilateral amblyopia. The term *visual deprivation syndrome* was introduced by Crawford (1978) to describe unilateral amblyopia. The syndrome comprises:

• decreased vision in the deprived eye;

• loss of binocular summation and stereopsis;

• a reduction in the number of cortical neurones receiving input from the deprived eye and loss of binocularly driven cells;

• a decrease in cell size in the relevant layers of the LGN.

Some of the changes in cell structure can be reversed, but only if use of the deprived eye is enforced within the critical period. Reverse suturing resulted in most of the LGN cells related to the deprived eye regaining their normal size (Blakemore *et al.* 1978). Swindale *et al.* (1981) reported fresh growth of afferent axons in layer IVc of the visual cortex. These changes correlated with an improvement in visual function. In contrast there is apparently no recovery of function of formerly binocularly driven cells.

Relevance of experimental amblyopia to amblyopia in humans

It must be stressed that all experimental work on amblyopia has been carried out on kittens and young monkeys within the critical period for these animals. The differences in the visual systems of cat and humans suggest that the findings in kittens may not be applicable to humans, but the visual systems of monkey and humans are very similar and it has been established that the findings in young monkeys apply equally to the human child. von Noorden (1985a) stated: 'There is no question now that the behavioural aspect of amblyopia in the monkey model is similar to human amblyopia in terms of aetiology, severity, reversibility and occurrence during a period early in life when the visual system is susceptible to abnormal influence'.

Proof of similar anatomical changes in humans has been provided by postmortem examination on a patient known to have had anisometropic amblyopia; shrinkage of the layers of the LGN receiving input from the amblyopic eye was found (von Noorden *et al.* 1983). The findings were comparable with those reported in monkeys with anisometropic amblyopia.

Influence of research on the management of amblyopia

The influence of the results of research on the management of amblyopia can be summarized as follows.
• The most important factor is the realization that severe stimulus-deprivation amblyopia should be treated within days of birth or at the latest within the first few weeks of life.
• Occlusion, penalization and the use of atropine all cause visual deprivation and can result in loss of vision if precautions are not taken.
• An orderly visual environment must be provided as soon as possible; therefore, early correction of refractive errors is of great importance, particularly when significant astigmatism is present, which could lead to meridional amblyopia.
• Loss of binocularly driven cells occurs in the presence of unilateral and alternating strabismus. Once it

has occurred the loss appears irreversible. Full-time total occlusion neither causes further loss of these cells nor prevents recovery of function, therefore its use is not contraindicated on these grounds.
• Bilateral simultaneous occlusion for a short period is considered less disruptive to the developing visual system than is a similar period of unilateral occlusion. It has been suggested that simultaneous occlusion should be used in infants with bilateral cataract during the interval before surgery is carried out on the second eye (Harcourt *et al.* 1988).

Influence of the normal eye on the visual function of the amblyopic eye

The best possible vision in an amblyopic eye is obtained when the normal eye is prevented from seeing. Vision decreases when both eyes are open (Pugh 1954), indicating that the normal eye has an inhibitory effect on the amblyopic eye. von Noorden and Leffler (1966) demonstrated that the greater the luminance of the stimulus to the normal eye the lower the vision in the amblyopic eye. It is believed that the inhibitory effect persists after recovery of visual acuity and elimination of the factors causing amblyopia.

Diagnosis

A detailed history should be taken in all cases, with particular reference to the parents' opinion of a child's vision, the age at onset and duration of any strabismus present and the family history.

The aim of the examination is the comparison of:
• the visual function of the two eyes;
• the patient's known or estimated vision with the norm for his age.

The diagnosis of amblyopia is based on:
• The estimation or, preferably, the measurement of visual acuity in each eye.
• The assessment of fixation in the amblyopic eye and on fixation preference in manifest strabismus. However, Calcutt (1995) showed that fixation preference for one eye does not necessarily indicate the presence of amblyopia although it is unlikely to occur if there is free alternation.
• Refraction and careful examination of the fundi and media.

Methods of assessing visual acuity, fixation and refraction have been described in Chapters 3 and 4. Contrast sensitivity may be assessed.

Accommodation amplitude appears to be reduced in amblyopic eyes on objective measurement. Whilst this is probably due to an afferent defect (Hokoda & Ciuffreda 1982), possibly related to lack of foveal function (Otto & Safra 1976), there is some evidence to suggest that the defect lies in the efferent system (Utsumi *et al.* 1984). Subjective testing of accommodation in the amblyopic eye is limited by the inability of the individual to assess target clarity and/or noticeable differences in target defocus (Hokoda & Ciuffreda 1982).

Clinically the inaccuracy in the accommodation response suggests that undercorrected hypermetropes may be disadvantaged during occlusion therapy. In addition, formerly amblyopic eyes may not have accurate accommodation (Chiesi *et al.* 1986).

Treatment

Selection of patients

The main factors to be considered in patient selection are:
• Age: amblyopia is treated in childhood. The younger the patient the better and more rapid the response. Treatment is rarely started after the age of 8 years, when the visual system has matured. Exceptions are mainly older children with anisometropic amblyopia who have demonstrable binocular single vision and good motivation. It can be worthwhile treating these patients up to the age of 14–16 years, as improvement in binocular function, particularly in the level of stereoacuity, results from improved visual acuity.
• General health: the patient's health should be reasonably good and any physical or mental handicap must have been considered. For example, a deaf child dependent on lip-reading may be very handicapped by occlusion, and children with defective locomotion may lose confidence or regress if occluded. Cooperation between all the therapists involved is essential in deciding on the priorities in these patients, but in general amblyopia therapy will still be advocated and the regime tailored for the individual's needs.

All patients must be wearing a correction for any significant refractive error. Constant spectacle wear can result in improvement of vision in some cases (see below).

Methods of treatment to restore visual acuity in amblyopia

The principle underlying the restoration of visual acuity is to promote the use of the amblyopic eye or eyes. This can be achieved by:
• occlusion of the better eye;
• cycloplegic drugs alone or in combination with optical penalization;
• CAM visual stimulator.

Pleoptic treatment (as conceived by Bangerter and Cüppers rather than in the wider sense in which this term is sometimes used) has largely been discontinued and is referred to only briefly later in this section.

The use of systemic drugs is as yet only in the experimental stage.

Occlusion

Occlusion may be of different degrees.
• *Total occlusion, excluding all light and form*, for example, adhesive occluders worn on the skin, made from proprietary and preferably nonallergenic materials. Hand-made or proprietary occluders attached to the spectacle frames also come into this category but are not always successful in excluding all light from the eye, however carefully they are fitted. An opaque black contact lens has also been used for this purpose (Summers *et al.* 1995).
• *Total occlusion, excluding form*, but allowing the passage of some light, comprising an opaque material adherent to the spectacle lens. Semi-opaque occlusion material such as Blenderm tape or frosted glass, is effectively total occlusion. It is possible to distinguish rather more than light through these but impossible to read even the largest Snellen letter at any distance. The occlusion should be attached to the back surface of the lens.
• *Partial occlusion*, allowing the appreciation of form but diminishing its acuity. Examples of this type of occlusion are translucent materials such as Fablon or Bangerter foils, which reduce visual acuity by a known amount. The term partial occlusion is also applied to occlusion covering only part of the spec-

tacle lens, such as the sector occlusions widely used in France, or occlusion on the lower half of a spectacle lens to promote the use of the other eye for close work.

Occlusion can be worn:
- full time, either 24 h a day or during waking hours;
- part time, for specific periods or for prescribed activities.

Cycloplegic drugs

The principle of the use of cycloplegia in this context is to blur the vision of the better eye by preventing accommodation and decreasing the depth of focus. Cycloplegia is more effective for near. The drug in common use is atropine 1% or 0.5% as drops or ointment.

Ointment is considered safer for use in infants as it is less likely to be swallowed via the nasolacrimal duct. Once the drug has taken effect its action can be maintained by instilling it once daily or on alternate days. The usual response is that the child will use his amblyopic eye for near fixation and will use the better eye for distance fixation. Atropine should be used for 1–2 weeks in the first instance and the effect assessed.

Optical penalization

The principle of penalization is the use of lenses to blur the visual acuity of the better eye and to augment the visual acuity of the amblyopic eye. Three types of penalization are used:
- distance penalization;
- near penalization;
- total penalization.

The choice depends mainly on the degree of amblyopia.

Distance penalization encourages the use of the amblyopic eye for distance. This is achieved by prescribing an optimum correction for the amblyopic eye and adding +3.00 DS to the better eye.

Near penalization encourages the use of the amblyopic eye for near. This is achieved using cycloplegia in the better eye with full correction and adding a convex lens (up to 3 DS) to the amblyopic eye.

Total penalization encourages the use of the amblyopic eye for all distances. This is achieved by adding a strong convex lens (or occasionally atropine and a strong concave lens) to the better eye, so that the amblyopic eye sees best for both near and distance.

The extra correction required is usually added by means of a Fresnel lens.

Total penalization is most commonly used when atropine alone does not reduce the acuity sufficiently. In this instance atropine is continued and a concave lens is used. Penalization is uneconomic compared with occlusion but it may be better tolerated by the child and his parents because of its advantages in comfort and cosmesis. It is possibly less dissociative than total occlusion and less likely to cause stimulus-deprivation amblyopia, although its use is probably better confined to an older age group less at risk from these factors.

Indications for use

Cycloplegia and/or optical penalization can be effective in:
- Children with moderate or mild amblyopia who do not cooperate well with occlusion. Neither method is effective if amblyopia is severe because the child will see better with the penalized eye at all distances and will have no incentive to change fixation to the amblyopic eye.
- When the level of visual acuity has improved to some extent with occlusion but has become static.
- When occlusion has been worn for a long period and the child has become tired of it.
- In older children with anisometropic amblyopia who are embarrassed by occlusion.
- When nystagmus with a latent component is present in addition to amblyopia. It was thought that occlusion would make the latent component manifest and would prevent improvement in vision. This view is no longer held by many clinicians.

Precautions

Ikeda and Tremain (1978) demonstrated that stimulus-deprivation amblyopia could result from the use of atropine or penalization. An infant or young child requires close supervision.

Some conditions can become more apparent when these methods are used; for example, the penalized eye may remain elevated and cause a cosmetic problem in DVD.

Value

Penalization and cycloplegia are rarely the first choice

in amblyopia treatment but are useful in supplementing or replacing occlusion. Penalization is an acceptable way of maintaining visual acuity in older children. Cycloplegia remains a useful method in younger children provided that adequate precautions are taken.

CAM visual stimulator

This apparatus was designed by Campbell and his co-workers to treat amblyopia by intense visual stimulation for short periods of time (Banks *et al.* 1978). Gratings of different spatial frequency are rotated in front of the amblyopic eye while the other eye is occluded. Concentration on the grating is better if the child draws on a transparent cover over the grating. This method was based on the knowledge that cortical cells respond to specific line orientations and to certain spatial frequencies; therefore rotation of gratings of different spatial frequencies ensured that a large range of cortical neurones was stimulated. Improvement was reported in nearly all patients by Banks *et al.* (1978). Lennerstrand and Samuelsson (1983) found that patients with anisometropic amblyopia responded slightly better to treatment using the CAM stimulator than they did to full-time occlusion, but those with strabismic amblyopia showed the same response to either method and occlusion was needed for maximum effect. However, it has been shown that nonlinear targets are equally effective, making it dubious whether there is any significance in the use of gratings (Keith *et al.* 1980; Mehdorn *et al.* 1981).

The CAM visual stimulator supplemented other forms of amblyopia treatment but did not supplant them. It is now rarely used.

Pleoptic treatment

In the past patients with eccentric fixation were treated differently from cases of amblyopia with central or wandering fixation. The underlying principle was that the eccentric point must first be disrupted and then the fovea retrained to resume normal fixation. Pleoptic treatment was used for this purpose. Apparatus based on the ophthalmoscope principle (the Euthyscope, the Projectoscope and the Pleotophore) was used to expose the peripheral retina to very bright light while protecting the macular area. This resulted in an after-image which, if negative, had a clear area corresponding to the macula, which the patient was then trained

to localize correctly. Other methods were used, including Haidinger's brushes to re-educate foveal fixation and exercises to overcome separation (crowding) difficulties. The pupil of the eccentrically fixing eye was kept dilated and the eye was occluded except during treatment. Pleoptic treatment was only suitable for older children and adults. Its use was gradually discontinued as patients were referred at a much younger age (see Douthwaite & Lee 1958; Douthwaite 1960).

Systemic drugs

Dopamine is a neurotransmitter which is involved in several visual functions. Levodopa given orally produces an increase in contrast sensitivity in an amblyopic eye but does not induce changes in the nonamblyopic eye (Gottlob & Stangler-Zuschrott 1990). These findings suggest an involvement of dopaminergic function in amblyopia, and support the association between amblyopia and neurotransmitters reported in the literature.

Leguire *et al.* (1993a,b) found dose levels of 0.95/0.24 mg kg^{-1} and 1.94/0.49 mg kg^{-1} levodopa/carbidopa to be well tolerated in a small group of amblyopic patients aged from 4 to 14 years. This was combined with occlusion therapy. A significant improvement in vision occurred in all age groups, with a better response from the use of the higher dose. The improvement was significantly greater in this group than in a control group using occlusion and a placebo, but the visual acuity was similar in the two groups one month after termination of the treatment. In a later study in which the treatment was prescribed over a period of 7 weeks, Leguire *et al.* (1995) reported a 5-week period of improvement which was maintained for 6 weeks following cessation of treatment. Campos *et al.* (1995) used citicoline, which has a similar action, and reported an improvement in visual acuity following 15 days of treatment.

This therapy is still undergoing research and is not yet a clinical option.

Choice of treatment

In our opinion full-time total occlusion is the method of choice in nearly all patients with manifest strabismus. It has the advantages that abnormal binocular interaction is prevented and the inhibiting effect of the sound eye is eliminated. If part-time occlusion is used, both these factors are reinforced whenever the occlusion is removed. Improvement is likely to be more rapid when occlusion is worn full time. However, part-time total occlusion may be preferable, at least initially when treating anisometropic amblyopia in children well into school age, when full-time total occlusion may be impractical. Penalization and atropine are useful alternative forms of treatment when occlusion is impractical or has limited success.

General guidelines

Certain general guidelines should be followed when embarking on treatment to restore visual acuity in amblyopia.

- The method to be used should be explained to the parents and to the child, unless he is too young to understand, and the importance of the treatment should be emphasized.
- The parents should be advised on the care of the child when he is wearing the occlusion and should be encouraged to devise ways of helping him to use the amblyopic eye.
- They should be asked to inform the school authorities if the child is at school, so that allowances can be made for his slower progress and the teacher's cooperation can be gained.
- An outline of future treatment should be given, stressing the need for regular attendance for some time to come.
- The younger the patient the more frequently the vision and fixation should be reviewed. With full-time total occlusion, the review time in weeks should equal the patient's age in years (e.g. 3-year-old, 3 week review).
- Occlusion should be discontinued or maintenance occlusion used if there is no further improvement on two consecutive visits and compliance has been good.

Treatment applied to different types of amblyopia

Stimulus-deprivation amblyopia

The cause of the deprivation must first be successfully treated. The child should be refracted and any necessary spectacles prescribed. Aphakia following surgical removal of congenital cataract must be adequately corrected, usually with a contact lens, which is generally tolerated. Moore (1993) reported that in his series most treatment failures were caused by problems related to amblyopia treatment rather than to the fitting or wearing of contact lenses.

Intraocular lenses are not yet widely used to correct aphakia in infants, due to the difficulty in assessing the necessary lens power and to lack of knowledge of the long-term prognosis. They are in common use in acquired cataract in children, particularly in those over 6 years of age.

Most patients treated for stimulus-deprivation amblyopia will be under 1 year of age, but the risk of occlusion amblyopia is remote.

If the stimulus deprivation dates from birth, for example if a unilateral cataract is truly congenital, the prognosis for improvement in vision is reasonable, but it improves if the cataract was acquired in early infancy. Hoyt *et al.* (1982) reported visual acuity as high as 6/9 in treated unilateral cataract after occlusion therapy, but this is not achieved in the majority of patients.

Intensive total occlusion should commence as soon as possible after optical correction. The limitations of preferential looking techniques in the measurement of visual acuity in amblyopic infants and young children make it difficult to be sure of the extent of the defect and the effectiveness of occlusion therapy. However, Lloyd *et al.* (1995) reported the successful use of the acuity card procedure to regulate amblyopia therapy by identifying the interocular acuity differences and prescribing the treatment regime accordingly. No long-term results for these patients are yet available.

Demonstrable stereopsis is rare in these patients but there is evidence that very early treatment is more likely to result in random dot stereopsis (Birch *et al.* 1993).

Strabismic amblyopia

In cases of strabismic amblyopia, occlusion remains the treatment of choice, in the first instance at any rate. Some form of total occlusion is nearly always indicated, the type depending on the known or estimated difference in vision between the two eyes.

If the visual acuity in the squinting eye is less than 6/60, full-time total occlusion is employed. Patients with very large-angle unilateral esotropia may respond badly to occlusion if the ipsilateral medial rectus is contracted, making it difficult to move the squinting eye into a fixing position. If there is no improvement after a trial period of occlusion, botulinum toxin or surgery to reduce the esotropia should be considered and occlusion resumed immediately postoperatively. The same considerations apply to the nystagmus blockage syndrome.

Eccentric fixation

Patients with eccentric fixation were at one time treated by occlusion of the squinting eye until fixation became unstable, when occlusion was changed to the fixing eye. This method is now rarely used, and direct occlusion of the fixing eye is the initial treatment of choice. Peripheral eccentric fixation can gradually approach the fovea as treatment progresses until it becomes central or, more usually, parafoveolar or parafoveal. Fixation should be regularly monitored during occlusion therapy. Established parafoveal fixation does not respond to further treatment but the visual acuity of the squinting eye can improve to 6/9–6/12, which is the level expected from this area of the retina. Eccentric fixation should not prohibit continuing occlusion until the best possible acuity is reached.

Supervision

Both distance and near visual acuity should be tested if possible, as improvement is sometimes first seen for near (von Noorden & Helveston 1970), although this view was not supported by Lennarson *et al.* (1984), who found that 47% of amblyopes had less good near visual acuity when comparable vision charts were used for distance and near. The state of fixation should be noted and the child's fixation preference for near and distance should be recorded.

The parents should be taught to observe the child's preferred eye 15–20 min after removal of the occlusion to assess whether or not fixation has changed to the previously strabismic eye. This observation is usually possible if the angle of deviation is moderate or large. If the better eye remains fixing they are instructed to continue the occlusion on that eye. If fixation has changed and the child continues to fixate with the strabismic eye the occlusion should be discontinued until the child is examined by an orthoptist.

As the visual acuity improves, the type of occlusion can be changed to occlusion on the spectacle lens instead of on the face, but it is our opinion that full-time total occlusion should be continued if possible, until the best possible vision has been obtained. If improvement has ceased and the child is still amblyopic it is worth trying an alternative form of treatment, for example distance or near penalization. Treatment should not be stopped until there has been no further improvement for at least 2 months.

The level of improvement reached should be maintained if binocular single vision can be restored by surgery or if the strabismus alternates with no preference for fixation with one eye. Fresnel prisms can be used in suitable cases to maintain binocular single vision whilst awaiting surgery, placing a stronger prism in front of the fixing eye and a weaker one in front of the squinting eye. When there is a persistent unilateral strabismus, recurrence of amblyopia must be prevented until the visual acuity becomes stable. It is difficult to know at what age stability occurs. Recurrence of amblyopia is much less likely in children over 8 years of age but it can occur up to 10–12 years of age. Part-time occlusion for a period of several months to prevent deterioration may be employed. von Noorden and Attiah (1986) reported good results using alternating penalization for at least 12 months as a preventive measure.

Anisometropic amblyopia

The majority of patients with anisometropic amblyopia are over the age of 5 years when treatment is commenced as this condition is frequently not detected until a school medical examination is carried out. However, with the increased use of preschool visual screening and photorefraction of young children, it is being detected earlier. Either way the prognosis for achieving good acuity is good.

Aim

The treatment aims to improve the visual acuity of the amblyopic eye to its optimum level. If central fixation is present an acuity of 6/6 or better can be reached, but this level is very unlikely to be achieved if there is parafoveolar fixation.

Management

Some spontaneous improvement in visual acuity

usually follows correction of the refractive error and constant spectacle wear, therefore time should be allowed for this to occur; a period of 4–6 weeks is usually sufficient. Treatment is not commenced until spontaneous improvement ceases.

TREATMENT

Treatment consists of:

- occlusion of the better eye;
- active use of the amblyopic eye.

Because binocular single vision is present and the child is likely to be at school, part-time occlusion is preferable. Although this is more effective if used for school work, many parents prefer the child to use occlusion out of school hours, only wearing it at school if this proves insufficient. Occlusion can be supplemented by home exercises. Older children can do much to help themselves and should be encouraged at all times. Atropine can be considered as an alternative to occlusion, with the advantage that it acts continuously and is socially less embarrassing. It is, however, quite disruptive to binocular single vision and patients may not tolerate the dilated pupil in the summer months. Occlusion is usually well tolerated.

If there is a marked degree of anisometropia, better vision may be obtained with contact lenses. However, few children in the 5–10 year-old age group will co-operate sufficiently to make their use practicable.

Amblyopia occurring in a highly myopic eye often responds less well to treatment than does amblyopia associated with anisohypermetropia, and the prognosis in many cases of myopia of high degree is not good.

Once the optimum visual acuity has been obtained and occlusion discontinued, the patient should be encouraged to continue wearing his spectacles constantly and his vision should be checked periodically. Amblyopia should not recur because binocular single vision is present. However, perhaps due to the aniseikonia, it can do so and resumption of part-time occlusion may be necessary until visual acuity is stable.

If a very low correction is needed in the better eye, spectacles may be discontinued after the age for visual maturity, but stereoacuity may then be reduced.

Ametropic amblyopia

Aim

The aim of treatment is to achieve useful vision with the refractive error corrected: normal visual acuity is very rarely obtained.

Management

The sole treatment is constant wear of spectacles or contact lenses which fully correct the refractive error. Tolerance of spectacles is good in younger children because of increased comfort as well as improvement in vision. Older patients are less able to accept a full correction, especially if astigmatic. Usually a gradual improvement in visual acuity takes place over a period of 2–3 years.

Amblyopia associated with ocular pathology

Defective vision due to pathological causes affecting one eye, or more marked in one eye, can lead to the development of a unilateral strabismus. Poor visual acuity can therefore be due to a combination of stimulus deprivation, strabismic amblyopia and possibly anisometropic amblyopia, as there is often an associated refractive error. Treatment for the amblyopia is indicated if careful ophthalmic examination suggests that the ocular pathology is insufficient to account for all the vision loss.

The refractive error should be corrected. Occlusion of the better eye is commenced as early as possible and continued until further improvement is considered unlikely.

The prognosis depends on the severity of the pathology as well as the age at which occlusion is begun. Patients with persistent hyperplastic primary vitreous or hypoplastic optic discs very seldom improve after occlusion, as vision is so badly affected by the pathology. More common causes of ocular pathology with a rather better prognosis for amblyopia therapy are:

- Congenital or early-onset cataract, which is discussed earlier in this chapter.
- Buphthalmos: the more affected eye will be myopic and this may contribute to the vision loss. These patients often respond better than expected to occlusion therapy (Clothier *et al.* 1979).

Amblyopia associated with nystagmus

It is necessary to test visual acuity with the patient's preferred head posture in order to assess the extent of the amblyopia. Near vision is often better than distance vision. If the patient demonstrates a null area in which nystagmus is absent or its amplitude much reduced, the response to conventional occlusion should be good. If there is a latent component to the nystagmus, atropine in the fixing eye may be used instead of occlusion, in the hope that the latent component will not become manifest. However, occlusion of the fixing eye is often more effective, and good results have been reported (von Noorden *et al.* 1987). It is the treatment of choice, at any rate in the first instance.

Problems arising during treatment

The main problems that can arise are described below.

Occlusion amblyopia

This is most likely to occur when total occlusion is used, but is seen after the instillation of atropine. Awaya (1978) reported that stimulus deprivation amblyopia resulted from one week's occlusion in children under 18 months of age and that visual acuity was not always recovered after occlusion of the previously affected eye. Occlusion amblyopia can certainly occur up to the age of 2 years and is occasionally seen at a later age. In the majority of cases visual acuity can be recovered with carefully supervised treatment.

Intractable diplopia

This is a relatively uncommon sequel to occlusion. If it occurs in older children without binocular vision, suppression of the unwanted image is unlikely to follow. Occlusion should be stopped at the first sign of diplopia, and the child's attention should not be drawn to it. Measurement of the density of suppression during treatment should ensure this does not occur.

Dissociation of latent or intermittent strabismus

Dissociation is most likely to occur in children under 5 years of age or in older children with inadequate motor fusion. If the strabismus becomes manifest, occlusion should be stopped and the patient observed. Binocular single vision may be restored spontaneously; if not, prisms can be used to fuse the diplopia and efforts made to reduce the prism strength. If a manifest strabismus persists, surgery can be considered. The prognosis for a functional result is good and the risk of dissociation should not deter from the aim of achieving the best possible visual acuity.

Recurrence of amblyopia

If binocular single vision is present or can be restored by surgery, visual acuity should be maintained. There is a risk of recurrence when a unilateral strabismus persists, especially in children under 8 years. It is widely believed that the visual acuity achieved by treatment can be restored in adult life if, for example, vision becomes defective in the better eye. However, there is little if any statistical evidence to support this belief and efforts should be made to prevent recurrence or to resume treatment if it occurs. Usually a short period of occlusion is sufficient to restore the level of vision. Treatment may have to be repeated several times until the visual acuity becomes stable.

Other less serious complications of treatment are:
• An increase in the angle of deviation seen when the occlusion is removed, which is usually temporary and soon decreases. For this reason, occlusion should always be removed a few days before strabismus surgery so that the true angle of deviation can be measured, although surgery for the increased angle may be required (Charney & Morris 1984). Holbach *et al.* (1991) reported both increase and decrease in angle following occlusion but found that these variations did not differ significantly from those in a control group of alternating esotropias who were not occluded.
• An eye with DVD may remain elevated for some time after removal of the occlusion.
• The patient may be allergic to the occlusion material.
• Any conjunctival or eyelid infection can be 'incubated' by total occlusion adherent to the skin.
• The physical risks involved, for example in traffic or going up and down stairs.
    Some of these risks should be explained to the parents so that precautions can be taken.

Results of amblyopia treatment

Ideally, treatment is discontinued when equal visual acuity is obtained, but in many cases this is not achieved and residual amblyopia remains.

Failure to obtain equal vision is often due to persistent parafoveal fixation, usually associated with some degree of anisometropia. In other cases it results from failure to carry out the treatment as directed or to persevere with it for a long enough period.

Compliance

It is recognized that compliance plays a key role in the successful outcome of occlusion therapy. Noncompliance is a common problem encountered in amblyopia treatment. Lithander and Sjöstrand (1991) followed 44 children aged 2–9 years undergoing occlusion therapy for strabismic and/or anisometropic amblyopia. Compliance with treatment proved to be the most crucial factor in predicting a successful outcome. Nucci *et al.* (1992) retrospectively reviewed the case notes of 496 amblyopes and found 18% of all subjects failed to comply fully with the occlusion prescribed. This figure rose to 37% noncompliance in the 1–2-year age range. Leach (1995) found accurate compliance with occlusion therapy in only 19 out of 59 children studied (32%). Factors which appeared to influence compliance unfavourably included treatment regimes of less than 3 h occlusion per day, prescription of occlusion for 2 years or more, and an initial visual acuity of less than 6/60 in the amblyopic eye.

Compliance is a complex issue, partly due to difficulties in assessing it and in obtaining meaningful and accurate data. Fielder *et al.* (1995) described an objective method of monitoring occlusion in which patch–skin contact was recorded using two miniature electrocardiogram electrodes attached under the occluder. The ability to measure compliance should facilitate the implementation of effective therapy.

Every effort should be made to convince the parents of the need for treatment and to gain their trust and cooperation. Treatment should not be stopped until alternative methods have been tried, for example a trial period using penalization instead of occlusion. Steps can be taken in an attempt to obtain better cooperation; for example, the health visitor or school authorities may help with supervision. Splinting the arms of young children is advocated by some so that they cannot remove the occlusion; others admit selected patients to hospital for supervision of treatment. If there has been little improvement and visual acuity remains low, further investigations to assess retinal and optic nerve function should be carried out, especially repeated careful fundoscopy. The Marcus Gunn swinging flashlight test should reveal any significant unilateral organic defect; however, small defects of 0.3–0.9 log units may occur in amblyopia (Portnoy *et al.* 1983). Small degrees of hypoplasia of the optic disc sufficient to cause defective central vision are particularly easy to overlook. In a study comparing the effects of full-time and part-time occlusion, Watson *et al.* (1985) reported that 23% of the patients studied showed no improvement despite very adequate and vigorous treatment. The high failure rate stresses the need for the prevention of amblyopia by early visual screening and detection of those at risk.

References

Awaya, S. (1978) Stimulation deprivation amblyopia in humans. In: *Strabismus* (ed. R.D. Reinecke), pp. 31–44. Grune & Stratton, New York.

Awaya, S., Miyake, S., Koizumi, E. & Hirai, T. (1987) The sensitive period of visual system in humans. In: *Orthoptic Horizons. Transactions of the Sixth International Orthoptic Congress, Harrogate* (eds M. Lenk-Schafer, C. Calcutt, M. Doyle & S. Moore), pp. 44–48. British Orthoptic Society, London.

Banks, R.V., Campbell, F., Hess, R.F. & Watson, P.G. (1978) A new treatment for amblyopia. *British Orthoptic Journal* 35, 1–12.

Birch, E.E., Swanson, W.H., Stager, D.R., Woody, M. & Everett, M. (1993) Outcome after very early treatment of dense congenital unilateral cataract. *Investigative Ophthalmology and Visual Science* 34 (13), 3687–3699.

Blakemore, C. & Cooper, G. (1970) Development of the brain depends on the visual environment. *Nature* 228, 477–478.

Blakemore, C. & Vital-Durand, F. (1983) Development of contrast sensitivity by neurones in the monkey striate cortex. *Journal of Physiology* 334, 18–19.

Blakemore, C., Garey, L.J. & Vital-Durand, F. (1978) The physiological effects of monocular deprivation and their reversal in the monkey's visual cortex. *Journal of Physiology* 283, 223–262.

Calcutt, C. (1995) Is fixation preference assessment an effective method of detecting strabismic amblyopia? *British Orthoptic Journal* 52, 29–31.

Campos, E.C., Schiavi, C., Benedetti, P., Bolzani, R. & Porciatti, V. (1995) Effect of citicoline on visual acuity in amblyopia: preliminary results. *Graefe's Archive for Clinical and Experimental Ophthalmology* 233 (5), 307–312.

Charney, K. & Morris, J.E. (1984) Decompensation of pre-existing esotropia during occlusion therapy. *American Orthoptic Journal* **34**, 83–86.

Chavasse, F.B. (1939) *Worth's Squint or the Binocular Reflexes and the Treatment of Strabismus*, pp. 115–116. Baillière-Tyndall, London.

Chiesi, C., Inzillo, G. & Campos, E. (1986) Accommodation and visual acuity in cured strabismic amblyopia. In: *Proceedings of the Fifth Meeting of the International Strabismological Association, Rome*, pp. 127–130. ETA, Italy.

Clothier, C.M., Rice, N.S.C., Dobinson, P. & Wakefield, E. (1979) Amblyopia in congenital glaucoma. *Transactions of the Ophthalmological Society of the United Kingdom* **99**, 427–431.

Crawford, M.L.J. (1978) The visual deprivation syndrome. *Transactions of the American Academy of Ophthalmology* **85**, 465–469.

Crawford, M.L.J. & von Noorden, G.K. (1979) Concomitant strabismus and cortical eye dominance in young rhesus monkeys. *Transactions of the Ophthalmological Society of the United Kingdom* **99**, 369–374.

Crawford, M.L.J., Blake, R., Cool, S.J. & von Noorden, G.K. (1975) Psychological consequences of unilateral and bilateral eye closure in macaque monkeys: some further observations. *Brain Research* **84**, 150–154.

Crawford, M.L.J., Smith, E.L., Harwerth, R.S. & von Noorden, G.K. (1984) Stereoblind monkeys have few binocular neurons. *Investigative Ophthalmology and Visual Science* **25**, 779–781.

Dobson, V. & Teller, D.Y. (1978) Visual acuity in human infants: a review and comparison of behavioural and electrical-physiological studies. *Vision Research* **18**, 1469–1483.

Douthwaite, C. (1960) Report on pleoptics. *British Orthoptic Journal* **17**, 74–81.

Douthwaite, C. & Lee, B. (1958) An investigation of pleoptics. *British Orthoptic Journal* **15**, 27–35.

Epelbaum, M., Milleret, C., Buisseret, P. & Dufier, J.L. (1993) The sensitive period for strabismic amblyopia in humans. *Ophthalmology* **100** (3), 323–327.

Fielder, A.R., Irwin, M., Auld, R., Cocker, K.D., Jones, H.S. & Moseley, M.J. (1995) Compliance in amblyopia therapy: objective monitoring of occlusion. *British Journal of Ophthalmology* **79**, 585–589.

Firth, A.Y. & Davis, H. (1994) Idiopathic amblyopia: The role of anisometropia in etiology. A case report. *Binocular Vision and Eye Muscle Surgery Quarterly* **9** (2), 129–132.

Gottlob, I. & Stangler-Zuschrott, E. (1990) Effect of levodopa on contrast sensitivity and scotomas in human amblyopia. *Investigative Ophthalmology and Visual Science* **31** (4), 776–780.

Gwiazda, J., Bauer, J., Thorn, F. & Held, R. (1986) Meridional amblyopia does result from astigmatism in early childhood. *Clinical Visual Science* **I**, 145–152.

Harcourt, R.B., Campos, E.C. & von Noorden, G.K. (1988) Discussion. In: *Strabismus and Amblyopia: Wenner Gren International Symposium Series* (eds G. Lennerstrand, G.K. von Noorden & E.C. Campos), p. 299. Macmillan Press, London.

Hardman Lea, S.J., Loades, J. & Rubinstein, M.P. (1989) The sensitive period for anisometropic amblyopia. *Eye* **3**, 783–790.

Harwerth, R.S., Smith, E.L., Duncan, G.C., Crawford, M.L.J. & von Noorden, G.K. (1986) Multiple sensitive periods in the development of the primate visual system. *Science* **232**, 235–238.

Held, R. (1988) Normal visual development and its deviations. In: *Strabismus and Amblyopia: Wenner Gren International Symposium Series* (eds G. Lennerstrand, G.K. von Noorden & E.C. Campos), pp. 247–258. Macmillan Press, London.

Hokoda, S.C. & Ciuffreda, K.J. (1982) Measurement of accommodative amplitude in amblyopia. *Ophthalmic and Physiological Optics* **2** (3), 205–212.

Holbach, H.T., von Noorden, G.K. & Avilla, C.W. (1991) Changes in ocular alignment after occlusion therapy in patients with strabismic amblyopia. In: *Advances in Amblyopia and Strabismus. Transactions of the 7th International Orthoptic Congress, Nürnberg* (eds G. Tillson, M. Doyle, M. Lonly & D. Verlohr), pp. 141–144. Fahner Verlag, Germany.

Hoyt, C.S., Jastrebski, G. & Marg, E. (1982) Long-term visual results in bilateral congenital cataracts. *American Journal of Ophthalmology* **93**, 615–621.

Hubel, D.H. & Wiesel, T.N. (1972) Laminar and columnar distribution of geniculo-cortical fibres in the macaque monkey. *Journal of Comparative Neurology* **146**, 421–450.

Ikeda, H. & Tremain, K.E. (1978) Amblyopia resulting from penalisation: neurophysiological studies of kittens reared with atropinisation of one or both eyes. *British Journal of Ophthalmology* **62**, 21–28.

Ikeda, H. & Tremain, K.E. (1979) Amblyopia occurs in retinal ganglion cells in cats reared with convergent squint without alternating fixation. *Experimental Brain Research* **35**, 559–582.

Ikeda, H. & Wright, M.J. (1974) Is amblyopia due to inappropriate stimulation of 'sustained' visual pathways during development. *British Journal of Ophthalmology* **58**, 168–175.

Jampolsky, A. (1978) Unequal visual inputs and strabismus management: a comparison of human and animal strabismus. In: *Symposium on Strabismus. Transactions of the*

New Orleans Academy of Ophthalmology (ed. J.H. Allen), p. 358. Mosby, St Louis.

Keith, C.G., Howell, E.R., Mitchell, D.E. & Smith, S. (1980) Clinical trial of the use of grating patterns in the treatment of amblyopia. *British Journal of Ophthalmology* **64**, 8–14.

Leach, C. (1995) Compliance with occlusion therapy for strabismic and anisometropic amblyopia: a pilot study. *Binocular Vision and Eye Muscle Surgery Quarterly* **10** (4), 257–266.

Leguire, L.E., Rogers, G.L., Bremer, D.L., Walson, P.D. & McGregor, M.L. (1993a) Levodopa/carbidopa for childhood amblyopia. *Investigative Ophthalmology and Visual Science.* **34** (11), 3090–3095.

Leguire, L.E., Walson, P.D., Rogers, G.L., Bremer, D.L. & McGregor, M.L. (1993b) Longitudinal study of levodopa/carbidopa for childhood amblyopia. *Journal of Pediatric Ophthalmology and Strabismus* **30** (6), 354–360.

Leguire, L.E., Walson, P.D., Rogers, G.L., Bremer, D.L. & McGregor, M.L. (1995) Levodopa/carbidopa treatment for amblyopia in older children. *Journal of Pediatric Ophthalmology and Strabismus* **32** (3), 143–151.

Lennarson, L.W., Portnoy, J.Z., Scott, W.E. & France, T.D. (1984) A comparison of distance and near vision in amblyopia. In: *Transactions of the Fifth International Orthoptic Congress, Cannes* (eds A.P. Ravault & M. Lenk), pp. 329–336. LIPS, Lyon.

Lennerstrand, G. & Samuelsson, B. (1983) Amblyopia in 4-year-old children treated with grating stimulating and full-time occlusion: a comparative study. *British Journal of Ophthalmology* **67**, 181–190.

Lithander, J. & Sjöstrand, J. (1991) Anisometropic and strabismic amblyopia in the age group 2 years and above: a prospective study of the results of treatment. *British Journal of Ophthalmology* **75**, 111–116.

Lloyd, I.C., Dowler, J.G.F., Kriss, A. *et al.* (1995) Modulation of amblyopia therapy following early surgery for unilateral congenital cataracts. *British Journal of Ophthalmology* **79**, 802–806.

Mehdorn, E., Mattheus, S., Schuppe, A., Hein, U. & Kommerell, G. (1981) Treatment for amblyopia with rotating gratings and subsequent occlusion: a controlled study. *International Ophthalmology* **3**, 161–166.

Moore, B.D. (1993) Pediatric aphakic contact lens wear: rates of successful wear. *Journal of Pediatric Ophthalmology and Strabismus* **30** (4), 253–258.

von Noorden, G.K. (1985a) Amblyopia, a multi-disciplinary approach. *Investigative Ophthalmology and Visual Science* **26**, 1704–1716.

von Noorden, G.K. (1985b) Idiopathic amblyopia. *American Journal of Ophthalmology* **100**, 214–217.

von Noorden, G.K. (1987) Correlation between human and animal research in amblyopia. In: *Orthoptic Horizons. Transactions of the Sixth International Orthoptic Congress, Harrogate* (eds M. Lenk-Schafer, C. Calcutt, M. Doyle & S. Moore), pp. 56–62. British Orthoptic Society, London.

von Noorden, G.K. & Attiah, F. (1986) Alternating penalization in the prevention of amblyopia recurrence. *American Journal of Ophthalmology* **102**, 473–475.

von Noorden, G.K. & Helveston, E.M. (1970) Influence of eye position on fixation behaviour and visual acuity. *American Journal of Ophthalmology* **70**, 199–204.

von Noorden, G.K. & Leffler, M.B. (1966) Visual acuity in strabismic amblyopia under monocular and binocular conditions. *Archives of Ophthalmology* **76**, 172–177.

von Noorden, G.K. & Middleditch, P.R. (1975) Histology of the monkey lateral geniculate nucleus after unilateral lid closure and strabismus: further observations. *Investigative Ophthalmology* **14**, 674–683.

von Noorden, G.K., Crawford, M.L.J. & Levacy, R.A. (1983) The lateral geniculate nucleus in human anisometropic amblyopia. *Investigative Ophthalmology and Visual Science* **24**, 788–790.

von Noorden, G.K., Avilla, C., Sidikaro, Y. & LaRoche, R. (1987) Latent nystagmus and strabismic amblyopia. *American Journal of Ophthalmology* **103**, 82–89.

Nucci, P., Alfarano, R., Piantanida, A. & Brancato, R. (1992) Compliance in antiamblyopia occlusion therapy. *Acta Ophthalmologica* **70**, 129–131.

Otto, J. & Safra, D. (1976) Methods and results of quantitative determination of accommodation in amblyopia and strabismus. In: *Orthoptics: Past, Present & Future. Transactions of the 3rd International Orthoptic Congress, Boston* (eds S. Moore, J. Mein & L. Stockbridge), pp. 45–58. Symposia Specialists, Miami, Florida.

Portnoy, J.Z., Thompson, H.S., Lennarson, L. & Corbett, J.J. (1983) Pupillary defects in amblyopia. *American Journal of Ophthalmology* **96** (5), 609–614.

Pugh, M. (1954) Foveal vision in amblyopia. *British Journal of Ophthalmology* **38**, 321–328.

Summers, C.G., Davis, L.K. & Egbert, J.E. (1995) Using an occluder contact lens for amblyopia management. In: *Update on Strabismus and Pediatric Ophthalmology. Proceedings of the Joint ISA and AAPOS and S Meeting, Vancouver, Canada* (ed. G. Lennerstrand), pp. 63–66. CRC Press, Boca Raton.

Swindale, N.V., Vital-Durand, F. & Blakemore, C. (1981) Recovery from monocular deprivation in the monkey. III. Reversal of anatomical effects in the visual cortex. *Proceedings of the Royal Society* B **213**, 435–450.

Utsumi, T., Sugasawa, J., Ishida, Y. & Nobe, Y. (1984) Accommodative response in anisometropic amblyopia with successfully recovered visual acuity. In: *Transactions of the 5th International Orthoptic Congress, Cannes* (eds A.P. Ravault & M. Lenk), pp. 337–342. LIPS, Lyon.

Watson, P.G., Sanac, A.S. & Pickering, M.S. (1985) A comparison of various methods of treatment of amblyopia. A block study. *Transactions of the Ophthalmological Society of the United Kingdom* **104**, 319–328.

Wiesel, T.N. & Hubel, D.H. (1963) Single-cell responses in striate cortex of kittens deprived of vision in one eye. *Journal of Neurophysiology* **26**, 1003–1017.

Wiesel, T.N. & Hubel, D.H. (1965) Comparison of the effects of unilateral and bilateral eye closure on cortical unit responses in kittens. *Journal of Neurophysiology* **28**, 1029–1040.

11
Introduction to Concomitant Strabismus

Classification
Classification of horizontal concomitant strabismus

Aetiology
Heredity
Refractive errors
Neurological defects
Innervational causes
Anatomical/mechanical effects
Febrile illness

Investigation
Aims
Use of +3.00 DS lenses
Measurement of the AC/A ratio
Diagnosis of the maximum angle of deviation
Diagnostic uses of botulinum toxin A

Management
Aims
Methods

References

The essential features of concomitant strabismus are that ocular movement is within normal limits at the time of onset of the strabismus, and that the angle of deviation is virtually the same whichever eye is used for fixation in the primary position.

Classification

Concomitant strabismus is predominantly horizontal. Vertical strabismus is almost invariably incomitant, caused by cranial nerve palsy or ocular muscle abnormality, including restrictive strabismus due to congenital abnormality or trauma. Secondary concomitance can develop in some long-standing cases of muscle palsy (see Chapter 19). Only horizontal concomitant strabismus is included in this introduction and in the following chapters.

Classification of horizontal concomitant strabismus

A consecutive strabismus occurs when the direction of the deviation reverses, either following surgery or with the passage of time. Horizontal concomitant strabismus can be classified into:

Primary manifest strabismus can be constant or intermittent. The angle of deviation can range from

Primary manifest strabismus ——————| Esotropia
| Exotropia

Tree 11.1 Classification of primary manifest strabismus.

Latent strabismus (heterophoria) ——————| Esophoria
| Exophoria

Tree 11.2 Classification of latent strabismus.

very small, resulting in microtropia with useful but not bifoveal binocular single vision (BSV), to very large. The onset can be in infancy, usually between 2 and 4 months of age (infantile strabismus), or later in childhood. Onset after 6 years of age is uncommon and suggests the possibility of a neurological or pathological cause, which must be excluded before considering treatment.

Consecutive strabismus, either spontaneous or postoperative: exotropia following primary esotropia or esotropia following primary exotropia.

Secondary strabismus following pathological visual loss in one or both eyes can result in esotropia or exotropia, largely depending on the age of onset. In general exotropia results if vision is lost at or very shortly after birth or in adult life; esotropia results if the loss occurs in childhood.

The differential diagnosis of concomitant and incomitant strabismus is not always clear-cut. For example, overaction of one or both inferior oblique muscles is a fairly common finding in primary constant esotropia, especially in those of early onset, while certain cases of consecutive strabismus show postoperative incomitance after liberal recession or resection of the horizontal rectus muscles.

Aetiology

Important early concepts of the aetiology of concomitant strabismus were based on the work of Worth (1901) and Chavasse (1939).

• Worth proposed that strabismus resulted from a defect of the 'fusion' faculty.

• Chavasse described the gradual development of the binocular reflexes during the first 5 years of life, reinforced by use until they became unconditionally fixed by 8 years. He considered that obstacles to their development during this period could disrupt reflex development and lead to strabismus. Chavasse's views revolutionized the management of childhood strabismus, resulting in much earlier surgery, which hitherto had rarely been carried out before the age of 8 years and often much later.

It is now generally accepted that there is a multifactorial aetiology. A number of factors, either singly, or more often in combination, can disrupt binocular vision during the developmental period. The main contributory factors are considered below.

Heredity

Manifest strabismus occurs in 3–4% of the population in the Western hemisphere: if either parent has strabismus the risk of the child being affected is four times greater than that of a child of parents without strabis-mus. Sixty per cent of affected children have a close relative with strabismus. The inheritance pattern is multifactorial. The type of strabismus varies among family members and it is thought likely that the predisposing factor is inherited rather than the strabismus itself.

Refractive errors

Uncorrected refractive error influences the development of several types of strabismus, most commonly accommodative esotropia associated with a moderate degree of hypermetropia. Anisometropia influences the development of vision, leading to central suppression and amblyopia, and is commonly found in patients with microtropia. High degrees of congenital myopia can result in esotropia, while high degrees of hypermetropia can lead to exotropia as well as ametropic amblyopia.

The majority of those with refractive error maintain BSV, supporting the view that more than one factor is responsible for strabismus.

Neurological defects

There is an abnormally high incidence of strabismus in brain-damaged children, particularly in those with cerebral palsy. Birth trauma may result in central damage due to an anoxic/ischaemic insult. Brain damage can occur during foetal life. Premature and low birthweight babies also show a high incidence of strabismus: the preterm baby is more susceptible to damage perinatally or later during the 'catching up' period in development.

Innervational causes

Evidence in support of an innervational cause comes from electromyographic studies. For example, the medial rectus muscles of a number of esotropic patients showed significant discharge while the patient was under general anaesthesia and the esotropic angle was reduced, whereas the medial recti of the anaesthetized control group were silent (Mitsui *et al.* 1981). Innervation is reduced by retrobulbar anaesthesia but at the same time increased innervation goes to the contralateral eye, suggesting an abnormal feedback loop for proprioception.

An abnormal AC/A (accommodative convergence/accommodation) ratio can also be considered an innervational anomaly. A high ratio is associated with strabismus and considered to be the main aetiological factor in esotropia of the convergence excess type. It is also an important diagnostic feature in intermittent distance exotropia.

Anatomical/mechanical effects

Exodeviations may be associated with conditions such as hypertelorism, where the interpupillary distance is wide, or craniofacial dystosis, when the origins of the extraocular muscles may be displaced or the orbits may be shallow. However, most patients presenting with anatomical or mechanical aetiologies have an incomitant strabismus.

Febrile illness

Strabismus is not infrequently reported after febrile illness such as measles and chickenpox in children under 6 years of age. In a few patients an encephalomyelitis occurs which could cause a manifest strabismus, but in most cases it is likely that the illness precipitates rather than causes the deviation.

The term *essential strabismus* is sometimes applied to those of unknown origin.

Investigation

Aims

Investigation has the following aims.
• To diagnose the presence and type of strabismus.
• To determine if binocular single vision is present all or some of the time or if the deviation is constant.
• To elicit whether a patient with a constant strabismus has the capacity to fuse images and therefore a good prognosis for restoration of binocular single vision.
• To investigate the area and density of suppression. This is important in patients with a good prognosis, when suppression can be safely treated, and in patients with a poor prognosis for BSV who require cosmetic surgery: these patients may be at risk of intractable postoperative diplopia, and this possibility must be fully investigated before surgery is performed.
• To measure and record the angle of deviation in the primary position for near (33 cm), at 6 m distance and in the far distance if necessary, for example in distance exotropia and esophoria of the divergence weakness type. Measurement should be repeated on two or three different visits to ensure that the findings are accurate and consistent. Further measurements may be needed, for example on up-gaze and down-gaze if a V- or A-pattern is seen.

The methods of measurement and of investigating binocular function are described in Chapters 5 and 7.

Additional methods of investigation are described below.

Use of +3.00 DS lenses

These lenses are used to relax the patient's accommodation for near. The angle of deviation is measured by the prism cover test without the lenses and repeated with the lenses in position ensuring that accommodation is relaxed by using a detailed fixation object which the patient must identify. This method is indicated in the differential diagnosis of:
• Convergence excess esotropia and near esotropia. The angle of deviation will be much reduced with the lenses in convergence excess but will remain the same in near esotropia.
• True and simulated intermittent distance exotropia. The near deviation in true distance exotropia will remain the same with the lenses but will increase significantly to approximately equal the distance deviation in simulated distance exotropia.

Measurement of the AC/A ratio

Measurement using the gradient method is indicated in patients with convergence excess esotropia and in most patients with intermittent exotropia. The findings influence both the treatment and its likely outcome, especially when the AC/A ratio is high. Methods of measuring the AC/A ratio can be found in Chapter 5.

Diagnosis of the maximum angle of deviation

The patient's ability to control a deviation can mask its size; either of the following methods can be useful in eliciting the maximum angle.
• Diagnostic occlusion: one eye is occluded for 1 h in order to prevent control and to relax the angle, which should be remeasured immediately after removing the occluder, ensuring there is no opportunity to regain fusion.
• Prism adaptation: this method is mainly applicable to children with acquired esotropia. The angle is measured by prism cover test and Fresnel prisms are used to correct or slightly overcorrect the deviation. The prisms are worn for 1–2 weeks and the deviation is remeasured. If it has increased the prism strength is

increased and the procedure repeated until there is no further increase in angle: this is taken to be the maximum angle and treated accordingly.

Diagnostic uses of botulinum toxin A

Injection of botulinum toxin A into the extraocular muscles can alter a manifest deviation by causing temporary weakness in the injected muscle; for example, an esotropia can be reduced in size by injection into a medial rectus muscle.

There are two main indications for use of botulinum toxin:

1 To assess the sensory status, which is often easier when the angle is reduced. This is useful to determine potential binocular single vision in patients with manifest deviations and variable or unreliable responses to clinical testing.

2 To predict if intractable diplopia will be present postoperatively and how well the patient can tolerate it.

Management

Aims

The aims of concomitant strabismus management are:

• To restore and maintain the best possible visual acuity by correction of the refractive error and treatment of amblyopia.

• To restore symptom-free binocular single vision whenever there is sufficient binocular potential.

• To restore a normal appearance.

Methods

Treatment can be conservative or surgical. Frequently the two are combined.

Conservative treatment
Optical measures

• Accurate and full correction of the refractive error.

• The use of supplementary convex and concave lenses or bifocal spectacles to relax or stimulate accommodation, thereby decreasing or increasing accommodative convergence.

• The use of prisms, in spectacles or as Fresnel prisms, either as a temporary measure—for example, to maintain binocular single vision pending surgery, or to control a residual postoperative deviation—or permanently in lieu of other treatment.

Orthoptic exercises

Exercises can be used to manage various features.

• Overcome suppression as a preliminary to further treatment. The orthoptist must be certain that the patient will be able to fuse the ensuing diplopia before starting treatment.

• Teach control of an intermittent deviation, for example in fully accommodative esotropia.

• Increase the fusion amplitude.

• Improve control of a latent or intermittent strabismus in order to relieve symptoms and/or maintain binocular single vision.

• Improve the binocular visual acuity by teaching negative relative convergence, mainly in fully accommodative esotropia with a low hypermetropic refractive error.

The role of exercises in constant manifest strabismus is limited to overcoming suppression preoperatively. Exercises are of value in the control of residual postoperative under- and overcorrections, especially when combined with the use of lenses and/or prisms, and in the management of intermittent strabismus, when they are combined with surgery in some cases. Exercises to increase the fusion amplitude and convergence are effective in most cases of symptom-producing heterophoria and in convergence insufficiency. Careful selection of patients is essential.

Therapeutic uses of botulinum toxin A

• As an alternative to surgery, mainly in patients where a general anaesthetic is contraindicated, or in those whose preferred option is botulinum toxin, often when previous surgery has not been successful.

• To restore fusion, especially in patients with decompensating strabismus or postoperative under- or overcorrections where the angle of deviation or age of patient prevent the use of orthoptic exercises.

Surgical treatment

The aim of surgery depends on whether it is used to restore binocular single vision or simply to obtain an acceptably normal appearance.

• To restore binocular single vision the surgeon aims either to place the visual axes parallel or to overcorrect the deviation to some extent. The latter is indicated mainly in the treatment of intermittent distance exotropia to ensure lasting stability.

• To improve the appearance, the surgeon usually aims to achieve an esotropia of up to 10 Δ in both esotropia and exotropia to guard against consecutive exotropia or redivergence, respectively.

The main factors to be considered when planning surgery are:

• The maximum angle of deviation: even in small angles it is more effective to perform less surgery on two muscles rather than attempt to correct the angle by, for example, a single recession.

• The difference in the near and distance measurement.

• The need to avoid:

1 postoperative diplopia in patients lacking fusion ability;

2 postoperative incomitance due to over-liberal recession or resection.

• Any previous extraocular muscle surgery.

The application of all these methods to different types of concomitant strabismus can be found in Chapters 12–16 inclusive.

References

Chavasse, F.B. (1939) *Worth's Squint or the Binocular Reflexes and the Treatment of Strabismus*, pp. 115–116. Baillière-Tindall, London.

Mitsui, Y., Tamura, O., Hirai, K., Akazawa, K., Ohga, M. & Masuda, K. (1981) An electromyographic study of esotropia. *British Journal of Ophthalmology* **65**, 161–166.

Worth, C. (1901) The orthoptic treatment of convergent squint in young children. *Transactions of the Ophthalmological Society of the United Kingdom* **21**, 245–258.

12
Esotropia

Classification

Esotropia of nonparalytic origin may be divided into four main groups for the purpose of investigation and management.
- primary
- consecutive
- secondary (sensory)
- residual.

Primary esotropia

Once refractive errors have been corrected and optimum visual acuity reached, the further management of primary esotropia depends firstly on whether there is an accommodative component, and secondly on the potential for binocular single vision.

Most primary esotropias with good potential for binocular single vision are acquired and begin as intermittent deviations, which can progress to a constant strabismus if left untreated, possibly risking the loss of potential binocularity.

Intermittent esotropia is related to:
- accommodative effort;
- the fixation distance;
- the time at which it occurs (cyclical).

This is the basis for the classification used in this section (Table 12.1).

Accommodative esotropia

Accommodative esotropia can result from an uncorrected hypermetropic refractive error, a high accommodative convergence to accommodation ratio (AC/A ratio) or a combination of the two.

The resulting deviation will depend on:

Table 12.1 Classification of primary esotropia.

Accommodative
INTERMITTENT
Fully accommodative esotropia
Convergence excess esotropia
CONSTANT
Partially accommodative esotropia

Nonaccommodative
INTERMITTENT
Near esotropia (nonaccommodative convergence excess)
Distance esotropia
Cyclical esotropia
CONSTANT
Infantile esotropia†
Acquired nonaccommodative esotropia
Esotropia associated with myopia
Nystagmus blockage syndrome†
Microesotropia†

† See Chapters 14 & 15 for main discussion.

- The magnitude of the hypermetropia: the higher this is the greater the resulting accommodative convergence.
- The patient's need for clear vision: high levels of uncorrected hypermetropia may exceed the limits of the accommodative system (insuperable hypermetropia): the visual acuity remains blurred and binocular single vision is maintained. Patients with lower degrees of hypermetropia may opt for blurred vision rather than the diplopia that follows accommodative convergence, but if the need for clear vision is paramount the patient will tolerate diplopia to obtain it. Persistent blurred vision can result in bilateral refractive amblyopia (ametropic amblyopia) (Werner & Scott 1985).
- The magnitude of the accommodative convergence to accommodation ratio: high ratios result in high levels of accommodative convergence for near.
- The fusional divergence amplitude (negative fusional amplitude): fusional divergence opposes any tendency for the accommodative convergence to result in an esotropia, thereby maintaining an esophoria. If the negative fusion amplitude is poor an accommodative esotropia may become manifest at a lower level of hypermetropia than would generally be expected.

Intermittent accommodative esotropia

See Tree 12.1.

Fully accommodative esotropia (refractive accommodative esotropia)

Description
This is an esotropia which occurs when accommodation is exerted to overcome uncorrected hypermetropia. Accommodation is accompanied by equivalent accommodative convergence, which is excessive for the distance of the fixation object. Binocular single vision is present for near and distance with the hypermetropia fully corrected.

Features
The main features are:
- An onset most commonly in children aged 2 to 5 years of age, rarely in children aged 6 months to 2 years and in those over 5 years of age.
- A degree of uncorrected hypermetropia, commonly 2–7 DS in both eyes.

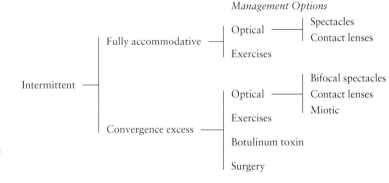

Tree 12.1 Classification and management options for intermittent accommodative esotropia.

- Associated signs at onset: the child may rub or close an eye, appear upset and quickly lose interest in what he is doing; the esotropia is generally more noticeable when the child is tired or unwell.
- An intermittent esotropia which may become constant if left untreated. Strabismic amblyopia may result in these cases.
- Bifoveal binocular single vision with the hypermetropia corrected, present in most cases (Wilson *et al.* 1993): a microtropia is seen in a small minority.

Management

Correction of the refractive error

A cycloplegic refraction is essential, and techniques which do not use cycloplegia should be avoided (Cruz *et al.* 1990). Caucasians can be adequately refracted under cyclopentolate; atropine should not be used routinely but may be required in patients who fail to respond to cyclopentolate, mainly those with dark irides. A general anaesthetic for the sole purpose of performing a refraction is rarely if ever justifiable, even in the most uncooperative child, although sedation may occasionally be required. The full hypermetropic correction should be prescribed, with allowance made for the refractionist's working distance. There is no need to allow for the cycloplegic used as most children accept the full prescription: it is a mistake routinely to prescribe lower strength lenses on the basis that tolerance is likely to be a problem, as this is rarely the case. A reduced strength prescription will simply complicate management and delay treatment. If the corrected visual acuity is less than 6/9 after 6 weeks constant wear and improves when the lens strength is reduced, we recommend repeating the refraction before reducing the prescription. Children requiring corrections higher than 5 DS, or older children wearing spectacles for the first time, should be told that it will take a few weeks before the correction is accepted. The family should be warned that the esotropia may be more noticeable once spectacles are worn: the child appreciates the advantage of clear vision with the correction and tries to attain the same level when the spectacles are removed, resulting in a more obvious or more frequent esotropia. The refraction should be repeated yearly or sooner if control of the deviation deteriorates. Hypermetropia in patients with accommodative esotropia appears to behave the same as it does in the normal population, gradually increasing until 7 years and thereafter showing a gradual decrease (Raab 1984).

Use of contact lenses

Calcutt (1984, 1989) reported improvement in the binocular visual acuity and a reduction in the angle of deviation in patients wearing contact lenses rather than spectacles. We prefer to wait until the child can safely handle daywear contact lenses before considering their use.

Restoration of visual acuity

Amblyopia is uncommon: if present it is usually mild and should be managed by part-time occlusion to minimize the risk of decompensation; this risk should not detract from providing effective occlusion treatment when amblyopia is more marked (Charney & Morris 1984). Improvement in the visual acuity and reduction in suppression should result in improved levels of binocular function and better overall control of the deviation. Some degree of anisometropia can be present with the possibility of a microtropia; equal visual acuity will not result if this is found.

Orthoptic treatment

Once the optimum level of visual acuity has been achieved, further treatment may not be required, and management is confined to regular review of the patient's refraction and continued spectacle wear. However, most patients are able to remove their corrections for sport or social events, and a small number can be helped to regain binocular single vision without spectacles by orthoptic exercises.

The aims of orthoptic treatment are:
- to overcome suppression and gain recognition of diplopia when the deviation is manifest;
- to achieve voluntary control of the esotropia without spectacles by extending the fusion amplitude;
- to improve the binocular visual acuity without spectacles to a useful level, enabling the patient to take off his correction for some activities.

The purpose of the treatment should be explained to the child and parents.

In the selection of patients for orthoptic treatment the following factors should be considered:
- The degree of hypermetropia: the most suitable patients are those with corrections of +3 Δ or less,

with no more than 1 D of astigmatism. Patients with higher errors can be taught to control the esotropia without the correction but are unlikely to obtain a good binocular visual acuity: this considerably lessens the value of treatment. These patients should not be taught diplopia recognition.

• Cooperation and motivation: the patient should be able to read in order to improve the binocular visual acuity; usually children under 7 years do not respond well. Older children are more concerned about their appearance and are therefore better motivated. The parents' cooperation is needed so that treatment can continue at home. They and the child must understand that spectacles will still be needed, at least for close work, if the correction exceeds +3 DS.

• Size of the deviation without spectacles: the angle of deviation is an important factor in predicting which patients can be taught to control the deviation with a good binocular visual acuity (Unwin & Rogers 1968). Treatment is less likely to succeed if the deviation exceeds 25 Δ.

The stages of orthoptic treatment are:

• Diplopia recognition: this can usually be obtained quite easily using a septum or coloured filters. It may be necessary to use an accommodative target as well as a spotlight to sustain accommodation and ensure that the strabismus remains manifest. It helps to show the patient where to look for the second image. If difficulty is experienced a vertical prism can be used to illustrate diplopia to the child, reducing the strength slowly once it is recognized, and proceeding to spontaneous appreciation of diplopia fixing with either eye whenever the deviation is manifest.

• Control of esotropia: spontaneous control without spectacles may follow the appreciation of diplopia. If not it can be achieved by fusing the images at the point of intersection of the visual axes, and gradually withdrawing the target. A spotlight can be used initially to minimize accommodation. The patient should be told that the fused image will be blurred. Holding the target above eye level sometimes aids control. Repeated rapid lifting up and replacement of the patient's spectacles will often show him the difference between a single blurred image and two clear images; the intervals without the correction can be increased until the patient is able to straighten his eyes voluntarily. Control of the deviation can be practised at home under close supervision, using fixation targets at near and distance. If the fusion amplitude is poor it can be improved using a horizontal prism bar, concentrating on the negative fusion amplitude but ensuring that the positive amplitude and convergence are both good.

• Improvement of the binocular visual acuity without the correction. It is usually easy to teach the patient to control the esotropia but improvement of the binocular visual acuity by increasing negative relative (fusional) convergence is more difficult. The stages involved are:

1 Near binocular visual acuity: this can be improved by using bar-reading (see Chapter 7), starting with the correction and adding concave lenses in 1 DS stages in the form of clip-on lenses on the spectacles. Large print should be used at first, reducing the size gradually at each stage until at least N8 print can be read with the addition of −3 DS in front of each eye (or without the correction if this is +3 DS or less).

2 Distance binocular visual acuity: concave lenses can be used in a similar way whilst the patient watches television; he must maintain a single fused image at all times, trying to improve the clarity. In

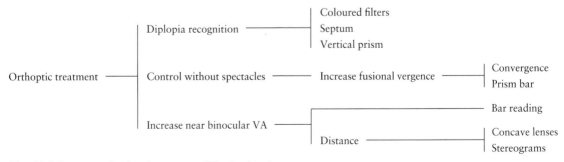

Tree 12.2 Summary of orthoptic treatment. VA, visual acuity.

the final stages of treatment, stereogram cards and the diploscope can be used at home by cooperative patients, concentrating on the positions based on crossed physiological diplopia.
• Reduction in the strength of the hypermetropic correction. It is common policy to reduce the strength of the spectacle lenses gradually during treatment, but if the patient cannot discard his spectacles more or less constantly a small reduction in their strength is of no advantage to him and this practice has little value. Most patients are more comfortable with a full correction, even if the spectacles are worn only for close work.

Surgical treatment

Although surgery has been advocated for selected cases of fully accommodative esotropia (Dyer 1971), an operation is not justified, whatever the strength of the refractive correction, unless decompensation with spectacles occurs.

Convergence excess accommodative esotropia with a high AC/A ratio (nonrefractive accommodative esotropia)

Description

This is an esotropia which occurs on near fixation with the refractive error corrected, due to the excessive accommodative convergence exerted for each dioptre of accommodation. Binocular single vision is present for distance fixation.

Features

The main features are:
• Onset commonly in the age range 2–5 years.
• All patients have a high AC/A ratio, often exceeding 8 : 1. The amount of accommodative effort and the AC/A ratio determine the size of the angle for near. The difficulty in controlling the accommodation exerted in young children can make precise quantification of the size of the deviation and the AC/A ratio difficult.
• Uncorrected hypermetropia is common, and esotropia is often present in the distance as well as for near until the hypermetropia has been corrected. The degree of uncorrected hypermetropia is commonly +1.5 to +5 DS; emmetropia and myopia are occasionally seen.

• An intermittent esotropia to an accommodative target for near, becoming more constant with time: a nonaccommodative target, for example a pen torch, may not produce a deviation for near.
• An esotropia first noticed when the child looks up from a book, or when eating; the child may close one eye or appear upset and quickly lose interest. The esotropia is more noticeable when the child is tired or unwell.
• Equal visual acuity; any amblyopia present is likely to be associated with uncorrected anisometropia.
• Microtropia, which is more commonly seen in this group compared with its incidence in fully accommodative esotropia, mainly in association with anisometropia (Wilson *et al.* 1993).
• Suppression is present in most patients when the deviation is manifest.
• A normal near point of accommodation.

Differential diagnosis

The differential diagnosis includes:
• Fully accommodative esotropia with undercorrected hypermetropia: differentiation is made by accurate refraction using cycloplegia and the prescription of the full cycloplegic refractive error.
• V-pattern esotropia: esotropia is often associated with underaction of the superior oblique muscles and overaction of the inferior oblique muscles. The V-pattern is more marked for near fixation and occasionally these patients present with an esotropia only for near. If the near cover test is performed in slight downward gaze the esotropia increases. The presence of a hypertropia on cover test and careful examination of ocular movements should clearly differentiate the two conditions.
• Near esotropia (nonaccommodative convergence excess): this form of intermittent esotropia has a normal AC/A ratio. Measurement of the AC/A ratio should allow differentiation of the two conditions (see later).
• Hypoaccommodative convergence excess: in this type of esotropia there is a remote near point of accommodation, which differentiates this type of convergence excess (see later).
• Partially accommodative esotropia with a high AC/A ratio: there is a constant esotropia after full correction of any hypermetropia present. The deviation

is significantly larger for near but a cover test at 6 m will show smaller esotropia, differentiating this condition from true convergence excess.

Management
Correction of the refractive error
Hypermetropia should be fully corrected. If myopia is present, the decision to correct or undercorrect it depends on the planned treatment for the strabismus and on the child's need for good vision at school. Low degrees of myopia can usually remain uncorrected if the child can manage without difficulty. If conservative treatment using bifocals with or without orthoptic exercises is planned then an undercorrection of the myopia will facilitate control of the deviation for near. Surgery should be delayed in these cases at least until it is established whether the myopia is progressive. Regular refraction is required. If surgery is planned then the myopia should be adequately corrected to uncover the maximum near deviation preoperatively.

Restoration of visual acuity
Amblyopia is occasionally found, either associated with anisometropia or resulting from constant strabismus, and should be managed in the same way as for fully accommodative esotropia. Microtropia usually results in an optimum visual acuity of 6/9 in the affected eye.

Treatment options
Both conservative and surgical options are available to treat the near deviation once any refractive error has been corrected and amblyopia treated. The decision to treat conservatively does not mean that surgery cannot be performed later if conservative treatment is found to be unsuccessful, or vice versa.

The main factors governing the choice of treatment are:

- The age of the patient: young patients may have difficulty cooperating with bifocal spectacles and orthoptic exercises, and may be managed by observation or early surgical intervention.
- The size of the deviation for both near and distance fixation: large near angles (greater than 30 Δ, where the eye is seen to 'zoom' towards the nose) are likely to require long-term bifocals or surgical intervention (Ludwig *et al.* 1989). Smaller angles for near in patients above 6 years of age may be suitable for short-term bifocals combined with orthoptic exercises. The risk of consecutive exotropia is minimized by the presence of binocular single vision, so a small distance deviation is not a contraindication for surgery.
- The size of the AC/A ratio: ratios larger than 8 : 1 are associated with large near deviations which are likely to require surgery or long-term bifocals.
- The level of binocular single vision: if there is subnormal binocular single vision with a microtropia or an inadequate fusion amplitude, there is some risk of postoperative consecutive exotropia.
- The difference of opinion in the USA and Europe on the relative value of bifocal spectacles and surgery: surgery may never be considered an option for patients who respond to bifocals, with this attitude predominating in the USA, where surgery for this type of strabismus is often frowned upon. In the UK, bifocals are less frequently used as a long-term treatment option and surgery is more often preferred.

Conservative treatment
BIFOCAL SPECTACLES

The aim of prescribing bifocal spectacles is to provide the patient with a reading correction of sufficient strength to enable him to maintain comfortable binocular single vision for all near activities, with an adequate binocular visual acuity; this should be related to the size of print used in his school books. The lenses

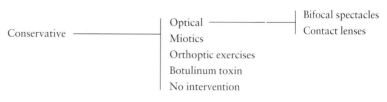

Tree 12.3 Summary of treatment options in convergence excess.

act by reducing the patient's need to accommodate, thereby decreasing the amount of accommodative convergence exerted through the AC/A ratio.

Bifocal spectacles can be considered for use in the short, medium or long term.

- Short-term use as an adjunct to other treatment:
  1 to maintain binocular single vision preoperatively;
  2 in conjunction with orthoptic treatment;
  3 in the postoperative management of residual deviations.
- Medium-term use as the primary treatment until the patient is around 10 years of age in the expectation that the bifocals can then be discontinued. Ludwig *et al.* (1989) reported that patients whose AC/A ratio is not too high can successfully discontinue bifocals without a recurrence of the near esotropia.
- Long-term use when surgery is not considered an option or when apparently adequate treatment by other means has failed to restore binocular single vision.

Although the ultimate aim is gradually to reduce the strength of the reading addition until the patient can maintain a good binocular visual acuity without it, this is not always possible and any attempt to reduce the correction leads either to asthenopic symptoms or to a recurrence of the esotropia (von Noorden *et al.* 1978). Ludwig *et al.* (1989) reported that the esotropia recurred or surgery was required to correct a distance esotropia in 40–60% of their patients when bifocals were discontinued. von Noorden and Jenkins (1995) commented on young adults unable to accommodate after long-term bifocal wear. Because the patient becomes so dependent on the bifocal spectacles many ophthalmologists prefer to treat the strabismus surgically. Patients unlikely to discard their bifocals are those who initially demonstrate an esotropia exceeding 30 Δ for near: we would recommend only short-term use of bifocals in these patients, with planned surgery around 6 years of age. We do not in general recommend the medium- or long-term use of bifocals for the reasons given above.

Indications for the short-term use of bifocals
- The patient is under 6 years of age and later surgical intervention is planned.
- The patient is myopic: any increase in myopia will increase the size and frequency of the esotropia and

because the final degree of myopia is unknown in young children, bifocal spectacles may be preferred to surgery, at least until the refraction is stable (Calcutt 1987).
- The deviation at 33 cm measures less than 20 Δ: these patients can usually dispense with bifocals.

Indications for the medium- and long-term use of bifocals
- If the parents are unwilling for surgery or the patient is unsuitable for it.
- When the over-convergence persists in spite of extensive treatment by other means.

Method
The minimal reading correction is assessed, using print comparable with the size used in the child's school work (a detailed fixation target can be used with younger children), starting with a 1 DS addition, increasing the strength in 0.5 DS steps until binocular single vision is maintained and the print is seen clearly. A trial period is advisable before spectacles are ordered: this can be achieved by using Fresnel lenses, cutting them to fit the patient's spectacles with a flat top either bisecting the pupil or just below. A month's trial is sufficient, giving a good indication that the lens strength is correct and that the patient will tolerate the addition in this form. Bifocal spectacles must be fitted very carefully (see Chapter 3).

Parks (1975) advocates bifocal spectacles for children under 4 years of age; however, they are more suitable for children who are old enough to read, when a more accurate assessment of lens strength can be made and correct use is more likely. We do, however, attempt to put all patients into bifocal spectacles in the short term prior to deciding on surgical intervention.

Problems with bifocal spectacles
- Poorly fitted reading segment.
- Keeping the lenses correctly centred. Children's spectacles are subject to rough treatment and it is difficult to ensure that the centration remains correct.
- Blurred vision leading to reading difficulties. Some children having difficulty with bifocals may prefer to maintain binocular single vision for near and accept the blurred images resulting from relaxation of

accommodation; this may lead to reading difficulties (Poole & Strachan 1986). The greatest problem is dependency on the bifocal spectacles, as discussed above. We have seen a number of patients with this difficulty, and therefore do not in general recommend their medium- or long-term use.

Advantages of bifocal spectacles

• Short-term bifocal spectacles are an effective method of treatment provided they are well fitted and used correctly. They allow binocular single vision to be maintained preventing further suppression and decompensation. Surgery can be deferred until a more suitable age or time.

• Medium- and long-term bifocals provide an alternative to surgery when this is refused or the patient is unfit. The patient and his family must be aware that he may be unable to discontinue bifocal wear without a recurrence of the esotropia or difficulty in accommodating.

It has been suggested that bifocals offer little advantage vs. single focus lenses in the management of an esotropia with a high AC/A ratio in which fusion is present in the distance (Pratt-Johnson & Tillson 1985).

CONTACT LENSES

Although Calcutt (1984, 1989) reported that contact lenses were of some benefit in this type of esotropia, they are not in widespread clinical use.

MIOTIC DRUGS

The purpose of miotic therapy is to allow sufficient accommodation to take place for clear vision without associated accommodative convergence. The miosis induced by the drug also increases the depth of focus so that less accommodation is needed.

Long-acting miotics are no longer available in the UK but are still obtainable in some other countries. Short-acting miotic drugs, usually pilocarpine 4%, are a safer but unsatisfactory alternative: the need for frequent instillation is impractical and unpleasant for children and this treatment is little used.

The patient should be wearing an appropriate refractive correction and the vision should be equal. It is advantageous if the patient appreciates diplopia when the strabismus is manifest and has some con-

scious control over it. For this reason miotic therapy is often usefully combined with orthoptic exercises, which can be used to ensure that the optimum conditions prevail.

Method

Initially the drug is used diagnostically and the patient reviewed after a 2–4-week period. If the miotic has been successful in allowing binocular vision to be maintained for near fixation with a useful binocular visual acuity, its use can be continued over a period of several weeks, with close supervision, looking particularly for any signs of ocular or systemic side-effects, which would necessitate immediate cessation of the treatment. If there are no side-effects, the drug should be gradually discontinued over a further 4–6-week period by instilling it at increasing intervals of 2, 4 and 7 days. The improvement gained is maintained in only a small minority of patients, whether the miotic is used alone or in combination with orthoptic treatment.

Problems with treatment

Problems may arise from the not infrequent side-effects described in Chapter 8. Hypermetropic patients sometimes find that they can see better when their spectacles are removed, and are therefore unwilling to wear them, which adversely affects the management of the strabismus.

Advantages of treatment

The main value of miotic therapy is probably in treating children between the ages of 2 and 5 years who may be considered too young for other forms of treatment. Repeated use of the miotic, at intervals spread over several months, may help to maintain binocular single vision most of the time, leading to a more stable binocular relationship and allowing other treatment to be deferred until cooperation improves. However, miotics have been shown to be a less effective form of treatment than bifocals (Hiatt *et al.* 1979).

ORTHOPTIC TREATMENT

Treatment may be considered as a primary option or used in combination with bifocal spectacles and in the management of postoperative residual deviations.

It is unrealistic to attempt orthoptic exercises if:

- the deviation is constant for near fixation;
- the distance deviation measures more than a few dioptres and the near deviation exceeds 20 Δ;
- the AC/A ratio is greater than 8–10 : 1.

Favourable cases are those with a small deviation and excellent cooperation, which usually means that the child must be at least 6 years of age but probably older.

Aims

The aims of orthoptic treatment are:
- recognition of diplopia for near fixation;
- control of the esotropia for near;
- improvement of the near binocular visual acuity (with spectacles if worn).

Methods

The stages of orthoptic treatment are:
- Overcoming suppression: diplopia can be taught for near using the methods described for fully accommodative esotropia. This part of the treatment does not usually present any difficulties.
- Control of the deviation: it should be possible to achieve control of the esotropia for near by:

  1 working from the position nearest the eyes at which binocular single vision is easily obtained, practising controlled binocular convergence or withdrawing the target from the point of intersection;

  2 using a prism bar to fuse the images, gradually reducing the strength of the prism until a single image can be maintained without it.

Control is achieved at the expense of accommodation; the near binocular visual acuity will therefore be very poor at this stage.
- Improvement of the near binocular visual acuity: improvement is obtained by increasing negative relative convergence (fusional divergence) with the patient's correction. This cannot usually be achieved by orthoptic exercises alone; in nearly every case treatment must be supplemented by optical aids.
- Optical aids: the effect on the deviation of additional convex lenses should first be assessed, aiming to find the minimum addition which will result in binocular single vision with a binocular visual acuity adequate for the patient's needs, related to the smallest size print he uses at school. This correction, in the form of clip-on lenses, can be used to teach the patient

bar reading. The strength of the addition can be reduced in stages and bar-reading exercises continued.

Advantages

Although orthoptic exercises alone can only rarely achieve a satisfactory near binocular visual acuity, they are useful as an adjunct to other conservative and surgical treatment. It is helpful if suppression can be overcome before other treatment is undertaken and improvement of the fusion amplitude can be invaluable in achieving comfortable binocular single vision after surgery.

BOTULINUM TOXIN

Botulinum toxin in our hands has not been effective as a primary form of treatment for this type of esotropia. Neither have we found it useful in the long-term management of postoperative residual angles. However, we would recommend it as an important option in the management of consecutive exotropia if used in the early postoperative period.

Surgical treatment

We consider that surgery has a role in patients with:
- esodeviations measuring more than 20 Δ for near;
- an AC/A ratio exceeding 8 : 1;
- a poor response to conservative treatment.

We prefer to carry out surgery after the age of 6 years because of the probable improved level of cooperation, which will facilitate the management of any residual deviation. Delay in carrying out treatment does not appear to have an adverse influence on successful alignment (Ludwig *et al.* 1988).

AIMS OF SURGERY

Surgery is directed at reducing the near deviation to allow fusion for both near and distance fixation with any refractive error fully corrected. The amount of surgery is calculated on the basis of the size of the deviation for near and the level of binocular single vision. The size of the deviation at distance is relatively unimportant when calculating the amount of correction (O'Hara & Calhoun 1990), although if the esophoria measures 10 Δ in the distance it shows that the negative fusional amplitude is healthy and the patient should be able to cope with any residual postoperative deviation. Esophoria measuring more than

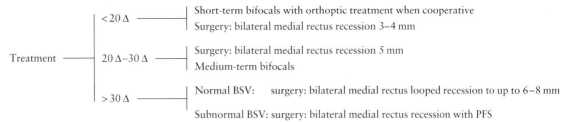

Tree 12.4 Preferred treatment options in relation to the size of the near deviation. BSV, binocular single vision; PFS, posterior fixation suture.

10 Δ in the distance makes the likelihood of consecutive exotropia remote.

Convergence excess accommodative esotropia is often classed in the literature with partially accommodative esotropia in which a high AC/A ratio results in a manifest deviation that is greater for near than distance. It is reported that patients with true convergence excess can develop a nonaccommodative component, which results in esotropia for distance (Ludwig *et al.* 1988). These patients are discussed under 'Partially accommodative esotropia' below.

SURGICAL OPTIONS

Important considerations are:

• A weakening procedure to both medial rectus muscles is the operation of choice. This can be achieved by conventional recession, by a supramaximal recession with or without the use of loops (West & Repka 1994), or by combining the recession with a posterior fixation suture (Poole & Strachan 1986; Leitch *et al.* 1990). We prefer not to use the posterior fixation suture as a primary procedure because of our preference for surgical procedures that can readily be reversed. The posterior fixation suture should be considered a nonreversible operation, whereas primary recessions and looped recessions can readily be reversed later if required.

• A single medial rectus muscle recession is not effective in reducing the size of the near deviation (O'Hara & Calhoun 1990).

• Bilateral medial rectus muscle recession of less than 4 mm is similarly ineffective (Rosenbaum *et al.* 1974).

• A medial rectus recession followed by a posterior fixation suture or enhanced looped recession performed as a two-stage procedure definitely has a smaller effect on the deviation than carrying out the two procedures

at one sitting. This needs to be taken into consideration when further surgery is being planned.

• Patients, especially older children, should be warned about the likelihood of crossed diplopia on lateral gaze in the immediate postoperative period, particularly if augmented looped recessions or recessions with posterior fixation suture are used. With both these techniques the variable limitation of adduction postoperatively causes incomitance on lateral gaze, which may persist.

RECOMMENDED PROCEDURES

We recommend the following surgical procedures for correction of convergence excess accommodative esotropia.

• Bilateral medial rectus recession of 5 mm:
    1 for near angles measuring from 20 to 30 Δ;
    2 as a first procedure for patients over the age of 10 years with near angles greater than 25 Δ.

• Augmented looped bilateral medial rectus recessions of 6–8 mm:
    1 for near angles exceeding 30 Δ;
    2 in patients who have failed to respond to 5 mm bilateral medial rectus recession.

• Bilateral medial rectus recession combined with posterior fixation suture: for near angles measuring more than 30 Δ, in patients with subnormal binocular function or poor fusion reserves.

Patients with near deviations measuring less than 20 Δ may respond to conservative management: bilateral medial rectus recession of 3–4 mm should be carried out should this be unsuccessful.

POSTOPERATIVE MANAGEMENT

Reoperation may be required for patients with surgical undercorrection or overcorrection when the residual deviation has failed to respond to conservative measures. Leitch *et al.* (1990) reported a reoperation rate of as high as 16%.

Residual esotropia

The refraction should always be rechecked to ensure that the hypermetropia is fully corrected. Important issues are:

• Residual near angles of less than 20 Δ may respond to short-term bifocals and orthoptic treatment. A temporary plus addition in the form of Fresnel lenses can be used.
• Residual near angles between 20 and 30 Δ: if further surgery is still an option, we prefer reoperation to other forms of treatment. Failing this, these patients may benefit from medium-term bifocal use with planned reduction in reading addition around 9–10 years of age.
• Residual near angles greater than 30 Δ will require either further surgery or long-term bifocals. Alternatively the patient can be electively left without further treatment if symptom free.

Overcorrection (consecutive exotropia)

Overcorrection has been reported in approximately 10% of cases in which the amount of surgery has been based on the size of the deviation for near (West & Repka 1994). The following factors should be considered.

Isolated overcorrection for distance: The management options depend on the size of the deviation and the extent to which it can be controlled:

• Exophoria at distance: this is usually well controlled and does not require further intervention.
• Large exophoria for distance, with crossed diplopia on lateral gaze: usually the diplopia will resolve within 2–3 months, but if there is limitation of adduction of –2 or greater which persists for 2–3 months there is a risk of a progressive increase in the exodeviation for distance. These patients will probably require further surgery.
• Intermittent exotropia or constant exotropia at distance: diplopia is usually present although a few patients will suppress. A reduction in a hypermetropic correction may help to control the exotropia in the short term but the long-term benefit is uncertain. Base-in prisms can be used to fuse the diplopia: we recommend reducing the prism strength as soon as

possible. A single botulinum toxin injection to both lateral rectus muscles can result in stable distance alignment if performed within two months of surgery. We would recommend this method when the prism strength cannot be reduced. Patients who fail to respond to a maximum of two botulinum toxin procedures or those presenting more than two months after surgery should be considered for recession of both lateral rectus muscles. If the exotropia is the result of the use of a posterior fixation suture, early intervention is recommended, before surgical dissection is complicated by rapid structural changes.

Isolated overcorrection for near: A persistent isolated overcorrection for near is rare and we have not seen any cases.

Overcorrection for both near and distance: This is unusual and we have only seen a few cases. Should it occur, this would suggest:

• an error in the original diagnosis of convergence excess esotropia with binocular single vision;
• an excessive amount of surgery has been performed;
• that the action of the medial rectus has been excessively compromised, which should be apparent as at least a –2 limitation of adduction.
• that either a pre-existing or postoperative vertical component to the esotropia has compromised binocular single vision.

Late overcorrection: We have not seen any late overcorrections. If present, possible causes are a compromised medial rectus action or poor binocular function.

TREATMENT OUTCOME

• Subnormal binocular single vision: Pratt-Johnson and Tillson (1985) reported that only 5% of patients with treated convergence excess esotropia demonstrated bifoveal binocular single vision. Many patients treated with bifocal spectacles or surgery show subnormal binocular single vision with a microtropia in spite of adequate treatment.
• Failure to improve: there exists a group of patients who either fail to comply with bifocal spectacles or remain unchanged following surgery. Those we have followed up continue to maintain binocular single vision in the distance with an esotropia and suppression for near. Although they cannot benefit from the visual rewards of binocular single vision for near viewing, they are unlikely to suffer in any other way.

It remains unclear whether near alignment is likely to improve with advancing years.

Hypoaccommodative convergence excess (convergence excess with defective accommodation)

This condition was first described by Costenbader (1958), who found an esotropia on near fixation in patients with a remote near point of accommodation. The increased accommodative effort required for clear vision is accompanied by commensurate accommodative convergence, which is excessive for the fixation distance. Orthophoria or a small esophoria is present on distance fixation. The AC/A ratio is low or normal, although Chin and Breinin (1967) suggested it might become high.

Management

The patient should first be refracted and even very small amounts of hypermetropia should be corrected. A small overcorrection should be considered providing that it does not reduce distance visual acuity by more than a line. Prescription of spectacles and use of a reading distance in excess of 33 cm may be sufficient to maintain comfortable binocular single vision. If convergence excess persists, bifocals can be effective in making the patient comfortable but should be avoided if possible, as it is unlikely that he will be able to dispense with them.

Early-onset accommodative esotropia

Accommodative esotropia with onset under 1 year of age is discussed in Chapter 14.

Constant accommodative esotropia

Constant accommodative primary esotropia contains just a single category, namely partially accommodative esotropia.

Partially accommodative esotropia (esotropia with an accommodative element)

Description

These patients have a nonaccommodative element to the esotropia that results in a manifest deviation for near and distance when the accommodative component is corrected. The accommodative element may be refractive—the result of uncorrected hypermetropia—or nonrefractive—due to a high AC/A ratio. Both may be present.

- Uncorrected hypermetropia. The esotropia decreases by at least 10 Δ with correction of the hypermetropic refractive error but remains manifest for near and distance fixation.
- High AC/A ratio. The esotropia at 33 cm is at least 10 Δ greater than the esotropia at 6 m. The addition of +3 Δ lenses equalizes the near and distance measurements. The higher the AC/A ratio the greater the difference between the near and distance angles. These patients are sometimes mistakenly classed with those with convergence excess accommodative esotropia.

Hypermetropia and high AC/A ratio

A larger deviation for near persists after correction of the hypermetropia but should be eliminated by bifocal spectacles with the correct near addition. If the larger near esotropia persists, the difference in angle may be due to proximal or tonic convergence rather than accommodative convergence. The prescription of bifocal spectacles is only really justified if binocular single vision can be obtained.

Aetiology

Partially accommodative esotropia can occasionally arise from a fully accommodative esotropia, or from convergence excess esotropia in which a nonaccommodative component has developed. These cases have the best potential for binocular single vision (Tree 12.5).

Most of the cases we see presumably arise from small-angle early-onset esotropia which later develops

Partially accommodative esotropia — Decompensation of an intermittent accommodative esotropia

A constant esotropia developing an accommodative component

Tree 12.5 Aetiology of partially accommodative esotropia.

an accommodative element, thus increasing the size of the deviation and bringing it to attention; these patients have poor potential for normal binocular single vision.

Features

The main features are:
• Onset most frequently between 1 and 3 years of age.
• Anisometropia and astigmatism are common.
• Amblyopia is commonly found at presentation and may be either strabismic or anisometropic (with or without a meridional component) or a combination of both types.
• Fusion potential is found in a minority of patients. The early identification of these patients will ensure treatment is delivered promptly.
• Associated vertical deviations are common and are often due to unilateral or bilateral overaction of the inferior oblique muscles, with or without a V-pattern. Less often A-patterns are seen with associated overaction of the superior oblique muscles and primary underaction of the inferior rectus muscles.
• Dissociated vertical deviation and latent nystagmus are associated with poor potential for binocular single vision, but are more frequently seen in infantile esotropia.

Management

Correction of the refractive error

A cycloplegic refraction with the prescription of the full hypermetropic refractive error is essential before categorizing the patient as having a partially accommodative esotropia. Bifocal spectacles have been used to reduce the near deviation in patients with a high AC/A ratio, but binocular single vision is rarely obtained.

LONG-TERM SPECTACLE REQUIREMENT

After the full hypermetropic prescription has been worn and the diagnosis of a partially accommodative esotropia has been confirmed, the decision whether or not to continue with spectacles can be made before embarking on further treatment. Spectacles that neither aid visual acuity nor serve a useful purpose in the management of the strabismus or amblyopia should be discarded.

The long-term use of spectacles is likely to be required in the following situations:
• in the management of anisometropic amblyopia;
• to correct anisometropia for optimum binocular single vision if demonstrable, for example in microtropia;
• if the strabismus has a large accommodative component;
• to achieve optimum visual acuity when the refractive error exceeds +3 DS in the fixing eye.

If the strabismus has a large accommodative element, spectacles are often required to provide a degree of stability. In other cases when the refractive error is symmetrical and less than +3 DS without significant astigmatism, and follow-up has shown that the hypermetropia is not increasing, spectacles can be electively discarded and the child's vision and angle of strabismus reassessed prior to planning further treatment. In this situation surgery aims to correct the angle without the correction in place.

Restoration of visual acuity

Full-time occlusion should be used in patients over 2 years of age. Part-time occlusion is advisable in younger patients.

Treatment

The decision whether or not to treat the non-accommodative component of the deviation depends firstly on the potential for binocular single vision and secondly on the patient's appearance. A minority of patients have good binocular potential: in the majority the residual angle is corrected for cosmetic reasons when necessary.

Early identification of patients with fusion potential is important in order to expedite treatment for those with a good prognosis for binocular single vision. Most patients are too young for subjective responses to some methods of sensory and motor testing; the best options available are considered below.

Prism adaptation test (see Chapter 7)

Correction of the nonaccommodative component with prisms is the preferred method of investigation and should be attempted in all patients from 3 years of age with visual acuity of 6/12 or better in the squinting eye. Factors which should be considered are:

• Patients wearing spectacles usually tolerate Fresnel prisms.

• If the deviation is greater for near than distance, the larger angle should be corrected, dividing the prism strength between the two eyes (Kutschke *et al.* 1992). If the vision is unequal, a higher-strength prism should be placed before the better eye, with a lower-powered prism in front of the amblyopic eye.

• The patient is re-examined after wearing the prisms for approximately 1 week, looking for evidence of binocular single vision.

• Confirmation of binocular single vision can be obtained from:

   1 a recovery movement on cover test;

   2 the presence of stereopsis on free-space testing. This may be impractical if high-powered prisms are required;

   3 sensory fusion shown with Bagolini striated glasses or Worth's four-lights test.

   4 motor fusion demonstrable with base-out and base-in prisms.

• The prism adaptation test provides information on the true size of the angle prior to surgery. A gradual increase in the size of the deviation is not infrequently found when prisms are worn (Prism Adaptation Study Research Group 1990).

Major amblyoscope

Usually only older children can cooperate sufficiently for a reliable sensory assessment to be made.

Botulinum toxin

Botulinum toxin injection into one or both medial rectus muscles is an effective means of reducing the size of the esotropia to facilitate the investigation of binocular potential.

   Important issues are:

• Ketamine anaesthesia is required for patients under 14 years of age. An induced vertical deviation or, rarely, complete ptosis, may complicate the investigation of binocular vision.

• Incomitance caused by the botulinum toxin may result in an abnormal head posture in patients with good binocular potential, suggesting the presence of fusion, which must be confirmed.

• Good visual acuity unimpeded by prisms facilitates free-space sensory testing.

• Patients with small nonaccommodative components who obtain binocular single vision after botulinum toxin injection may sometimes remain straight and show no sign of recurrence of the esotropia.

Treatment to restore binocular single vision

Early treatment is recommended in patients who demonstrate the potential for binocular single vision. If treatment has to be delayed, then prisms that restore binocular single vision should be used to help consolidate and maintain binocular function. Treatment is aimed at aligning the visual axes to achieve stable binocular single vision, with most patients showing control to a microtropia postoperatively. Many patients are too young to cooperate with preoperative orthoptic treatment to overcome suppression and promote the recognition of diplopia.

The principal treatment choices are botulinum toxin and surgery.

Botulinum toxin

This is an option in patients when the angle of strabismus is less than 20 Δ. We have had success with long-term binocular alignment in this group.

Surgery

Important issues are:

• The basic surgical goal is the alignment of the visual axes with the correction of any incomitance that may arise from an associated alphabet pattern. Incomitance arising from these patterns should be managed according to the individual situation, with treatment of any associated oblique muscle overactions taking priority over the option of vertical transposition of the horizontal recti.

• Horizontal alignment of the visual axes can be achieved with either a recession of both medial rectus muscles, or a medial rectus recession and lateral rectus resection. If the angle of strabismus is greater than 45 Δ three or occasionally four horizontal muscles have to be operated on at one sitting.

• Esotropia which is larger for near than distance, associated with a high AC/A ratio, should be managed with surgery based on the size of the deviation for near (West & Repka 1994).

• Accompanying vertical strabismus exceeding 4 Δ in the primary position should also be corrected as binocular potential can be compromised in the presence of postoperative hypertropia.

Further information can be found in Chapter 9.

Treatment for cosmetic purposes

Surgery is indicated if the appearance is poor and it is the wish of the patient, or of the parent of a young child. A postoperative diplopia assessment should be performed in children aged 5 years and older, and the patient and family warned about any diplopia risk (see Chapter 9): in general this is unlikely to occur if the esotropia is left undercorrected. The risk of consecutive divergence, perhaps developing years after initial surgery, should also be discussed. Risk factors include lack of binocular potential, intractable amblyopia and postoperative limitation of adduction.

The treatment choices include botulinum toxin and surgery.

Botulinum toxin

Important issues are:
- Long-term stability with the use of botulinum toxin is unlikely in patients who lack binocular potential; repeated injections will be required to maintain a normal appearance, which is unacceptable in this age group. We mainly reserve botulinum toxin for adult patients who are either unsuitable for surgery or decline it.
- We have used botulinum toxin before performing surgery in patients with combined horizontal and vertical deviations to determine if simply correcting the horizontal angle would be sufficient to restore a normal appearance.

Surgery

Important issues are:

- The basic surgical goal is to leave a residual esotropia of around 10 Δ and to correct any incomitance arising from an associated alphabet pattern.
- The horizontal surgical options are the same as those listed earlier for patients with good binocular potential, except that a smaller amount of surgery should be performed for a given angle.
- Associated vertical deviations are treated on their merit; we find that most of those measuring less than 8 Δ in the primary position do not require treatment.
- Incomitance arising from alphabet patterns should be managed according to the individual situation, with the treatment options the same as for the binocular potential group. Treatment is especially important in these patients as associated A- and V-patterns can result in exotropia with diplopia on down-gaze or up-gaze, respectively. In addition, an A- or V-pattern may be the driving force behind the later development of a consecutive divergence (Bradbury & Doran 1993).

Nonaccommodative esotropia

Intermittent esotropia related to distance or time

Intermittent esotropia comprises near esotropia, distance esotropia and cyclical esotropia.

Near esotropia (nonaccommodative convergence excess)

Description

The term nonaccommodative convergence excess was first used by von Noorden *et al.* (1978) to describe patients with binocular single vision for distance fixation and an esotropia for near fixation which could

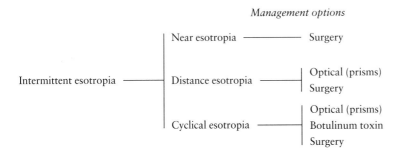

Management options

Intermittent esotropia ———|— Near esotropia ——————— Surgery

|— Distance esotropia ——|— Optical (prisms)
|— Surgery

|— Cyclical esotropia ——|— Optical (prisms)
|— Botulinum toxin
|— Surgery

Tree 12.6 Management options in intermittent esotropia related to distance and time.

not be explained by a high AC/A ratio or by defective accommodation.

Aetiology

It was thought that high proximal convergence accounted for the near esotropia. However, von Noorden and Avilla (1986) found the mean value of proximal convergence to be 2.5 Δ and therefore insufficient to explain the degree of esotropia. They proposed high tonic convergence as a more probable cause. There is no means of measuring tonic convergence in humans, and the diagnosis is arrived at by exclusion of a high AC/A ratio and hypoaccommodation.

Features

The main features are:
• orthophoria or a small esophoria on distance fixation;
• a moderate or large esotropia on near fixation;
• equal visual acuity;
• often no significant refractive error;
• a normal or even a low AC/A ratio;
• a normal near point of accommodation;
• minimal reduction in the degree of esotropia with convex lenses;
• normal sensory and motor fusion for distance and when the deviation is neutralized for near;
• no amblyopia.

Management

Conservative treatment

Bifocal spectacles, miotic drugs and orthoptic treatment have no effect on this type of esotropia. However, the patient should be refracted and any significant refractive error corrected. Prisms may be used to maintain binocular single vision for near as a temporary measure.

Surgical treatment

Treatment is essentially surgical. As in accommodative convergence excess, bilateral medial rectus recession of a full 5 mm is the operation of choice in most cases, with looped sutures for added effect if warranted by the degree of esotropia. Alternatively, a posterior fixation suture can be performed on both medial rectus muscles, with or without added recession. von Noorden and Avilla (1986) found no difference in the results obtained after conventional recession and recession with posterior fixation suture and therefore preferred the simpler recession operation. Reoperation may be necessary, making recession the first choice, leaving the posterior fixation suture procedure in reserve.

Distance esotropia

Description

Initially there is an intermittent esotropia for distance fixation, becoming more constant with time. Binocular single vision is present for near with any refractive error fully corrected.

Features

The main features are:
• no deviation or a small esophoria on near fixation;
• a small to moderate esotropia on distance fixation;
• suppression at distance, although diplopia may be present in the early stages;
• no significant refractive error in most cases, with equal visual acuity and full extraocular movement.

Differential diagnosis

Distance esotropia is an uncommon entity which is often simulated by other conditions.

The differential diagnosis includes:
• Mild sixth nerve palsy. The presence of limitation of abduction strongly suggests this alternative diagnosis. The patient's age is an important consideration, as an adult patient is unlikely to present with a recent-onset distance esotropia, making a sixth nerve palsy the likely diagnosis.
• Mechanical restriction of abduction associated with thyroid eye disease. Lid lag and lid retraction may support this diagnosis.
• Convergence and accommodative spasm. Patients with spasm will have a variable esotropia: measurement of the angle of deviation in the primary position and on horizontal gaze may show an increase on lateral versions. Distance visual acuity will be reduced in accommodative convergence spasm.
• Decompensating distance esophoria. Patients usually present after childhood with symptoms related to the effort to control the deviation or diplopia when it becomes manifest.

- Divergence palsy. Patients with this condition have little or no negative fusion amplitude (fusional divergence), but this sign may also apply to a few patients with distance esotropia.
- Childhood myopia. Esotropia is sometimes found in children with moderately high degrees of myopia. Binocular convergence develops, allowing clear binocular single vision at the far point, but is not relaxed on looking into the distance. In time the esotropia can become constant.

Further information on the conditions discussed in this section can be found in Chapters 16, 19 and 21.

Management

Distance esotropia is difficult for the patient to control even when the angle of deviation is small. Treatment can be:

- Conservative. Base-out prisms are effective in controlling the deviation in the distance: they are more acceptable if the patient is already wearing spectacles.
- Surgical. The distance deviation can be corrected by an asymmetrical lateral rectus resection and ipsilateral medial rectus recession; for example, a moderate resection of the lateral rectus muscle in the order of 5–6 mm is combined with a 1–2 mm recession of the medial rectus, using adjustable sutures if possible. This choice avoids the need to consider a unilateral or bilateral lateral rectus resection, which can have an unpredictable long-term effect on the deviation in the primary position. An initial overcorrection is likely to lead to better long-term alignment: the patient's positive fusional convergence amplitude enables him to tolerate the temporary exodeviation.

Cyclical esotropia (alternate-day strabismus)

Description

Cyclical esotropia is defined as an esotropia for near and distance which occurs at regular intervals, with binocular single vision present at other times.

Features

The main features are:

- an alternate-day cycle (48 h) is usual, and the condition is sometimes known as alternate-day strabismus.
- the manifest phase lasts 24 h and is followed by a straight phase of similar duration; other time intervals can occur and the phases may not be so regular;
- onset around 4–6 years of age is most common;
- most patients are emmetropic with equal vision;
- binocular single vision is present on straight days with no significant latent component. Suppression prevents diplopia when the strabismus is manifest.

Cyclical esotropia has been reported following successful strabismus surgery (Muchnick *et al.* 1976; Metz & Jampolsky 1979). It can be associated with central nervous system disease (Pillai & Dhand 1987). Rarely it can occur without demonstrable binocular single vision, when the eyes appear straight but fusion is not present (Riordan-Eva *et al.* 1993).

The frequency of the manifest phase usually increases with time until a constant strabismus develops. Roper-Hall and Yapp (1968) reported periods of intermittency ranging from 4 to 11 months in a series of 12 patients.

Differential diagnosis

Cyclical esotropia is easily differentiated from other forms of intermittent esotropia by the regularity of the squinting phase, which is unrelated to any particular form of visual activity, and by the absence of a significant latent deviation when binocular single vision is present.

Management

Important points in the management of cyclical esotropia are:

- once the diagnosis has been made and reproducible measurements during the manifest phase are available, there is no need to defer surgical intervention until the esotropia becomes constant as was once thought necessary;
- when planning surgery the full manifest angle of deviation should be corrected;
- a bilateral medial rectus recession or unilateral medial rectus recession and lateral rectus resection are equally effective;
- binocular single vision should be restored after surgery with little risk of permanent overcorrection;
- botulinum toxin has been used with a successful outcome;
- prisms have been used and surgery thereby avoided (Woodruff 1995).

Constant nonaccommodative esotropia

Constant nonaccommodative primary esotropia contains the following categories:
- infantile esotropia;
- acquired nonaccommodative esotropia;
- esotropia associated with myopia;
- nystagmus blockage syndrome;
- microesotropia.

Infantile esotropia

Infantile esotropia is dealt with in Chapter 14.

Acquired nonaccommodative esotropia

Description

This is a nonaccommodative esotropia with an onset after 6 months of age. Two main subtypes are recognized, depending on the age at onset:
- esotropia occurring between 6 and 24 months of age;
- esotropia with onset from 2 to 8+ years of age (normo-sensorial late-onset esotropia).

Patients with onset of esotropia between 6 months and 2 years of age

Previous binocular experience implies that the potential for binocular single vision should be good; however, this is rarely the case. Associated strabismic amblyopia is usually present, requiring early effective management prior to surgical treatment.

Assessment of binocular potential

Botulinum toxin used diagnostically offers the only real option of aligning the visual axes to allow assessment of binocular potential in this age group. We would not recommend the therapeutic use of botulinum toxin as early surgical intervention after amblyopia has been treated offers the best long-term option for stable alignment.

Prism adaptation can be used on patients presenting after the age of 3 years.

Surgical treatment

Surgical management depends on the potential for binocular single vision. Important issues are:

- Good potential for binocular single vision. This is assumed to be present in patients with unilateral esotropia who have nearly equal vision or who responded favourably to prism adaptation or diagnostic botulinum toxin. An intentional surgical overcorrection of up to 10 Δ of exotropia has been suggested to provide the best environment for postoperative binocular single vision to become established (Dankner *et al.* 1978). We prefer to fully correct the esotropia, rather than overcorrect these patients.
- Poor potential for binocular single vision. Binocular potential is assumed to be defective in amblyopic patients whose visual acuity fails to improve beyond 6/18, or in those unresponsive on prism adaptation. Surgery can be performed to improve the appearance when necessary: it is rarely indicated unless the deviation measures more than 15–20 Δ. We prefer to undercorrect these patients, leaving a residual esotropia of 10 Δ to reduce the risk of later consecutive exotropia.

Normo-sensorial late-onset esotropia (acute-onset concomitant esotropia)

The term 'normo-sensorial late-onset esotropia' was introduced by Lang (1981) to describe constant esotropia with onset from 2 to 8 years of age, or sometimes slightly later.

Features

- The esotropia may be intermittent for a short period but rapidly becomes constant and of large angle.
- Diplopia is usually present in the early stages, either the child complains of it or is seen to close one eye.
- There is no significant accommodative component.
- Normal retinal correspondence and sensory and motor fusion are present.
- A full range of eye movements and clinically normal lateral rectus muscle saccadic velocities are always found.
- A minor injury or a short period of uniocular occlusion may precipitate the onset.

Differential diagnosis

This condition may be seen in association with a brain tumour, which may involve the brainstem, cerebellum or pituitary (Williams & Hoyt 1989; De Young Smith & Baker 1990). The exact mechanism for the concomitant esotropia in this setting remains unknown.

Important features that necessitate further neuroradiological investigation include:
• any evidence of lateral incomitance suggesting subtle lateral rectus weakness, especially if associated with a V-pattern;
• any neurological symptoms or signs, in particular papilloedema;
• nystagmus, in particular dissociated nystagmus on lateral gaze;
• failure to obtain binocular single vision with prisms or surgery.

An acute-onset esotropia may also be seen in hydrocephalus as a result of raised intracranial pressure. Although in the early stages there is lateral incomitance with limited abduction, with time a more concomitant horizontal deviation develops; it is usually associated with an A-pattern (Wybar & Walker 1980).

Management
Once the diagnosis has been made, all patients should initially be prescribed prisms to restore binocular single vision. In some patients spontaneous improvement occurs, which eventually allows the prisms to be discarded (Elhatton & Repka 1994; Burke & Firth 1995). Those patients who fail to improve after using prisms may respond successfully either to botulinum toxin (Schiavi et al. 1995) or to early surgery aimed at aligning the visual axes, with an excellent prognosis for the restoration of binocular single vision.

Esotropia associated with myopia

Myopia is seen in association with most types of strabismus. In general, the prevalence of myopia in these conditions does not differ from that of the normal population. There are however, two types of esotropia which are characteristically seen in association with moderate and high levels of myopia:

Moderate level of myopia (6–12 DS)
This degree of myopia can be associated with a gradual onset of esotropia with diplopia, occurring characteristically in young adults. The esotropia develops first for distance fixation, and eye movements are usually full. Although prisms are useful in the initial management of the diplopia, most of the patients seen by us have worn contact lenses and were unwilling to

change to prismatic glasses. Surgery, usually a bilateral medial rectus recession, is successful in restoring alignment.

High level of myopia (greater than 15 DS)
This degree of myopia can result in an esotropia associated with mechanical restriction of movement. There is often a history of esotropia with onset in adult life, and the deviation has sometimes been present for a number of years when first seen by an ophthalmologist. Diplopia is rarely present. The level of myopia is generally higher than 15 DS in both eyes, and the range of abduction is limited; sometimes the eye is unable to cross the mid-line. Myositis has been suggested as a cause for the esotropia (Hugonnier & Clayette-Hugonnier 1969); however, histological examination has shown atrophy and fibrosis of the medial rectus muscle with no evidence of inflammation (Kaynak et al. 1994; Remón et al. 1996). Kaynak et al. (1994) have proposed that the esotropia seen in this condition is a direct result of the enlarging globe compressing the lateral rectus, resulting in atrophy of that muscle. Long-standing esotropia may lead to medial rectus fibrosis that both increases the deviation and causes mechanical restriction of abduction. These authors do not consider that the limitation of abduction is due to the contact between the globe and the medial wall of the orbit, as suggested by Demer and von Noorden (1989).

Differential diagnosis
The differential diagnosis is:
• Thyroid eye disease. The large globe and limitation of abduction seen in pathological myopia are similar to the findings in thyroid eye disease. However, laboratory studies of thyroid function will be normal and the lid lag and lid retraction typical of thyroid eye disease will be absent. Orbital ultrasonography will show normal-sized extraocular muscles, although this can also be the finding in the late cicatricial stages of thyroid eye disease.
• Lateral rectus palsy.
• Congenital extraocular muscle fibrosis.
• Orbital trauma.

Management
Botulinum toxin to both medial rectus muscles was

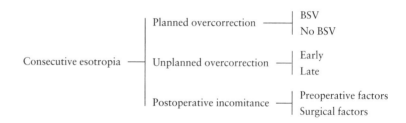

Tree 12.7 Classification of
consecutive esotropia. BSV,
binocular single vision.

effective in producing short-term alignment in two of
our patients (unpublished results) and it is also useful
for exploring binocular potential in this condition.

Surgery, comprising recession of the tight medial
rectus and resection of the lateral rectus, has resulted
in both improved alignment and a better range of
ocular movement (Remón *et al.* 1996). However, the
esotropia may recur (Frilling & Kowal 1996).

Swan's blind-spot mechanism

Swan (1948) first described the condition in which the
image of the fixation object falls on the optic disc of
the deviating eye in an esotropia measuring 30–35 Δ.
Suppression of the diplopic image is not needed and
normal retinal correspondence should be retained. It
is difficult to be certain that this mechanism is maintained for all distances of fixation and therefore we
doubt if it is an entity.

Nystagmus blockage syndrome

Nystagmus blockage syndrome is dealt with in
Chapter 14.

Microesotropia

Microesotropia is dealt with in Chapter 15.

Consecutive esotropia

Description

Consecutive esotropia is an esotropia occurring in a
patient with a previous history of exotropia or, less
usually, exophoria. Consecutive esotropia most commonly results from surgical overcorrection of a primary exotropia. It occasionally develops spontaneously.

Spontaneous consecutive esotropia

Unlike spontaneous consecutive exotropia, spontaneous consecutive esotropia is rare. Mein (1981)
reported on a small number of young children with
this condition who first presented with apparently
constant infantile exotro-pia without evidence of ocular pathology. The esotropia was of gradual onset.
DVD was present in all cases.

Postoperative consecutive esotropia following surgery for intermittent or constant exotropia

Overcorrection may be planned or unplanned. It can
occur as the immediate result of surgery or develop
later. A subgroup can be identified in which significant postoperative incomitance results in consecutive
esotropia in one or more gaze directions. Management depends on the potential for binocular single
vision, on whether the esotropia occurred very soon
after surgery or was delayed, and on the degree of any
incomitance present.

Planned overcorrection

Overcorrection is planned with a view to obtaining
the best possible long-term result. It is indicated:
• In patients with intermittent distance exotropia: the
esotropia is expected to resolve spontaneously and
rarely requires treatment. Diplopia is almost invariably
present and the patient is encouraged to fuse the images.
Temporary prisms may be needed in a few cases.
• In patients with poor binocular potential who
undergo surgery for cosmetic reasons, particularly
those with consecutive or secondary exotropia, when
a small overcorrection is planned to guard against the
postoperative drift towards exotropia which is commonly seen. If the patient is comfortable, no further

treatment is required. Overcorrection is contraindicated if the preoperative simulation of overcorrection can demonstrate diplopia.

Unplanned overcorrection

Early marked postoperative esotropia

If a large esotropia is present with a −3 or more limitation of abduction, slippage of the lateral rectus muscle should be suspected. If the eye can abduct past the mid-line, the lateral rectus is likely to be still attached to the globe at some point. The ophthalmologist should be aware of this possibility: early exploratory intervention is recommended.

Smaller degrees of consecutive esotropia with better abduction can be treated using botulinum toxin. We, like others, have found this a useful method in the management of early postoperative overcorrection, especially in patients with potential binocular single vision (McNeer 1990).

Late postoperative consecutive esotropia

A distance esotropia can slowly develop some weeks after surgery has been performed to correct an intermittent exotropia. The esotropia often continues to increase despite the use of prisms to control the patient's diplopia. Intervention with botulinum toxin or further surgery is indicated.

Postoperative incomitance resulting in consecutive esotropia in some gaze positions

Consecutive esotropia can be expected in patients with marked preoperative limitation of ocular movement, when the aim of surgery is to achieve a useful field of binocular single vision, accepting that diplopia will occur outside this area. In other cases consecutive esotropia can result from:
• surgically induced incomitance, resulting in limitation of abduction and esotropia in lateral gaze;
• when there is failure to treat preoperative incomitance, usually caused by A- and V-patterns.

Further discussion of the management of consecutive esotropia can be found in Chapters 8, 9 and 13.

Secondary (sensory) esotropia

Description

Secondary esotropia results from visual loss which is so severe that it completely disrupts the fusion mechanism: usually there is loss of foveal function. The visual loss is unilateral in most cases, although bilateral visual loss can result in esotropia in the worst affected eye.

The age at which the visual loss occurs appears to influence whether the eye diverges or converges.
• Visual loss at or shortly after birth can result in either an esotropia or an exotropia.
• Visual loss in childhood more often results in an esotropia, probably due to the very active accommodation and convergence mechanism at this age.
• Visual loss in later childhood and adulthood results in an exotropia in most instances.

It is of utmost importance that all patients presenting with strabismus undergo a full ocular examination: retinoblastoma in particular can result in secondary strabismus, which may be the first sign of the disorder.

Management

The cause must first be identified and treatment offered if possible.

Surgical treatment

Surgery is indicated to restore a normal appearance in most cases: the timing of surgery is influenced by the stability of the alignment, the age of the patient and whether the strabismus is causing psychosocial problems. Some deviations reduce in size with increasing age, although this has not occurred in most of our cases.

Surgery is best carried out on the affected eye: a combined medial rectus recession and lateral rectus resection is the operation of choice. Judgement of the amount of surgical correction is difficult when a significant degree of microphthalmos is associated with a congenital visual defect.

Botulinum toxin

We have used repeated botulinum toxin injections to treat patients with small but cosmetically unacceptable deviations when we were uncertain whether or not the angle would increase in size. Several of these patients subsequently underwent strabismus surgery. The need for general anaesthesia and repeat injections in children has to be explained to the family and the patient before commencing treatment.

Residual esotropia

Description

Residual esotropia is an esotropia remaining after surgery for a larger primary esotropia.

The residual esotropia may be planned, in which case no further treatment is required providing that the appearance is satisfactory and the patient is symptom-free. In other cases, in which the aim of surgery was to achieve a smaller residual angle or parallelism of the visual axes (unplanned residual esotropia), further treatment is generally indicated if:
• the esotropia exceeds 15 Δ in patients with poor binocular function whose deviation remains cosmetically unacceptable;
• the esotropia cannot be controlled by the motor fusion reserves in patients expected to achieve binocular single vision.

Planned residual esotropia

It is advisable to leave a small angle esotropia in the following groups of patients:
• Patients at risk of developing consecutive exotropia, particularly those with high hypermetropia and/or dense amblyopia who are particularly likely to diverge in time. A residual angle of 5–10 Δ should result in a long-term satisfactory appearance.
• Patients likely to be left with insuperable diplopia if the esotropia is more fully corrected, as demonstrated by the preoperative investigation using prisms or botulinum toxin.
• Patients for whom the surgeon elects to carry out surgery for a large-angle esotropia in two stages, partially correcting the deviation by maximal recessions of the medial rectus and resection of the lateral rectus of one eye, with the intention of operating on the other eye later. We prefer to correct the esotropia by a single-stage procedure whenever possible, operating on three or possibly four muscles if necessary, believing that this approach gives a better result and is more acceptable to the patient.

Unplanned residual esotropia

Early postoperative management aims to reduce the size of the deviation if possible by:
• Ensuring that hypermetropic patients wear their spectacles all waking hours. The refraction should be checked to ensure that the error is fully corrected. Patients with good binocular potential may be helped by temporary overcorrection, which can be achieved using Fresnel lenses, usually no stronger than 1 DS, in an attempt to obtain binocular single vision.
• The use of botulinum toxin injected into the recessed medial rectus muscle. This can be effective in the early postoperative period if the esotropia measures less than 20 Δ.
• The use of base-out Fresnel prisms when there is good binocular potential, assuming that the patient is wearing spectacles. If the ability to fuse is in doubt, the prism adaptation test should first be used. If prisms are successful in achieving binocular single vision, an attempt should be made to reduce their strength over the next 2 or 3 months. In a few cases, it may be appropriate eventually to incorporate prisms in the spectacles for permanent wear.

Longer-term management
Further management
This depends on:
• the success or failure of the measures described above;
• whether or not there is potential for binocular single vision;
• the residual angle of deviation, once it has stabilized, and the patient's appearance.

Treatment options
The treatment options are:
• the use of bifocal spectacles in hypermetropic patients who can obtain binocular single vision at distance but show a manifest esotropia for near;
• permanent use of prisms incorporated in the patient's spectacles providing binocular single vision is achieved and the prism strength required is relatively low;
• further surgery, performed to improve the patient's appearance if binocular potential is poor, or to obtain binocular single vision if it is good.

Factors influencing the choice of surgery
• The size of the deviation for near and distance: residual esotropia of 15–20 Δ is an awkward size to manage surgically.
• A better and more concomitant result is obtained by operating on previously unoperated muscles. When a bilateral medial rectus recession has already been performed, reoperation should comprise resection of both lateral rectus muscles (King *et al.* 1987).
• The duration of the residual esotropia. In our experience more consistent results are achieved if a second procedure is performed within 3 months of the original surgery.
• Other factors which influence the patient's appearance, which are of particular relevance when reoperation is undertaken for cosmetic reasons. These include:
  1 a positive or negative angle kappa;
  2 the size of the intercanthal and interpupillary distance;
  3 facial asymmetry;
  4 an associated vertical deviation;
  5 the size of the refractive error.
The influence of these factors is fully discussed in Chapter 5 (see 'Pseudostrabismus') and below.
• The presence of a subconscious face turn which improves the appearance of the strabismus. There appears to be no other explanation for the head posture. Binocular single vision is not achieved. No attempt should be made to interfere with the patient's preferred head position.
  The use of prism adaptation is important to identify those patients with binocular potential and to uncover the maximum underlying deviation prior to any further surgery.
  Mechanical components must be identified by an intraoperative forced duction test and any significant restrictive factors released at surgery.

TREATMENT OF PATIENTS WITH NO
BINOCULAR POTENTIAL
Each patient must be assessed on an individual basis, and the decision to proceed with further treatment is based on discussion with both the patient and his family. Important considerations are:
• The size of the deviation for near and distance. Residual esotropic angles between 15 and 20 Δ are

an awkward size to manage surgically, especially if a single muscle procedure is planned. We have generally found that the response to a single medial rectus recession of 5–6 mm is unpredictable, and falls short of the desired correction. In the early postoperative period, some patients have responded to botulinum toxin injected into the recessed medial rectus muscle. Residual esotropic angles larger than 20 Δ with poor cosmesis can generally be managed by surgery on the previously unoperated muscles. Resection of the lateral rectus muscles is planned in patients initially treated by a bilateral medial rectus recession. In our experience more consistent results are achieved if a second procedure is performed within 3 months of the original surgery.
  Other factors that may influence the appearance of the residual esotropia include:
• An associated vertical deviation, which usually worsens the appearance of any horizontal strabismus.
• Angle kappa: a positive angle kappa with nasal displacement of the corneal reflection will result in pseudodivergence and is often an important factor in explaining why some 15–30 Δ residual esotropias do not look as large as the measurements suggest. The opposite situation is occasionally seen, where a negative angle kappa worsens the appearance of a small-angle esotropia.
• Intercanthal and interpupillary distance. A wide displacement of the eyes tends to improve the appearance of esotropia and worsen the appearance of exotropia, with a narrow interpupillary distance having the opposite effect.
• Facial asymmetry can also enhance or improve the effect of any strabismus.
• Head posture. We have been aware that a number of patients appear to adopt a subconscious face turn which improves the appearance of the strabismus. There appears to be no other reason for the head posture.
• Enophthalmos and asymmetrical lid fissure changes may further degrade the appearance of a strabismus.
• Conjunctival scarring and inflammation are not infrequently seen, especially following reoperations.
• High refractive errors. The magnification associated with high-powered convex lenses can enhance any defect, especially if the refractive error is unilateral.

TREATMENT OF PATIENTS WITH BINOCULAR
POTENTIAL

Important issues to consider include:
• Further treatment should be expedited in patients
under 7 years of age to establish and consolidate
binocular single vision as soon as possible. If this can
be achieved during the period of visual maturation, the
risk of developing strabismic amblyopia is minimized.
• Correction of hypermetropia is occasionally sufficient to re-establish binocularity in children with deviations less than 20 Δ. Older children and adults may
tolerate the long-term use of prisms, especially if spectacles are already worn.

OPTIONS AVAILABLE IN PATIENTS WITH POOR
COSMESIS AFTER MAXIMAL CONVENTIONAL
SURGERY TO BOTH EYES

Particular problems arise when the patient's appearance is still unsatisfactory after bilateral medial rectus
recession of 5–6 mm and bilateral lateral rectus resection of 7+ mm. Usually the primary esotropia has
been corrected in two stages, first on one eye, then on
the other.

Before deciding on further surgery the ophthalmologist must consider:
• The range of extraocular movement. Adduction may
already be limited in one or both eyes or will become
limited if the medial rectus muscle is weakened and
the ipsilateral lateral rectus muscle is strengthened
by further conventional surgery. The 'trade-off' for
improvement in alignment in the primary position is
often a worsening of ductional eye movement. Pre-
existing limitation of adduction should be viewed
with caution, since further surgery is likely to worsen
it. If one eye demonstrates a better range of adduction
than the other, the more mobile eye should be operated on; but whenever possible, surgery should be
divided between the eyes to minimize incomitance.
• The result of the forced duction test. A positive
forced duction test on abduction necessitates that a
further recession of the ipsilateral medial rectus muscle, with or without conjunctival recession, should be
performed before the lateral rectus is resected.
• Relative enophthalmos. If this is present in one eye,
recession of the medial rectus in that eye should
reduce it.

• Conjunctival inflammation and scarring. Further
surgery will aggravate inflammation. Significant conjunctival scarring may warrant its removal, combined
with conjunctival recession, which can be carried out
at the same time as any necessary extraocular muscle
surgery.
• The patient's viewpoint. A patient who has undergone surgery on an amblyopic eye is often reluctant
to agree to surgery on the 'good' eye. The risk of late
development of consecutive exotropia should be explained to the patient or to the parents of a child.

A further recession of the medial rectus, using
either the conventional technique or on loops, is probably the operation of choice in most cases, but the
decision is influenced by the factors outlined above
and, of course, by the size of the residual esotropia.
These problems are discussed further in Chapter 9.

References

Bradbury, J.A. & Doran, R.M.L. (1993) Secondary exotropia: a retrospective analysis of matched cases. *Journal of
Pediatric Ophthalmology and Strabismus* 30, 163–166.

Burke, J.P. & Firth, A.Y. (1995) Temporary prism treatment of acute esotropia precipitated by fusion disruption.
British Journal of Ophthalmology 79, 787.

Calcutt, C. (1984) The use of contact lenses in the treatment
of accommodative esotropia. In: *Transactions of the
Fifth International Orthoptic Congress, Cannes* (eds A.P.
Ravault & M. Lenk), pp. 311–315. LIPS, Lyon.

Calcutt, C. (1987) The treatment of convergence excess
esotropia in the myopic patient. *British Orthoptic Journal*
44, 55–58.

Calcutt, C. (1989) Contact lenses in accommodative
esotropia therapy. *British Orthoptic Journal* 46, 59–65.

Charney, K. & Morris, J.E. (1984) Decompensation of pre-
existing esotropia during occlusion therapy. *American
Orthoptic Journal* 34, 83–86.

Chin, N.B. & Breinin, G.M. (1967) Ratio of accommodative
convergence to accommodation. *Archives of Ophthalmology* 77, 752–756.

Costenbader, F.D. (1958) Clinical course and management
of esotropia. In: *Strabismus Ophthalmic Symposium.
Transactions of the New Orleans Academy of Ophthalmology* (ed. J.H. Allen), p. 355. Mosby, St Louis.

Cruz, A.A.V., Sampaio, N.M.V. & Vargas, J.A. (1990) Near
retinoscopy on accommodative esotropia. *Journal of
Pediatric Ophthalmology and Strabismus* 27, 245–249.

Dankner, S.R., Mash, A.J. & Jampolsky, A. (1978) Intentional surgical overcorrection of acquired esotropia. *Archives of Ophthalmology* 96, 1848–1852.

Demer, J.L. & von Noorden, G.K. (1989) High myopia as an unusual cause of restrictive ocular motility disturbance. *Survey of Ophthalmology* 33, 281–284.

De Young Smith, M. & Baker, J.D. (1990) Esotropia as the presenting sign of brain tumor. *American Orthoptic Journal* 40, 72–75.

Dyer, J.A. (1971) Non-surgical treatment of esotropia. In: *Symposium on Strabismus. Transactions of the New Orleans Academy of Ophthalmology*, pp. 154–159. Mosby, St Louis.

Elhatton, K. & Repka, M.X. (1994) Prism treatment of acute esotropia following interruption of fusion. *American Orthoptic Journal* 44, 76–79.

Frilling, R. & Kowal, L. (1996) Letter. *Binocular Vision and Strabismus* 11, 176–177.

Hiatt, R.L., Ringer, C. & Cope-Troupe, C. (1979) Miotics vs glasses in esodeviation. *Journal of Pediatric Ophthalmology and Strabismus* 16, 213–217.

Hugonnier, R. & Clayete-Hugonnier, S. (1969) *Strabismus, Heterophoria, Ocular Motor Paralysis: Clinical Muscle Imbalance*, p. 305. Mosby, St Louis.

Kaynak, S., Durak, I., Özaksoy, D. & Canda, T. (1994) Restrictive myopic myopathy: computed tomography, magnetic resonance imaging, ecography, and histological findings. *British Journal of Ophthalmology* 78, 414–415.

King, R.A., Calhoun, J.H. & Nelson, L.B. (1987) Reoperations for esotropia. *Journal of Pediatric Ophthalmology and Strabismus* 24, 136–140.

Kutschke, P.J., Scott, W.E. & Stewart, S.A. (1992) Prism adaptation for esotropia with a distance-near disparity. *Journal of Pediatric Ophthalmology and Strabismus* 29, 12–15.

Lang, J. (1981) Normo-sensorial late convergent squint. In: *Orthoptics, Research and Practice. Transactions of the Fourth International Orthoptic Congress, Berne* (eds J. Mein & S. Moore), pp. 230–233. Kimpton, London.

Leitch, R.J., Burke, J.P. & Strachan, I.M. (1990) Convergence excess esotropia treated with faden operation and medial rectus muscle recessions. *British Journal of Ophthalmology* 74, 278–279.

Ludwig, I.H., Parks, M.M., Getson, P.R. & Kammerman, L.A. (1988) Rate of deterioration in accommodative esotropia correlated to the AC/A relationship. *Journal of Pediatric Ophthalmology and Strabismus* 25, 8–12.

Ludwig, I.H., Parks, M.M. & Getson, P.R. (1989) Long-term results of bifocal therapy for accommodative esotropia. *Journal of Pediatric Ophthalmology and Strabismus* 26, 264–270.

McNeer, K.W. (1990) An investigation of the clinical use of botulinum toxin A as a postoperative adjustment procedure in therapy of strabismus. *Journal of Pediatric Ophthalmology and Strabismus* 27, 3–9.

Mein, J. (1981) La divergence verticale dissociée (DVD). *Journal Français D'orthoptique* 13, 151–153.

Metz, H.S. & Jampolsky, A. (1979) Alternate day esotropia. *Journal of Pediatric Ophthalmology and Strabismus* 16, 40–42.

Muchnick, R.S., Sanfilippo, S. & Dunlap, E.A. (1976) Cyclic esotropia developing after strabismus surgery. *Archives of Ophthalmology* 94, 459–460.

von Noorden, G.K. & Avilla, C. (1986) Non-accommodative convergence excess. *American Journal of Ophthalmology* 100, 70–73.

von Noorden, G.K. & Jenkins, R.H. (1995) Accommodative amplitude in children wearing bifocals. In: *Update on Strabismus and Pediatric Ophthalmology. Proceedings of Joint ISA and AAPOSS Meeting, Vancouver* (ed. G. Lennerstrand), pp. 201–204. CRC Press, Boca Raton.

von Noorden, G.K., Morris, J. & Edelman, P. (1978) Efficacy of bifocals in the treatment of accommodative esotropia. *American Journal of Ophthalmology* 85, 830–834.

O'Hara, M.A. & Calhoun, J.H. (1990) Surgical correction of excess esotropia at near. *Journal of Pediatric Ophthalmology and Strabismus* 27, 120–123.

Parks, M.M. (1975) *Ocular Motility and Strabismus*, p. 104. Harper & Row, Hagerstown, Md.

Pillai, P. & Dhand, U.K. (1987) Cyclical esotropia with central nervous system disease: report of two cases. *Journal of Pediatric Ophthalmology and Strabismus* 24, 237–241.

Poole, M. & Strachan, I. (1986) The surgical treatment of convergence excess. In: *Proceedings of the Fifth International Strabismological Association, Rome* (ed. Emilio C. Campos), pp. 339–344. ETA, Italy.

Pratt-Johnson, J.A. & Tillson, G. (1985) The management of esotropia with high AC/A ratio (convergence excess). *Journal of Pediatric Ophthalmology and Strabismus* 22, 238–242.

Prism Adaptation Study Research Group (1990) Efficacy of prism adaptation in the surgical management of acquired esotropia. *Archives of Ophthalmology* 108, 1248–1256.

Raab, E.L. (1984) Hypermetropia in accommodative esodeviation. *Journal of Pediatric Ophthalmology and Strabismus* 21, 64–68.

Remón, L., Palomar, T., Gabas, M. & Dominguez, M. (1996) Acquired convergent strabismus fixus associated with high myopia: a case report. *Binocular Vision and Strabismus Quarterly* 11 (1), 41–47.

Riordan-Eva, P., Vickers, S.F., McCarry, B. & Lee, J.P. (1993) Cyclical strabismus without binocular function.

Journal of Pediatric Ophthalmology and Strabismus **30**, 106–108.

Roper-Hall, M.J. & Yapp, J.M.S. (1968) Alternate day squint. In: *Transactions of the First International Congress of Orthoptics*, pp. 262–271. Kimpton, London.

Rosenbaum, A.L., Jampolsky, A. & Scott, A.B. (1974) Bimedial recession in high AC/A esotropia. *Archives of Ophthalmology* **91**, 251–253.

Schiavi, C., Scorolli, L. & Campos, E.C. (1995) Long-term follow-up of botulinum toxin treatment in essential infantile esotropia and in late-onset normosensorial esotropia. In: *Transactions of the 22nd ESA Meeting, Cambridge* (ed. M. Spiritus), pp. 159–163. Aeolus Press, The Netherlands.

Swan, K.C. (1948) The blind-spot syndrome. *Archives of Ophthalmology* **40**, 371–388.

Unwin, M.B. & Rogers, J.M. (1968) Some aspects of orthoptic treatment in cases of fully accommodative strabismus. *British Orthoptic Journal* **25**, 37–41.

Werner, D.B. & Scott, W.E. (1985) Amblyopia case reports – Bilateral hypermetropic ametropic amblyopia.

Journal of Pediatric Ophthalmology and Strabismus **22**, 203–205.

West, C.E. & Repka, M.X. (1994) A comparison of surgical techniques for the treatment of acquired esotropia with increased accommodative convergence/accommodative ratio. *Journal of Pediatric Ophthalmology and Strabismus* **31**, 232–237.

Williams, A.S. & Hoyt, C.S. (1989) Acute comitant esotropia in children with brain tumours. *Archives of Ophthalmology* **107**, 376–378.

Wilson, M.E., Bluestein, E.C. & Parks, M.M. (1993) Binocularity in accommodative esotropia. *Journal of Pediatric Ophthalmology and Strabismus* **30**, 233–236.

Woodruff, G. (1995) Abolition of cyclical esotropia following retention of binocular function by optical correction of the deviation on squinting days. In: *Transactions of the 22nd ESA Meeting, Cambridge* (ed. M. Spiritus), p. 117. Aeolus Press, The Netherlands.

Wybar, K. & Walker, J. (1980) Surgical management of strabismus in hydrocephalus. *Transactions of the Ophthalmological Society of the UK* **100**, 457–458.

13
Exotropia

Classification

Primary exotropia

Intermittent exotropia
Intermittent distance exotropia and nonspecific exotropia
Intermittent near exotropia
Constant exotropia
Decompensated intermittent exotropia

Consecutive exotropia

Spontaneous consecutive exotropia
Postoperative consecutive exotropia following surgery for
    primary esotropia

Planned overcorrection
Unplanned overcorrection
Early postoperative exotropia
Late postoperative consecutive exotropia
Consecutive exotropia and vertical muscle imbalance

Secondary (sensory) exotropia

Residual exotropia

References

Classification

Exotropia is an outward deviation of the visual axes.
Nonparalytic exotropia is classified in the same way
as nonparalytic esotropia:
• primary
• consecutive
• secondary
• residual.

Primary exotropia

Primary exotropia is more commonly intermittent
than constant. Duane (1897) described three types:

divergence excess, convergence weakness and basic
exotropia, based mainly on the imbalance between
the convergence and divergence mechanisms, and
although there is little evidence to support this concept of the aetiology, the classification has been
useful. The classification of intermittent exotropia
included below, which is in general use, is based on
whether the deviation is manifest for distance or for
near, or for near and distance without preference.
Intermittent distance and near exotropia can be subdivided into true and simulated types after the use of
diagnostic occlusion or prism adaptation and measurement of the AC/A ratio.

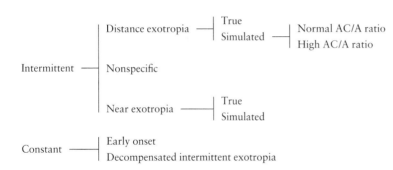

Tree 13.1 Classification of primary
exotropia.

Intermittent exotropia

Description

Intermittent exotropia is an exotropia that is intermittently manifest, when there is either suppression of the deviating eye or, less usually, diplopia. At other times the eyes are aligned and binocular single vision is maintained.

Classification

Intermittent exotropia is classified on the basis of whether it is manifest for distance or near fixation and whether the measurements are significantly more for one distance than the other. A significant difference is taken to be in excess of 10 Δ. We prefer to use the terms:
• intermittent distance exotropia instead of 'divergence excess';
• intermittent near exotropia instead of 'convergence insufficiency/weakness'.

There are three main types of intermittent exotropia, which are considered below.

Intermittent distance exotropia

This is when the exotropia is manifest in the distance and an exophoria is present for near fixation. The prism cover test measurement in the distance is at least 10 Δ larger than the measurement for near.

Distance exotropia can be further subdivided into three groups, mainly on the response to occlusion and on the size of the AC/A ratio:
• True intermittent distance exotropia: there is no significant increase in the near deviation after uniocular occlusion or when +3.00 DS lenses are used to relax accommodation.
• Simulated intermittent distance exotropia with high AC/A ratio: the near deviation increases to approximate the distance deviation when measured with +3.00 DS lenses but is unchanged after occlusion.
• Simulated intermittent distance exotropia with normal AC/A ratio: the near deviation increases to approximate the distance deviation after uniocular occlusion but is unchanged by +3.00 DS lenses.

Nonspecific intermittent exotropia (basic exotropia)

This is when the exotropia may be intermittently manifest at any fixation distance, although usually at distance, and the difference between the prism cover test measurements for near and distance fixation does not exceed 10 Δ.

Intermittent near exotropia

This is when an exotropia is present at near and an exophoria at distance fixation. The prism cover test measurement at near is at least 10 Δ greater than the measurement for distance.

Two types are recognized:
1 True intermittent near exotropia: there is no significant change in the size of the distance angle following a period of uniocular occlusion.
2 Simulated intermittent near exotropia: the distance angle increases to approximate that of the near angle following a period of uniocular occlusion.

Intermittent distance exotropia is the commonest of the three main types; most cases are of the simulated form with a normal AC/A ratio or are nonspecific.

This classification of intermittent exotropia is based on the behaviour of the strabismus and the prism and cover test measurement at near and distance fixation. Some cases with intermittent exotropia are difficult to categorize using this classification, particularly patients with apparent intermittent distance exotropia, with a manifest deviation on distance fixation but with a prism and cover test measurement which is significantly more on near fixation. These patients are sometimes classified as having intermittent near exotropia, but their clinical behaviour is that of a patient with intermittent distance or nonspecific exotropia.

Intermittent distance exotropia and nonspecific exotropia

Intermittent distance exotropia and nonspecific exotropia differ chiefly in their prism and cover test measurements at near and distance fixation. To all intents and purposes they are otherwise the same and will therefore be considered together.

Features

The features include:
• Onset after the age of 6 months.
• Women are affected more frequently than men (Cass 1937; Gregersen 1969).

• There may be some control over the deviation on distance fixation. The manifest phase may be precipitated by:

1 Inattention: the parents of children with this condition often state that they see the deviation when the child is 'day-dreaming'. In a clinical setting when the child is anxious and alert, the deviation may appear better compensated than is suggested by the family.

2 Poor health or excessive fatigue: this is likely to lessen the patient's control over the deviation.

3 Alcohol: adult patients find that even small amounts of alcohol cause the strabismus to become manifest.

4 Bright light: a high level of illumination is well recognized as a decompensating factor in intermittent exotropia (Eustace *et al.* 1973) and it apparently accounts for the large number of exotropias seen in areas with high sunlight hours, such as Australia and the west coast of the USA (Holt 1951; Berg 1982). The reason for the divergence in bright light is not fully understood. It has been suggested that the dazzling effect of light on the retina disrupts fusion; Wirtschafter and von Noorden (1964) reported that bright light can adversely affect fusional convergence. Plenty (1988) suggested that pupillary constriction in response to light increases the depth of focus, resulting in less accommodative demand and so less accommodative convergence, increasing the likelihood of the deviation becoming manifest. Closure of the deviating eye in bright light is a common but not invariable sign, strongly suggestive of this type of intermittent exotropia; it is occasionally observed before other evidence of the strabismus can be found and is sometimes the presenting sign when the exotropia itself has not been noticed. It has been suggested that eye closure is a response to the manifest deviation and so avoids diplopia; however, it has been shown to occur prior to the deviation becoming manifest, and patients with intermittent exotropia do not in general perceive diplopia when exotropic. If the patient is exposed to long periods of bright sunlight, closure of the eye is a further dissociating factor likely to make the strabismus manifest. Patients are not consistently aware when the eye diverges, despite outward signs of blinking and partial eyelid closure.

However, the occasional patient who reports he can 'feel' the eye diverge is often accurate in his observations.

• The presence of panoramic vision, when the image seen by the deviating eye is projected from the fovea but is not superimposed on the fixation object, as it is in confusion. It is more common in patients with large-angle constant exotropia than it is in intermittent exotropia.

• The purposeful manipulation of accommodation, which is occasionally used by adult patients to control the exotropia for distance or near; the patient is sometimes aware of blurred vision when accommodating. If allowed to persist, convergence or accommodative spasm may follow.

Several authors have discussed the natural history of untreated intermittent exotropia. Jampolsky (1954) proposed that there is a natural progression from exophoria decompensating to intermittent distance exotropia in early childhood, becoming a constant exotropia as suppression increases. This view is supported to some extent by the infrequency of intermittent exotropia in later life (Burian & Franceschetti 1970). Burian (1966) stated that true divergence excess generally remained stable until the onset of presbyopia, whereas the near deviation gradually increased in simulated divergence excess until it approximated to the distance deviation. However, von Noorden (1996) reported that 25% of exotropic patients in a series of 51 either remained unchanged or even showed improvement. This possibility suggests that patients should be kept under observation for a time before treatment is undertaken.

Differential diagnosis of intermittent exotropia and decompensating exophoria (Table 13.1)

The differences between intermittent exotropia and exophoria are often overlooked, leading to confusion over the management of the two disorders. Both conditions are frequently present in the same patient; for example, there can be an intermittent exotropia for distance and an exophoria for near. An important difference is that suppression occurs in intermittent exotropia but not in exophoria: the suppression is more dense in intermittent exotropia of early onset, and the vergence system may fail to mature in these cases, resulting in dissociation between the sensory

Table 13.1 Differential diagnosis of decompensating exophoria and intermittent exotropia.

Diagnostic feature	Exophoria	Intermittent exotropia
Awareness of deviation	Aware when BSV lost	Unaware
Reason for attendance	Asthenopia	Exotropia
Binocular single vision	Symptomatic BSV	Asymptomatic BSV when XT controlled
Stability	Stable throughout life	XT can increase with age
Suppression	None or minimal	Dense and widespread
Retinal correspondence	Normal	Normal, abnormal or no correspondence when manifest
Prism fusion amplitude	Reliable measurements obtained. Positive amplitude defective	Often unreliable or not repeatable
Management directed to:	Motor problem	Sensory and motor problem
Response to treatment	Good	Poor

BSV, binocular single vision; XT, exotropia.

and motor aspects of vergence control, which explains why some patients with intermittent exotropia can appreciate diplopia but cannot make an appropriate motor response to fuse the images. The motor response is intact in decompensating exophoria but has become increasingly fatigued. Most patients with intermittent exotropia do not have symptoms when the deviation is manifest, although some are aware of diplopia or blurred vision. Asthenopic symptoms are common in poorly compensated exophoria.

Investigation

Routine tests are carried out as described in Chapters 6 and 7. It is important that there should be uniformly good illumination in the examination room, and access to a far distance fixation target. There are various special points that influence the management of the strabismus and should be noted. These are discussed below.

Visual acuity

Vision is usually equal in all types of intermittent exotropia (Simpson *et al.* 1962; Krzystkowa & Pajakowa 1972), although Smith *et al.* (1995) found approximately one-third of their series had unequal vision, with 13% showing a difference of two or more lines. If amblyopia is present it is more likely to be anisometropic than strabismic; however, the presence of even mild strabismic amblyopia suggests that the exotropia is manifest most of the time. The binocular visual acuity (BVA) should be tested at 33 cm and 6 m if binocular single vision can be obtained. A reduced distance BVA is more often found in adult patients and older children and indicates that accommodative convergence is being used to control the exotropia.

Cover test

Patients should be routinely assessed in the far distance as well as at 6 m and 33 cm. The deviation often increases at distances greater than 6 m; this increase is not confined to intermittent distance exotropia but is a feature of exotropia in general, apparently in up to 33% of patients. A smaller deviation at 6 m either indicates that accommodation is still active at this distance or that loss of sensory fusion at a greater distance is sufficient to increase the deviation. It is still unclear how much weight should be placed on the far distance measurement when planning surgery. Associated vertical deviations are common, usually only apparent on full dissociation, particularly on distance fixation. A minority show evidence of oblique muscle dysfunction (Davies 1971).

Measurement of the deviation

The prism and cover test is the best method of measuring the angle in distance and nonspecific intermittent exotropia. The deviation should be measured at 33 cm, 6 m and in the far distance. It should also be routinely recorded on lateral gaze at distance fixation. This is more easily achieved by moving the patient's head rather than the fixation target. It should be measured on up-gaze and down-gaze if an A- or V-pattern is present.

Ocular movements

Moore (1969) has reported that a decrease in the size of the deviation frequently occurs on lateral gaze because of an underaction of the abducting eye. Subsequently, Kushner (1988) found that only 5% of his group of patients demonstrated lateral incomitance. Repka and Arnoldi (1991) proposed that many reported cases of lateral incomitance are due to errors in positioning the prism when carrying out measurements in lateral gaze, and maintained that it is uncommon to find primary lateral incomitance in these patients.

Care should be taken when performing the prism and cover test on lateral gaze: if the adducted eye is used for fixation, the prisms placed in front of the abducting eye can prevent it from reaching the physiological limit of abduction and can thus reduce the angle of deviation. This can be avoided by measuring the deviation with the abducting eye fixing, placing the prism in front of the adducted eye: this method should be used whenever possible but may be hampered by a prominent nasal bridge. Alternatively, measurements can be made using a major amblyoscope.

V-patterns are commonly found in association with distance exotropia. However, many patients with this type of exotropia cannot control the strabismus on up-gaze, thus simulating a V-pattern, but without a significant change in the size of the deviation. The increase in deviation on up-gaze must be confirmed by cover test, and the prism and cover test performed on up-gaze and down-gaze at distance fixation and for near fixation using an accommodative target.

Convergence

Most patients with distance exotropia have good convergence. The near point should be measured at each visit since deterioration is a sign of increasing decompensation and may indicate the need for early treatment. In a few cases of constant exotropia the eyes may appear straight when accommodation is exerted,

simulating an intermittent exotropia. Careful observation will show that consistent convergence is not maintained, the eye position fluctuates and a variable but constant exotropia is present. Near visual acuity will vary and pupillary constriction may provide evidence of accommodation. These patients are sometimes found to have DVD, which is a further indication that binocular single vision is improbable.

Binocular function

Patients with distance or nonspecific exotropia may show one of several different sensory responses when the deviation is manifest, largely depending on the stimulus used and the test environment. The following findings have been reported:
• an extensive suppression scotoma involving temporal and nasal retina (Pratt-Johnson & Wee 1969);
• both hemiretinal and smaller suppression scotomas (Melek *et al.* 1992);
• hemiretinal suppression which prevents normal retinal correspondence (Jampolsky 1955);
• abnormal retinal correspondence when the deviation is manifest (Bielschowsky 1934);
• very occasionally the patient claims to see both images simultaneously and equally clearly when using a major amblyoscope but is unable to superimpose them; the images do not cross each other when moved over a large range.

Suppression

Suppression and absence of diplopia are characteristics of intermittent distance and nonspecific exotropia. It is widely held that suppression is hemiretinal, extending over the whole temporal retina. However, Pratt-Johnson *et al.* (1981) and Pratt-Johnson and Tillson (1984) plotted the suppression scotoma using fusion targets placed within a 10° radius of the fovea, using first a Lees screen and later an Aimark perimeter, and were able to demonstrate suppression of images falling on both temporal and nasal retina. They concluded that there was little difference in the characteristics of suppression in exotropia and esotropia. Melek *et al.* (1992), using a Goldmann bowl perimeter and Bagolini striated glasses, found 52% had temporal suppression whilst the remainder showed more localized suppression scotomata. Campos (1988) has stressed the need to use nondissociating fusion targets in the assessment of suppression, otherwise retinal rivalry and experimental artefacts can give misleading results.

We believe that true hemiretinal suppression is rare and consider that suppression of the overlapping visual fields in the nasal and temporal retina occurs whenever one eye deviates, with only the monocular temporal crescent of the deviating eye remaining unsuppressed. The temporal crescent can be quite extensive when the angle of deviation is large and is responsible for the enlarged binocular visual field that is sometimes demonstrable in these patients. This may also be the reason why panoramic vision is more common in large-angle exotropia.

Retinal correspondence

There are differences of opinion in the literature as to whether some form of retinal correspondence exists when the deviation is manifest, and on the possible coexistence of normal and abnormal retinal correspondence, which has been reported by Burian (1966) and colleagues, but is considered to be very rare. These differences may be explained by the criteria that have been applied and the methods used to make the diagnosis. In the past, for example, the presence of abnormal retinal correspondence (ARC) was assumed in some centres if normal retinal correspondence could not be demonstrated. Normal retinal correspondence is more likely to be found using near-normal seeing conditions: Melek *et al.* (1992) reported that all 21 patients in their series showed normal retinal correspondence using Bagolini striated glasses. Tests using an artificial environment, mainly the after-image test, have indicated a higher incidence of ARC. Orthoptic treatment to overcome suppression will only succeed if normal retinal correspondence is present.

The role of the vergence system in intermittent exotropia

There is now a clearer understanding of the mechanisms contributing to the difference in near–distance prism and cover test measurements and the role of the vergence system in keeping the near deviation latent. One of the vergence system's component parts, fusional, accommodative, proximal or tonic convergence, usually plays a dominant role in any one patient.

• Fusional convergence is stimulated by retinal disparity, and consists of two components, a fast and a slow response. The fast response reacts to rapid changes in retinal disparity and feeds into the slow component, which acts as a vergence storage system: a negative feedback loop then reduces the signal generated by the fast vergence system, leaving it effectively 'zeroed' and able to react optimally to change when required. The fast and slow responses react differently during the prism and cover test: the amount of dissociation used in the test will break down only the fast fusional vergence control. Either prolonged dissociation using uniocular occlusion or prism adaptation is required to break down the slow component.

• Accommodative convergence is a synkinetic response linking the convergence and accommodative systems. The relationship is expressed as the AC/A ratio: high ratios are associated with excess convergence at near fixation and are responsible for the near–distance disparity in some cases of intermittent distance exotropia. An apparently high AC/A ratio is often found at near in these cases, with a normal or even low ratio at distance fixation. The high near ratio may be due to the influence of other vergence mechanisms that are inactive at 6 m, but it is also influenced by dissociation. If the near measurement with a +3.00 DS lens is repeated after a period of uniocular occlusion, it may equate with the normal distance measurement.

• Proximal convergence is stimulated by the individual's awareness of the proximity of the fixation object and results in increased fusional convergence. Its effect may explain the differences in measurements obtained when using the major amblyoscope and prism and cover test, and be the mechanism responsible for the near–distance disparity in nonaccommodative near esotropia and true intermittent distance exotropia.

• Tonic convergence arises from the resting state activity of the extraocular muscles and explains changes not accounted for by the above three mechanisms, mainly the increase in divergence seen under general anaesthesia.

Differential diagnosis of true and simulated intermittent distance exotropia

True and simulated intermittent distance exotropia must be differentiated in order to ensure that appropriate treatment is given. Differentiation is based on the use of occlusion or the prism adaptation test and the measurement of the AC/A ratio.

Occlusion

The squinting eye should be occluded for approximately 45 min; a shorter time is insufficient to ensure full dissociation. Its use is indicated:

• in all cases of intermittent distance exotropia after initial prism and cover test measurements for near, 6 m and far distance;

• before measuring the near AC/A ratio with +3.00 DS lenses, otherwise a falsely high ratio may be recorded.

RESULTS

• No significant change in the prism and cover test measurements indicates either a true intermittent distance exotropia or a simulated intermittent distance exotropia with a high AC/A ratio.

• An increase in the near deviation to approximate the distance measurement indicates a simulated intermittent distance esotropia with a normal AC/A ratio.

Prism adaptation test

This method can be used as an alternative to occlusion. The angle is corrected with prisms, which are increased at each visit until the deviation is static, leaving an interval of 1 week between visits.

AC/A ratio

The AC/A ratio should be measured at 6 m in all patients with intermittent exotropia using the gradient method (see Chapter 5). The measurement should be repeated for near after uniocular occlusion.

RESULTS

• A normal ratio is found in true intermittent distance exotropia and in simulated distance exotropia with excessive fusional convergence, as indicated by an increase in the near exotropia after uniocular occlusion.

• A high AC/A ratio is found in other cases of simulated distance exotropia, in which the angle of deviation does not increase after occlusion.

Management

Correction of the refractive error

Most patients have no significant refractive error. Hypermetropia of less than +3 DS is best left uncorrected unless it shows signs of increasing. Levels of hypermetropia greater than +3 DS are uncommon but spectacle prescription may occasionally result in improved control (Iacobucci *et al.* 1993). Myopia of more than −0.5 DS and any significant anisometropia should be corrected.

Restoration of visual acuity

Anisometropic and strabismic amblyopia should be managed by occlusion. The risk of decompensating a latent deviation should not detract from providing effective occlusion treatment. In most cases improved visual acuity and consequent reduction in suppression leads to improvement in binocular function and better control of the deviation. A microexotropia is a possibility in anisometropic patients and makes it unlikely that equal visual acuity can be obtained.

Observation

Control of the exotropia is often variable and no decision should be taken on the management until the patient has been seen at least three times, recording binocular function, the size of the deviation and how often it becomes manifest. The parents should be instructed to record how frequently they see the exotropia and bring their findings to the clinic. These observations are particularly helpful in children as the strabismus is often better controlled in the clinic than it is at home. Although most intermittent exotropias become more constant, some will remain unchanged and others even improve.

The main features that should be monitored on each visit are:

• Uniocular and binocular visual acuity: the development of amblyopia implies that the strabismus is manifest much of the time. A reduced distance binocular visual acuity results from the use of accommodation to control the deviation. Early treatment is indicated in both circumstances.

• Convergence: deterioration of convergence results in poor control for near fixation and can lead to a constant exotropia if not treated.

• Angle of deviation: an increase in the angle of deviation is an adverse sign suggesting that the exotropia will become more difficult to control if not treated.

Most patients will require surgery to restore constant binocular single vision. Possible exceptions are:

• Small deviations measuring 15 Δ or less. In our experience, it is unusual to see such small angles in intermittent exotropia, and the possibility that the patient has a decompensating exophoria should be considered.

• The manifest phase is infrequent, and the exotropia is not causing concern to the patient or his family.

Treatment

Treatment is indicated if the deviation is manifest sufficiently often to cause concern or affect binocular function.

Conservative treatment

Conservative treatment comprises orthoptic exercises and optical measures. It has limited value as an alternative to surgery but can be given in selected cases where the angle of deviation is small or the manifest phase is only infrequently seen. It is indicated, however, in the early management of postsurgical undercorrection and overcorrection or when delaying surgical intervention in the visually immature child.

ORTHOPTIC TREATMENT

The aims of treatment are to make the patient aware of the manifest deviation and to improve his control over it. Cooperation and understanding are key issues in the success of any orthoptic treatment, which is unlikely to succeed in children aged less than 6 years. Treatment comprises:

• Antisuppression treatment, which is only possible if normal retinal correspondence can be demonstrated. Treatment is mainly directed to diplopia recognition. Voluntary control may follow if diplopia is appreciated but it is impossible to teach diplopia recognition in a number of patients. Although alternate occlusion has been shown to be effective in improving control, the improvement is usually temporary and the dissociation caused may worsen the condition, so we do not routinely recommend its use.

• Binocular single vision can be strengthened by extension of the positive fusion amplitude and by teaching the patient relative convergence. However, it is unwise to encourage control of a large-angle exotropia by convergence, as success in such cases is unlikely to last and may lead to complications when surgery is eventually performed, particularly if the deviation is overcorrected and the patient tries to fuse the ensuing diplopia by using convergence.

The methods used are described in Chapter 8.

Orthoptic treatment alone will succeed in very few cases. There is no evidence that preoperative orthoptic treatment enhances the surgical result; however, we believe that it has an important role in the management of postsurgical undercorrection and overcorrection (see 'Surgical treatment' below).

OPTICAL TREATMENT

Optical treatment consists of the use of concave lenses, prisms or tinted glasses. Its main roles are:

• to provide improved, albeit temporary control over an intermittent exotropia which is progressively deteriorating in a visually immature child and therefore allow surgery to be delayed in this age group;

• to allow early treatment of postsurgical undercorrection and overcorrection.

Unfortunately, optical treatment is often handicapped by poor patient compliance, especially where there is no refractive error, making acceptance of spectacles less likely.

Concave lenses

Up to −3 DS lenses have been used to stimulate convergence by inducing accommodation, thus aiding control of the exotropia. The management option is:

• Definitive treatment. Caltrider and Jampolsky (1983) reported on a group of 35 children with intermittent distance exotropia treated with overcorrecting concave lenses. In approximately half, the deviation changed from a poorly controlled distance exotropia to a well-controlled distance exophoria, which was maintained after the lenses were gradually reduced and discontinued. The median period of concave lens wear was 18 months. In contrast, Reynolds *et al.* (1994) reported that although 56% of their series of 74 patients responded well initially, they were able to discard the lenses or reduce their strength in only 14%. The best response was obtained in deviations measuring less than 20 Δ.

Patients who initially have a high AC/A ratio are likely to show the largest reduction in angle with concave lenses. Since a high AC/A ratio is uncommon in this condition, success with concave lenses is likely to be limited to those who initially present with angles less than 25 Δ. Most of our patients have angles greater than this amount on presentation and we have not found this treatment particularly useful.

• Management of postsurgical undercorrection. Early management is advocated. Residual manifest distance deviations are not infrequently left untreated because the patient and his family are satisfied with the improvement in appearance and symptoms are unusual. However, the residual angle is likely to be small and therefore of a size that responds well to concave lens therapy, early use of which is recommended (Reynolds *et al.* 1994).

Prisms

Base-in prisms can be used in children to compensate the strabismus and allow the continued use of binocular single vision, providing that the angle of deviation is not too large.

The management options with prisms are:

• definitive treatment;
• the management of postsurgical undercorrection;
• the management of postsurgical overcorrection.

Pratt-Johnson and Tillson (1979) found that using prisms as a definitive treatment for up to $2^1/_2$ years resulted in a long-term improvement in 8 out of 12 patients with exodeviations of less than 20 Δ. In our experience deviations of this size most commonly occur postoperatively and we strongly support the early use of optical treatment in these cases.

Tinted glasses

It is well recognized that bright light is a dissociating factor in exotropia; the use of tinted glasses to reduce the amount of light entering the eye can improve the patient's control of the exotropia, providing the tint is sufficiently strong.

Surgical treatment

PREOPERATIVE INFORMATION

Before embarking on surgery the patient, and his family if a child, need to be made aware of the expectations and likely outcome of surgical intervention.

• The surgical aim is initial overcorrection and is likely to result in diplopia, which often resolves spontaneously within 2 weeks of surgery.

• The management of surgical undercorrection and overcorrection should be clearly explained.

• Persistent diplopia may necessitate the use of prisms, which are fitted on plano glasses if spectacles are not worn.

• Additional forms of treatment may be required, including botulinum toxin injection, and further surgery may be indicated. An observation period of at least 6 months may be necessary before a final decision on reoperation is made.

AIMS OF SURGERY

Our surgical aim is to achieve:

• stable binocular alignment for both near and distance fixation;

• a residual deviation which does not exceed 10 Δ and is well compensated.

Evidence clearly supports a planned initial overcorrection as the best way of achieving long-term stability (Raab & Parks 1969; Scott *et al.* 1978). Suppression is the main barrier to a binocular result and unless it can be overcome, any undercorrection tends to deteriorate with time, with a significant number requiring further surgery. Ideally, an overcorrection of 5–15 Δ should be obtained: overcorrection of less that this amount can prove insufficient in the long term. It is not easy to obtain a large enough overcorrection, and a significant number of our patients have remained undercorrected, in spite of apparently adequate surgery.

AGE FOR SURGERY

We prefer to perform surgery after 6 years of age, when visual maturity has been reached, considering that the safe management of undercorrection or overcorrection is possible at this age. In our experience earlier surgery is indicated only if there is evidence of decompensation, as suggested by:

• an increase in the size and frequency of the manifest phase;

• reduction in the near point of convergence;

• strabismic amblyopia.

Early surgery has been advocated for the following reasons:

• the habit of squinting is not reinforced over a long period;

• sensory changes are prevented or do not become intractable.

However, the overriding disadvantage of early

operation is that children who are overcorrected whilst visually immature are at serious risk of developing amblyopia and losing stereoacuity, as reported by Edelman *et al.* (1988) and Pratt-Johnson *et al.* (1977). In Edelman's series, amblyopia did not develop in patients operated on after 6 years of age. Jampolsky (1986) reported a lower reoperation rate when surgery was carried out between 6 and 16 years of age: 32% of those operated on before 3 years and 21% of those operated on between 3 and 6 years needed further surgery. The reoperation rate was reduced to 7% when surgery was delayed until 6 years or older. There was less consecutive esotropia in older patients in Jampolsky's series. Similar findings were reported by Richards and Parks (1983), who found a 12% incidence of consecutive esotropia in patients operated on before 3 years of age, which reduced to 3% if surgery was carried out later.

In contrast, Pratt-Johnson *et al.* (1977) reported a higher success rate in patients operated on before 4 years of age compared with those undergoing later surgery: 61% of patients in their series were aligned to within 10 Δ when early surgery was performed, compared with 28% of those operated on late. These authors did not aim to overcorrect the deviation, a factor that may have influenced the success rate, especially in those undergoing late surgery.

When early surgery is necessary, the surgeon has to accept that the postoperative conservative management of undercorrection and overcorrection will be limited by poor compliance. The aims of surgery are:
• to convert a poorly compensated exotropia into a well-compensated exophoria, avoiding overcorrection where possible;
• the early use of prisms or botulinum toxin when overcorrection occurs.

CHOICE OF SURGERY

Symmetrical bilateral lateral rectus recessions are widely performed, with many surgeons electing to use this procedure on both true and simulated intermittent distance exotropia and on nonspecific intermittent exotropia. We prefer to restrict symmetrical surgery to true intermittent distance exotropia. A unilateral lateral rectus recession and medial rectus resection is the preferred option for both simulated and nonspecific intermittent exotropia.

There does not appear to be any significant difference between unilateral surgery and bilateral symmetrical surgery in terms of achieving an initial satisfactory alignment. However, unilateral surgery has the advantage of allowing the surgeon the more straightforward option of operating on the other eye should this be necessary.

RECOMMENDED PROCEDURES

• True intermittent distance exotropia—bilateral lateral rectus recession.
• Simulated intermittent distance exotropia—unilateral lateral rectus recession and medial rectus resection.
• Nonspecific intermittent exotropia—unilateral lateral rectus recession and medial rectus resection.

We routinely recommend operating on three muscles in one sitting when the angle exceeds 35 Δ: adjustable sutures should be used in all suitably co-operative patients.

If there is a V-pattern without overaction of the inferior oblique muscles, both lateral rectus muscles can be transposed upwards or, if unilateral surgery is performed, the lateral rectus transposed upwards and the medial rectus downwards. A-patterns are nearly always associated with overaction of the superior oblique muscles, which should be weakened at the same sitting.

PRECAUTIONS

• Large recession of the lateral rectus muscle and resection of the medial rectus muscle can both easily induce incomitance, limiting abduction of the operated eye or eyes and giving rise to uncrossed diplopia on lateroversion. Small amounts of incomitance can usually be tolerated provided the fusion amplitude is adequate, but larger amounts of 10 Δ or more can cause insuperable diplopia, possibly with a face turn, and can prevent spontaneous reduction in an overcorrection, resulting in persistent esotropia. Particular care should be taken when resecting the medial rectus as mechanical restriction can be caused by as little as 5 mm resection. Incomitance should be avoided whenever possible by performing a smaller amount of surgery on three or even four muscles if necessary.
• Severe limitation of abduction of −3 or −4 may indicate partial or complete detachment of the lateral

rectus muscle. Early surgical intervention is essential to resecure the affected muscle.

POSTOPERATIVE MANAGEMENT

Satisfactory alignment

Our surgical aim is to achieve stable binocular alignment for both near and distance fixation. Any residual deviation should be entirely latent and measure no more than 10 Δ, requiring only observation. Patients operated on late should be monitored for one year postoperatively to check stability; those operated on early need regular checks until the age of 7 years. Treatment is not required unless convergence is poor and the fusion amplitude inadequate.

Overcorrection

An overcorrection may be present for near fixation only or for both near and distance fixation, resulting in diplopia.

Most resolve spontaneously within 2–4 weeks. Providing the patient has been made aware that postoperative diplopia is both expected and beneficial, tolerance is usually good and the diplopia can be left untreated. If tolerance is poor, alternate-day occlusion or temporary prisms can be used. Persistent diplopia should be treated conservatively to restore binocular single vision, make the patient comfortable and to avoid the behavioural problems which sometimes occur in children as a probable manifestation of their discomfort.

The methods used are:

• Fresnel prisms. We prefer to use Fresnel prisms mounted on spectacle lenses to correct the diplopia. All hypermetropia is corrected and the minimum strength of prism that restores binocular single vision is used. The patient is seen weekly and an attempt to reduce the strength of prism is made at each visit. In most patients the prism strength can be rapidly reduced, although larger overcorrections take a longer period. Binocular single vision will first be restored in the distance in most cases; prism use can then be limited to close work, or fitted on the lower segment of bifocal spectacles.

• Bifocal lenses. Patients with a high AC/A ratio who are overcorrected only for near should respond to bifocal spectacles, using the minimum strength of convex lens which results in binocular single vision for near fixation.

• Botulinum toxin. This is indicated:

1 when the patient does not respond to prisms or bifocal spectacles;

2 if it proves impossible to reduce the overcorrection after 2 months' continuous use of prisms or bifocal spectacles in patients over 6 years of age, or after 1 month in younger children.

Young children should not be left with an esotropia for longer than 1 month because suppression and amblyopia can quickly develop. We prefer to use half our standard dose of botulinum toxin, as the aim is to reduce the size of the esotropia without causing an exotropia thus preventing any re-establishment of the suppression mechanism.

• Surgery. Early surgery is indicated if a detached muscle is suspected, otherwise we defer any further surgery until conservative measures have failed to re-establish normal binocular single vision, or botulinum toxin has proved unsuccessful, usually waiting 6 months. Further surgery should be based on the findings at the time of the preoperative assessment and note should be made of lateral incomitance and near–distance variation in the angle. We generally prefer to reoperate on the previously operated eye, especially if lateral incomitance is significant. The surgical options are:

1 near esotropia equals distance esotropia: a medial rectus muscle recession and lateral rectus muscle advancement are performed;

2 near esotropia with distance esophoria: a bilateral medial rectus muscle recession is used.

Care should be taken in children under 6 years of age to ensure that binocular single vision does not deteriorate and amblyopia does not develop whilst conservative treatment is carried out. Occlusion treatment or prisms may be needed.

Undercorrection

We define undercorrection as either any tendency for manifest exotropia for near or distance or an exophoria exceeding 10 Δ. Not all undercorrections require treatment: the majority fall under the heading of well-compensated intermittent exotropia; the patient and his family are satisfied with the improvement gained and an offer of further treatment is usually declined.

Management option for undercorrection
• Conservative treatment: all patients with an exodeviation of 10–25 Δ for near or distance at 4–8 weeks postoperatively are offered concave lenses aiming to correct the maximum deviation.
• Botulinum toxin treatment: our experience with botulinum toxin injected into both lateral rectus muscle as a primary treatment for intermittent exotropia is that it is not successful when the effect of the toxin has worn off, so we do not recommend its use.
• Surgery: further surgery is offered if the exotropia exceeds 20 Δ and is manifest sufficiently often to pose a cosmetic problem or affect developing binocular function. The offer is often refused because most patients have improved control and remain symptom-free.

Results of treatment
The prognosis for the restoration of binocular single vision should be good because the strabismus is intermittent, often with well-maintained convergence and a normal fusion amplitude. However, although near-constant binocular single vision is obtained in many cases, the results are sometimes disappointing. Overconservative surgery, lateral and vertical incomitance and a V-pattern, or less commonly an A-pattern, are all factors which may contribute to failure to achieve a perfect result.

Intermittent near exotropia

Description
An exotropia is present at near and an exophoria at distance fixation; the prism cover test measurement at near is at least 10 Δ greater than the measurement for distance. Two types are recognized, depending on the reaction to a period of uniocular occlusion:
1 True intermittent near exotropia: there is no significant change in the size of the distance angle after occlusion.
2 Simulated intermittent near exotropia: the distance angle increases to approximate that of the near angle after occlusion.

Simulated near exotropia is rare and its management is the same as for nonspecific intermittent exotropia. The discussion that follows refers to true intermittent near exotropia.

Features
Intermittent near exotropia is much less common than either intermittent distance exotropia or nonspecific exotropia. Exotropia for near fixation is less obvious and this may be one reason why it is rarely seen in young children; most patients are older children or young adults. The nature of any presenting symptoms can vary, some patients remain asymptomatic and are only identified following routine optometric assessment; others are aware of panoramic vision, are concerned over their 'lack of control' over the deviation, or, more commonly, they complain of general asthenopic symptoms and diplopia.

The main features are:
• equal visual acuity;
• very poor binocular convergence;
• normal retinal correspondence and sensory and motor fusion, with a poor positive fusion amplitude;
• asthenopic symptoms and headaches caused by the effort to control the strabismus;
• diplopia, which can be the presenting symptom or else can easily be elicited with coloured filters, in contrast to distance exotropia.

It has been suggested that near exotropia is associated with a low AC/A ratio, but Plenty (1988) found a ratio of less than 2 : 1 in many normal adults and children acting as controls in a study of intermittent exotropia, implying that this level is not significant.

Differential diagnosis
• Convergence palsy. A patient with near exotropia can converge his eyes to some extent, and to targets held beyond 1 or 2 m will show a fusional response to a small base-out prism. A patient with convergence palsy will not converge and will not demonstrate a fusional response to a base-out prism unless only a mild paresis is present.
• Primary convergence insufficiency. Near exotropia can be differentiated from primary convergence insufficiency by the presence of an exotropia at near fixation.

• Decompensating near exophoria. Near exotropia can be differentiated from decompensating near exophoria by the presence of a normal to enlarged positive fusion amplitude and diplopia when the deviation is manifest. The positive fusion amplitude is poor in decompensating exophoria. Both conditions are associated with convergence insufficiency and it may not always be possible to differentiate between them.

• Accommodative convergence insufficiency. Accommodative convergence insufficiency can be distinguished from near exotropia by the presence of a reduced amplitude of accommodation.

• Acquired loss of motor fusion. Loss of horizontal vergence movement has been described after head trauma and encephalitis but can also occur idiopathically (Shah *et al.* 1995). There is often a long history of treatment for convergence insufficiency but some present relatively acutely. An exotropia is present for near and an exophoria at distance fixation. Correction of the near exotropia results in sensory fusion, but the defective vergence system prevents stable motor alignment. Measurement of the prism fusion range in the distance confirms the markedly reduced positive and negative amplitude. The amplitude of accommodation may also be reduced.

Management

Correction of the refractive error

This type of exotropia may be associated with acquired myopia. Near exotropia may occur in teenage children when the onset of myopia or an increase in the degree of myopia decompensates a pre-existing exophoria. Correction of the refractive error can result in compensation of the deviation and no further treatment is required.

Conservative treatment

The response to conservative treatment is better than it is in distance and nonspecific exotropia. Treatment can take the form of orthoptic exercises or prisms.

ORTHOPTIC EXERCISES

These should be successful in small deviations in which the near measurement does not exceed 25 Δ; however, it may be difficult to maintain improvement with near angles greater than 15 Δ. Treatment is dir-

ected to teaching recognition of diplopia if it is not already present, fusion of the images and extension of the fusion amplitude, emphasizing the positive amplitude and binocular convergence. The patient should have good positive relative convergence. Exercises based on physiological diplopia, particularly stereogram cards and bar reading, are useful in this respect.

PRISMS

Base-in prisms can be used as a method of treatment and to relieve the patient's symptoms. The prism strength should be just sufficient to enable binocular single vision to be maintained at near: usually this amount is tolerated for distance fixation. The strength should be reduced in stages until the patient can maintain binocular single vision for near unaided. This treatment can be combined with orthoptic exercises. If prisms cannot be discarded without a return of symptoms, small amounts can be incorporated into spectacles.

Surgical treatment

Surgery is indicated only if the deviation is too large to respond to conservative measures or if there has been a poor response to exercises or prisms.

CHOICE OF SURGERY

The surgical options are resection of:
• a single medial rectus muscle;
• both medial rectus muscles;
• one medial rectus combined with a recession of the antagonist lateral rectus muscle;
• both medial rectus muscles combined with recession of one lateral rectus muscle if the deviation is exceptionally large.

Because the angle of deviation is greater for near fixation, resection of both medial rectus muscles has been recommended; however, the results of surgery can be variable. In von Noorden's (1976) series of six patients with convergence insufficiency a resection of the medial rectus of 4–6 mm was performed for near deviations ranging from 14 to 30 Δ. All patients developed a temporary esotropia in the distance, lasting up to 5 months and requiring prisms. In four out of the six patients the near postoperative angle was less than 10 Δ base-in. Kraft *et al.* (1995) reported a series of 14 cases of exotropia with convergence weakness in which all patients had a near–distance disparity of 8 Δ or more and distance deviations of at least 8 Δ base-in. The amount of surgery performed was based on the size of the deviation at near and consisted of a unilateral medial rectus resection and lateral rectus recession, with more surgery performed on the medial rectus than on the lateral rectus muscle. Postoperatively the near angle was below 10 Δ base-in in all cases and no patient had troublesome diplopia in the distance.

We prefer to perform an asymmetrical medial rectus resection and lateral rectus recession rather than operate on both medial rectus muscles: to be successful the latter procedure requires initial overcorrection that we find difficult to quantify. However, deviations smaller than 10 Δ base-in in the distance should undergo a bilateral medial rectus resection, with adjustable sutures if possible. Care should be taken to avoid inducing significant lateral incomitance from over-liberal resection.

Constant exotropia

Description

An exotropia is present for near and distance fixation.

The classification of primary constant exotropia is based on age at onset and whether or not there was a preceding intermittent deviation. A constant exotropia with an onset in the first 12 months of life is termed infantile exotropia and is discussed in Chapter 14. Patients with an onset after this age usually have a history of an intermittent deviation of the distance or nonspecific type that has decompensated.

Decompensated intermittent exotropia

Decompensation of distance or nonspecific exotropia resulting in a constant strabismus can happen at any age. When it occurs in adult life a diminished amplitude of accommodation is a likely contributory factor.

Features

- A constant unilateral exotropia.
- Equal visual acuity is usual: any amblyopia present generally results from anisometropia.

- There is marked suppression and diplopia cannot readily be elicited.
- It may be impossible to demonstrate any retinal correspondence.
- It is often impossible to demonstrate any binocular vision at the divergent angle.

In spite of these apparently adverse signs, the prognosis for the restoration of binocular single vision is quite good.

Differential diagnosis

It may be difficult to differentiate infantile exotropia from an intermittent exotropia that has decompensated in early childhood if the patient first presents in adult life. Early photographs should be examined looking for closure of one eye, which is common in intermittent exotropia but rare in infantile exotropia.

The presence of strabismic amblyopia implies an early onset of constant and probably unilateral exotropia; if combined with DVD and latent nystagmus, as it can be in infantile exotropia, there is a poor prognosis for the restoration of binocular single vision. Care should be taken to differentiate a primary exotropia with severe amblyopia from a secondary exotropia with visual loss due to ocular pathology. All patients with an apparently constant exotropia should be assessed using a test for stereoscopic vision at near, such as the TNO or Wirt tests, to differentiate constant and intermittent exotropia. Retinal image disparity is the strongest stimulus to the vergence system in exotropia: the deviation may remain manifest using an accommodative target but demonstrate binocular single vision when presented with a stereoscopic target.

Management

All patients should be refracted, using cycloplegia in children. The potential for binocular single vision should be investigated in cooperative patients, although significant strabismic amblyopia indicates a poor prognosis for fusion. Diagnostic Fresnel prisms placed base-in can sometimes be used to correct the exotropia and assess fusion potential, but this method is often impractical because of the large angle of deviation. The major amblyoscope frequently shows a suppression response at the corrected angle, even in patients who later develop binocular single vision after surgery, and is therefore not a reliable method of investigating fusion in this group of patients. The diagnostic use of botulinum toxin to one or both lateral rectus muscles can temporarily correct the exotropia and help differentiate patients with or without the potential for binocular single vision. Patients older than 6 years of age without the potential for fusion should be assessed for postoperative diplopia. Goldstein and Schneekloth (1993) found that 9 out of 10 cases of constant exotropia showed the presence of fusion after surgery, in spite of lack of evidence of it preoperatively.

Surgical treatment

Surgery is the main treatment in constant exotropia. Patients with the craniofacial abnormalities sometimes associated with this type of strabismus should not undergo strabismus surgery until the completion of any necessary reconstructive surgery. In other forms of constant exotropia, the timing of surgery depends on the age at presentation and the potential for binocular single vision. Decompensating intermittent exotropia presenting in childhood with a constant strabismus requires early surgical intervention to restore fusion. Although early surgery is recommended in infantile exotropia on the basis that a delay is likely to result in a failure to develop fusion (Biedner *et al.* 1993), evidence that binocular single vision can be obtained by early treatment is presently lacking.

CHOICE OF SURGERY

Surgery is performed on the nonfixing eye. A unilateral lateral rectus recession and medial rectus resection is our preferred option in constant exotropia, although symmetrical bilateral lateral rectus recessions are also widely used. There does not appear to be any significant difference between the two methods in terms of achieving an initial satisfactory alignment; however, unilateral surgery has the advantage of allowing the surgeon the more straightforward option of operating on the other eye should this be necessary.

We routinely recommend operating on three muscles in one sitting when the angle exceeds 35 Δ: adjustable sutures should be used in all suitably cooperative patients.

If there is a V-pattern without overaction of the inferior oblique muscles, both lateral rectus muscles can be transposed upwards or, if unilateral surgery is performed, the lateral rectus transposed upwards and the medial rectus downwards. In A-patterns there is nearly always an association with overaction of the superior oblique muscles, which should be weakened at the same sitting.

POSTOPERATIVE MANAGEMENT

The aim of surgery is to achieve a stable cosmetically acceptable alignment and to restore binocular single vision in those with fusion potential. Further treatment may be indicated when overcorrection or undercorrection occurs: the treatment options are discussed under consecutive and residual exotropia.

Consecutive exotropia

Consecutive exotropia is an exotropia occurring in a patient with a previous history of esotropia or, less commonly, esophoria. It occasionally develops spontaneously but more usually results from surgical overcorrection of a primary esotropia.

Spontaneous consecutive exotropia

This condition occurs when there is weak or absent sensory or motor fusion. The onset is gradual and diplopia does not usually occur. Factors that contribute to its development are early-onset esotropia, hypermetropia of 5 Δ or more and amblyopia. Consecutive exotropia can develop in childhood or much later in adult life as the amplitude of accommodation decreases. Onset is sometimes precipitated by late correction of hypermetropia. It can be managed conservatively or surgically. If there is a low degree of hypermetropia, spectacles can be discontinued in younger patients. Reduction in a moderate to high hypermetropic correction is neither advisable nor practical: it is unlikely to improve the appearance significantly and will not be tolerated by older children and adults. Surgery is indicated if the exotropia is cosmetically unacceptable, aiming at slight overcorrection. Suppression affecting the nasal retina should ensure that postoperative diplopia will not occur; this can be confirmed preoperatively using base-in prisms.

Postoperative consecutive exotropia following surgery for primary esotropia

The incidence in reported series of consecutive exotropia range from 4% to 20% (Dunnington & Regan 1950; Bietti & Bagolini 1965). These patients can be classified on the basis of whether the overcorrection was planned, if it occurs in the early or late postoperative period and the potential for binocular single vision. A further subgroup of patients exists where significant postoperative incomitance results in a consecutive exotropia in one or more directions of gaze.

Planned overcorrection

The planned overcorrection of some primary esotropia has been recommended as the best way of achieving a stable long-term result:
• Dankner *et al.* (1978) reported that an initial overcorrection in patients with acquired nonaccommodative esotropia resulted in a greater number demonstrating fusion 6 months or more after surgery.
• Scott *et al.* (1986) advised overcorrection in congenital esotropia and reported that postoperative exotropia resolved spontaneously provided that full adduction was retained.

Although we aim to correct fully the esotropia when binocular potential is present, caution is required in those with uncertain fusion and these patients are best left slightly undercorrected.

Unplanned overcorrection

Most consecutive exotropia is the result of an unplanned overcorrection of an esotropia. Two subgroups have been described, those occurring in the immediate or early postoperative period and a more common late-onset group. Significant factors for the development of a postoperative consecutive exotropia are a preoperative A- or V-pattern, postoperative limitation of adduction and the absence of fusion (Bradbury & Doran 1993). Lee *et al.* (1995) reviewed patients who underwent surgery for esotropia and divided them into three groups based on the postoperative alignment at least 6 months after surgery. Their results agreed with those of Bradbury and

Doran except that patients with exotropia of at least 9 Δ by 6 months after surgery had significantly more V-patterns but, interestingly, less A-patterns than the other two groups, who maintained alignment to within ±8 Δ of orthotropia or were undercorrected by at least 9 Δ. They also found that patients with an initial postoperative exotropia of at least 15 Δ had a four times greater chance of remaining significantly exotropic compared to those with angles between 0 and 14 Δ exotropia, and a 26 times greater risk than patients with postoperative deviations between 1 and 8 Δ esotropia. Their data also suggest that a near–distance disparity predisposes to both significant overcorrection and undercorrection.

Early postoperative exotropia

In cases of early postoperative exotropia, Bradbury and Doran (1993) found that patients presented within the first few weeks after surgery and that the exotropia could be associated with malpositioning or slippage of the extraocular muscles, suggesting poor technique at the time of surgery.

Features
• An exotropia present for distance and or near fixation.
• Diplopia may occur in older patients if the image falls outside the suppression scotoma or if the angle of deviation exceeds the motor fusion reserves. Monocular eye closure is seen, especially in bright light.
• There may or may not be a limitation of adduction in the operated eye.

Management
Early surgical intervention is indicated if a detached muscle is suspected, otherwise a period of observation is recommended. A detached medial rectus muscle is likely to cause a moderate to marked exotropia with limitation of the range of adduction by −2 or more; some patients may adopt a face turn to avoid diplopia. Further details on the management of detached muscles can be found in Chapter 9. Other patients should be kept under observation as consecutive exotropia can resolve spontaneously, suggesting that it resulted from tissue trauma during surgery. It is important to recheck the refraction in all patients, and small

amounts of myopia should be corrected. Hypermetropic spectacles can be reduced but although this may result in an initial reduction in the exotropia, most increase with time and require other forms of treatment. If the exotropia persists, further treatment depends on the potential for binocular single vision and the patient's appearance. In the absence of fusion a moderate to large exotropia will require surgical intervention, while smaller deviations that are cosmetically acceptable do not require treatment. We have used botulinum toxin injection into one or both lateral rectus muscles in early consecutive exotropia and found it to be successful in restoring alignment in the long term: to be effective we recommend its use within 3 months of the original procedure. A more aggressive approach is indicated when binocular single vision is present. Prisms should be worn if possible, and can be reduced or incorporated into spectacles. If prisms are unsuccessful, the deviation can be treated with either botulinum toxin or further surgery.

Late postoperative consecutive exotropia

In our experience most patients with consecutive exotropia present in adult life many years after the original surgery. Knapp (1958) has postulated that the absence of normal binocular reflexes—the consequence of early-onset esotropia—prevented the eyes moving into the divergent position of rest as the hyperconvergent tonus of childhood decreased, accounting for the apparently late onset of consecutive exotropia.

Features
The characteristics have been described by ourselves and colleagues (Folk *et al.* 1983; Quere *et al.* 1989; Heaven & Ansons 1995). The main features of patients in our series were:
• most patients were aged between 20 and 30 years at presentation with an age range from 4 to 64 years;
• large-angle exotropia, averaging 45 Δ with a range of 10–90 Δ; the older the patient at presentation the larger the exotropia;
• amblyopia, defined as a difference of two lines or more in Snellen acuity, was present in 58%;

• 25% of patients were wearing spectacles to correct hypermetropia;
• 25% were aware of diplopia;
• adduction was limited in one or both eyes in 92%;
• an alphabet pattern was present in 44%.

Bradbury and Doran (1993) proposed that late postoperative consecutive exotropia could be classified according to its aetiology as due to:
• mechanical factors when adduction is limited;
• loss of fusion when adduction is full.

They found late postoperative consecutive exotropia without limitation of adduction was less likely to require surgical intervention, which agrees with our findings that most patients with consecutive exotropia we operate on demonstrate an adduction deficiency.

Management
All patients should be refracted and significant myopia corrected. Hypermetropic refractive errors are corrected on an individual basis, depending on the needs of the patient and the magnitude of the hypermetropia. Anisometropia is common in this group of patients and should be corrected if the patient benefits from improved visual acuity or binocular single vision. Most patients seek cosmetic improvement, although a few cite diplopia as their main concern. Both these groups of patients need to be assessed for fusion potential using prisms, a major amblyoscope or botulinum toxin. Although less than 5% of patients showed fusion potential, its presence facilitates further treatment using prisms or surgery. In the absence of fusion potential, the risk of postoperative diplopia should be assessed with prisms or botulinum toxin. We recommend using botulinum toxin for this purpose as the visual blur and distortion caused by temporary prisms frequently impedes the evaluation of diplopia risk.

Possible postoperative diplopia is not a contraindication for surgery as most patients are able to tolerate it if made aware of the risk before surgery. In our experience the best predictor of postoperative diplopia is whether double vision is present at presentation; 77% of patients with diplopia will continue to have it postoperatively. Twenty-five percent of those without diplopia develop it after surgery (Spencer *et al.* 1997).

Conservative treatment

If the main complaint is diplopia, a reduction of hypermetropic lenses or a trial of prisms may be effective, although we have found these methods useful only in small-angle exotropia. Most patients request an improvement in appearance and can be treated successfully with botulinum toxin or strabismus surgery.

BOTULINUM TOXIN

Botulinum toxin is a therapeutic option for patients unwilling for surgery or medically unfit for it. Despite the need for repeat injections, patients opt to continue with this form of treatment. Small-angle exotropia, especially if gradually increasing in size, can be managed with repeat injections rather than by early surgery, which is unlikely to be successful in the medium to long term in this group.

Surgical treatment

AIMS

The aims of surgery are to:
• achieve a small postoperative overcorrection of 5–10 Δ in anticipation of the tendency for postoperative recurrence of this type of exotropia;
• improve any adduction deficiency by relieving mechanical factors and restoring medial rectus action;
• cause a mild abduction restriction in the operated eye—we believe that this reduces the recurrence rate of the exotropia.

The results of postoperative diplopia assessment can influence the surgical goal. Patients with a risk of diplopia if overcorrected should be left with a small residual exotropia and should not be made esotropic.

CHOICE OF SURGERY

The surgical correction of consecutive exotropia comprises a lateral rectus recession, usually combined with a strengthening procedure to the medial rectus muscle. Advancement of the medial rectus muscles to the original insertions has been suggested as an alternative to a recession and resection procedure (Ohtsuki *et al.* 1993), but this is unlikely to relieve the contraction present in the lateral rectus muscle and conjunctiva and has not been successful in our hands. An exotropia which increases for near is likely to respond poorly to simply recessing the lateral rectus

muscles (Kushner 1992), and in these cases and in those with limitation of adduction an additional strengthening procedure to the medial rectus muscle is required. Bilateral surgery is indicated for bilateral adduction limitation greater than −1 and for angles larger than 60 Δ. A decision on the amount of surgery should be reserved until the findings at operation are known. The intraoperative forced duction test and the location and condition of the extraocular muscles can influence the surgical procedure.

Intraoperative findings

• A positive forced duction test on adduction was present in 40% of our study group. This is the result of contraction in the lateral rectus muscle and conjunctiva, and can be relieved with a recession of both muscle and the overlying conjunctiva.
• An anomaly affecting the medial or lateral rectus muscles was found in 73% of our patients. The insertion of the medial rectus muscle was significantly narrowed in 56%: there was a statistically significant correlation between the width of the medial rectus muscle and the amount of preoperative limitation of adduction, the less the width the greater the adduction limitation. In most cases the limitation of adduction was due to a compromised action of the medial rectus muscle; strengthening this muscle resulted in improvement in adduction.

RECOMMENDED PROCEDURES

For small exotropia of 15 Δ or less a single lateral rectus recession of 5–8 mm may be sufficient. Patients with angles greater than 15 Δ require surgery on two or more horizontal muscles. We routinely perform a 5–7 mm lateral rectus recession, using adjustable sutures when possible, and a medial rectus advancement, deciding on the amount of advancement intraoperatively. With the eye held in an abducted position the detached medial rectus muscle is advanced towards its original insertion until it develops sufficient tension to prevent any further movement; the muscle is then secured to the sclera at this site. This puts the medial rectus on maximum stretch, thus optimizing its force of contraction without causing a significant mechanical restriction of abduction. The amount of advancement is measured and recorded. Occasionally the extent of advancement required moves the insertion anterior to its original position. If this occurs, advancement is combined with medial rectus resection. The conjunctiva is recessed if the intraoperative forced duction test indicates that significant contracture is present.

POSTOPERATIVE MANAGEMENT
Overcorrection
A small postoperative overcorrection of up to 10 Δ esotropia is preferred, and should be achievable in most patients if adjustable sutures are used. The overcorrection tends to reduce by 2 months; however, in a minority the esotropia will increase postoperatively and require further treatment. Patients with diplopia and potential binocular single vision should be managed initially with base-out prisms, aiming to reduce the prism strength in stages. Low-strength prisms can be incorporated into spectacles. Surgery may be required if prisms are not tolerated. In the absence of fusion, a cosmetically unacceptable esotropia persisting longer than 2 months without spontaneous resolution requires treatment with botulinum toxin injection to the operated medial rectus muscle. Botulinum toxin can achieve a long-term improvement after one or two injections in patients with acute surgical overcorrection. Patients not responding to botulinum toxin require further surgery, usually a combined medial rectus recession and lateral rectus advancement.

Undercorrection
Significant undercorrection of the exotropia requires further surgery, usually to the muscles of the fellow eye.

Consecutive exotropia on lateral gaze
Lateral incomitance resulting in a small consecutive exotropia on side gaze is seen frequently following surgery for esotropia, in particular after large bilateral medial rectus muscle recession and when posterior fixation sutures are used. The features are a limitation of adduction in one or both eyes and an abnormal head posture, usually a face turn, to maintain fusion or avoid diplopia. If a detached medial rectus muscle is suspected early re-exploration is indicated; otherwise in the absence of symptoms no treatment is required. Diplopia on lateral gaze is initially managed conservatively, with reassurance and ductional eye movement exercises. Persisting disabling diplopia on lateroversion can be managed with sector occlusion on spectacles, with botulinum toxin injection to the lateral rectus muscle or by further surgery.

Consecutive exotropia and vertical muscle imbalance

Vertical muscle imbalance is seen as oblique muscle overaction or as concomitant vertical deviation.

Oblique muscle overaction
The superior oblique muscles most commonly overact, with the greatest overaction usually on the side of the deviating eye. Unless there is a significant A-pattern exotropia we do not recommend treatment to the superior oblique muscle as the overaction may decrease after correction of the exotropia. When the A-pattern is significant we recommend weakening both superior oblique muscles by a posterior tenotomy. Inferior oblique overaction is managed in the same way as superior oblique overaction: inferior oblique weakening is indicated if the V-pattern is significant.

Concomitant vertical deviation
A concomitant vertical deviation is commonly seen. Most do not require treatment and the exotropia is managed by horizontal muscle surgery or botulinum toxin when indicated. Vertical muscle surgery is performed if the deviation prevents restoration or maintenance of satisfactory binocular single vision or if it causes a cosmetic problem. Hypertropia is usually more unsightly than hypotropia of the same amount; however, correction of a hypotropia associated with a significant pseudoptosis will improve the position of the upper eyelid. If uncertain about the need to correct the vertical deviation, botulinum toxin can be injected into the lateral rectus muscle to correct the exotropia and the significance of the vertical component is re-evaluated.

The choice of surgery for the vertical component depends on its aetiology. If it is due to overaction of an oblique muscle this can be weakened. When there is no cyclovertical muscle dysfunction, treatment of the vertical deviation entails combining surgery for the exotropia with infraplacement or supraplacement of the horizontal rectus muscle insertions.

Secondary (sensory) exotropia

Description

Secondary exotropia results from visual loss sufficiently severe to completely disrupt fusion: usually there is loss of foveal function. The visual loss is unilateral in most cases, although bilateral visual loss can result in exotropia in the worse affected eye. Severe aniseikonia and the resulting image distortion can also disrupt fusion.

Secondary exotropia occurs in some infants with pathological visual loss dating from birth or occurring in infancy; it may affect one eye or is more marked in the deviating eye. If the visual loss occurs in childhood, secondary esotropia is likely to develop, but these patients may become consecutively exotropic later in life. More commonly, it occurs in adult life when disease or injury severely affects visual acuity in one eye: the onset is gradual.

Aetiology

Secondary exotropia can result from congenital or acquired loss of vision that may be irreversible or reversible.

Congenital causes include:

* microphthalmos;
* congenital glaucoma and cataract;
* persistent hyperplastic primary vitreous;
* retinal dysplasia;
* optic nerve hypoplasia.
  Acquired causes include:
* severe blunt or penetrating eye injury;
* corneal disease;
* glaucoma;
* cataract and uncorrected aphakia;
* retinal detachment;
* retinoblastoma;
* optic neuropathy.

Management

All patients presenting with strabismus must undergo a full ocular examination to establish and treat the underlying cause. Retinoblastoma in particular can result in secondary strabismus, which may be the first sign of the disorder. Further management comprises restoration of vision if possible, assessment of the potential for binocular single vision, and realignment of the visual axes, either for functional or cosmetic purposes.

Restoration of visual acuity

Before treating the cause of the visual loss the patient should be warned that diplopia may occur or existing diplopia worsen. Removal of a childhood-onset cataract in later life can result in intractable diplopia: if diplopia is a risk then the cataract should be removed and aphakia initially corrected with a contact lens to assess the sensory status prior to considering secondary intraocular lens implantation. If intractable diplopia occurs the aphakia can be left uncorrected. Secondary exotropia due to traumatic uncorrected aphakia should be managed in the same way. Surgery for cataract associated with an exotropia in an adult can result in diplopia postoperatively, although this is unlikely if the deviation measures less than 20 Δ.

Investigating the potential for binocular single vision

Secondary exotropia due to traumatic unilateral uncorrected aphakia is a common indication for assessing the fusion potential prior to further treatment. There is frequently a history of correction of the aphakia using a contact lens which was later discontinued; the patient then attends several years later requesting treatment of an exotropia. All patients should be refracted and the visual potential in the aphakic eye recorded. Those with poor visual potential or who do not wish the aphakia to be corrected should be investigated for postoperative diplopia risk using prisms or botulinum toxin before undertaking strabismus surgery. All other patients should have the aphakia corrected with a contact lens and their sensory potential investigated using the same method. We have found botulinum toxin particularly effective in this group in investigating fusion potential and in assessing the risk of postoperative diplopia when binocular single vision cannot be obtained. If fusion is not demonstrable the contact lens is removed and the postoperative diplopia test repeated.

After correction of the exotropia with botulinum toxin the outcome and further management can be summarized as follows:
• Stable binocular single vision with contact lens—surgery is planned to correct the exotropia with post-operative contact lens use or secondary intraocular lens implant.
• No fusion potential with contact lens and no post-operative diplopia risk—the exotropia is corrected surgically and the contact lens can be used if necessary.
• No fusion potential with contact lens, diplopia with the contact lens and none without it—the exotropia is treated and aphakia left uncorrected.

Botulinum toxin can be used therapeutically if surgery is contraindicated or refused; repeat injection will be required.

Surgical treatment

Operating on the extraocular muscles of a degenerate eye runs the risk of anterior segment ischaemia, chronic inflammation and pain. A painted contact lens is not usually a satisfactory alternative. Surgery should be deferred in young children to allow time for change; the angle of deviation usually increases but occasionally decreases when accommodation has developed and is used. It is, however, advisable to correct the exotropia before the child starts school and is made aware of the defect. Adult patients can be treated surgically if it is their wish.

AIMS

In patients with fusion potential we aim for a small undercorrection of about 5 Δ; if fusion is absent a small overcorrection of about 5–10 Δ esotropia is recommended.

RECOMMENDED PROCEDURES

A lateral rectus recession and medial rectus resection, with adjustable sutures if possible, is the procedure of choice. We recommend that surgery is confined to the defective eye whenever possible. A liberal amount of surgery on this eye can be performed in patients without fusion potential, even if it results in some restriction of ocular movement. Significant lateral incomitance should be avoided in those with binocular potential by restricting the amount of surgery performed on the defective eye and operating on three or more horizontal muscles if necessary. Vertical deviations should be managed on an individual basis; correction by vertical transposition of the horizontal recti selected for horizontal muscle surgery is the usual choice.

POSTOPERATIVE MANAGEMENT

Postoperative inflammation can be severe and prolonged in eyes that have suffered previous damage, so close follow-up is recommended. Acute overcorrection and undercorrection can be managed conservatively with prisms if fusion is present, or by botulinum toxin and further surgery. There may be a recurrence of the exotropia in the long term in the absence of fusion.

Residual exotropia

This is an exotropia remaining after surgery for a larger primary exotropia. Postoperative residual exotropia may be planned or unplanned; however, unlike residual esotropia, which is frequently planned to prevent the development of consecutive exotropia, most cases of residual exotropia are unplanned.

Indications for planned residual exotropia

It is advisable to leave a small-angle exotropia or an exophoria in:
• adults with decompensating exophoria or intermittent exotropia as persistent overcorrection is poorly tolerated;
• patients who demonstrate insuperable diplopia when tested with prisms or botulinum toxin preoperatively; this occasionally applies to those with consecutive exotropia.

Residual exotropia is also encountered when surgery for large-angle exotropia is carried out in two stages. We prefer to correct the exotropia by a single-stage procedure whenever possible, operating on three or possibly four muscles if necessary: we find that this approach is more acceptable to the patient and gives a better result.

Management

The management of both planned and unplanned residual exotropia depends on:
• The prognosis for binocular single vision: if this

is good, treatment should be directed at helping the patient to control the residual angle.

• The patient's appearance if surgery was performed for cosmetic reasons. If the patient is symptom-free and his appearance is acceptable to him, further treatment is not required.

In general treatment is indicated if:

• the exotropia cannot be controlled by the motor fusion reserves;

• the exotropia exceed 15–20 Δ in patients with poor binocular function.

Early postoperative management

Early management aims to reduce the size of the deviation by the use of:

• Concave lenses in patients with good binocular single vision or a residual deviation of 10–25 Δ.

• Botulinum toxin injected into the recessed lateral rectus muscle. In our hands this has proved to be less effective in obtaining a cure for residual exotropia compared to residual esotropia. Repeat injections are required to maintain alignment, which may prove to be acceptable in adults with small residual deviations but is not justified in children.

• Base-in Fresnel prisms: this method is rarely effective in residual primary exotropia, but may be effective in consecutive exotropia and certain secondary exotropias that show binocular potential following surgery. If prisms are successful in achieving binocular single vision, efforts should be made to reduce the prism strength in stages whenever possible. Eventually it may be appropriate to incorporate prisms in the spectacles for permanent wear.

Long-term management

Further management depends on:

• potential for binocular single vision;

• the success or failure of the measures described above;

• the residual angle of deviation, once it has stabilized, and its effect on the patient's appearance.

Treatment options

The treatment options are:

• Permanent use of prisms incorporated in the patient's spectacles providing binocular single vision is achieved and the prism strength required is relat-

ively low. Prisms can also be effective in moving the image back into a suppression scotoma.

• Repeat injection of botulinum toxin into the lateral rectus muscle if binocular potential is not present.

• Further surgery, performed to improve the patient's appearance if binocular potential is poor, or to obtain binocular single vision if it is good.

Surgical treatment

Factors influencing the choice of surgery:

• The size of the deviation for near and distance: it is difficult to obtain a stable result with surgery on residual exotropia between 15 and 20 Δ when binocular potential is poor. Adult patients, concerned about their cosmesis, are offered repeat botulinum toxin injections with an option of further surgery later if the angle increases in size.

• The muscles previously operated on: a better and more concomitant result is usually obtained by selecting previously unoperated muscles but this is not always possible.

• The duration of the residual exotropia:

1 Resection of both medial rectus muscles is indicated when further surgery is required within 3 months following recession of both lateral rectus muscles. If a longer period has elapsed, re-recession of one lateral rectus can be combined with resection of the ipsilateral medial rectus.

2 Contracture of the lateral rectus muscles and overlying conjunctiva can develop with time in large residual exotropias: if this is confirmed by the forced duction test, recession of the tight tissues is indicated.

• The surgeon should consider other factors which influence the patient's appearance, including the angle kappa, the intercanthal and interpupillary distances, facial asymmetry, the strength of the lenses worn and any associated vertical deviation. The effect of these factors is fully discussed in the section on pseudostrabismus (see Chapter 5).

• A subconscious face turn can mask the residual exotropia: Binocular single vision is not achieved and no attempt should be made to interfere with the patient's preferred head position.

Diagnostic occlusion should always be used to uncover the maximum underlying deviation before further surgery is performed.

TREATMENT OF PATIENTS WITH BINOCULAR
POTENTIAL

Important issues to consider include:

• Most primary exotropia is intermittent: patients with residual deviations usually continue to maintain binocular single vision for at least part of the time, therefore further treatment is less urgent than it is for residual esotropia.

• Older children and adults may tolerate the long-term use of prisms, especially if spectacles are already worn.

TREATMENT OF PATIENTS WITH NO
BINOCULAR POTENTIAL

Each patient must be assessed on an individual basis and the decision to proceed with further treatment based on discussion with both the patient and his family. The main consideration is the size of the deviation for near and distance. As discussed earlier, adults with residual exotropic angles of between 15 and 20 Δ are offered repeat botulinum toxin injection. Residual exotropia larger than 20 Δ with poor cosmesis can generally be managed by surgery on the previously unoperated muscles.

OPTIONS FOR PATIENTS WITH POOR COSMESIS
AFTER MAXIMAL CONVENTIONAL SURGERY
TO BOTH EYES

This situation is seen less often in residual exotropia compared with residual esotropia. However, the important factors to consider are similar for both conditions, and are summarized below.

Before deciding on further surgery the ophthalmologist must consider:

• The range of extraocular movement: abduction may already be limited in one or both eyes or will become limited if the lateral rectus muscle is weakened and the ipsilateral medial rectus muscle is strengthened by further conventional surgery. The 'trade-off' for improvement in alignment in the primary position is often a worsening of ductional eye movement. Pre-existing limitation of abduction should be viewed with caution, since further surgery is likely to worsen it. If one eye demonstrates a better range of abduction than the other, the more mobile eye should be operated on, but whenever possible, surgery should be divided between the eyes to minimize incomitance.

• The result of the forced duction test: a positive forced duction test on adduction necessitates that a further recession of the ipsilateral lateral rectus muscle, with or without conjunctival recession, should be performed before the medial rectus is resected.

• Relative enophthalmos: if this is present in one eye, recession of the lateral rectus in that eye should reduce it.

• Conjunctival inflammation and scarring: further surgery will aggravate inflammation. Significant conjunctival scarring may warrant removal, combined with conjunctival recession, which can be carried out at the same time as any necessary extraocular muscle surgery.

• The patient's viewpoint: a patient who has undergone surgery on an amblyopic eye is often reluctant to agree to surgery on the 'good' eye.

A recession of the lateral rectus, using either the conventional technique or with adjustable sutures, is probably the operation of choice in most cases, but the decision is influenced by the factors outlined above and, of course, by the size of the residual exotropia. These problems are discussed further in Chapter 9.

References

Berg, P.H. (1982) Effect of light intensity on the prevalence of exotropia in strabismus populations. *British Orthoptic Journal* **39**, 55–56.

Biedner, B., Marcus, M., David, R. & Yassur, Y. (1993) Congenital constant exotropia: surgical results in six patients. *Binocular Vision* **8**, 137–140.

Bielschowsky, A. (1934) Divergence excess. *Archives of Ophthalmology* **12**, 157–166.

Bietti, G.B. & Bagolini, B. (1965) Problems related to surgical overcorrection in strabismus surgery. *Journal of Pediatric Ophthalmology* **2**, 11–14.

Bradbury, J.A. & Doran, R.M.L. (1993) Secondary exotropia: a retrospective analysis of matched cases. *Journal of Pediatric Ophthalmology and Strabismus* **30**, 163–166.

Burian, H.M. (1966) Exodeviations: their classification, diagnosis and treatment. *American Journal of Ophthalmology* **62**, 1161–1166.

Burian, H.M. & Franceschetti, A.T. (1970) Evaluation of diagnostic methods for the classification of exodeviations. *Transactions of the American Ophthalmology Society* **68**, 56–67.

Caltrider, N. & Jampolsky, A. (1983) Overcorrecting minus lens therapy for treatment of intermittent exotropia. *Ophthalmology* 90, 1160–1165.

Campos, E.C. (1988) Visual perception in strabismus. In: *Strabismus and Amblyopia: Wenner Gren International Symposium Series 49* (eds G. Lennerstrand, G.K. von Noorden & E.C. Campos), pp. 311–318. Macmillan Press, London.

Cass, E.E. (1937) Divergent strabismus. *British Journal of Ophthalmology* 21, 538–559.

Dankner, S.R., Mash, A.J. & Jampolsky, A. (1978) Intentional surgical overcorrection of acquired esotropia. *Archives of Ophthalmology* 96, 1848–1852.

Davies, G.T. (1971) Vertical deviations associated with exodeviations. In: *A Symposium on Horizontal Ocular Deviations* (ed. D.R. Manley), pp. 149–156. C.V. Mosby, St Louis.

Duane, A. (1897) A new classification of the motor anomalies of the eyes based upon physiological principles. *Annals of Ophthalmology* 6, 84–122.

Dunnington, J.H. & Regan, E.F. (1950) Factors influencing the postoperative result in concomitant convergent strabismus. *Archives of Ophthalmology* 44, 813–822.

Edelman, P.M., Broan, M.H., Murphree, L.H. & Wright, K.W. (1988) Consecutive esodeviation . . . then what? *American Orthoptic Journal* 38, 111–116.

Eustace, P., Wesson, M.E. & Drury, D.J. (1973) The effect of illumination on intermittent divergent squint of the divergence excess type. *Transactions of the Ophthalmological Society of the United Kingdom* 93, 559–570.

Folk, E.R., Miller, M.T. & Chapman, L. (1983) Consecutive exotropia following surgery. *British Journal of Ophthalmology* 67, 546–548.

Goldstein, J.H. & Schneekloth, B.B. (1993) The potential for binocular single vision in constant exotropia. *American Orthoptic Journal* 43, 67–70.

Gregersen, E. (1969) The polymorphous exo patient. Analysis of 231 consecutive cases. *Acta Ophthalmologica* 47, 579–590.

Heaven, C.J. & Ansons, A.M. (1995) Operative findings in patients with consecutive divergent strabismus. In: *Transactions of the 22nd Meeting of the European Strabismological Association, Cambridge* (ed M. Spiritus), pp. 216–221. Aeolus Press, The Netherlands.

Holt, R. (1951) A study of divergent strabismus in Australia. *British Orthoptic Journal* 8, 95–100.

Iacobucci, I.L., Archer, S.M. & Giles, C.L. (1993) Children with exotropia responsive to spectacle correction of hyperopia. *American Journal of Ophthalmology* 116, 79–83.

Jampolsky, A. (1954) Differential diagnostic characteristics of intermittent exotropia and true exophoria. *American Orthoptic Journal* 4, 48–55.

Jampolsky, A. (1955) Characteristics of suppression in strabismus. *Archives of Ophthalmology* 54, 683–696.

Jampolsky, A. (1986) Treatment of exodeviations. In: *Pediatric Ophthalmology and Strabismus: Transactions of the New Orleans Academy of Ophthalmology* (ed. J.H. Allen), pp. 201–234. Raven Press, New York.

Knapp, P. (1958) Divergent deviations. In: *Strabismic Ophthalmic Symposium II* (ed. J.H. Allen), pp. 354–363. Mosby Year Book, St Louis.

Kraft, S.P., Levin, A.V. & Enzenauer, R.W. (1995) Unilateral surgery for exotropia with convergence weakness. *Journal of Pediatric Ophthalmology and Strabismus* 32, 183–187.

Krzystkowa, K. & Pajakowa, J. (1972) The sensorial state in divergent strabismus. In: *Orthoptics, Proceedings of the Second International Orthoptic Congress* (eds J. Mein, J.J.M. Bierlaagh & T.E. Brummelkamp-Dons), pp. 72–76. Excerpta Medica, Amsterdam.

Kushner, B.J. (1988) Exotropic deviations: a functional classification and approach to treatment. *American Orthoptic Journal* 28, 81–93.

Kushner, B.J. (1992) Surgical pearls for the management of esotropia. *American Orthoptic Journal* 42, 65–71.

Lee, W.R., Keech, R.V. & Kim, J. (1995) Predictive factors for exotropia following esotropia surgery. In: *Update on Strabismus and Pediatric Ophthalmology. Proceedings of the Joint ISA and AAPOS and S Meeting, Vancouver* (ed. G. Lennerstrand), pp. 252–255. CRC Press, Boca Raton.

Melek, N., Shokida, F., Dominguez, D. & Zabalo, S. (1992) Intermittent exotropia: a study of suppression in binocular visual field in 21 cases. *Binocular Vision* 7, 25–30.

Moore, S. (1969) The prognostic value of lateral gaze measurements in intermittent exotropia. *American Orthoptic Journal* 19, 69–71.

von Noorden, G.K. (1976) Resection of both medial muscles in organic convergence insufficiency. *American Journal of Ophthalmology* 81, 223–226.

von Noorden, G.K. (1996) *Binocular Vision and Ocular Motility: Theory and Management of Strabismus*, 5th edn, p. 344. Mosby, St Louis.

Ohtsuki, H., Hasebe, S., Tadokoro, Y., Kobashi, R., Watanabe, S. & Okano, M. (1993) Advancement of medial rectus muscle to the original insertion for consecutive exotropia. *Journal of Pediatric Ophthalmology and Strabismus* 30, 301–305.

Plenty, J. (1988) A new classification for intermittent exotropia. *British Orthoptic Journal* 45, 19–22.

Pratt-Johnson, J.A. & Tillson, G. (1979) Prism therapy in intermittent exotropia: a preliminary report. *Canadian Journal of Ophthalmology* **14**, 243–245.

Pratt-Johnson, J.A. & Tillson, G. (1984) Suppression in strabismus, an update. *British Journal of Ophthalmology (B)* **68**, 174–178.

Pratt-Johnson, J.A. & Wee, H.S. (1969) Suppression associated with exotropia. *Canadian Journal of Ophthalmology* **4**, 136–144.

Pratt-Johnson, J.A., Barlow, J.M. & Tillson, G. (1977) Early surgery in intermittent exotropia. *Archives of Ophthalmology* **84**, 689–694.

Pratt-Johnson, J.A., Pop, A. & Tillson, G. (1981) The complexities of suppression in intermittent exotropia. In: *Orthoptics, Research and Practice. Transactions of the Fourth International Orthoptic Congress, Berne* (eds J. Mein & S. Moore), pp. 172–173. Kimpton, London.

Quere, M.A., Toucas, S., Lavenant, F. & Pechereau, A. (1989) Les strabismes divergents secondaires post-chirurgicaux. Analyse statistique de 160 exotropies consecutives. *Journal Français D'Ophthalmologie* **12**, 3–10.

Raab, E.L. & Parks, M.M. (1969) Recession of the lateral recti. *Archives of Ophthalmology* **82**, 203–208.

Repka, M.X. & Arnoldi, K.A. (1991) Lateral incomitance in exotropia: fact or artifact. *Journal of Pediatric Ophthalmology and Strabismus* **28**, 125–128.

Reynolds, J.D., Wackerhagen, M. & Olitsky, S.E. (1994) Overminus lens therapy for intermittent exotropia. *American Orthoptic Journal* **44**, 86–91.

Richards, J.M. & Parks, M.M. (1983) Intermittent exotropia – surgical results in different age groups. *Ophthalmology* **90**, 1171–1177.

Scott, W.E., Keech, R.V. & Marsh, J.A. (1978) The postoperative results and stability of exodeviations. *Archives of Ophthalmology* **96**, 268–274.

Scott, W.E., Reese, P.D., Hirsch, C.R. & Flabetich, C.A. (1986) Surgery for large-angle congenital esotropia. *Archives of Ophthalmology* **104**, 374–377.

Shah, S., Spencer, A.L. & Ansons, A.M. (1995) Intractable diplopia due to non-traumatic loss of motor fusion. In: *Transactions of the 22nd Meeting of the European Strabismological Association, Cambridge* (ed. M. Spiritus), pp. 73–78. Aeolus Press, The Netherlands.

Simpson, D.G., Matheson, D.C. & Lunn, C.T. (1962) An analysis of one hundred cases of divergent strabismus. *Transactions of the Canadian Ophthalmological Society* **25**, 5–19.

Smith, K., Kaban, T.J. & Orton, R. (1995) Incidence of amblyopia in intermittent exotropia. *American Orthoptic Journal* **45**, 90–96.

Spencer, A.L., Ansons, A.M., Denning, A. & Kranemann, C. (1997) The post-operative diplopia test and botulinum toxin as predictors of post-operative sensory outcome. In: *Transactions of the 24th Meeting of the European Strabismological Association, Vilamoura, Portugal* (ed. M. Spiritus), pp. 69–74. Aeolus Press, The Netherlands.

Wirtschafter, J.D. & von Noorden, G.K. (1964) The effect of increasing luminance on exodeviation. *Investigative Ophthalmology* **3**, 549.

14

Infantile Strabismus

Classification

Incidence

Infantile esotropia

Essential infantile esotropia

Dissociated vertical deviation (DVD; dissociated vertical divergence)

Dissociated horizontal deviation

Nystagmus blockage syndrome (nystagmus compensation syndrome)

Accommodative esotropia

Sixth nerve palsy

Infantile exotropia

References

The term 'infantile strabismus' is used to describe a persistent manifest deviation of the visual axes with an onset in the first 6 months of life. Most patients have a form of esotropia as shown below; persisting exotropia is relatively uncommon.

Classification

The classification for infantile strabismus is shown in Tree 14.1.

Incidence

The reported incidence of infantile strabismus in the population is between 1% (Friedman *et al.* 1980) and 0.1% (Nixon *et al.* 1985). Following studies by Nixon *et al.* (1985) and by Friedrich and de Decker (1987), most if not all cases should be considered acquired with a probable age at onset of 2–6 months. Nixon

et al. (1985) found that 32.7% of 1219 neonates were exotropic and 3.2% were esotropic. All those with exotropia and three of those with esotropia became orthotropic by the age of 3 months. Friedrich and de Decker (1987) reported a 50% incidence of exotropia; only one of 1024 infants developed an esotropia that was still present at 3 months. Archer *et al.* (1989) found three out of 4211 infants developed esotropia between 2 and 4 months of age having been exotropic from birth. Horwood (1993), in a smaller study of 75 infants, reported 80.4% with esotropia, 4.4% with exotropia and 15.2% who varied from esotropia to exotropia. By 6 months 9.3% (seven subjects) had some form of strabismus but in six of them the deviation was rarely seen. These reports demonstrate the instability of eye alignment within the first 6 months of life and emphasize the unreliability of the given age at onset. A period of 'straight' eyes may, however, be significant for the prognosis for binocular potential.

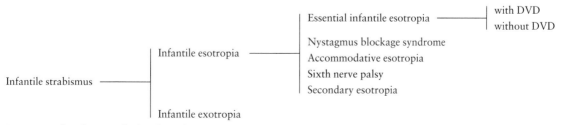

Tree 14.1 Classification of infantile strabismus.

Infantile esotropia

This is the more common presentation of infantile strabismus. It may take various forms:

- essential infantile esotropia;
- accommodative esotropia;
- nystagmus blockage syndrome;
- sixth nerve palsy;
- secondary esotropia.

Secondary esotropia is discussed further in Chapter 12.

Essential infantile esotropia

This is an infantile esotropia in which the aetiology is largely unknown but is probably multifactorial.

Features

The features of essential infantile esotropia are:

- A stable esotropia which in most cases exceeds 30 Δ and is usually considerably larger. In some, the angle is unstable and a progressive increase in size occurs: in Ing's series (Ing 1995) 60% of a group of 41 patients demonstrated this response over a 3-month follow-up period from the time of diagnosis. More rarely, there is a substantial decrease in the angle; this may sometimes occur when the presenting angle is small or variable (Robb & Rodier 1987). The size of the deviation in essential infantile esotropia is typically similar for near and distance: the patient is usually emmetropic and convex lenses have little or no effect on the deviation.
- The onset is before 6 months of age, usually occurring from 3 to 4 months.
- The esotropia is usually alternating and although there is often a fixation preference, gross amblyopia is rare: mild to moderate degrees are fairly common; Costenbader (1961) found amblyopia in 41%, and von Noorden (1988a) in 35%. Amblyopia tends to be more common postoperatively, when patients often develop a fixation preference that was not present preoperatively. Murray and Calcutt (1990) found only a 19% incidence of amblyopia in long-standing untreated infantile esotropia.
- Crossed fixation, although present in most cases, does not necessarily preclude the development of amblyopia: when visual acuity is equal, alternation

of fixation takes place at the mid-line with each eye; if there is amblyopia the eye with better vision will follow the target beyond the mid-line into the field of abduction before fixation is taken up by the amblyopic eye (Dickey *et al.* 1991). Crossed fixation is usually associated with bilateral limited abduction.

- There is a poor prognosis for binocular single vision, either normal or anomalous.

In addition there are likely to be some, or possibly all, of the following findings:

- *Latent nystagmus:* Essential infantile esotropia is commonly associated with latent and manifest latent nystagmus. This apparently contradictory term was introduced by Dell'Osso *et al.* (1979) to describe a type of childhood nystagmus in which the intensity increased when one or other eye was covered and decreased when both eyes were open but remained manifest. In true latent nystagmus, there is no nystagmus when both eyes are open, otherwise the characteristics of manifest latent nystagmus and latent nystagmus are the same, and therefore the term 'latent nystagmus' will be used. There may also be a rotary component at this stage making differentiation from congenital nystagmus difficult. Mein and Johnson (1981) reported that 30% of infants under 1 years of age seen by them had manifest rotary nystagmus, which became predominantly horizontal and latent with time. Latent nystagmus frequently becomes manifest on lateroversions.
- *Associated vertical deviations:* There is a high incidence of dissociated vertical deviation (DVD) associated with essential infantile esotropia. von Noorden (1988a) reported 51% whilst Lang (1968) suggested it was as high as 90%. DVD presents after the onset of strabismus and nystagmus, usually after 2 years of age and often after surgery for the esotropia. Oblique muscle overaction is a common finding, usually affecting both inferior oblique muscles with or without superior oblique underaction. Overaction of the superior obliques is more rarely seen (Helveston 1980). Hiles *et al.* (1980) reported primary inferior oblique overaction in 78% of their patients and von Noorden (1988a) found 68% in his series. DVD and inferior oblique overaction can coexist.
- *Asymmetry of optokinetic nystagmus (OKN):* Atkinson (1979) reported on the asymmetry of uniocular horizontal OKN seen in normal infants up to the

age of 3–4 months. When vertical stripes are presented and moved in a temporal to nasal direction a normal optokinetic response is seen but when moved in a nasal to temporal direction either there is no response or weak irregular eye movements occur. Symmetry develops between 4 and 6 months of age. Persistent asymmetry of OKN is seen in nonbinocular animals such as the rabbit (Collewijn 1975), leading Atkinson to postulate that asymmetry of OKN might indicate the absence of binocular vision. Several authors have investigated uniocular horizontal OKN in early-onset strabismus and have reported persistent asymmetry in a significant number (van Hof-van Duin & Mohn 1986; Bourron-Madignier *et al.* 1987). Kommerell (1988) emphasized the connection between asymmetry and latent nystagmus. Mein (1983) reported that asymmetry occurred in patients with DVD. More recently, asymmetry has been reported as a defect of motion processing (Norcia 1996). Patients show a spectrum of abnormalities in ocular following responses, visual perception and visual evoked potentials (VEPs), suggesting a failure to develop a normal complement of motion processing mechanisms. Similar asymmetries have been shown in patients with unequal visual input of congenital or early onset. Shawkat *et al.* (1995) found that asymmetry did not persist if the vision of the affected eye was negligible, implying that lack of interocular competition allows symmetry to develop, contradicting the view that lack of binocular function leads to the asymmetry.

Horizontal OKN can be assessed clinically using a hand-held drum with vertical black-and-white stripes. The drum should be held at eye level and rotated at a speed of at least 20° s^{-1}. If the drum moves too fast, the patient cannot fixate on each stripe and if it moves too slowly, the smooth pursuit system takes over. OKN should first be tested with both eyes open, when a normal response should be elicited. Each eye is then tested in turn, moving the drum first in a temporal to nasal direction and then in a nasal to temporal direction, observing the eye movements. Demer and von Noorden (1988) have stated that if asymmetry is present there is an 85% likelihood that the strabismus developed in the first 6 months of life, therefore OKN can be used to confirm or possibly indicate the age of onset. Mein (1983) found asym-

metry in nearly all patients who had or subsequently developed DVD. Although Demer and von Noorden found asymmetry in the majority of their patients with DVD it was by no means present in all of them.

• *Abnormal head position:* An abnormal head posture was reported in 70% of patients with essential infantile esotropia by Lang (1968) and in 65% by Harcourt and Mein (1982). A head tilt, often combined with a face turn, was the predominant feature in Lang's series, but a face turn to fix with the adducting eye was prevalent in the series of Harcourt and Mein. The head posture may be adopted for the following reasons:

1 to compensate for nystagmus, which is abolished or reduced when the face is turned to the side of the fixing eye; it may be present only when needed to see detail, for example when the visual acuity is tested;

2 to compensate for limitation of abduction by turning the face to the side of the fixing eye;

3 in the presence of DVD, when the head may be tilted, most commonly to the side of the fixing eye; the reason for this is unknown.

These features can occur in combination: Ciancia (1962) first described the association of essential infantile esotropia, horizontal jerky nystagmus and an abnormal face turn to adduct the fixing eye, referred to as *Ciancia's syndrome*. Lang (1968) used the term *congenital strabismus syndrome* to describe patients with esotropia, latent nystagmus and DVD. Kommerell (1988) has defined the *infantile strabismus syndrome* as strabismus, latent nystagmus and asymmetry of OKN.

Relationship between essential infantile esotropia and associated signs

The aetiology of essential infantile esotropia and its associated features are not yet understood. Tychsen *et al.* (1985) found that patients with infantile strabismus showed an impairment of temporally directed pursuit when a moving target was viewed monocularly, and suggested that patients with infantile strabismus have a defect of cerebral pursuit control. Kommerell (1988) postulated that the onset of esotropia impairs the development of cortical binocularity, which in turn prevents the maturation of the ocular motor system: OKN remains asymmetrical and asymmetry of the pursuit system leads to nystagmus.

Lang (1982) proposed an imbalance between the primitive extrageniculate system, referred to as the ambient pathway, in which nasal retina is dominant, and the retinogeniculate system, the focal pathway, in which the fovea is dominant. Nystagmus results from a rhythmic alternation between the slow fixation drift on the nasal retina and the rapid recovery to foveal fixation.

There is a close link between the optokinetic and vestibular systems. Hoyt (1982) demonstrated that the vestibulo-ocular reflex (VOR) was defective in patients with essential infantile esotropia. Flynn *et al.* (1984) reported that subjects with asymmetry of OKN failed to suppress the VOR when rotated while fixating a target which rotated with them. However, a later study showed that the VOR is normal in these patients, casting doubt on any link between essential infantile esotropia and the vestibulo-ocular system (Tychsen *et al.* 1985).

Tsutsui and Fukai (1978) reported evidence suggesting that misrouting of the visual pathway might be present in essential infantile esotropia. Fitzgerald and Billson (1984) used patterned stimuli to record the visual evoked potential in patients with essential infantile esotropia, DVD and OKN asymmetry: they reported that 78% of those tested demonstrated contralateral cortical projection, comparable with the projection found in albinism, in which it is known that up to 30% of temporal retinal fibres cross at the chiasm (Creel *et al.* 1974). Hoyt and Caltrider (1984) could not confirm these findings. Boylan *et al.* (1988) using full-field flash stimuli compared the visual evoked potentials of patients with strabismus and DVD with those of age- and sex-matched groups of albino and normal subjects. They reported that only albino subjects showed evidence of misrouting and concluded that there was no visual pathway abnormality in squinting patients with DVD. Ciancia *et al.* (1988) reported asymmetrical visual evoked potentials in 22 out of 25 patients with congenital esotropia but found that misrouting took several forms.

Management

The management of essential infantile esotropia consists of the correction of significant refractive error, treatment of amblyopia and the surgical alignment of the visual axes.

Correction of the refractive error

All patients should be refracted. Essential infantile esotropia by definition does not have a significant accommodative component but this cannot be confirmed until after refraction and, when necessary, a trial wear of spectacles has shown this to be the case. Patients are unlikely to benefit from the correction of hypermetropia of +2.00 DS or less, the exception being a small variable esotropia that may respond to a low level of hypermetropic correction. Larger degrees of hypermetropia and significant amounts of astigmatism and myopia should be corrected to ensure normal visual development and to identify patients with accommodative esotropia, which can present very early and may be missed if spectacles are not ordered. The effect of any correction on the deviation should be assessed before proceeding with surgery.

Restoration of visual acuity

Acuity card procedures allow the measurement of acuity in infants but are not sensitive to small degrees of amblyopia (see Chapter 3, Refraction) therefore the results should be compared with the fixation pattern (Zipf 1976).

If visual acuity is reduced or amblyopia suspected due to fixation preference, occlusion of the preferred eye should be used, taking care to avoid occlusion amblyopia; details of occlusion therapy are given in Chapter 10. Occlusion should be used whether or not nystagmus is present. It can help improve abduction, and alternate occlusion can be used for this purpose in the absence of amblyopia.

Some patients with large-angle nonalternating esotropia do not tolerate occlusion of the fixing eye, possibly because of low visual acuity combined with the need to adopt a large face turn to fix with the squinting eye. These patients may benefit from botulinum toxin injection into the medial rectus muscle to align the visual axes and facilitate effective amblyopia management.

Botulinum toxin

Magoon (1984) and Scott (1987) have used botulinum toxin injection of the medial rectus muscles to treat essential infantile esotropia. Scott reported an average correction of 65% of the esotropia. Both authors considered that botulinum toxin could provide an alternative to strabismus surgery. Repeat injections are likely to be needed and muscle surgery appears to us a more predictable and safer method. Large-angle essential infantile esotropia exceeding 70 Δ is difficult to treat surgically, requiring either supramaximal medial rectus recession or simultaneous surgery of four rectus muscles. These procedures carry the risk of severely compromising the range of adduction in the first instance, or a high failure rate in the second; therefore we initially manage these very large esotropias with botulinum toxin injection of the medial rectus muscles: one or two toxin injections result in a stable, significantly smaller esotropia that can be managed by more conventional surgery. The important role of the toxin in the treatment of postoperative undercorrection and overcorrection is discussed later.

Surgical treatment

The majority of patients with essential infantile esotropia require surgery to correct the horizontal deviation. A significant number will need surgery on overacting oblique muscles and a minority will require surgery to reduce DVD. Careful assessment of ocular movements should identify an associated sixth nerve palsy. Infantile esotropia associated with a neurological abnormality should be managed in the same way as it is in a normal patient unless the neurological disorder is unstable, when surgery should be delayed. We are usually less aggressive in the amount of surgery performed in this subgroup in view of the higher incidence of postoperative undercorrection and overcorrection (Holman & Merritt 1986).

AIMS OF SURGERY

The main aim of surgery is to achieve stable ocular alignment by correcting the esotropia and eliminating incomitance, taking care that the surgery itself does not induce it. Carefully planned surgery should overcome or modify an abnormal head posture. The optimum outcome to facilitate the development of binocular single vision is considered to be alignment to within 10 Δ either side of orthotropia. We believe that up to 15 Δ esotropia is acceptable, whereas 10 Δ exotropia could result in persistent consecutive exotropia (Caputo *et al.* 1991). We prefer to undercorrect esotropia rather than take this risk.

AGE FOR SURGERY

A large strabismus is unsightly, embarrassing to the parents and can lead to muscle and conjunctival contracture if left untreated, therefore early correction is desirable. It can also help parents accept the appearance of a multiply handicapped child. Despite the increasing trend towards earlier surgery on essential infantile esotropia, the ideal age has yet to be established. The term 'early' usually refers to surgery performed before 2 years of age although 'very early' has been used for surgery before 6 months of age; 'late' refers to surgery undertaken after the age of 2 years. These terms are inadequately defined in the literature and it is better to state clearly the age at which surgery is performed.

Important factors influencing this decision are:
• The patient's age on presentation to the ophthalmologist. This is an important limiting factor when striving for earlier surgery, and in our practice a patient's late presentation is one of the main reasons why surgery is delayed.

• Reliability of the diagnosis and findings. It is important to obtain consistent repeated measurements of the deviation, which may necessitate a number of visits. Unstable small-angle esotropia is typically seen in the neurologically impaired infant, and time should be allowed for spontaneous improvement; surgery may not be required in these cases (Robb & Rodier 1987). Amblyopia treatment should be given preoperatively and may be protracted in some children with large-angle unilateral esotropia, delaying surgery. It is more difficult to detect and treat amblyopia postoperatively, especially when relying on preferential looking for detection. Moreover, parents who are satisfied with their child's appearance may fail to keep follow-up appointments.

• Potential for binocular single vision. Taylor (1963) reported that 50% of children operated on for congenital esotropia at an average age of 12 months showed evidence of binocular single vision. Failure to achieve this standard was attributed to unsatisfactory alignment or an untreated vertical deviation. There is now sufficient scientific evidence to support the view that patients are more likely to develop a form of binocular single vision if surgery is performed before rather than after 2 years of age. Ing *et al.* (1966) reported on 50 patients operated on before 18 months of age and followed-up for 2 years: fusion was investigated using Worth's lights, the major amblyoscope, the 4 Δ prism test and Wirt stereotest. Forty-four per cent gave a positive response to two or more tests. Those aligned to within 10 Δ of orthotropia showed better results when operated on before 12 months of age. However, re-examination of Ing's results by Fisher *et al.* (1969) showed that there was no significant difference in the number demonstrating binocular single vision, whether surgery was performed at 6–12 months or between 12 to 18 months. Taylor (1967) reviewed the outcome in 140 patients operated on from 6 to 23 months or after the age of 2 years. Seventeen out of 45 patients operated on early showed that the tropia had been converted to a phoria, compared with 5 out of the 95 patients operated on later and therefore recommended early surgery, but Fisher *et al.* (1969),who also reanalysed these results, found there was no statistical difference in the number of functional results obtained in the two groups. Fisher did agree with Taylor's finding that a functional result was less likely when surgery was performed after 24 months of age.

The improved potential for binocular single vision resulting from surgery before 2 years of age is further supported by Foster *et al.* (1976) and by a multicentre study by Ing (1981), which showed that alignment after 2 years of age resulted in a significantly lower percentage with fusion: the sensory outcome was not statistically different among children operated on at 6 months, 12 months and 24 months of age. Helveston *et al.* (1983) reported results suggesting that fusion can still be obtained when surgery is performed after 2 years of age: 12 out of 55 patients demonstrated stereopsis postoperatively, 10 of whom were operated on after 2 years of age; in contrast, stereopsis was not found in the 13 patients operated on before 12 months of age. A more recent study by Helveston *et al.* (1990) reported satisfactory alignment in children operated on as early as 4 or 5 months: sensory data were not included.

• Anatomical factors, including the effect of the growth of the eye on the position of the muscle insertions. In neonatal eyes the distance of the rectus insertions from the limbus is approximately 80% of that of the adult eye but because of the poorly developed posterior segment they may lie at or close to the equator;

therefore a recession of even 3–4 mm could place the insertion posterior to it (Swan & Wilkins 1984). The implication of this remains uncertain, and it is not yet known whether a posterior shift of a recessed muscle actually occurs with posterior growth of the globe. The rapid enlargement of the eye in infancy principally takes place in the posterior segment, so by 6 months of age the insertions of the muscles lie close to the adult position.

• Stability of any underlying medical or neurological condition and the risk of anaesthesia. Patients recovering from hydrocephalus, intracerebral haemorrhage and epilepsy are likely to have changing patterns of ocular motility as the neurological disorder evolves, necessitating a delay in performing strabismus surgery. General anaesthesia does not pose a significant risk to the normal infant, but the presence of a general medical or neurological disorder may significantly increase the risk.

• The effect of misalignment on social, behavioural and psychomotor development. The presence of a squint in infancy may affect parent-child bonding and interaction and can result in wider problems that affect the rest of the family. Occasionally a child's problems with behaviour or co-ordination are put down to the presence of the squint and, in some, these problems appear to resolve after surgery.

Advantages and disadvantages of early vs. late surgery

The advantages and disadvantages of surgery performed before the age of 2 years or after that age can be summarized as follows:

Surgery performed before 2 years of age:
• Advantages:
  1 greater potential for binocular single vision;
  2 improved child–parent interaction;
  3 reduced mechanical component from muscle and connective tissue contracture.
• Disadvantages:
  1 problems with assessment and obtaining reliable measurements in the young child;
  2 changing anatomical landmarks in the infant eye;
  3 difficulty with amblyopia management after surgery.

Surgery performed after 2 years of age:

- Advantages:

  1 reliable measurement and assessment of alphabet patterns and DVD is usually possible;

  2 amblyopia management facilitated by improved cooperation;

  3 anatomical relationships approaching adult dimensions.

- Disadvantages:

  1 reduced potential for binocular single vision;

  2 increased mechanical component from muscle and connective tissue contracture;

  3 potential problems with child–parent bonding.

CHOICE OF SURGERY

The horizontal deviation in essential infantile esotropia can be corrected surgically by a symmetrical bilateral medial rectus muscle recession or an asymmetrical unilateral medial rectus recession and lateral rectus resection. Important considerations influencing intervention in this group of patients include:

- Bilateral medial rectus recession, which is the more usual procedure and is our preferred option. Recessions to a maximum of 6 mm are successful in correcting deviations up to 45 Δ in our hands. There are three main options available for the treatment of larger angles:

  1 *conventional surgery:* the maximum amount of surgery on two muscles is performed initially, comprising either bilateral medial rectus recession of 5–6 mm or unilateral recession and resection. Further surgery on unoperated muscles is carried out later to correct the remaining deviation. The disadvantages of conventional surgery are that more than one reoperation may be required to achieve the desired result, and that surgery performed in stages results in a smaller amount of correction overall compared with surgery carried out as a single procedure.

  2 *graded bilateral medial rectus recession* in excess of 6 mm, with a maximum of 8 mm. Although the successful use of graded bilateral medial rectus recession in excess of 6 mm was reported by Hess and Calhoun (1979) and later by Weakley *et al.* (1991), long-term follow-up has shown a higher incidence of consecutive exotropia following 7 mm recession as well as a severely compromised range of adduction (Stager *et al.* 1994).

Table 14.1 Graded recession of the medial rectus muscles.

Angle (Δ)	Bilateral medial rectus recession (mm)
35	5
40	5.5
45	6
55–70	6.5
>70	7

3 *selective surgery:* an attempt is made to correct the strabismus with a single procedure by operating on two, three or four rectus muscles, depending on the size of the deviation. Scott *et al.* (1986) reanalysed the previous literature and concluded that selective surgery is superior to conventional surgery in essential infantile esotropia. We prefer this approach, operating on a maximum of three muscles in one sitting, confining medial rectus recession to a maximum of 6 mm and aiming to undercorrect the esotropia by 5 Δ. On the rare occasions when the deviation measures 70 Δ or more, we first treat the patient with botulinum toxin injection of both medial rectus muscles. This results in a long-term reduction in the size of the angle after one or two injections, making the surgical intervention on the residual angle relatively straightforward. A surgical plan is presented, based either on graded recession of the medial rectus muscles (Table 14.1) or on selective surgery on two or three muscles (Table 14.2). The amount of surgery is based on the angle of deviation: measurements are taken from the muscle insertion.

- Measurement of the amount of recession: measurement can be made from the corneoscleral limbus or from the muscle insertion. We prefer to use the corneoscleral limbus as the reference point for recession in children under 18 months in order to reduce the incidence of undercorrection arising from the relative anterior position of the muscle insertion (Kushner & Morton 1984). After 18 months the relationship between the muscle insertion and limbus approximates to adult dimensions and the position of the insertion is the appropriate landmark.

- Graded or standard amount of recession: graded recessions from the corneoscleral limbus were used by

Table 14.2 Selective surgery on the rectus muscles.

Angle (Δ)	Bilateral medial rectus recession (mm)	Unilateral lateral rectus resection (mm)
35	5	
40	5.5	
45	6	
50	5	5
55	5	6
60–65	5	7

Helveston *et al.* (1983) to treat early-onset esotropia: alignment within 10 Δ of orthotropia was achieved in 84% of patients. Kushner and Morton (1984) found that a standard recession of 10.5 mm was equally effective. We prefer to grade the amount of recession to the nearest 0.5 mm, using the corneoscleral limbus as the reference point only in young children.

• Dose–response curve: a standard amount of surgery is known to result in greater correction of large angles of deviation compared with its effect on small deviations: this observation has led to the concept of a variable dose–response curve for different-sized angles of squint. The dose–response relationship is expressed as the amount of correction per millimetre of surgery. The relationship is generally nonlinear, larger amounts of surgery resulting in proportionally more correction per millimetre than smaller amounts of surgery (Mims *et al.* 1985). A dose–response curve should be used only as a guide and should be open to modification according to intraoperative findings. We calculate the effect of bilateral medial rectus recession as follows:

  1 a surgical recession of 3–5 mm corrects approximately 3 Δ esotropia per mm;

  2 a 5.5 mm recession corrects 3.2 Δ esotropia per mm;

  3 a 6 mm recession corrects 3.4 Δ esotropia per mm.

• Fixed or loop sutures: Repka and Guyton (1988) have advocated loop sutures, also termed hang-back or hang-loose sutures, and found them simple to insert and effective in achieving satisfactory alignment. We restrict their use to adjustable sutures and supramaximal recessions (see Chapter 9). We see no advantage

in using loop sutures in essential infantile esotropia, preferring to fix the muscle securely to the sclera whenever possible.

• Forced duction test: an intraoperative forced duction test should be repeated at each stage of surgery and on its completion. If passive abduction is restricted in both eyes, recession of the medial rectus muscles is indicated together with the medial conjunctiva. If passive movement is full there is no need to perform a conjunctival recession and the surgeon can decide whether to operate on one or both eyes.

• Inferior oblique overaction: when indicated, surgery for overacting inferior obliques should be performed at the same time as surgery to correct the esotropia. Weakening the inferior oblique muscles does not have a significant effect on horizontal alignment in the primary position and we make no allowance for this when carrying out such surgery. We treat A-pattern associated with overaction of the superior oblique muscles by a posterior tenotomy of the muscle and believe this procedure has a minimal effect on the horizontal alignment in the primary position. A V-pattern without inferior oblique muscle overaction can be managed by inferior placement of both medial rectus muscles.

RECOMMENDED PROCEDURES BASED ON SIZE OF DEVIATION

• Deviations measuring 25–45 Δ: bilateral medial rectus recession of 3–6 mm.

• Deviations measuring 50–65 Δ: bilateral medial rectus recession of 5 mm and a single lateral rectus resection of 5–7 mm.

• Esotropia measuring 70 Δ or more: this is initially treated with botulinum toxin injection of both medial recti.

POSTOPERATIVE MANAGEMENT

Further treatment is unnecessary if the postoperative appearance is satisfactory and the best possible level of visual acuity is maintained. Although we aim for a small residual esotropia of 5–10 Δ, an alignment between 15 Δ esotropia and 10 Δ exotropia is acceptable and should allow fusion in the few cases in which binocular single vision develops. Scott *et al.* (1986) advised purposeful overcorrection and reported that postoperative exotropia resolved spontaneously provided that full adduction was retained. We do not recommend deliberate overcorrection.

Patients with previously alternating esotropia usually show a strong preference for fixation with one eye and cease to cross-fixate after surgical correction, with a high risk of strabismic amblyopia (Harcourt *et al.* 1980). Part-time or even full-time occlusion may be indicated. The importance of regular postoperative follow-up should be stressed to the parents, and regular cycloplegic refraction continued as recurrence of the esotropia is frequently the result of an accommodative component. In a series by Freeley *et al.* (1984), 61% of 23 cases of recurrent esotropia were successfully managed by correction of hypermetropia alone. Binocular function should be assessed as soon as cooperation allows.

Reoperation may be required for patients with surgical undercorrection or overcorrection.

Undercorrection (residual esotropia)

Residual angles greater than 15 Δ may require further treatment. Treatment options include:
• Spectacle correction: this is only likely to be successful when the residual angle is between 15 and 25 Δ and the hypermetropia exceeds +1 DS. Prisms are useful in the older child with a small residual angle and binocular potential.
• Botulinum toxin: toxin injection of the medial rectus muscles may be successful in the treatment of residual angles up to 20 Δ. We have found it needs to be administered in the early postoperative period, and that more than one injection may be required.
• Further surgery: the type and amount is influenced by the nature of the original procedure and the postoperative findings. Surgical options include:
  1 a resection of the lateral rectus muscles if the medial rectus muscles have previously been recessed or if the esotropia measures significantly more at distance fixation. This is best performed within 3 months of the original procedure as the muscles have not yet readjusted their length–tension relationships and there appears to be sufficient slack present for an isolated resection procedure to take up. Delaying surgery after this time gives a less predictable result.
  2 a unilateral medial rectus recession and a lateral rectus resection if this procedure has already been performed on the other eye.

3 further recession of the medial rectus muscles, with or without loop sutures, if the esotropia measures significantly more for near fixation.

The potential for binocular single vision should be assessed where possible and if the child is at least 3 years old, a period of prism adaptation should be considered in suitable cases. We are more aggressive in treating small residual angles if binocular potential can be demonstrated.

See Chapter 12 for further details on the treatment of residual esotropia.

Overcorrection (consecutive exotropia)

Consecutive exotropia can occur as the immediate result of surgery or can develop later. Management depends on the potential for binocular single vision, on whether the exotropia occurred very soon after surgery or was delayed, and on the degree of any incomitance present. It is discussed in detail in Chapter 13.
• Early marked postoperative exotropia: if a large exotropia is present with a −3 or more limitation of adduction, slippage of the medial rectus muscle should be suspected. If the eye can adduct past the mid-line, the medial rectus is likely to be still attached to the globe at some point. The ophthalmologist should be aware of this possibility and early exploratory intervention is recommended.
• Smaller degrees of consecutive exotropia with better adduction can simply be observed or treated conservatively by reducing the strength of hypermetropic lenses or with concave lenses if fusion is present. Some consecutive exotropias may resolve spontaneously; however, in our experience most show a gradual increase in size, first in the distance then for near. If conservative measures fail to correct the exotropia we recommend using botulinum toxin injection of both lateral rectus muscles. We, like others, have found this a useful method in the management of early postoperative overcorrection, especially in patients with potential binocular single vision. If toxin is not effective, surgery is indicated for cosmetic purposes or to restore fusion.
• Late postoperative consecutive exotropia: in the absence of any useful binocular single vision an exotropia can slowly develop weeks, months or years after initial surgery. Caputo *et al.* (1991) reported

on a series of 142 patients with successfully aligned congenital esotropia who were followed-up for 6 years postoperatively. Nineteen per cent developed a consecutive exotropia after 4 years and a further 26% were exotropic after 6 years. Intervention with botulinum toxin at this late stage is rarely successful and further surgery is usually indicated for cosmetic reasons.

Results of treatment

The success rate of surgery in achieving a satisfactory early postoperative alignment, usually reported as within ±10 Δ of orthotropia, ranges from 50% (Ing *et al.* 1966) to 85% (Mims & Wood 1989a) after a single operation. Hiles *et al.* (1980) stressed the need for regular postoperative follow-up; additional surgery was required in 69% of their group. They identified three broad categories of patients with infantile esotropia based on the postoperative findings:

• 39% in whom the alignment remained stable following early surgery;
• 31% who were initially stable but later decompensated and required additional surgery;
• 30% who had unstable ocular alignment throughout the follow-up period.

They suggested that fusion was an important stabilizing factor in their patients but also stressed the importance of additional conservative and/or surgical therapy in maintaining alignment.

It is generally agreed that bifoveal binocular single vision is not obtained after successful surgery for infantile strabismus (Taylor 1967; Freeley *et al.* 1983). At best, patients may develop subnormal binocular single vision, microtropia or small-angle esotropia with abnormal binocular single vision.

There is evidence that patients whose visual axes are aligned show binocular responses on testing in the immediate postoperative period but subsequently lose binocularity. This was reported by Hiles *et al.* (1980), and we have seen similar cases. Archer *et al.* (1986) tested stereopsis in infants by recording eye movements in response to dynamic random dot stereograms. They were able to demonstrate stereopsis immediately postoperatively in infants under 1-year-old who had good ocular alignment but found that stereopsis was quickly lost and the eyes did not remain straight. von Noorden (1988a) gave subnormal binocular single vision as the optimum treatment result in infantile

esotropia and microtropia as a desirable treatment result, but included absent or reduced stereopsis among the characteristics. In contrast, patients with primary microtropia may have stereoacuity as good as 60 seconds of arc.

The inference from these findings is that while satisfactory alignment can be obtained, stable binocular single vision is rare.

Dissociated vertical deviation (DVD; dissociated vertical divergence)

Helveston (1980) listed 16 synonyms for DVD: the term most widely used in the recent past was 'alternating sursumduction'. DVD describes the condition in which either eye, or occasionally only one eye, elevates when the amount of light entering it is reduced, for example by an occluder during the cover test. The elevated eye returns to its original position when the cover is removed. The cover test must be performed slowly, covering each eye long enough to allow elevation of the covered eye to occur. Each eye must be covered in turn even if one is densely amblyopic, otherwise the diagnosis can be missed. DVD is often easier to see when the patient fixes on a distance target.

Features

The features of DVD are detailed below.
• The eye under cover progressively elevates with continued dissociation but returns to its original position on removal of the cover. The upper eyelid position does not change.
• Unsightly hypertropia, usually during a period of inattention, poor health or fatigue.
• The vertical deviation is nearly always bilateral but often asymmetrical, usually but not invariably more marked in the squinting eye and generally greater in size in the distance.
• The degree of elevation of the covered eye remains approximately the same when the eye is adducted and abducted, although in rare cases elevation consistently occurs when the eye is abducted.
• In most patients the covered eye extorts as it elevates and intorts as it resumes its habitual position. Extorsion is occasionally observed before other signs of DVD become apparent and may be the only feature

in some patients. It is often easier to see intorsion on removal of the cover than it is to observe the initial extorsion.

• Either an A- or a V-pattern may be present but in our experience an A-pattern is more common, occurring in 46% of reported cases, whereas a V-pattern occurred in 21% (Mein & Johnson 1981).

• A head tilt is sometimes present. It has been suggested that the head is tilted to compensate for cyclotropia of the fixing eye (Crone 1954; Dahan & Spielmann 1985). However, this may not be the only explanation since the head is tilted to the side of the nonfixing eye in some cases.

• There is a high incidence of latent nystagmus, reported as high as 100% in some series (Billet & Ehrlich 1966; Helveston 1980). DVD is commonly associated with infantile esotropia but can coexist with other constant and intermittent esodeviations or exodeviations and has been reported as an isolated phenomenon.

• In some patients the horizontal angle of deviation increases or decreases when either eye is covered, and when this is the main feature it is referred to as dissociated horizontal deviation (Wilson & McClatchey 1991). When the cover is removed the eye returns to its original position, simulating esophoria or exophoria. Dissociated horizontal deviation is discussed further at the end of this section.

• Binocular vision is likely to be weak. Cohen and Moore (1980) found DVD in association with normal binocular single vision but this has not been our experience. The exception is intermittent exotropia, when DVD is occasionally present in association with stereoacuity of 60 seconds of arc or better. It should be stressed that the 'recovery' movement which occurs on cover/uncover test is not evidence of motor fusion.

• There are rarely any symptoms of diplopia.

No theory gives a satisfactory explanation of the phenomena and it is clear that DVD is unlike any latent or manifest concomitant or incomitant deviation.

Development

DVD is an acquired condition that usually develops between the ages of 18 months and 3 years. It is rarely seen under 1 year of age but can occur as late as 5 or 6 years. Its onset is therefore later than the associated strabismus and nystagmus. The onset is gradual,

sometimes preceded by a unilateral or bilateral alternating hypertropia (Mein & Johnson 1981). Several weeks or even months of observation may be needed before the diagnosis can be confirmed. Harcourt *et al.* (1980) found no significant decrease in DVD over a long follow-up period.

Important factors in the investigation

• Case history: DVD is associated with infantile esotropia and often occurs after treatment of the horizontal deviation.

• Abnormal head posture: a head tilt to the side of the fixing eye is often present. Bechtel *et al.* (1996) found an incidence of 35% in patients with predominantly unilateral esotropia but reported that it did not occur in alternating deviations, although we have seen an alternating head tilt when fixation spontaneously changed. The mechanism for the head posture is unknown but DVD is often seen to increase on forced tilt to the contralateral side.

• Cover test: a cover/uncover test will reveal a hypertropia in each eye, which increases as the test is prolonged. Any hypotropia present will change to hypertropia under cover. Careful observation of the occluded eye as the cover is removed can reveal intorsion as the eye resumes its usual position: this sign may provide conclusive evidence of the presence of DVD. In a few patients the horizontal or torsional element may be predominant on occlusion, in which case the condition is referred to as dissociated horizontal deviation or dissociated torsional deviation; the underlying anomaly is probably the same.

Ocular movements

DVD can be associated with all types of motility defects, including limited elevation, although infantile esotropia is the most common. Inferior oblique overaction is a common finding and although the two may coexist it is important that they are not confused (see Table 14.3). Observation of corneal reflections is particularly important as sudden elevation of the adducted eye can occur on contralateral version when the nose acts as an occluder and reveals the DVD. Inferior oblique overaction occurs gradually as the eye moves from the primary position into adduction. An alternating cover test in the diagnostic positions of gaze can confuse the diagnosis by eliciting DVD.

Both A- and V-patterns can be seen in DVD; however, A-patterns are more common and this can help to differentiate DVD from inferior oblique overaction, when a V-pattern would be expected.

Measurement of the deviation

Accurate measurement is difficult to obtain because of the progressive nature of DVD. The manifest part of the deviation should first be measured using a simultaneous prism cover test, preferably at 6 m. Measurement of the DVD can be obtained using an alternate prism cover test with each eye fixing in turn to record the degree of asymmetry: it may be impossible to reverse the deviation to check the accuracy of the measurement but the maximum amount of elevation can be recorded. Alternatively DVD can be measured using the major amblyoscope.

Bielschowsky darkening wedge test

This test was designed specifically to diagnose the presence of DVD. The principle is gradually to reduce the amount of light entering the eye: a graded wedge was originally used but a neutral-density filter bar or Sbisa bar are suitable alternatives. The patient fixates a light and the nonfixing eye is occluded, hence the eye behind the occluder will elevate. The filter is introduced in front of the fixing eye, starting with the lowest filter, and the density is slowly increased. As the light entering the eye is reduced the eye under the cover will be seen to move down, possibly dropping below the mid-line. As the filter density is reduced the eye under the cover will progressively elevate again. (Bielschowsky phenomenon; Fig. 14.1). The cover and occluder can be reversed to observe the phenomenon in each eye. The test requires quite prolonged fixation, which makes it difficult to use with young children, and it can only be demonstrated in approximately 50% of patients with DVD (Raab 1970).

Differential diagnosis of DVD and bilateral inferior oblique overaction

The differential diagnosis of DVD and bilateral inferior oblique overaction is summarized in Table 14.3.

Management

Hypertropia in DVD that is only evident intermittently and is small in size does not require treatment.

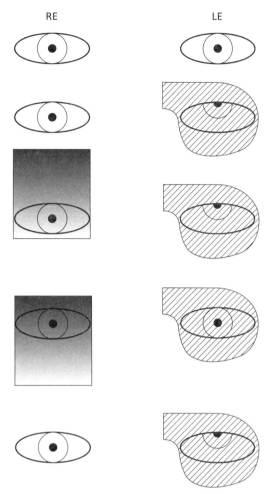

Fig. 14.1 The Bielschowsky phenomenon. The patient's right eye fixates a light and the left eye is occluded and will elevate behind the occluder. The filter is introduced in front of the right eye and the density is slowly increased. As the light entering the right eye is reduced the left eye under the cover will be seen to move down, possibly dropping below the mid-line. The filter is removed and the eye behind the occluder returns to the elevated position.

Correction of the refractive error

Occasionally DVD first becomes a problem in adult life, and we have had some success in manipulating the refractive error to change fixation to the more affected eye.

Table 14.3 Differential diagnosis of DVD and inferior oblique overaction.

Diagnostic feature	DVD	Inferior oblique overaction
Cover test	Progressive elevation	Constant degree of elevation
	Intorsion on refixation	No torsion noted
Ocular movements	Elevation under cover equal in all positions of gaze	Greatest elevation on adduction
	May become manifest on versions	
	V- or A-pattern possible	V-pattern often present
	A-pattern predominant	
	Superior oblique overaction possible	Superior oblique underaction possible
Latent nystagmus	Usually present	Less often present
Bielschowsky darkening wedge test	Positive	Negative

Surgical treatment

Surgery is indicated if there is frequent and persistent spontaneous elevation of one or both eyes, which can be very unsightly: it is required in relatively few cases. Helveston (1986) reported operating on 10% of patients with DVD. The purpose of the surgery is to reduce the frequency and size of the manifest phase and it is performed for cosmetic purposes. Surgery aims to weaken the eye's elevating force or strengthen the depressing force by operating on the relevant cyclovertical muscles.

The choice of surgery is influenced by

• associated inferior oblique overaction;
• whether DVD is bilateral or unilateral;
• the degree of asymmetry in bilateral DVD;
• the presence of an A-pattern with overacting superior oblique muscles.

DVD WITH OVERACTION OF THE INFERIOR OBLIQUE MUSCLES

A V-pattern with overaction of both inferior oblique muscles was present in 10% of the cases of DVD that we treated surgically. Mims and Wood (1989b) reported on a series of 61 children with inferior oblique overaction who underwent bilateral recession with antero-positioning procedures. The procedure was not only successful in the treatment of the inferior oblique overaction but also resulted in a substantial reduction in any DVD present, obviating the need for surgery specifically for DVD.

Kratz *et al.* (1989) also reported on the effect of anterior positioning of the inferior oblique tendon in DVD. In most of their cases, overaction of the inferior oblique was present: the procedure was performed bilaterally in the majority and was successful in treating the DVD. We have also found it effective in reducing the amount of inferior oblique overaction and in correcting any V-pattern. If a truly unilateral DVD is present which measures at least 15–20 Δ of hypertropia in the primary position, then a unilateral procedure can be performed on the overacting inferior oblique muscle.

Caution is required when operating on patients without inferior oblique overaction as torsional diplopia can result or an A-pattern may develop. Unilateral procedures may result in a significant hypotropia of the operated eye (Bremer *et al.* 1986), and we do not recommend surgery if the DVD measures less than 15 Δ.

BILATERAL OR UNILATERAL DVD WITHOUT INFERIOR OBLIQUE OVERACTION

DVD is likely to affect both eyes if there is no strong fixation preference. This was the most frequent finding in patients we treated for DVD. Most require surgery on both eyes: we reserve unilateral surgery for patients whose visual acuity in the affected eye is three or more lines lower than that of the other eye. Surgery comprises a bilateral superior rectus recession of 10–13 mm in bilateral symmetrical DVD, securing the muscle firmly to the sclera with fixed sutures. We do not use posterior fixation sutures for these patients. Lesser amounts of recession are rarely effective in our hands. In unilateral cases the amount of superior rectus recession can be graded according to the size of the hypertropia. Freeman and Rosenbaum (1989) reported on a series of persistent and incomitant DVD after large superior rectus recession: the vertical deviation measured more on adduction and less on abduction. We have not observed this in our patients and it may be a problem that occurs when the superior rectus recession is performed using loop sutures.

DEGREE OF SYMMETRY

Magoon *et al.* (1982) recommended surgery on both eyes even if the DVD was markedly asymmetrical. If only one eye is operated on, the DVD in the other eye will almost certainly increase and cause a new cosmetic problem. We reduce the amount of superior rectus recession in the less affected eye in asymmetrical cases.

DVD WITH OVERACTION OF THE SUPERIOR OBLIQUE MUSCLES

An A-pattern with overaction of both superior oblique muscles was present in 30% of cases of DVD which we treated surgically. The A-pattern is managed by weakening the action of the superior oblique muscles, usually with a posterior tenotomy, and the DVD is managed by superior rectus recession as described above, performing both procedures in one sitting. The superior oblique posterior tenotomy removes the tendon from the posterior sclera, facilitating the scleral placement of the recessed superior rectus muscle.

Postoperative management

The effect of surgery can be disappointing. Early results often show improvement in the DVD but recurrence is common and long-term follow-up is required to judge the effects of treatment. Residual postoperative DVD is a relatively common finding, but most patients do not require further surgery at this stage. When further treatment is required, management depends on the surgery originally performed:

• DVD following bilateral inferior oblique anterior positioning: the superior rectus muscle should be recessed unilaterally or bilaterally.

• DVD occurring in the fellow eye following a unilateral procedure: either the contralateral inferior oblique or superior rectus muscle can be operated on.

• DVD after bilateral superior rectus recession: if a further recession is possible this should be the operation of choice. An ipsilateral inferior rectus resection, using adjustable sutures if possible, is an alternative option (Knapp & von Noorden 1994); 6 mm resections have been effective in our hands.

Dissociated horizontal deviation

Dissociated horizontal deviation is an asymmetrical or unilateral slow outward deviation that occurs spontaneously or following dissociation of the eyes.

Features

• An exotropia which develops spontaneously or only after dissociation.
• Marked asymmetry of the deviation. An alternating cover test reveals a greater angle when one eye is fixing compared to the other.
• Difficulty in neutralizing the deviation during the prism cover test.
• Response to the Bielschowsky dark wedge test: the eye behind the cover progressively moves towards the mid-line and may become esotropic as the fixing eye is progressively darkened.
• Other components of DVD are present, albeit to a lesser degree.

Differential diagnosis

A dissociated horizontal deviation can be superimposed on an esotropia or exotropia. A dissociated horizontal deviation should be distinguished from:

• An intermittent exotropia: in some the two conditions may coexist; however, differentiation is helped by other components of DVD being evident, the asymmetry of the deviation and the response to the dark wedge test.
• Uncorrected anisometropia causing a smaller exodeviation when fixing with the less myopic or more hypermetropic eye can be readily detected after refraction.
• Overcorrection of hypermetropia: we have seen two patients who developed a typical dissociated horizontal deviation following an increase in the hypermetropia

prescription for accommodative esotropia; the intermittent slow unilateral exodeviation disappeared after the hypermetropia was reduced.

• Paralytic strabismus in which the secondary deviation exceeds the primary deviation should be easily identified by testing ocular movements.

Management

All patients should be refracted and significant refractive errors corrected, including anisometropia. Dissociated horizontal deviation does not require treatment if the angle is small and not causing concern. Surgical management involves a unilateral lateral rectus recession of 4–8 mm, and the amount of recession is based on the size of the deviation and the presence of superimposed esotropia or exotropia (Wilson & McClatchey 1991).

Nystagmus blockage syndrome (nystagmus compensation syndrome)

Adelstein and Cüppers (1966) first described this condition to explain an esotropia that results from the use of the convergence mechanism to block or abolish manifest nystagmus and improve visual acuity. This condition is rare compared with essential infantile esotropia.

Features

• A congenital horizontal nystagmus is present which remains the same whether both eyes open or if one eye is covered. It increases in intensity as the eye is abducted and is blocked when the eye is adducted.

• The esotropia is nonaccommodative and variable. Visual attention is associated with an increase in esotropia and a decrease in nystagmus; conversely at times of visual inattention the esotropia decreases and the intensity of the nystagmus increases.

• The patient adopts a face turn to the side of the fixing eye: in combination with the convergence mechanism used to maintain the fixing eye in an adducted position, this gives the impression of both eyes being convergent.

• The esotropia is usually unilateral, and strabismic amblyopia is common.

• Adelstein and Cüppers reported pseudo-sixth nerve palsy with full passive movement on abduction. However, contracture of the medial rectus muscles and/or the medial conjunctiva may result in a positive forced duction test.

• Pupil miosis may occur during the esotropic phase.

• The squinting eye remains adducted when a base-out prism is introduced in front of the fixing eye.

• There is a high incidence of neurological disorders (Hoyt 1977). von Noorden (1988b) diagnosed the nystagmus blockage syndrome in 12 out of 15 esotropic patients with ocular or oculocutaneous albinism.

• DVD is rare.

• The results of strabismus surgery are unpredictable.

Differential diagnosis

Some similarities between cases of essential infantile esotropia and the nystagmus blockage syndrome, notably a face turn to the side of the fixing eye and congenital horizontal nystagmus, have led to confusion and probably to misdiagnosis. This is reflected in the wide variation in the reported incidence of the nystagmus blockage syndrome, which ranges from 12% (von Noorden & Avilla 1984) to 72% (Mühlendyck 1976). The differential diagnosis is based in the features listed in Table 14.4. The essential difference is the type of nystagmus, which is latent in essential infantile esotropia and congenital in the blockage syndrome. The wave forms of the two types are different, but can only be distinguished by electro-oculographic tracings (see Chapter 23). Since this investigation is impractical in all cases, clinical differentiation of the nystagmus blockage syndrome must depend on careful observation of the other characteristics. Aligning the eyes temporarily with botulinum toxin enhances the nystagmus waveform in the nystagmus blockage syndrome but diminishes it in essential infantile esotropia, helping to differentiate the two conditions.

Management

Significant refractive errors should be corrected with spectacles, although these may prove unsatisfactory when the compensatory head posture results in eccentric viewing through the spectacle lens. Contact lenses should be considered in these cases, especially if the refractive error is high or significant levels of astigmatism are present. Occlusion for amblyopia should be

Table 14.4 Differential diagnosis of infantile esotropia and the nystagmus blockage syndrome.

Diagnostic feature	Essential infantile esotropia	Nystagmus blockage syndrome
Amblyopia	Uncommon	Common
Angle of deviation	Static and large angle	Variable, may show spasmodic increase in angle
Type of nystagmus	Latent	Congenital
Passive movement	May be limited	Usually full
Reason for compensatory head posture	Limitation of abduction or nystagmus	Nystagmus compensation
DVD	Common	Rare
Neurological anomalies	Not usually present	Common
Results of strabismus surgery	Predictable	Unpredictable

the mainstay of therapy, and a head posture serving to dampen the nystagmus and improve visual acuity will often be present when the occlusion is worn.

Surgery is indicated if the esotropia is constant and cosmetically poor. Surgical procedures routinely used to treat essential infantile esotropia are usually ineffective in the nystagmus blockage syndrome. The preferred option is a bilateral medial rectus recession and posterior fixation sutures to prevent the initiating effect of the convergence mechanism.

Accommodative esotropia

Fully accommodative esotropia with a moderate degree of hypermetropia and onset before 6 months of age is seen only very occasionally. Baker and Parks (1980) reported on patients with early-onset esotropia which was only present on near fixation (the accepted definition of convergence excess) or became more pronounced for near. Most were hypermetropic and half of them were judged to have a high AC/A ratio (accommodative convergence/accommodation ratio). Binocular vision was weak and unstable compared with that in most accommodative esotropia of later onset. There was a high incidence of strabismic amblyopia and the esotropia recurred after apparently successful surgical treatment in half the patients studied.

Management
The weak binocular vision found in these patients makes them particularly prone to consecutive exotropia. Surgery should not be considered if the appearance is

reasonably good. The patients should be observed and treatment confined to obtaining and maintaining good visual acuity in both eyes and to ensuring that hypermetropia remains fully corrected. Surgery can be performed to improve alignment when the child is older should it be necessary.

Sixth nerve palsy

Sixth nerve palsy is one explanation for limited abduction in esotropia but it is difficult to ascribe the strabismus to this cause with certainty. There were no infants with persistent sixth nerve palsy among the large number of neonates examined by Nixon *et al.* (1985), Friedrich and de Decker (1987) and Archer *et al.* (1989). An isolated palsy should be considered rare, although the sixth nerve can be affected in neurological disorders such as hydrocephalus.

Management
The surgical treatment for esotropia with sixth nerve palsy is discussed in Chapter 19.

Infantile exotropia

Description
Infantile exotropia is an exotropia present for near and distance fixation, with an onset usually in the first year of life.

Essential infantile exotropia is comparatively rare. Although exotropia is common in neonates, it generally resolves by 3 months of age (Nixon *et al.* 1985).

Symptomatic exotropia can occur in early childhood because of ocular pathology either affecting one eye or worse in one eye. Pathology should always be suspected if there is a constant unilateral exotropia. Early-onset exotropia is also associated with severe craniofacial abnormality. Moore and Cohen (1985) reported on 150 patients with exotropia that developed in infancy. Only 10 patients had essential infantile exotropia, the rest had craniofacial anomalies or neurological disease.

The characteristics of essential infantile exotropia are:

• A large-angle alternating exotropia in nearly every case.
• A possible decrease in the exotropia on accommodation thereby simulating an intermittent exotropia. However, if the eyes are observed whilst the patient attempts to maintain fixation on an accommodative target held at 15–20 cm, a small fluctuating exotropia will be seen rather than steady binocular convergence.
• DVD is probable. Helveston (1980) reported that 20% of patients with DVD were exotropic, and Mein and Johnson (1981) found an incidence of 12%. All but one of Cohen and Moore's (1980) patients had DVD.

Management

Significant refractive error should be corrected with spectacles and occlusion treatment started if alternation does not occur. The angle of deviation may change, and Mein reported patients who developed spontaneous consecutive esotropia in early childhood (Mein 1981), while in other patients the exotropia may increase. A period of observation is therefore recommended, but surgical intervention should not be delayed if the condition is stable.

The aim of surgery is to leave the visual axes slightly convergent to guard against redivergence. As most infantile exotropias are large, extensive surgery is required. The choice is usually a unilateral recession of the lateral rectus muscle combined with a resection of the medial rectus muscle or, if the angle is larger than 35 Δ, then this is combined with surgery on the other eye.

References

Adelstein, F.E. & Cüppers, C. (1966) Zum problem der echten und scheibaren Abducenslahmung (das sogenannte 'Blockierungs syndrom'). In: *Buch der Augenarzt*, pp. 271–278. Enke, Stuttgart.

Archer, S.M., Helveston, E.M., Miller, K.K. & Ellis, F.D. (1986) Stereopsis in normal infants and infants with congenital esotropia. *American Journal of Ophthalmology* **101**, 591–596.

Archer, S.M., Sondhi, N. & Helveston, E.M. (1989) Strabismus in infancy. *Ophthalmology* **96** (1), 133–137.

Atkinson, J. (1979) Development of optokinetic nystagmus in human infant and in monkey infant: an analogue to development in kittens. In: *Developmental Neurobiology of Vision* (ed. R.D. Freeman), pp. 277–287. Plenum Press, New York.

Baker, J.D. & Parks, M.M. (1980) Early onset accommodative esotropia. *American Journal of Ophthalmology* **90**, 11–18.

Bechtel, R.T., Kushner, B.J. & Morton, G.V. (1996) The relationship between dissociated vertical divergence (DVD) and head tilts. *Journal of Pediatric Ophthalmology and Strabismus* **33** (6), 303–306.

Billet, E. & Ehrlich, M. (1966) Occlusion hypertropia – a contralateral fixation phenomenon. *Journal of Pediatric Ophthalmology* **3**, 39–43.

Bourron-Madignier, M., Ardoin, M.L., Cypres, C. & Vettard, S. (1987) Study of optokinetic nystagmus in children. In: *Orthoptic Horizons. Transactions of the Sixth International Orthoptic Congress, Harrogate* (eds M. Lenk-Schafer, C. Calcutt, M. Doyle & S. Moore), pp. 134–139. British Orthoptic Society, London.

Boylan, C., Element, R.A. & Howrie, A. (1988) Normal visual pathway routing in dissociated vertical deviation. *Investigative Ophthalmology and Visual Science* **29**, 1165–1167.

Bremer, D.L., Rogers, G.L. & Quick, L.D. (1986) Primary-position hypotropia after anterior transposition of the inferior oblique. *Archives of Ophthalmology* **104**, 229–232.

Caputo, A.R., Guo, S.G., Wagner, R.S. & Picciano, M.V. (1991) Long term follow-up of extraocular muscle surgery for congenital esotropia. *American Orthoptic Journal* **41**, 67–71.

Ciancia, A. (1962) La esotropia en la lactante, diagnostico y tratamiento. *Archives of Chilean Ophthalmology* **9**, 117.

Ciancia, A.O., Borrone, R., Schuarzberg, D.E. & Garcia, H.A. (1988) Asymmetric visual evoked potentials (VEP) in congenital esotropia with bilateral limitation of abduction. *Binocular Vision* **3**, 15–22.

Cohen, R.L. & Moore, S. (1980) Primary dissociated vertical deviation. *American Orthoptic Journal* **30**, 107–108.

Collewijn, H. (1975) Direction sensitive units in the rabbit nucleus of the optic tract. *Brain Research* **100**, 489–509.

Costenbader, F.D. (1961) Infantile esotropia. *Transactions of the American Ophthalmological Society* **59**, 397–429.

Creel, D., Witkop, C.J. & King, R.A. (1974) Asymmetric visual evoked potentials in human albinos: evidence of visual system anomalies. *Investigative Ophthalmology and Visual Science* **13**, 430–440.

Crone, R.A. (1954) Alternating hyperphoria. *British Journal of Ophthalmology* **38**, 591–604.

Dahan, A. & Spielmann, A. (1985) Double torticollis and surgical artificial divergence. In: *Acta Strabologica*, pp. 187–192. CERES, Paris.

Dell'Osso, L.F., Schmidt, J.P. & Daroff, R.B. (1979) Latent, manifest latent and congenital nystagmus. *Archives of Ophthalmology* **97**, 1877–1885.

Demer, J.L. & von Noorden, G.K. (1988) Optokinetic asymmetry in esotropia. *Journal of Pediatric Ophthalmology and Strabismus* **25**, 286–292.

Dickey, C.F., Matx, H.S., Stewart, S.A. & Scott, W.E. (1991) The diagnosis of amblyopia in cross-fixation. *Journal of Pediatric Ophthalmology and Strabismus* **28**, 171–175.

Fisher, N.F., Flom, M.C. & Jampolsky, A. (1969) Early surgery of congenital esotropia. *American Journal of Ophthalmology* **65**, 439–443.

Fitzgerald, B.A. & Billson, F.A. (1984) Dissociated vertical deviation: evidence of abnormal visual pathway projection. *British Journal of Ophthalmology* **68**, 801–806.

Flynn, J.T., Pritchard, C. & Lasley, D. (1984) Binocular vision and OKN asymmetry in strabismus patients. In: *Strabismus II* (ed. R. Reinecke), pp. 35–44. Grune & Stratton, New York.

Foster, R.S., Paul, T.O. & Jampolsky, A. (1976) Management of infantile esotropia. *American Journal of Ophthalmology* **82**, 291–299.

Freeley, D.A., Nelson, L.B. & Calhoun, J.H. (1983) Recurrent esotropia following early successful surgical correction of congenital esotropia. *Journal of Pediatric Ophthalmology and Strabismus* **20**, 68–71.

Freeley, D.A., Nelson, L.B. & Calhoun, J.H. (1984) Recurrent esotropia following early successful surgical correction of congenital esotropia. In: *Strabismus II* (ed. R.D. Reinecke), pp. 143–147. Grune & Stratton, New York.

Freeman, R.S. & Rosenbaum, A.L. (1989) Residual incomitant DVD following large bilateral superior rectus recession. *Journal of Pediatric Ophthalmology and Strabismus* **26**, 76–80.

Friedman, Z., Neumann, E., Hyams, S.W. & Peleg, B. (1980) Ophthalmic screening of 38,000 children age one to two and a half years in child welfare clinics. *Journal of Pediatric Ophthalmology and Strabismus* **17**, 261.

Friedrich, D. & de Decker, W. (1987) Prospective study of the development of strabismus during the first 6 months of life. In: *Orthoptic Horizons. Transactions of the Sixth International Orthoptic Congress, Harrogate* (eds M. Lenk-Schafer, C. Calcutt, M. Doyle & S. Moore), pp. 21–28. British Orthoptic Society, London.

Harcourt, R.B. & Mein, J. (1982) Early onset esotropia. In: *Documenta Ophthalmologica Proceedings Series* (eds A.Th.M. van Balen & W. Houtman), pp. 79–81. Junk, The Hague.

Harcourt, B., Mein, J. & Johnson, F. (1980) Natural history and associations of dissociated vertical divergence. *Transactions of the Ophthalmological Society of the United Kingdom* **100**, 495–497.

Helveston, E.M. (1980) Dissociated vertical deviation: a clinical and laboratory study. *Transactions of the American Ophthalmological Society* **78**, 734–779.

Helveston, E.M. (1986) Esotropia in the first year of life. In: *Pediatric Ophthalmology and Strabismus. Transactions of the New Orleans Academy of Ophthalmology* (ed. J.H. Allen), pp. 419–429. Raven Press, New York.

Helveston, E.M., Ellis, F.D., Schott, J., Mitchelson, J. & Weber, J.C. (1983) Surgical treatment of congenital esotropia. *American Journal of Ophthalmology* **96**, 218–228.

Helveston, E.M., Ellis, F.D., Plager, D.W. & Miller, K.K. (1990) Early surgery for essential infantile esotropia. *Journal of Pediatric Ophthalmology and Strabismus* **27**, 115–119.

Hess, J.B. & Calhoun, J.H. (1979) A new rationale for the management of large angle esotropia. *Journal of Pediatric Ophthalmology and Strabismus* **16**, 345–348.

Hiles, D.A., Watson, B.A. & Biglan, A.W. (1980) Characteristics of infantile esotropia following early bimedial rectus recession. *Archives of Ophthalmology* **98**, 697–703.

van Hof-van Duin, J. & Mohn, G. (1986) Monocular and binocular optokinetic nystagmus in humans with defective stereopsis. *Investigative Ophthalmology and Visual Science* **27**, 574–583.

Holman, R.E. & Merritt, J.C. (1986) Infantile esotropia: results in the neurologic impaired and 'normal' child at NCMH (six years). *Journal of Pediatric Ophthalmology and Strabismus* **23**, 41–44.

Horwood, A.M. (1993) Maternal observations of ocular alignment in infants. *Journal of Pediatric Ophthalmology and Strabismus* **30** (2), 100–105.

Hoyt, C.S. (1977) The nystagmus compensation syndrome (correspondence). *American Journal of Ophthalmology* **83**, 423.

Hoyt, C.S. (1982) Abnormality of the vestibulo-ocular response in congenital esotropia. *American Journal of Ophthalmology* **93**, 704–708.

Hoyt, C.S. & Caltrider, N. (1984) Hemispheric visually evoked responses in congenital esotropia. *Journal of Pediatric Ophthalmology and Strabismus* 21, 19–21.

Ing, M.R. (1981) Early surgical alignment for congenital esotropia. *Transactions of the American Ophthalmological Society* 79, 625–663.

Ing, M.R. (1995) Progressive increase in the angle of deviation in congenital esotropia. In: *Update on Strabismus and Pediatric Ophthalmology. Proceedings of the Joint ISA and AAPO and S Meeting, Vancouver* (ed. G. Lennerstrand), pp. 211–213. CRC Press, Boca Raton.

Ing, M., Costenbader, F.D., Parks, M.M. & Albert, D.G. (1966) Early surgery for congenital esotropia. *American Journal of Ophthalmology* 61, 1419–1427.

Knapp, M.R.E. & von Noorden, G.K. (1994) Treatment of residual dissociated vertical deviation with inferior rectus resection. *Journal of Pediatric Ophthalmology and Strabismus* 31, 262–264.

Kommerell, G. (1988) Ocular motor phenomena in infantile strabismus. In: *Strabismus and Amblyopia: Wenner Gren International Symposium Series* (eds G. Lennarstrand, G.K. von Noorden & E.C. Campos), pp. 99–110. Macmillan Press, London.

Kratz, R.E., Rogers, G.L., Bremer, D.L. & Leguire, L.E. (1989) Anterior tendon displacement of the inferior oblique for DVD. *Journal of Pediatric Ophthalmology and Strabismus* 26, 212–217.

Kushner, B.J. & Morton, G.V. (1984) A randomized comparison of surgical procedures for infantile esotropia. *American Journal of Ophthalmology* 98, 50–61.

Lang, J. (1968) Squint dating from birth or with early onset. In: *Transactions of the First International Congress of Orthoptics, London*, pp. 231–237. Kimpton, London.

Lang, J. (1982) A new hypothesis on latent nystagmus and on the congenital squint syndrome. In: *Documenta Ophthalmologica Proceedings Series* (eds A.Th.M. van Balen & W. Houtman), pp. 83–86. Junk, The Hague.

Magoon, E.H. (1984) Chemo-denervation for strabismus in infants and children. *Journal of Pediatric Ophthalmology* 21, 110–112.

Magoon, E., Cruciger, M. & Jampolsky, A. (1982) Dissociated vertical deviation. An asymmetric condition treated by large bilateral superior rectus recession. *Journal of Pediatric Ophthalmology and Strabismus* 19, 152–156.

Mein, J. (1981) La divergence verticale dissociée (DVD). *Journal Français D'Orthoptique* 13, 151–153.

Mein, J. (1983) The OKN response in early onset strabismus. *Australian Orthoptic Journal* 20, 13–17.

Mein, J. & Johnson, F. (1981) Dissociated vertical divergence and its association with nystagmus. In: *Orthoptics,*

Research and Practice (eds J. Mein & S. Moore), pp. 14–16. Kimpton, London.

Mims, J.L. & Wood, R.C. (1989a) Verification and refinement of surgical guidelines for infantile esotropia: a prospective study of 40 cases. *Binocular Vision* 4, 7–14.

Mims, J.L. & Wood, R.C. (1989b) Bilateral anterior transposition of the inferior obliques. *Archives of Ophthalmology* 107, 41–44.

Mims, J.L., Treff, G., Kincaid, M., Schaffer, B. & Wood, R. (1985) Quantitative surgical guidelines for bilateral medial recession for infantile esotropia. *Binocular Vision* 1, 7–22.

Moore, S. & Cohen, R.L. (1985) Congenital exotropia. *American Orthoptic Journal* 35, 68–70.

Mühlendyck, H. (1976) Diagnosis of convergent strabismus with nystagmus and its treatment with Cüppers faden operation. In: *Orthoptics, Past, Present and Future. Transactions of the Third International Orthoptic Congress, Boston* (eds S. Moore, J. Mein & L. Stockbridge), pp. 143–154. Symposia Specialists, Miami.

Murray, A.D.N. & Calcutt, C. (1990) The incidence of amblyopia in longstanding untreated infantile esotropia. In: *Strabismus and Ocular Motility Disorders. Proceedings of the 6th International Strabismological Association, Surfers Paradise, Australia* (ed E.C. Campos), pp. 45–49. MacMillan Press, Basingstoke.

Nixon, R.B., Helveston, E.M., Miller, M., Archer, S.M. & Ellis, F.D. (1985) Incidence of strabismus in neonates. *American Journal of Ophthalmology* 100, 798–801.

von Noorden, G.K. (1988a) Current concepts of infantile esotropia. *Eye* 2, 343–357.

von Noorden, G.K. (1988b) A reassessment of infantile esotropia. *American Journal of Ophthalmology* 105, 1–10.

von Noorden, G.K. & Avilla, C. (1984) Nystagmus blockage syndrome revisited. In: *Strabismus II* (ed. R.D. Reinecke), pp. 75–82. Grune & Stratton, New York.

Norcia, A.M. (1996) Abnormal motion processing and binocularity: infantile esotropia as a model system for effects of early interruptions of binocularity. *Eye* 10, 259.

Raab, E.L. (1970) Dissociative vertical deviation. *Journal of Pediatric Ophthalmology and Strabismus* 7, 146–151.

Repka, M.X. & Guyton, D.L. (1988) Comparison of hangback medial rectus recession with conventional recession. *Ophthalmology* 95, 782–787.

Robb, R.M. & Rodier, D.W. (1987) The variable clinical characteristics and course of early infantile esotropia. *Journal of Pediatric Ophthalmology and Strabismus* 24, 276–281.

Scott, A.B. (1987) Botulinum injection treatment in congenital esotropia. In: *Orthoptic Horizons. Transactions of the Sixth International Orthoptic Congress, Harrogate* (eds M. Lenk-Schafer, C. Calcutt, M. Doyle & S. Moore), pp. 294–299. British Orthoptic Society, London.

Scott, W.E., Reese, P.D., Hirsch, C.R. & Flabetich, C.A. (1986) Surgery for large-angle congenital esotropia. *Archives of Ophthalmology* **104**, 374–377.

Shawkat, F.S., Harris, C.M., Taylor, D.S., Thompson, D.A., Russell Eggitt, I. & Kriss, A. (1995) The optokinetic response differences between congenital profound and nonprofound unilateral visual deprivation. *Ophthalmology* **102** (11), 1615–1622.

Stager, D.R., Weakley, D.R., Everettt, M. & Birch, E.E. (1994) Delayed consecutive exotropia following 7-millimeter bilateral medial rectus recession for congenital esotropia. *Journal of Pediatric Ophthalmology and Strabismus* **31**, 147–150.

Swan, K.C. & Wilkins, J.H. (1984) Extraocular muscle surgery in early infancy – anatomical factors. *Journal of Pediatric Ophthalmology and Strabismus* **21**, 44–49.

Taylor, D.M. (1963) How early is early surgery in the managment of strabismus. *Archives of Ophthalmology* **70**, 752–756.

Taylor, D.M. (1967) Congenital strabismus: the common sense approach. *Archives of Ophthalmology* **77**, 478–484.

Tsutsui, J. & Fukai, S. (1978) Human strabismus cases suggestive of asymmetric projection of the visual pathway. In: *Strabismus* (ed. R.D. Reinecke), pp. 79–88. Grune & Stratton, New York.

Tychsen, L., Hurtig, R.R. & Scott, W.E. (1985) Pursuit is impaired but the vestibulo-ocular reflex is normal in infantile strabismus. *Archives of Ophthalmology* **103**, 536–539.

Weakley, D.R., Stager, D.R. & Everett, M.E. (1991) Seven-millimeter bilateral medial rectus recessions in infantile esotropia. *Journal of Pediatric Ophthalmology and Strabismus* **28**, 113–115.

Wilson, M.E. & McClatchey, S.K. (1991) Dissociated horizontal deviation. *Journal of Pediatric Ophthalmology and Strabismus* **28**, 90–95.

Zipf, R.F. (1976) Binocular fixation pattern. *Archives of Ophthalmology* **94**, 401–404.

15

Microtropia and Allied Conditions

Imperfect binocular single vision is usually associated with a small-angle strabismus but it can also occur in patients who have no manifest strabismus. Modern methods of investigation, with an emphasis on testing in relatively normal seeing conditions, have revealed the high incidence of variants of normal binocular single vision and have led to their differentiation and classification, as shown in Tree 15.1.

Phenomena associated with binocular single vision

Panum's fusional area

Panum's fusional area is essential for the maintenance of binocular single vision. Stimulation of disparate retinal elements within the area allows fusion of the images and gives rise to stereopsis. Fender and Julesz (1967) and Crone *et al.* (1978) have shown that the normal Panum's area is larger than the original concept, measuring from 2° to 2°40'. Pasino and Maraini (1966) demonstrated that Panum's area was further enlarged in apparently 'cured' squint. Bagolini and

Capobianco (1965) demonstrated an enlarged area in patients with abnormal retinal correspondence.

Fixation disparity

Ogle *et al.* (1949) described fixation disparity as a physiological sensory phenomenon occurring in heterophoria, in which a deviation of the visual axes of 6–10 minutes of arc is compatible with bifoveal binocular single vision. They demonstrated fixation disparity by presenting the eyes with fusional targets containing centrally placed and dissimilar monocularly seen features. When the targets were fused, the dissimilar features were seen displaced, revealing the fixation disparity which could then be measured. The amount of fixation disparity increases if the degree of heterophoria increases or if binocular single vision is placed under stress by the introduction of base-in or base-out prisms of increasing strength. A curve can be plotted showing the degree of fixation disparity against the strength of each prism (Fig. 15.1).

Fixation disparity is dependent on Panum's fusional area. Crone (1981) and de Decker *et al.* (1976) have

Tree 15.1 Variants of normal binocular single vision.

Abnormal BSV —— Subnormal BSV
Microtropia
Monofixation syndrome
Abnormal retinal correspondence with angle > than 10 Δ

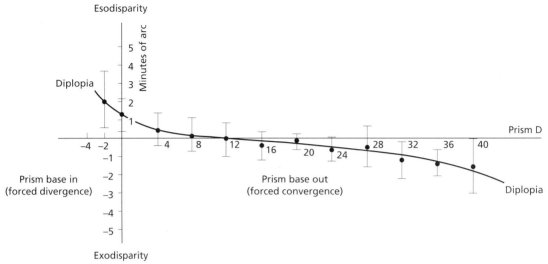

Fig. 15.1 Fixation disparity curve in a normal person (de Decker *et al.* 1976).

demonstrated that a pathological or 'obligate' fixation disparity can exist in patients with anomalous binocular single vision and that it is larger than the normal fixation disparity. It has been hypothesized that disparity is the first stage in the development of the different forms of anomalous binocular single vision, with or without abnormal retinal correspondence (Crone 1969).

Binocular single vision

Binocular single vision is present if images of the fixation object fall on corresponding retinal areas and are fused to give a single unified image.

Normal binocular single vision is present when there is normal retinal correspondence and bifoveal fusion. Abnormal binocular single vision is present when there is a single unified image in the presence of foveal suppression, with or without a small-angle strabismus. Binocular single vision in free space can be classified as shown in Tree 15.2.

Abnormal binocular single vision

The main aim of investigation is to differentiate abnormal from bifoveal BSV. The principal differentiating features are shown in Table 15.1.

Subnormal binocular single vision

Precise diagnosis of the type of retinal correspondence associated with anomalous binocular single vision is extremely difficult due to the limitations of the tests available. Where no manifest deviation is seen in the presence of central fixation but a central suppression scotoma is demonstrable, it is usually assumed that normal retinal correspondence is present and the condition is referred to as subnormal BSV. This finding follows successful surgical alignment of childhood strabismus. von Noorden (1988) reported that 20% of patients with surgically treated infantile esotropia demonstrated subnormal BSV postoperatively.

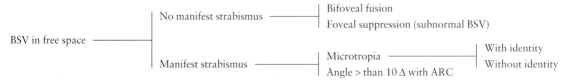

Tree 15.2 Classification of binocular single vision in free space.

Table 15.1 Differentiation between normal and abnormal binocular single vision.

Diagnostic feature	Bifoveal BSV	Abnormal BSV
Visual acuity	Equal in most cases	Unequal
Refractive error	Approximately the same in each eye	Anisometropia
Fixation	Central	Central or parafoveal/ parafoveolar
Cover test	No manifest deviation	Small deviation may be detected
Stereoacuity	40 seconds of arc or better	Worse than 40 seconds
4 Δ prism test	Bifoveal fusion	Central suppression

Microtropia (microstrabismus)

The term microtropia was first used by Lang (1968) to describe small-angle unilateral strabismus with binocular single vision in which the manifest deviation did not exceed 10 Δ. This is the most common form of abnormal binocular single vision.

Characteristics

The features of microtropia are:
• A monocular manifest strabismus of 10 Δ or less, often with an associated heterophoria.
• A foveal suppression scotoma in the affected eye.
• Abnormal binocular single vision with sensory and motor fusion.
• Reduced visual acuity in the deviating eye.
• Anisometropia in nearly all cases, commonly with hypermetropia or hypermetropic astigmatism.
• Parafoveolar fixation in the affected eye in many cases.
• Reduced or, more rarely, absent stereopsis.

Types of microtropia

Microtropia is more prevalent in esotropia (microesotropia) than it is in exotropia (microexotropia). Vertical microtropia is rare but has been reported (Shortland 1978) and may be seen in patients with congenital vertical muscle palsies, when it provides further confirmation of the early onset of the palsy.

Microtropia can be classified into cases with or without identity:

• Identity is present when the deviation is associated with eccentric fixation which is coincident with the angle of deviation. No manifest deviation is detected. Factors which suggest the presence of a microtropia are reduced unilateral visual acuity and demonstrable binocular single vision.
• Microtropia without identity is present when a very small manifest deviation is seen on cover test. It may be associated with central fixation or with eccentric fixation which is not coincident with the angle of deviation.

The quality of binocular single vision in microtropic patients is less good than it is in those with bifoveal binocular single vision. Hill *et al.* (1976) showed that a correlation exists between the angle of deviation and the degree of stereoacuity attained: those with angles measuring 4 Δ or less had significantly higher stereoacuity than those measuring from 5 to 9 Δ, when assessed using stereotests other than the TNO test.

Microtropia may also be classified as primary or secondary:
• Primary: when microtropia is the initial defect and there is no history of a larger angle of strabismus. It may also accompany other concomitant intermittent deviations, for example microtropia with fully accommodative characteristics.
• Secondary or residual: when a microtropia is demonstrated following treatment for a larger angle manifest deviation.

The differential diagnosis of primary and secondary microtropia is made difficult by the frequent presence of anisometropia in apparently secondary cases, suggesting that there was a primary microesotropia which decompensated to a larger deviation and required treatment to restore binocular single vision. It is also possible that the concomitant deviation preceded the microtropia. For the purposes of management it is sufficient to identify the presence of a microtropia.

Incidence

Lang (1976) reviewed 33 644 patients with ocular defects and reported an incidence of microtropia of 2.84%; the large majority had microesotropia, with only 3.6% of the group having microexotropia. In contrast, Boyd and Budd (1976) reported finding 39% with exotropia among their microtropic patients.

Aetiology

Anisometropia

All but a very few patients with microtropia have some degree of anisometropia, resulting in a defocused image to the more ametropic eye. This could explain:
- the foveal suppression scotoma;
- amblyopia;
- eccentric fixation on the border of the scotoma;
- peripheral binocular single vision with defective stereopsis.

Anisometropia with bifoveal binocular single vision is less common, especially when there is anisohypermetropia or hypermetropic astigmatism.

Conversely, Lang (1969) suggests that anisometropia may develop secondary to microtropia due to a lack of emmetropization of the affected eye.

Hereditary factors

It has been shown that members of different generations as well as siblings of microtropic patients have other types of strabismus and/or microtropia (Lang 1984). However, parents and siblings of microtropic children were found to have an increased incidence of refractive error as well as squint, suggesting that a genetically determined refractive error may be the fundamental anomaly.

Investigation

The aims of the investigation are to diagnose the microtropia and to assess the quality of binocular single vision by measuring the fusional amplitude and stereoacuity.

History

Patients may present with constant or intermittent strabismus or because defective vision in one eye has been discovered by chance or by routine visual screening.

Visual acuity

The difference in visual acuity between the two eyes can vary from part of a Snellen's line to a much larger difference. The optimum vision after amblyopia treatment is often one line lower than that of the better eye. Linear vision testing is necessary to detect small differences in visual acuity, which may appear equal when tested with single optotypes. The speed of reading letters should be noted for near and distance and is often slower when the affected eye is tested.

Cover test

- A small manifest deviation is usually seen, although none is present in microtropia with identity.
- The alternate cover test may reveal an associated heterophoria; the speed of recovery indicates the degree of compensation.
- According to Lang (1984) the fourth Purkinje image, the reflection produced at the posterior surface of the lens, is displaced nasally in cases of microtropia and can be observed using a spotlight, but slit-lamp examination is often required to see this image.

Fixation

Examination with a fixation ophthalmoscope such as the Visuscope is essential to diagnose the state of fixation. Stable parafoveolar fixation is seen in many cases of microtropia, usually situated nasal and often slightly superior to the fovea in microesotropia. In microexotropia fixation is still parafoveolar but may be sited temporal, superior or nasal to the fovea (Johnson *et al.* 1981).

Suppression scotoma

Objective testing: the scotoma is most easily detected using the 4 Δ prism test. The test is best performed using a detailed target whenever possible. If a suppression scotoma is present there will be no movement of either eye when the prism is placed in front of the eye with the suspected scotoma: when the prism is placed in front of the other eye that eye will move to fixate the target and the other eye will make a simultaneous conjugate movement but there will be no corrective disjugate movement to achieve bifoveal fusion.

Subjective testing: the suppression scotoma can be detected subjectively using;

- Bagolini striated glasses (see below);
- the Polaroid four dot test.

Lang (1976) demonstrated monocular visual disturbance during visual acuity testing or when using the Amsler grid. The scotoma can be measured using the Amsler grid monocularly or binocularly if Lang's Amsler major amblyoscope slides are used.

A patient with a right microtropia may notice that the right-hand letters disappear or fade when reading the Snellen chart. The left-hand letters disappear with a left microtropia. This he attributed to a temporally displaced scotoma.

All these methods demand considerable powers of observation on the patient's part and are usually only successful in older patients.

Confirmation of binocular single vision

This may be obtained by using the following techniques.

Bagolini striated glasses

A symmetrical cross is the usual response in microtropia. The presence of a suppression scotoma may be indicated subjectively as a central or paracentral gap in the line seen by the affected eye, but few patients observe this phenomenon even if its presence is suggested to them.

Although a suppression response is almost invariably seen in microtropia, Bagolini (1985) has reported that some patients maintain a perfect cross with Bagolini glasses during the 4 Δ prism test, indicating sensory adaptation rather than suppression.

Worth's four-lights test

A patient with microtropia should see four lights unless a large heterophoria or intermittent strabismus becomes decompensated by the test. Parks (1996) reported fusion using the near Worth lights test at 1/3 metre but if the distance from the patient was increased, the macular scotoma became apparent, usually at approximately 2/3 metre.

Fusion amplitude

Measurement of the fusion amplitude using base-out and base-in prisms can indicate whether or not any latent component is well compensated. A control such as Bagolini glasses may be required to confirm when fusion is lost, since peripheral suppression can prevent the appreciation of diplopia.

Stereotests

The majority of patients with microtropia demonstrate some degree of stereoacuity. Some patients have difficulty in obtaining a response from pure random dot tests and a few are stereoblind. Lang (1984) reported that patients with microtropia were unable to appreciate depth using the uncontoured Lang stereotest but this is not borne out by our experience. It is advisable to test patients using both a contoured and random dot test. The standard reached is only rarely as good as 40 seconds of arc.

Measurement of the deviation

The manifest part of the deviation in microtropia without identity can be measured using the simultaneous prism cover test (see Chapters 5 and 7). A conventional prism cover test will measure the total amount of deviation (i.e. manifest plus latent component).

In making a diagnosis of microtropia it is essential to relate visual acuity, fixation, the response to the 4 Δ prism test and the level of stereoacuity. It is usually accepted that retinal correspondence is abnormal in microtropia. However, Panum's fusional area is enlarged in microtropia and Parks (1971) believed that this allowed normal retinal correspondence with peripheral fusion. Reports of a small number of patients with apparently normal retinal correspondence are common.

Management of microtropia

Management is directed to obtaining and maintaining the best possible visual acuity. Restoration of binocular single vision may be necesary if the microtropia coexists with other types of strabismus.

Visual acuity
- The first stage is the correction of any significant refractive error and the constant wearing of spectacles.
- Occlusion: part-time total occlusion is preferable unless visual acuity is unusually low, for example 6/60, when constant total occlusion may be necessary. Occlusion is continued until there is no further improvement over two or three visits. Fixation should be checked at intervals, but in the authors' experience eccentric fixation remains unchanged and equal visual acuity does not result from treatment. Lang (1974) recommended the use of Bangerter graded filters, which he continued to use up to the age of 10 years in some cases, partly to obtain equal visual acuity, which he believed could be achieved, and partly to prevent monocular reading difficulties later. Our practice is to occlude for a much shorter period, using total occlusion (see Chapter 10).
- It may be necessary to use intermittent part-time occlusion or possibly penalization in young children until stability is obtained.

Restoration of constant binocular single vision
If a microtropia is associated with a concomitant deviation, for example a fully accommodative esotropia, treatment follows conventional lines depending on the characteristics of any intermittent deviation present. It is, of course, accepted that the microtropia will persist after treatment, and no effort is made to overcome it.

Influence of microtropia

Microtropia may influence compensation of a latent deviation, and also affect orthoptic treatment.

Compensation of a latent deviation
Although symptom-producing heterophoria with microtropia is rarely seen, there is a belief that young children with microtropia are more likely to develop a manifest strabismus in the presence of other factors, such as uncorrected hypermetropia; the reason given is the relatively poor quality of binocular single vision. The microtropia may then be diagnosed retrospectively after surgery for a constant strabismus.

Orthoptic treatment
It is claimed that the results of treatment of fully accommodative esotropia and esotropia with convergence excess are less good if the condition is associated with microtropia. Difficulties are found in improving the patient's binocular visual acuity as these patients do not readily appreciate physiological diplopia and the central suppression scotoma may prevent a fused central picture when using stereograms.

Monofixation syndrome

The term monofixation syndrome, introduced by Parks (1971), is sometimes used synonymously with microtropia. The monofixation syndrome describes patients with nonbifoveal binocular single vision who show the following characteristics:
- straight or near straight eyes;
- a suppression scotoma in the affected eye;
- motor fusion.

In addition, some of the following features are likely to be present:
- a history of strabismus;
- anisometropia;
- amblyopia;
- parafoveal fixation;
- a unilateral macular lesion;
- orthophoria or heterophoria;
- a small manifest strabismus of 8 Δ or less.

Thus it can be seen that the monofixation syndrome is a less specific diagnosis covering a wider spectrum of conditions, including microtropia but also subnormal binocular single vision and patients with macular pathology in one eye who can maintain binocular single vision.

The investigation and management is the same as for microtropia.

Esotropia with abnormal retinal correspondence

Demonstrable binocular function in free space in a patient with a strabismus, usually esotropia, which measures at least 10 Δ indicates the presence of abnormal retinal correspondence. Only gross binocular function is demonstrable in these patients. Binocular single vision may be indicated using Bagolini glasses, and rudimentary stereopsis may be present with a positive two-pen test or appreciation of the Fly on the Wirt stereotest, but fine random dot stereopsis is not achieved. The angle of anomaly can be further investigated by use of the Synoptophore, demonstrating a minimal subjective angle and a larger objective measurement. After-images can be employed to determine the projection of the foveae under binocular conditions; patients with normal retinal correspondence will see a symmetrical cross and those with abnormal retinal correspondence will see a displaced cross.

Paradoxical diplopia may occur after surgical correction, usually as crossed diplopia in the presence of a residual esotropia: this emphasizes the need to investigate the sensory status preoperatively and determine the likelihood of postoperative diplopia either with prisms or botulinum toxin, although paradoxical diplopia is often transitory.

There is a risk that the patient will reconverge to the original angle of deviation postoperatively in order to use binocular single vision, but since abnormal retinal correspondence is most often associated with relatively small angles of deviation, surgery is rarely required.

References

Bagolini, B. (1985) Objective evaluation of sensorial and sensorimotor status in esotropia: their importance in surgical prognosis. *British Journal of Ophthalmology* **69**, 725–728.

Bagolini, B. & Capobianco, N.M. (1965) Subjective space in comitant squint. *American Journal of Ophthalmology.* **50**, 430–442.

Boyd, T.A.S. & Budd, G.E. (1976) Monofixation exotropia and asthenopia. In: *Orthoptics, Past, Present and Future. Transactions of the Third International Orthoptic Congress, Boston* (eds S. Moore, J. Mein & L. Stockbridge), pp. 173–178. Symposia Specialists, Miami.

Crone, R.A. (1969) From orthophoria to microtropia. *British Orthoptic Journal* **26**, 45–51.

Crone, R.A. (1981) Anomalous binocular vision redefined. In: *Orthoptics, Research and Practice. Transactions of the Fourth International Orthoptic Congress, Berne* (eds J. Mein & S. Moore), pp. 160–161. Kimpton, London.

Crone, R.A., Vrooland, J.L., Hardjowito, S. (1978) Proportionregelung der Fusion. Integralregelung der willkurlichen konvergenz. In: *Disorders of Ocular Motility* (ed. G. Kommerell), pp. 323–327. Bergmann, Munich.

de Decker, W., Scheffel, T. & Baenge, J. (1976) Fixation disparity and the origin of microstrabismus. In: *Orthoptics, Past, Present and Future. Transactions of the Third International Orthoptic Congress, Boston* (eds S. Moore, J. Mein & L. Stockbridge), pp. 155–165. Symposia Specialists, Miami.

Fender, D.H. & Julesz, B. (1967) Extension of Panum's fusional area in binocularly stabilised vision. *Journal of the Optical Society of America* **57**, 819–825.

Hill, M., Perry, J. & Wood, I.C.J. (1976) Stereoacuity in microtropia. In: *Orthoptics, Past, Present and Future. Transactions of the Third International Orthoptic Congress, Boston* (eds S. Moore, J. Mein & L. Stockbridge), pp. 25–29. Symposia Specialists, Miami, Florida.

Johnson, F., Cunha, L.A.P. & Harcourt, R.B. (1981) The clinical characteristics of micro-exotropia. *British Orthoptic Journal* **38**, 54–59.

Lang, J. (1968) Evaluation in small angle strabismus or microtropia. In: *International Strabismus Symposium* (University of Giessen, 1966) (ed A. Arruga), pp. 219–222. Karger, Basle.

Lang, J. (1969) Microstrabismus. *British Orthoptic Journal* **26**, 30–37.

Lang, J. (1974) Management of microtropia. *British Journal of Ophthalmology* **58**, 281–292.

Lang, J. (1976) Lessons learned from microtropia. In: *Orthoptics, Past, Present and Future. Transactions of the Third International Orthoptic Congress, Boston* (eds S. Moore, J. Mein & L. Stockbridge), pp. 183–190. Symposia Specialists, Miami.

Lang, J. (1984) *Strabismus* [trans. C.W. Cibis], pp. 90–97. Slack, Thorofare, N.J.

von Noorden, G.K. (1988) A reassessment of infantile esotropia. *American Journal of Ophthalmology* **105**, 1–10.

Ogle, K.N., Mussey, F. & Pranger, A. (1949) Fixation disparity and fusional processes in binocular single vision. *American Journal of Ophthalmology* **32**, 1069–1087.

Parks, M.M. (1971) The monofixation syndrome. In: *Symposium on Strabismus. Transactions of the New Orleans Academy of Ophthalmology* (ed. J.H. Allen), pp. 121–153. Mosby, St Louis.

Parks, M.M. (1996) Small angle esotropia/monofixation: avoid the traps. *American Orthoptic Journal* **46**, 34–35.

Pasino, L. & Maraini, G. (1966) Area of binocular vision in anomalous retinal correspondence. *British Journal of Ophthalmology* **50**, 646–650.

Shortland, J.A. (1978) A case of vertical microtropia. *British Orthoptic Journal* **35**, 118–120.

16

Heterophoria and Anomalies of Convergence and Accommodation

Heterophoria

Definition

Heterophoria is a latent strabismus in which the visual axes are normally directed to the fixation object but deviate when the eyes are dissociated.

• Binocular single vision is maintained by motor fusion, and providing the motor fusion amplitude is adequate, the heterophoria remains symptom-free and is said to be compensated. If the fusion amplitude is insufficient the heterophoria becomes decompensated and gives rise to symptoms and/or a manifest deviation.

• There is no fixed dividing line separating an intermittent strabismus in which the deviation is very rarely manifest from a heterophoria in which the strabismus is nearly always controlled.

Orthophoria, the opposite of heterophoria, is present when there is no deviation of the visual axes when the eyes are dissociated and fusion suspended. In comparison it is rarely seen.

Heterphoria may be incomitant or concomitant.

Incomitant heterophoria

Most incomitant heterophorias are seen in the setting of paralytic or mechanical strabismus. For diagnostic purposes any strabismus should be classified according to the underlying cause; for example, paralytic strabismus due to fourth nerve palsy, which may be well compensated or showing signs of decompensating in certain gaze directions.

With incomitant heterophoria the dissociated deviation:

• increases when the paretic eye is made to fixate (secondary deviation);

• decreases when the fellow eye fixates (primary deviation);

• varies when the eyes are dissociated in different positions of gaze.

Large vertical heterophorias are principally seen in association with:

• congenital vertical muscle palsies, in particular fourth nerve palsy;

• thyroid eye disease.

In most cases the hyperphoria is incomitant.

In cases of acquired vertical muscle imbalance the small vertical fusional amplitude does not have time to expand, therefore significant hyperphorias are uncommon in acquired conditions and most vertical deviations are therefore poorly controlled.

Incomitance can be due to:

Table 16.1 Classification of concomitant horizontal heterophoria (N = near; D = distance).

Esophoria			Exophoria		
Divergence weakness	Convergence excess	Nonspecific	Divergence excess	Convergence weakness	Nonspecific
D > N	N > D	N = D	D > N	N > D	N = D

• Underaction of one or more of the extraocular muscles as a result of cranial nerve palsy or mechanical or myogenic factors.

• Uncorrected or undercorrected spherical anisometropia, requiring more accommodation and therefore more convergence when one eye fixates than when the other eye fixates. Accurate correction of anisometropia should result in restoration of concomitance.

In general, hyperphoria, hypertropia, hypophoria, hypotropia, cyclophoria and cyclotropia are nearly always incomitant in origin. For this reason vertical and torsional phorias are not included in the classification of concomitant heterophoria which follows.

Concomitant heterophoria

In concomitant heterophoria the dissociated deviation remains the same whichever eye is made to fixate and is virtually unchanged in the cardinal positions of gaze. Concomitant horizontal heterophoria is classified according to the nature and comparative size of the deviation for near and distance fixation, as shown in Table 16.1. In most cases there is a significant difference between the near and distance angles of deviation. Nonspecific heterophoria, in which the deviation measures approximately the same for both distances, is more rarely seen.

Decompensation of heterophoria

If decompensation of heterophoria occurs in childhood, the relative instability of binocular single vision makes it more likely that a manifest strabismus will develop. If it becomes decompensated in adult life, binocular single vision is retained in the great majority of cases but at the expense of symptoms.

Causes of decompensation

The causes of decompensation should be related to the age of the patient when the decompensating factor intervenes. For example:

• a short period of occlusion will disrupt binocular vision and lead to amblyopia and strabismus in a child but not in an adult;

• uncorrected refractive errors may produce a strabismus in a child but will most likely result in symptoms in an adult.

Decompensation may result from:

• optical causes;
• medical causes;
• others.

OPTICAL CAUSES

• Uncorrected or undercorrected spherical refractive errors. These may arise from planned undercorrection or the refusal to wear the spectacles prescribed. This can result in disturbance of the normal accommodative –convergence relationship as follows:

1 an esophoria, decompensated by uncorrected hypermetropia;

2 an exophoria, decompensated by uncorrected myopia.

• Wrongly corrected refractive errors. This may reduce visual acuity, and thus dissociate the eyes, especially if one is affected more than the other. Reduction in visual acuity from other causes has the same effect.

• Ill-fitting spectacles. These can result in a prismatic effect if the lenses are decentred, and can increase the degree of heterophoria and make control more difficult. A vertical prismatic effect is particularly disruptive to comfortable binocular single vision.

• Aniseikonia. The most obvious example is the difference in image size which occurs when unilateral aphakia is corrected by spectacle lens, when the aniseikonia is insuperable. Even when it is reduced to 6–8% with a contact lens the size difference is not always overcome. The most frequently encountered situation in clinical practice is following cataract extraction with intraocular lens implantation where a miscalculation of intraocular lens power has resulted in significant anisometropia postoperatively.

MEDICAL CAUSES

• Poor general health. This may cause fatigue, making it harder to exert enough motor fusion, or it may adversely affect the patient's accommodation, disturbing the relationship with convergence. Infectious mononucleosis is a recognized cause of defective accommodation in young people.
• Head trauma. Severe head trauma may result in loss of motor and sensory fusion, which may be temporary or permanent (Pratt-Johnson 1973). In some instances selective reduction in motor fusion may occur in the presence of normal sensory fusion. Lesser degrees of injury may temporarily reduce the fusion and accommodative amplitudes.
• Medication. Therapeutic drugs may affect accommodation and make heterophoria more difficult to control. Both centrally acting antihypertensive agents and antidepressant drugs commonly decrease the amplitude of accommodation.
• Alcohol. Quite small amounts of alcohol can temporarily decompensate heterophorias and intermittent strabismus, resulting in diplopia.

OTHERS

• Demand on vision during binocular viewing. An increase in ocular activity can place additional strain on control of the heterophoria, for example:
  1 when a patient with exophoria of the convergence weakness type is required to undertake increasing amounts of close work;
  2 when a patient with esophoria of the divergence weakness type has to drive a motor vehicle for long periods;
  3 prolonged use of video display units—a European directive is now in place requiring video display unit operators to undergo an ocular examination.
• Demand on vision during monocular viewing. In certain occupations, such as those involving the use of a jeweller's glass or a monocular microscope, excessive demands on one eye may result in decompensation of a pre-existing heterophoria. Therapeutic occlusion or atropinization of one eye in a child for any reason may rarely result in a manifest strabismus. Acquired loss of vision in one eye often leads to the development of a secondary form of manifest strabismus in children and adults.

Symptoms in heterophoria

The symptoms resulting from decompensation may be due to:
• the effort to maintain binocular single vision;
• failure to maintain binocular single vision.

Effort to maintain binocular single vision

The symptoms consist of:
• bilateral headache, which is usually located in the frontal region;
• eye strain and asthenopia.
In most cases the symptoms can be related to a particular ocular activity. Typically they are absent on awakening, and occur later in the day. During periods when the eyes are used less, for example at weekends and during holidays, the patient may be symptom-free. However, heterophoria which increases on distance fixation gives rise to more indefinite symptoms, which can occur at any time, although they may be associated with leisure activities, such as watching sport and attending the cinema.

Failure to maintain binocular single vision

This can result in:
• Transitory diplopia, usually noticed when the patient is tired or unwell. The diplopia can be controlled by blinking or by changing the fixation distance.
• Blurred vision due to manipulating accommodation in an attempt to control the deviation by accommodative vergence.
• Less specific symptoms, such as jumbling of the letters on reading.
  The patient may volunteer that he carries out certain activities, for example reading, with one eye shut.

Investigation of heterophoria

The investigation is directed to:

- the detection and measurement of the heterophoria, including the differential diagnosis of concomitant and incomitant heterophoria;
- assessment of the extent of compensation;
- ensuring that the patient's symptoms are attributable to the heterophoria.

History

Important questions are:
- the exact nature of the symptoms;
- when they occur;
- when the symptoms were first experienced and the average duration of each episode;
- if they can be relieved in any way, for example by closing one eye or stopping reading.
- the general health of the patient, in particular a history of recent illness or change of medication;
- any previous ophthalmic treatment, change in spectacle prescription or past orthoptic exercises;
- a change in occupation or leisure activities.

Clinical investigation

DETECTION AND MEASUREMENT OF THE HETEROPHORIA

Heterophoria is detected initially by the cover test, using the alternate cover test to dissociate the eyes and the cover/uncover test to observe recovery to binocular single vision. The speed of any recovery movement should be noted:
- a rapid recovery implies good compensation;
- a slow recovery implies that decompensation is probable.

The patient should also be asked about symptoms of blurring or diplopia during testing.

If the deviation is seen to increase from near fixation to fixation at 6 m, the cover test should be repeated with the patient fixing on a far distance object.

Methods used to measure and record the heterophoria must fully dissociate the eyes for both near and distance fixation in order to reveal the maximum angle of deviation. Methods include:
- Alternating prism cover test: this is the method of choice in most cases. Small amounts of esophoria are sometimes difficult to detect.
- Maddox rod: small amounts of esophoria are often easier to measure using this method. Plenty of time should be allowed to achieve maximum dissociation.

- Hess chart: this should only be plotted if there is any suspicion that the deviation is incomitant and it is indicated in symptom-producing esotropia with divergence weakness, especially in adults because of the possibility of a lateral rectus palsy.

MEASUREMENT OF CONVERGENCE

This is tested using the near point rule. The patient fixates a dot in the centre of a vertical black line. The examiner should measure the near point of convergence several times, either subjectively if the patient recognizes when his convergence fails, or objectively, making the following observations:
- The near point in centimetres on the first and subsequent measurements: the near point typically recedes on retesting.
- Which eye diverges and whether diplopia or suppression occurs on failure of convergence.
- Whether the patient finds it easy or difficult to converge: if diplopia is present he should be encouraged to rejoin the images, noting the effort required to do so.

MEASUREMENT OF THE HORIZONTAL FUSION AMPLITUDE

This is tested using the prism bar.
- The patient fixates an accommodative target for near. The prisms are introduced in front of one eye and gradually increased in strength, asking the patient to keep the image single as long as possible and report when it becomes double. The observer watches the patient's eyes, concentrating on the nondominant eye if known, to note when binocular single vision is lost.
- It is important that the distance of the target remains static so that the only variable is the disparity caused by the prism.
- The break point is recorded when diplopia occurs. The strength of prism should then be reduced until fusion is regained: this is recorded as the recovery point.
- The test can also be used to assess positive and negative relative convergence by asking the patient to report when the image blurs prior to the break point.
- The test is repeated for distance and then the same procedure used with the prisms in the opposite direction.

MEASUREMENT OF ACCOMMODATION

Heterophoria and anomalies of accommodation are closely connected, making it important to measure the near point of accommodation uniocularly and binocularly in all cases.

• The near point of accommodation can conveniently be measured using the near point rule, asking the patient to read the smallest print visible to each eye.

• Testing is entirely subjective.

• The patient must state when he no longer sees the print clearly.

• The test should be repeated several times, noting if the near point recedes or remains the same.

• The print should be changed on retesting, and it is useful to check the measurements by holding the text very close to the eyes, when it will be blurred, withdrawing it slowly until it can be seen clearly again.

• The pupil reactions should be noted during testing and give an objective sign that accommodative effort is being used.

COMPENSATION OF HETEROPHORIA

This is assessed by:

• the speed of recovery to binocular single vision after dissociation, best seen when using the cover test;

• the near point of convergence and the extent of the fusion amplitude.

Compensation of heterophoria is good if there is:

• Rapid recovery to binocular single vision.

• A well-maintained near point of convergence and a normal fusion amplitude. The size of the positive fusion amplitude is more important in exophoria and that of the negative fusion amplitude in esophoria.

Compensation of heterophoria is poor if there is:

• Slow or delayed recovery to binocular single vision.

• A remote near point of convergence, or poorly maintained convergence.

• A poor positive fusion amplitude in exophoria or a poor negative fusional amplitude in esophoria.

Heterophoria and the significance of any symptoms

Usually the correlation between the patient's symptoms and the type of heterophoria indicates whether or not the deviation is likely to be responsible, but in a few cases the issue is not clear, especially in small degrees of esophoria which can produce severe symptoms, not always related to the use of the eyes. In doubtful cases the significance of the symptoms can be assessed by:

• Diagnostic prisms to compensate the heterophoria. If the symptoms are relieved over a 2–3-week period they can be attributed to the deviation.

• Diagnostic occlusion, worn as much as possible over the same period. Symptoms due to the heterophoria should disappear when only one eye is used.

The use of prisms is more practical than occlusion, especially for adults, and is preferable because binocular single vision is maintained.

Management of heterophoria

Principles of management

Treatment may be directed to:

• increasing the fusion amplitude to facilitate control of the heterophoria;

• reducing the deviation so that the fusion amplitude can control it more easily.

The methods which can be used are:

• conservative treatment;

• orthoptic exercises;

• prisms;

• botulinum toxin;

• surgery.

Selection of patients

• Treatment is not given unless symptoms are present, with the possible exception of poorly controlled heterophorias in children in order to prevent later decompensation. The examiner must be satisfied that the symptoms are caused by the deviation.

• Refraction must have been carried out, and spectacles prescribed if required. Cycloplegia should be used in children when there is esophoria of the convergence excess type, which may be associated with a significant degree of hypermetropia. Lenses should be correctly centred. Time should be allowed to assess the effect of optical correction on compensation of the heterophoria.

• The patient's general health should be stable. If an undiagnosed physical cause for the symptoms is suspected further investigation is indicated.

• The patient must be cooperative, willing to have treatment and able to carry it out. This applies particularly to orthoptic exercises, which require more active participation than do other methods.

Conservative treatment

ORTHOPTIC EXERCISES

The success of orthoptic exercises in cooperative patients depends on:

- the type of heterophoria;
- the size of the angle of deviation.

Suitable patients are those with:

- concomitant heterophoria;
- exophoria less than 15–20 Δ: symptom-producing exophoria exceeding this amount is unlikely to respond to orthoptic exercises in the long term;
- esophoria of less than 10 Δ: symptom-producing esophoria exceeding 10 Δ is unlikely to respond to orthoptic exercises in the long term.

Although measurements are given as a criterion of selection for treatment they are intended only as guidelines and exceptions are found in all types of heterophoria. Treatment (see Chapter 8) is mainly directed at:

- improving the fusional amplitude, the positive amplitude in exophoria and the negative amplitude in esophoria;
- convergence, using exercises based on physiological diplopia to improve control and exercise relative (fusional) convergence, using positive relative convergence in exophoria and negative relative convergence in esophoria.

PRISMS

Prisms effectively reduce the amount of heterophoria which the patient has to control. Suitable patients for treatment with prisms include:

- elderly patients with incomitant or concomitant heterophoria, when prisms are often the first-choice treatment;
- patients with small amounts of heterophoria who have failed to respond to exercises or whose symptoms have recurred after initial improvement from orthoptic treatment;
- patients with small vertical phorias.

In general the lowest strength prism which allows comfortable control of the heterophoria is used; this is generally less than the dissociated measurement. More of the deviation needs to be corrected in esophoria than in exophoria. The amount of esophoria may apparently increase after a short period of wearing the prisms; this phenomenon is part of prism adaptation and is discussed in more detail in Chapter 7. Temporary Fresnel prisms should be used until the patient's response is known, as the amount of deviation which needs to be corrected varies from one patient to another.

BOTULINUM TOXIN

Botulinum toxin is effective in the management of decompensating esophoria and exophoria, and results in a decrease in the magnitude of the deviation and better overall control. Most patients require repeat injection for the improvement to be maintained, although in some a cure has followed a single injection of the toxin. Small decompensating phorias respond best to botulinum toxin; in particular exophoria responds so well that in our practice botulinum toxin is the first-line treatment for this condition. For long-term improvement in control of the phoria it is probably necessary for the ipsilateral antagonist of the injected muscle to become contracted, usually secondary to a significant consecutive deviation (see Chapter 8). Stable long-term changes in alignment are facilitated by the potential for fusion in this group of patients.

Surgical treatment

Patients requiring surgery to reduce the angle of deviation comprise those with a large-angle heterophoria of any type, in particular:

- distance exophoria;
- near esophoria with a high AC/A ratio;
- distance esophoria: most patients in this group require surgery for lasting improvement.

Others likely to require surgery include:

- heterophoria which has not responded to other forms of treatment or when the patient is unwilling to try conservative treatment;
- incomitant heterophoria due to underaction of the extraocular muscles.

CHOICE OF SURGERY

The choice of surgery depends on:

- whether the heterophoria is concomitant or incomitant;
- the size of the deviation for near and distance fixation.

Surgery for incomitant heterophoria is carried out according to the principles outlined in Chapter 9, aiming to restore concomitance and relieve symptoms.

In general, adjustable sutures should be used where possible.

Decompensating exophoria

Surgery should aim to leave the deviation slightly undercorrected.

• Distance exophoria: bilateral lateral rectus recession is the operation of choice. When the patient has used accommodative convergence to help control the deviation preoperatively, it may be difficult to get sufficient relaxation of accommodation postoperatively to allow accurate suture adjustment. The use of fixed sutures may be preferred.

• Nonspecific exophoria: unilateral lateral rectus recession and medial rectus resection. Deviations greater than 45 Δ will require surgery to three or four rectus muscles.

• Near exophoria: most near exophoria is associated with convergence insufficiency. Using conservative management of the exophoria whilst providing orthoptic exercises for the convergence insufficiency often results in long-term improvement of the exophoria. Patients with near exophoria need to be differentiated from patients with acquired near exotropia with loss of motor fusion who do not respond to surgical intervention. Patients with near exophoria respond to a medial rectus resection and lateral rectus recession, performing a greater amount of resection than recession. Alternatively, a bilateral medial rectus resection is performed; an initial reversal of the deviation results in the best long-term stability. A temporary overcorrection with diplopia in the distance is common, and the patient should be warned of this.

Decompensating esophoria

Long-term stability often results from heterophorias which have been fully or slightly overcorrected, as most patients have good positive fusion amplitudes.

• Distance esophoria: we prefer to perform a unilateral small medial rectus recession and a lateral rectus resection.

• Nonspecific esophoria: unilateral medial rectus recession and lateral rectus resection.

• Near esophoria: either a unilateral medial rectus recession, or bilateral medial rectus recession depending on the size of the deviation.

Some patients may still require the use of prisms to ensure that comfortable binocular single vision is maintained. Convergence insufficiency may require orthoptic exercises, especially following surgery for near exophoria.

Special problems in heterophoria

The types of heterophoria which are particularly difficult to manage are:

• distance esophoria;
• esophoria associated with convergence insufficiency.

Distance esophoria

The negative fusion amplitude in these patients is not infrequently extremely small; occasionally the patient can overcome 1 or 2 Δ placed base-in when fixing on a distant target. Simple exercises using crossed physiological diplopia dissociate the deviation and result in uncrossed diplopia which the patient has difficulty in fusing. Methods of treatment which may help are:

• Low-strength prisms loaned to the patient to use base-in at home, marking the prism base to avoid error in placement. He is instructed to hold the prism base-in in front of one eye while fixing on a near target. Once the images are fused he can increase the distance between himself and the fixation target until he can maintain binocular single vision at 6 m and eventually in the far distance. The procedure is then repeated with a stronger prism.

• Crossed physiological diplopia can be taught using a coloured vertical stripe on a clear plastic background to avoid dissociation. The patient is instructed to 'frame' a distance target between the two stripes. Detail can then be added to the plastic until the patient can proceed to use conventional stereograms.

These exercises are sometimes successful in significantly improving the patient's control of the esophoria. If exercises are unsuccessful, prisms, botulinum toxin and surgery can be used.

Esophoria associated with convergence insufficiency

Although this type of esophoria is not classified as an entity it is occasionally encountered. Two types can be recognized.

• Primary esophoria: patients with primary esophoria of moderate or large degree may be afraid to attempt to converge, possibly because this results in overconvergence with diplopia. If the esophoria is reduced by surgery, spontaneous improvement in convergence may follow. If it does not, postoperative exercises can be given as for primary convergence insufficiency.

• Primary convergence insufficiency: the esophoria is of much smaller degree and may be the result of the effort required to bring about convergence. Convergence can be treated routinely but particular attention must be paid to relaxation exercises and to ensuring that the negative fusion amplitude is adequate. Care should be taken not to increase the esophoria and the measurement should be regularly checked.

Anomalies of convergence

Convergence insufficiency

Definition

Convergence insufficiency is present if the near point of convergence is less than 10 cm or if it can be maintained at this level only with effort.

Convergence insufficiency may be primary or secondary. Secondary convergence insufficiency may be associated with primary intermittent exotropia, heterophoria, neurological disease, and mechanical and paralytic strabismus, and is discussed later in this section.

Primary convergence insufficiency

Primary convergence insufficiency is present when other causes for convergence insufficiency have been excluded, including a significant degree of heterophoria.

Features
The main feature are:
• frontal headaches and eyestrain associated with close work, caused by the effort needed to converge;
• blurred vision and intermittent diplopia for near fixation due to failure to maintain convergence.

Investigation
• Cover test: this will show a slight exophoria for near fixation in most cases, with no significant heterophoria for distance fixation. The speed of recovery for near should be noted.

• Convergence: convergence should be assessed as described for heterophoria. Convergence insufficiency is present if the near point of convergence is less than 10 cm or if it can be maintained at this level only with effort and if it deteriorates on repeated testing.

• Accommodation: the near point of accommodation should be measured as already described and related to the patient's age. Blurred vision for close work can result from convergence insufficiency or accommodative insufficiency. If uniocular accommodation appears significantly better than binocular accommodation, convergence insufficiency is the likely diagnosis. If accommodative insufficiency is present both uniocular and binocular accommodation will be below normal for the patient's age. The accommodative amplitude should also be measured for both near and distance.

• Fusional amplitude: this is measured at 33 cm using a horizontal prism bar. The positive fusion amplitude is deficient in convergence insufficiency but the negative amplitude should be normal. Sometimes the amplitude appears abnormal because the patient does not understand what he must do to maintain a single image. The test should be explained to him and the amplitude can often be improved by moving the target nearer to his eyes so that he can use accommodation to stimulate convergence. Once the images are joined the target can be withdrawn to the previous distance and the test repeated. An accommodative target is preferable to a spotlight.

Differential diagnosis
The symptoms of convergence insufficiency, exophoria with convergence weakness, acquired near exotropia, accommodative anomalies and even convergence paresis and paralysis can be similar. The differentiating signs and symptoms are shown in Table 16.2.

Management of convergence insufficiency
Correction of the refractive error
Any significant refractive error should be corrected if it is likely to account for the patient's symptoms or result in compensation of the convergence defect. Management should include:
• a cycloplegic refraction;
• correction of acquired myopia, which may compensate the condition by restoring a normal accommodative–convergence relationship;

Table 16.2 Differentiating symptoms and signs of convergence insufficiency, exophoria, accommodative defects and convergence palsies.

Condition	Symptoms	Signs
Primary convergence insufficiency	Headache; asthenopia; blurred vision relieved by closing one eye	Small exophoria for near only
Exophoria of the convergence weakness type	Similar	Exophoria for distance increasing for near
Accommodative insufficiency or fatigue	Blurred near vision, not relieved by closing one eye; asthenopia and headaches; possible micropsia	Exophoria for near likely
Convergence paralysis	Diplopia for distance closer than infinity	Exotropia within infinity
Convergence paresis	Intermittent diplopia for near; headache and eye strain (very difficult to distinguish from gross convergence insufficiency), does not respond to orthoptic exercises	Exotropia/phoria for near

• correction of low degrees of astigmatism, which can cause symptoms similar to those of convergence insufficiency especially if oblique;
• correction of a low or moderate degree of hypermetropia, which does not necessarily make convergence more difficult; it may have the opposite effect by providing a clearer stimulus and can result in improved convergence.

Orthoptic exercises
Provided they are carefully selected, most patients with convergence insufficiency respond to orthoptic exercises. Patients are suitable for treatment if:
• the condition is symptom-producing and the symptoms are related to the use of the eyes for close work;
• there is sufficient cooperation and motivation;
• the patient is in good general health.

Although it is an advantage if the patient can attend the clinic regularly, inability to do so is no bar to treatment since much of it can be carried out at home, providing that clear instructions are given.

The stages in orthoptic treatment are:
1 Treatment to overcome suppression and obtain spontaneous recognition of diplopia on failure of convergence if this is not already present. This step is usually easily achieved by using coloured filters.

2 Improvement of convergence and extension of the positive fusion amplitude. Simple convergence exercises can be given and the fusion amplitude extended using a prism bar base-out.
3 Appreciation of physiological diplopia, which can then be used in the uncrossed position to improve relative convergence, and in the crossed position to ensure that relaxation of convergence is easy to obtain. Stereograms and the dot card are useful methods based on physiological diplopia.
4 Voluntary convergence. Not all patients can achieve this stage.

The methods used in all stages of treatment are described in detail in Chapter 8.

GENERAL GUIDELINES
• The patient should be warned that his symptoms may become worse in the early stages of treatment and will only improve when convergence becomes easier to maintain.
• He must be able to recognize diplopia reliably before being given convergence exercises to practise at home. Very occasionally it is impossible to obtain diplopia recognition. If this happens the patient can usually learn to appreciate uncrossed physiological diplopia and can use this to control convergence.

• Detailed instruction on home exercises should be given, emphasizing the time which should be spent on each. New skills should be added at each visit to the clinic to encourage the patient and maintain his interest.

• Relaxation exercises must be practised at the end of every clinic or home exercise session.

OUTCOME

Patients with primary convergence insufficiency should respond well to orthoptic exercises. Even in those patients with an associated moderate exophoria an overall cure rate of 72% has been reported, lasting at least 2 years (Grisham 1988).

PROBLEMS

The problems which can arise are mostly the result of over-eager treatment, notably convergence spasm. This rare condition very occasionally results from overexuberant convergence exercises. Early indications are:

• inability to relax convergence, for example failure to obtain crossed physiological diplopia although it had been appreciated previously;

• blurred distance vision: even a small reduction in visual acuity is significant;

• esophoria for distance fixation;

• immediate blurring of the image when convergence is tested using a major amblyoscope.

If any of these signs are seen, convergence exercises should be stopped at once and treatment should be directed to increasing the negative fusion amplitude and using exercises based on crossed physiological diplopia.

Alternative forms of treatment

Gross convergence insufficiency does not always respond to orthoptic treatment and other measures may be required. Persisting symptoms in spite of well-maintained convergence is another problem sometimes encountered. It may reflect poor selection of patients. Other causes for the symptoms should be sought.

• Prisms: it is common practice to decentre convex lenses in reading spectacles to give a base-in effect, thus relieving some of the effort needed to converge. A larger prism can be incorporated into the spectacles. Indications for the use of prisms are:

1 Elderly patients who may be unwilling to attend for orthoptic treatment. Exercises are limited since accommodation cannot be used as effectively to aid convergence in this age group.

2 Patients whose convergence has not been sufficiently improved by exercises or those who are unwilling to undergo other treatment.

It is advisable to use a trial Fresnel prism first in order to assess the correct strength and ensure that symptoms are relieved.

• Surgery: surgery is not indicated for primary convergence insufficiency. There is no evidence that surgical treatment can improve the effectiveness of the convergence mechanism. Patients with convergence insufficiency associated with significant exophoria for near fixation occasionally require surgery to reduce the size of the exophoria before improvement in the convergence insufficiency can be achieved. Prior to considering surgery in this group of patients we recommend a trial of prisms; those patients who do not respond to prisms may prove to have defective motor fusion and may be poor candidates for surgery.

Secondary convergence insufficiency

Secondary convergence insufficiency is associated with certain recognized conditions. It differs from primary convergence insufficiency in that treatment of the underlying condition may result in its improvement. Subsequent treatment of convergence insufficiency may prove difficult in those who fail to improve following treatment for the underlying condition.

Those disorders which are frequently complicated by convergence insufficiency include:

• Parkinson's disease
• thyroid eye disease
• internuclear ophthalmoplegia.

Convergence palsy

Definition

The ability to converge is totally lost in convergence paralysis, some ability to converge is retained in convergence paresis.

Aetiology

Convergence palsy may be primary or secondary.

- In primary convergence palsy there is no significant past history, and examination confirms the convergence palsy as an isolated phenomenon.
- Convergence palsy may arise secondary to head trauma or encephalitis and is a feature of Parinaud's syndrome. If the intraocular muscles are involved, neurological disease is likely and a lesion in the region of the third nerve nucleus in the midbrain seems probable.

Features

- The absence of fusional convergence will result in the patient having crossed diplopia for distances nearer than infinity. The maximum distance at which diplopia is present is influenced by any pre-existing heterophoria therefore diplopia may be constant if there was exophoria before the onset of the convergence palsy.
- Fusional divergence is preserved, which provides a degree of stability to the alignment at distance fixation.
- Accommodation may or may not be affected; if it is, the symptoms are generally more severe due to the lack of associated accommodative vergence. The pupil may or may not be involved.
- Ocular movements are normal in primary convergence palsy, but may be affected if the palsy is secondary to an underlying neurological disease.
- Convergence paralysis can be simulated if the patient deliberately refuses to converge. True convergence paralysis can be differentiated from simulated paralysis by assessing the patient's horizontal fusional amplitude at 6 m. If true paralysis is present, then interposing a base-out prism in front of one eye will result in diplopia (as the patient fails to overcome the increasing prism strength). The patient should not be able to overcome even a 5 Δ base-out prism if true convergence paralysis is present.

Management

The underlying cause should be first investigated and treated in cases of secondary convergence paralysis. Treatment is conservative, and surgery offers no benefit in this condition. Botulinum toxin is useful in temporarily correcting the exodeviation present for near fixation in order to confirm the absent fusional convergence. We have not found botulinum toxin to be useful in the long-term management.

- Isolated convergence paralysis: if the accommodative system is functioning normally, base-in prisms can be used to correct the exodeviation for near.
- Combined accommodative and convergence paralysis: the minimum hypermetropic prescription to allow comfortable vision at near is combined with base-in prisms.

Treatment is usually ineffective in relieving the patient's symptoms. Patients either seem to learn to live with their symptoms or find their vision is more comfortable if one eye is occluded.

Divergence palsy

Definition

In divergence paralysis the negative fusion amplitude is totally lost. In divergence paresis some ability to diverge is retained.

Divergence palsy is a rare acquired condition first described by Parinaud (1883). It can occur in isolation or in association with other neurological signs.

Aetiology

The presence of a divergence 'centre' in the brainstem was suggested by Duane in the 19th century. This theory has received some scientific support from the work of Mays (1984), who demonstrated discharge from the mesencephalic reticular formation in monkeys during divergence movements. Further proof of the existence and site of a divergence 'centre' is awaited.

If divergence palsy exists as a separate entity it implies that divergence must be an active process, subject to damage by disease. Tamler and Jampolsky (1967) demonstrated active divergence by recording increased electromyographic activity in the lateral rectus muscles on divergence movements. Krohel *et al.* (1982) argued on the basis of 11 patients with divergence palsy and a variety of associated disorders that divergence palsy was a distinct entity which could be separated from bilateral lateral rectus weakness. However, Kirkham *et al.* (1972) reported on three patients with apparent divergence palsy and raised intracranial pressure; slowing of abducting saccades was recorded in each eye, suggesting mild bilateral lateral rectus weakness as a cause, although no limitation of abduction could be demonstrated clinically.

Reported causes of divergence palsy include trauma, intracranial tumour and vascular disease (Roper-Hall & Burde 1987).

Features
- The patient usually presents with uncrossed diplopia, sometimes of sudden onset.
- There is a concomitant esotropia, measuring more for distance than for near.
- Ocular movements are normal, with full abduction of either eye.
- The negative fusion amplitude is defective in divergence paresis and absent in divergence paralysis.
- Associated convergence weakness has been reported by Roper-Hall and Burde (1987).

Differential diagnosis
Divergence palsy resembles several more common conditions and must be differentiated from:
- Acquired sixth nerve palsy: occult unilateral or bilateral sixth nerve palsy can easily be mistaken for divergence palsy. Differentiation is based principally on careful examination of ocular movements: the esotropia should increase on lateroversion in sixth nerve palsy and limitation of abduction should be apparent on the outer field of the Hess chart. A slow abducting saccadic velocity may be observed in the presence of a full range of ocular movement. The negative fusion amplitude should be normal. These signs may become apparent even if they are not observed initially.
- Convergence spasm: the esotropia is variable in convergence spasm but static in divergence palsy. There is often an associated accommodative spasm with miosis and pseudomyopia.
- Early mechanical restriction of abduction in thyroid eye disease: other eye signs, notably lid-lag and proptosis, may be present. Tests for thyroid function may confirm the diagnosis.
- Esophoria with divergence weakness: the esophoria measures more for distance than near but remains controlled. The negative fusion amplitude enables the patient to maintain binocular single vision, whereas in divergence palsy there is an esotropia in the distance.

Management
Patients with an acquired divergence palsy should always be suspected of having an underlying neuro-logical disorder and should be appropriately investigated along the same lines as for acquired sixth nerve palsy (see Chapter 18). It may be possible to relieve the symptoms with base-out prisms.

Convergence and accommodative spasm

Because of the synkinesis between convergence, accommodation and miosis, spasm of either convergence or accommodation is usually accompanied by spasm of the other and by constriction of the pupils. In convergence spasm the medial rectus muscles can become contracted. In accommodative spasm the ciliary muscle is contracted in both eyes and cannot be relaxed. It is not always possible to decide which function was primarily affected. For these reasons accommodative spasm is discussed here rather than under accommodative anomalies.

Aetiology
Rare cases are seen in which an organic cause can be found. Convergence spasm can follow injudicious treatment for convergence insufficiency. Possible causes of accommodative spasm are:
- Uncorrected hypermetropia of moderate or high degree, in which the patient exerts a constant accommodative effort on an attempt to see clearly. In time, he is unable to relax the ciliary muscle.
- In intermittent distance exotropia, when the patient uses convergence and accommodation to control the exotropia at the expense of clear vision. If this state persists a spasm develops.
- Organic: cholinergic drugs, ocular inflammation, morphine and alcohol can all cause accommodative spasm.
- Nonorganic: no cause can be found for most cases and it is believed that the spasm is a functional disturbance, usually affecting young adults of a highly strung disposition, most commonly female. In these cases there is probably a primary convergence spasm.

Features
The patient usually presents complaining of symptoms, their severity depending on the degree of spasm. If the spasm is marked the symptoms comprise:
- Uncrossed diplopia, with increased separation of the images on distance fixation, caused by the

convergence spasm: this results in a variable esotropia, more marked on distance fixation and on lateral gaze. Spasm on lateral gaze gives rise to pseudolateral rectus palsy.

• Blurred vision, more marked in the distance, due to the accommodative spasm. This is accompanied by constriction of both pupils, which fail to dilate in scotopic conditions.

• Headache and facial pain which is localized in the eyes.

• Macropsia, in which objects appear larger than their actual size. Because the eyes are accommodating the object is judged to be closer than it is, resulting in an illusion of increased size. The spasm gives rise to pseudomyopia, which can be differentiated from true myopia by cycloplegic refraction.

Micropsia, the opposite of macropsia, may occur in accommodative paralysis or severe accommodative fatigue: the object is thought to be further from the eyes and therefore appears smaller. In practice patients rarely complain of or comment on macropsia or micropsia.

If the associated convergence spasm is mild the eyes may appear straight at the start of the ophthalmic examination but overconvergence occurs when the patient is asked to fixate an object or on testing visual acuity.

Differential diagnosis

Both convergence and accommodative spasm can mimic bilateral sixth nerve palsy. The conditions have in common a large esotropia and failure to abduct either eye when ocular movements are tested by conventional methods. They can be differentiated by:

• Pupil size: constriction occurs in spasm but normal pupils are seen in bilateral sixth nerve palsy.

• Doll's head manoeuvre, performed with either eye covered in turn. Abduction should result in either eye in spasm but movement will remain limited in bilateral sixth nerve palsy.

• Visual acuity, which should not be affected in sixth nerve palsy.

Investigation

Accommodative spasm should be suspected if there is an apparent late onset of myopia or if existing myopia suddenly increases. A careful history should be taken, with particular reference to the patient's medical history and to any previous treatment for refractive error or strabismus. Refraction should be carried out using cycloplegia. Further investigation to establish the cause of the spasm may be indicated.

Management

The cause of the spasm should be treated if known and if an intermittent distance exotropia is present this should be treated after the spasm has been completely relaxed. All patients should undergo a cycloplegic refraction and any significant refractive error should be corrected. Treatment can be directed at the accommodative component of the spasm by using atropine 1% instilled daily to relax the ciliary muscle, and should be continued for several weeks. This treatment necessitates the patient ceasing all close work, unless temporary convex lenses are prescribed to mitigate the effect of the drug. Treatment directed at the convergence spasm may be effective in some patients and consists of uniocular occlusion to abolish the diplopia; this often has to be continued for several weeks. Botulinum toxin can be injected into the medial rectus muscles in convergence spasm to align the visual axes and relieve the symptom of diplopia; repeat injections are often required. As most patients have a nonorganic cause for the spasm, treatment may not be effective and symptoms can recur once treatment is stopped. A few patients may be helped by psychiatric counselling.

Anomalies of accommodation

Anomalies of accommodation are rare compared with heterophoria and convergence insufficiency. They can give rise to very similar symptoms and must be differentiated in order that the correct management can be planned. Accommodation may be defective (accommodative insufficiency, fatigue, inertia or paralysis), or excessive (accommodative spasm: see above under convergence and accommodative spasm).

Accommodative insufficiency

Description

In accommodative insufficiency the patient's amplitude of accommodation is consistently below the level expected for his age. Both eyes are affected in nearly every case, the exception being those due to local trauma. The condition may be temporary or apparently permanent.

Aetiology

Possible causes of accommodative insufficiency are:
• Ophthalmic: accommodative insufficiency may result from disuse of accommodation and can occur in patients with high hypermetropia or in myopia of moderate or high degree, when it is noticed by the patient after correction of the refractive error. It is important to note that it can be an early symptom of glaucoma in prepresbyopic patients.
• Medical: accommodation may be affected by poor general health. Cases are seen after virus infections, especially mumps and infectious mononucleosis (glandular fever).
• Trauma: local trauma to the eye may result in loss of accommodation, usually only temporary, although recovery may not be complete.
• Drugs: certain drugs adversely affect accommodation, especially centrally acting antihypertensive agents and antidepressants.

Features

The features are:
• Blurred vision for near. Hypermetropic patients will also have blurred distance vision; myopes have less difficulty.
• A remote near point of accommodation.
• Asthenopic symptoms due to the effort required to bring about accommodation. Occasionally the patient may be aware of micropsia.
• A secondary convergence insufficiency is common.
• Rarely an esophoria or esotropia for near fixation caused when the extra effort needed to bring about accommodation results in excess convergence.

Investigation

The near point of accommodation should be measured uniocularly and binocularly on a near point rule, using the smallest sized print which the patient can read. Low-powered convex lenses can be used to confirm the diagnosis and should result in clear vision when accommodative insufficiency is present. If the accuracy of the patient's response is doubted, it is useful to assess the effect on the near point of both concave and convex lenses. The positive amplitude of accommodation can be measured by the strongest concave lens which can be tolerated while clear vision is maintained. The amplitude of accommodation should be measured in the distance. The patient should be refracted.

Management

The cause of the accommodative insufficiency should be treated if possible. Any significant amount of hypermetropia should be corrected; even half or three-quarters of a dioptre may make the patient comfortable. If no refractive error is present, further treatment is directed to providing temporary convex lenses up to +2.00 Δ to use for essential close work. Fresnel lenses can be used for a trial period, keeping the power as low as possible. It may be necessary to prescribe permanent spectacles if the condition persists and prevents the patient from following his work or leisure activities.

Accommodative fatigue

Description

In this condition accommodation is initially sufficient for the patient's needs but deteriorates with continued use.

The signs and symptoms are similar to those due to accommodative insufficiency but are less severe and can be relieved by rest.

Management

Any refractive error should be corrected and attention paid to the patient's general condition if necessary. Accommodative fatigue usually resolves spontaneously as the patient's health improves. If there is also convergence insufficiency this can be treated and, if improved, will possibly help to improve the accommodation.

Accommodative inertia

Description

Inertia is characterized by delay in exerting accommodation and in relaxing it once it is exerted. Both eyes are affected. Inertia may be a prepresbyopic condition occurring in patients aged 35–45 years. It is also seen in association with developing cataract.

Features

The patient's main complaint is one of blurred vision on changing focus from distance to near or from near to distance. With time the visual acuity improves at the distance fixated but vision becomes blurred again when the fixation distance is altered.

Management

Correction of even a small degree of hypermetropia or astigmatism can make the patient comfortable. A small reading correction up to +1.00 Δ should be considered. Any underlying condition should be treated. Orthoptic exercises have been suggested, using methods based on physiological diplopia, trying to clear the diplopic images more rapidly when changing from crossed to uncrossed diplopia (or vice versa), but the success of this treatment is not assured.

Holmes–Adie pupil

The Holmes–Adie pupil is described in Chapter 2. This condition has some similarity with accommodative inertia but usually only one eye is affected: occasionally the condition can be bilateral. The affected pupil is dilated and reacts very slowly, and once constricted it is slow to dilate again. Accommodation is similarly affected: near vision is initially blurred due to delayed accommodation. Once accommodation is achieved distance vision may be blurred until relaxation occurs. In long-standing cases the pupil frequently becomes constricted.

Accommodative paralysis

Description

Paralysis is present when no accommodation can be exerted, resulting in blurred vision for all distances nearer than infinity (assuming that the patient is emmetropic).

One or both eyes can be affected, depending on the cause. The paralysis can be an isolated condition or may be associated with convergence paralysis, and is an important feature of total third nerve palsy.

Aetiology

Causes of accommodative paralysis include:
• Trauma: blunt trauma to the eye can cause paralysis of the ciliary muscle, usually associated with traumatic mydriasis. Closed head injuries, including whiplash injuries, may cause true paralysis of accommodation, but this must be distinguished from the functional weakness of accommodation which particularly affects asthenic patients as one aspect of a postconcussional syndrome.
• Drugs: parasympathetic agents cause cycloplegia and may accidentally be introduced into the conjunctival sac, especially from preparations containing atropine.
• Neurological conditions: paralysis of accommodation was a classical late feature of diphtheria. It also occurs sometimes as an early or presenting feature of progressive midbrain disorders which later lead on to convergence paralysis and pupillary abnormalities; a pineal tumour in particular may present in this way.

Management

The cause of the accommodative paralysis must first be found and treated if possible. Correction of any degree of hypermetropia or astigmatism may help to improve the visual acuity. This condition is very difficult to treat. In unilateral paralysis it may be possible to match the near points of the two eyes in young patients by the use of a multifocal reading addition. These lenses may also be helpful in bilateral cases, when base-in prisms will also be needed.

References

Grisham, J.D. (1988) Visual therapy results for convergence insufficiency: a literature review. *American Journal of Optometry and Physiological Optics* **65**, 448–454.

Kirkham, T.H., Bird, A.C. & Sanders, M.D. (1972) Divergence paralysis with raised intracranial pressure. An electrooculographic study. *British Journal of Ophthalmology* **56**, 776–782.

Krohel, G.B., Tobin, D.T., Hartnett, M.E. & Barrows, N.A. (1982) Divergence paralysis. *American Journal of Ophthalmology* **94**, 506–510.

Mays, L.E. (1984) Neural control of vergence in eye movements: convergence and divergence neurons in the midbrain. *Journal of Neurophysiology* **51**, 1091–1108.

Parinaud, H. (1883) Paralysie des movements associés des yeux. *Archives of Neurology* 5, 145–172.

Pratt-Johnson, J.A. (1973) Central disruption of fusional amplitude. *British Journal of Ophthalmology* 57, 347–350.

Roper-Hall, G. & Burde, R.M. (1987) The diagnosis and management of divergence paresis. *American Orthoptic Journal* 37, 113–121.

Tamler, E. & Jampolsky, A. (1967) Is divergence active?: an electromyographic study. *American Journal of Ophthalmology* 63, 452–459.

17
Alphabet Patterns

The terms V-pattern and A-pattern are used to describe significant changes occurring in the horizontal angle of deviation as the eyes move from up-gaze to down-gaze. A V-pattern is present when there is relative divergence of the visual axes on up-gaze and relative convergence on down-gaze. An A-pattern is present when there is relative convergence of the visual axes on up-gaze and relative divergence on down-gaze.

Classification

A primary horizontal strabismus is present in many patients with V- and A-patterns but in others the patterns are associated with congenital or acquired paralytic strabismus or with mechanical restriction of ocular movement. Whatever the nature of the strabis-

mus, it is customary to classify the V- and A-patterns according to the horizontal deviation in the primary position as V-pattern esotropia or exotropia and A-pattern esotropia or exotropia.

In primary V- and A-patterns there is typically a gradual increase or decrease in the horizontal angle of deviation on changing from up-gaze to down-gaze. Variations have been described in which the change in horizontal angle follows a different pattern. These are termed:
• Y-pattern, when there is relative divergence on up-gaze but no significant change in angle from the primary position to down-gaze.
• Inverted Y (λ)-pattern, in which there is relative divergence on down-gaze but no significant change from the primary position to up-gaze.
• X-pattern, in which there is relative divergence on

both up-gaze and down-gaze compared with the angle of horizontal deviation in the primary position.
- ◊ pattern, in which there is relative convergence on both up-gaze and down-gaze compared with the primary position.
- V-pattern only on down-gaze, where there is a relative convergence, but no significant change from the primary position to up-gaze.
- A-pattern only on up-gaze, where there is a relative convergence, but no significant change from the primary position to down-gaze.

Criteria for diagnosis

A quantitative diagnosis is based on the amount of difference in measurement of the horizontal angle of deviation:
- V-pattern, measuring a minimum difference of 15 Δ from up-gaze to down-gaze.
- A-pattern, measuring a minimum difference of 10 Δ from up-gaze to down-gaze.

There is a physiological tendency to relative divergence on up-gaze, therefore the minimum standard demanded for a V-pattern is larger than that for an A-pattern.

However, these measurements are arbitrary as variations occur in the excursion from the primary position to the point of measurement.

Incidence

Alphabet patterns are a common occurrence in otherwise 'concomitant' strabismus, with V-pattern significantly more common than A-pattern. These patterns are also seen in many vertical muscle palsies, due to loss of adducting or abducting action of the affected muscles. A V-and-A pattern is especially prevalent in certain conditions; in some the pattern can have diagnostic value or pose particular management problems.

Aetiology

Most V- and A-patterns can be explained by:
- abnormalities of vertical or horizontal muscle action;
- anatomical anomalies involving either configuration of the orbits or insertion of the muscle tendons.

Anomalies of vertical muscle action

The horizontal angle of deviation is changed on up-gaze and down-gaze by the secondary abducting and adducting actions of the vertically acting muscles. The abducting action of the oblique muscles has a greater influence than the adducting action of the vertical rectus muscles, which is comparatively very slight unless there is a marked underaction or overaction. An acquired underaction of the inferior rectus muscle is more likely to give rise to an alphabet pattern than a similar underaction of the superior rectus muscle. Most acquired V- or A-patterns are associated with muscle underaction: this may be less obvious in alphabet patterns occurring with primary horizontal strabismus, when the predominant feature is usually overaction of one or both oblique muscles.

Related to V-pattern (Figs 17.1 & 17.2)
V-esotropia
The most frequent cause of V-pattern in esodeviations is underaction of one or, more commonly, both superior oblique muscles, either congenital or acquired. If the muscle sequelae has developed, the horizontal angle is influenced as follows:
- Down-gaze: the esodeviation is increased by:
  1 loss of abduction by the underacting superior obliques;
  2 increased adduction by the overacting inferior recti.
- Up-gaze: the esodeviation is decreased by:
  1 increased abduction by the overacting inferior obliques;
  2 decreased adduction by the inhibited superior recti.

A greater increase in the angle of deviation from the primary position to depression indicates superior oblique dysfunction. Inferior oblique dysfunction predominates if the angle of deviation increases from the primary position to elevation. If the change is gradual from up-gaze to down-gaze, the oblique muscles contribute to the same extent.

In primary esotropia with V-pattern the amount of inferior oblique overaction usually exceeds the amount of superior oblique underaction. In other cases, either the superior oblique underaction or the inferior oblique overaction can often predominate.

Field of Left Eye (fixing with right eye)   Field of Right Eye (fixing with left eye)

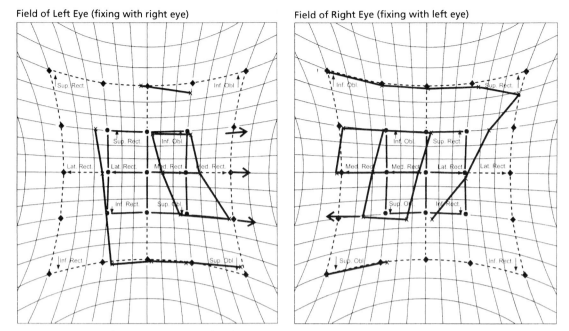

Fig. 17.1 Hess chart of a patient with bilateral sixth nerve palsy showing a V-pattern esotropia.

Field of Left Eye (fixing with right eye)   Field of Right Eye (fixing with left eye)

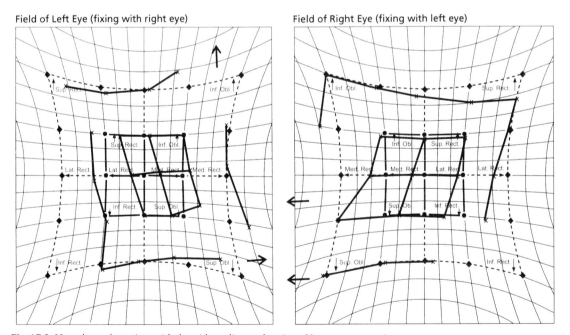

Fig. 17.2 Hess chart of a patient with thyroid eye disease showing a V-pattern esotropia.

V-exotropia

V-pattern with an exodeviation may be due to under-action of one, or usually both superior rectus muscles, of probable congenital origin. The change in horizontal angle is brought about as follows:

- Down-gaze: the exodeviation is decreased by:

  1 decreased abduction by the inhibited superior oblique muscles;

  2 increased adduction by the overacting inferior rectus muscles.

- Up-gaze: the exodeviation is increased by:

  1 increased abduction by the overacting inferior oblique muscles;

  2 decreased adduction by the underacting superior rectus muscles.

The common finding in V-exotropia is overaction of the inferior oblique muscles.

A subgroup has been described in which the eye movements resemble but are different from true bilateral inferior oblique overaction (Kushner 1991).

Despite the marked abduction of either eye when elevated in adduction this condition differs from true inferior oblique overaction in that:

- there is no elevation of the adducting eye on horizontal gaze;
- the superior oblique muscles are not underacting;
- no objective excyclotorsion can be observed on fundus photography;
- there is no response to weakening the inferior oblique muscles.

Related to A-pattern (Figs 17.3 & 17.4)

A-esotropia

The common cause for A-pattern with esodeviation is underaction of one, or more often both, inferior oblique muscles of congenital origin. The change in horizontal angle is brought about as follows:

- Down-gaze: the esodeviation is decreased by:

  1 increased abduction by the overacting superior obliques;

  2 decreased adduction by the inhibited inferior recti.

- Up-gaze: the esodeviation is increased by:

  1 loss of abduction by the underacting inferior obliques;

  2 increased adduction by the overacting superior recti.

Field of Left Eye (fixing with right eye)

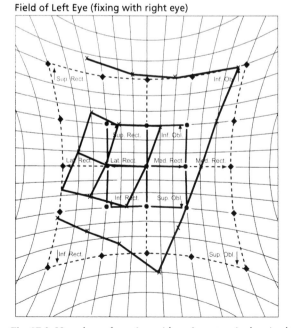

Field of Right Eye (fixing with left eye)

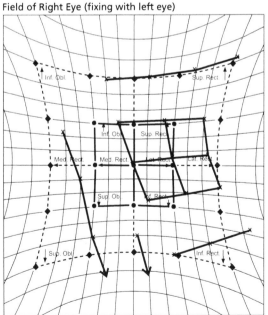

Fig. 17.3 Hess chart of a patient with an A-exotropia showing bilateral overaction of the superior obliques and underaction of the inferior recti.

Field of Left Eye (fixing with right eye)   Field of Right Eye (fixing with left eye)

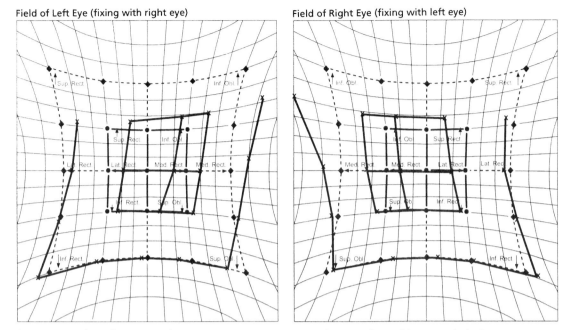

Fig. 17.4 Hess chart of a patient with a primary A-pattern esotropia without significant oblique muscle dysfunction.

In primary esotropia with A-pattern, the overaction of the superior oblique muscles usually predominates. Acquired forms associated with mechanical disorders of ocular motility, in particular thyroid eye disease, are frequently seen (see Chapter 21).

A-exotropia

Most A-pattern exotropia is caused by underaction of one or both inferior rectus muscles. The change in horizontal angle is brought about as follows:

- Down-gaze: the exodeviation is increased by:
  1 loss of abduction by the underacting inferior recti;
  2 increased abduction by the overacting superior obliques.
- Up-gaze: the exodeviation is decreased by:
  1 loss of abduction by the inhibited inferior obliques;
  2 increased adduction by the contracted superior recti.

Superior oblique overaction predominates in both primary and acquired forms of A-pattern exotropia.

Anomalies of horizontal muscle action

According to Urist (1958) the medial rectus muscles act more effectively on down-gaze and the lateral rectus muscles are more effective on up-gaze, therefore underaction and overaction of these muscles can influence the angle of deviation on up-gaze and down-gaze.

Related to V-pattern

V-esotropia may be due to overaction of the medial rectus muscles and V-exotropia to overaction of the lateral rectus muscles, although there is no evidence to suggest these occur. Bilateral lateral rectus palsy is associated with V-esotropia.

Related to A-pattern

An esotropia may be due to underaction of the lateral rectus muscles. The common incidence of A-pattern esotropia in children with hydrocephalus who develop bilateral sixth nerve palsy may give some support to this view, although acquired bilateral lateral rectus palsy is more often associated with a V-pattern esotropia.

An A-pattern exotropia can theoretically be due to underaction of the medial rectus muscles but there is little or no supporting clinical evidence.

Tendon insertion

Horizontal rectus muscles

If the muscle insertions are higher or lower than the normal position, abduction or adduction is increased on up-gaze or down-gaze. As a rule a displacement of a horizontal rectus muscle vertically weakens its action in that direction and strengthens it in the opposite direction. Using the lateral rectus muscle as an example, a high insertion favours abduction in depression of gaze and makes abduction in elevation less effective, resulting in an A-pattern. A low insertion has the opposite effect, resulting in a V-pattern.

Oblique muscles

The normal muscle axes of the superior and inferior oblique muscles are approximately parallel and make an angle of 51° with the anterior-posterior axis of the globe. If one insertion is more posterior than the normal, the muscle axis lies in a more sagittal plane, i.e. it is closer to the anterior-posterior axis of the globe. Gobin (1968) maintained that sagittalization reduced the muscle's torsional action, causing torsional imbalance, followed by muscle contraction to correct it. Consequently, both the horizontal and vertical balance was disturbed. It is simpler to view sagittalization as increasing the vertical and horizontal action of the muscle whilst decreasing the torsional action, and desagittalization as having the opposite effect.

Related to V-pattern

V-pattern results from sagittalization of the inferior oblique muscle, resulting in an overaction of the muscle and increasing abduction on up-gaze.

Related to A-pattern

A-pattern results from sagittalization of the superior oblique muscle, resulting in an overaction of the muscle and increasing abduction on down-gaze.

Sensory torsion

A loss of fusion appears to predispose the eyes to the development of V- or A-patterns (Guyton & Weingarten 1994). The normal sensorimotor control mechanisms fail to keep the eyes aligned and either extorsion or intorsion occurs, usually bilateral and often asymmetrical. It is proposed that this 'sensory' torsion with rotation of the planes of action of the rectus muscles leads to the clinical appearance of V- and A-patterns.

Anatomical anomalies

Orbital configuration

It is well recognized that mongoloid and antimongoloid palpebral fissures are associated with V- and A-patterns, respectively. Urrets-Zavalia *et al.* (1961) stated that:

• mongoloid fissures favoured the production of A-pattern esotropia and V-pattern exotropia;
• antimongoloid fissures favoured the production of A-pattern exotropia and V-pattern esotropia.

It is our experience that mongoloid fissures are mainly associated with A-pattern and that antimongoloid fissures are only associated with V-pattern. A-pattern esotropia is common in patients with Down's syndrome.

A shallow orbit results in proptosis and can alter the relationship between the vertically acting muscles, in particular superior oblique underaction causes a V-pattern, for example in Crouzon's syndrome.

Anomalies of muscle pulleys

Abnormalities in pulley position have been shown to be present in patients with V- and A-pattern strabismus (Clark *et al.* 1997), and may be important in the aetiology of some alphabet patterns as well as other types of strabismus. See Chapter 9 for further details.

Mechanical limitations

V- or A-patterns in mechanical defects are often different in nature from those related to neurogenic or anatomical features. These patients often only demonstrate a change in horizontal angle when the limitation of movement has been reached. The increase can be great and sudden and may be missed if extremes of gaze are not tested: it may not be evident on the Hess screen or major amblyoscope due to the limited excursions tested on these instruments. An X-pattern exotropia is frequently seen if the condition is long-standing, and is common in consecutive exotropia; it is usually the result of contracture of the lateral rectus.

The majority of V- and A-patterns can be explained by vertical muscle underaction and overaction.

Disorders commonly associated with alphabet patterns

Infantile strabismus

Lang (1968) reported a high incidence of V- and A-patterns in esotropia with onset before 6 months of age and commented on the prevalence of A-pattern. Mein and Johnson (1981) found an A-pattern in 44% of patients with infantile esotropia or exotropia, compared with a 21% incidence of V-pattern. Many patients with infantile strabismus develop DVD, which can simulate inferior oblique overaction. It is important to differentiate these two conditions, since surgical weakening of the inferior oblique muscles would increase the A-pattern. Inferior oblique overaction is very unlikely if an A-pattern is present.

Duane's retraction syndrome

Mein (1968) reported a high incidence of V- and A-patterns in Duane's retraction syndrome. A series of 77 patients included 36 with V-pattern and 14 with A-pattern. The reason for the pattern was not always clear. Jampolsky (1984) described how the lateral rectus muscle could slip over the globe, producing an up-shoot on attempted adduction if it slipped up and a down-shoot on adduction if it slipped down. An up-shoot would be expected to result in a V-pattern and a down-shoot in an A-pattern. Surgery on the lateral rectus muscle, planned to prevent slippage, should reduce the up-shoot or down-shoot and lessen the V- and A-pattern (see Chapter 21).

Brown's syndrome

The majority of patients with Brown's syndrome have a V-pattern, explained by the increased abduction that results when the mechanically inhibited inferior oblique muscle attempts to elevate the eye. This sign is not invariable; Fells (1975) reported a significant incidence of A-pattern in esotropic patients with Brown's syndrome. Nevertheless, it remains a useful sign in the differential diagnosis of this condition and isolated inferior oblique palsy.

Acquired bilateral fourth cranial nerve palsy

This condition is characterized by underaction of both superior oblique muscles, usually with bilateral excyclotropia, giving rise to insuperable diplopia. If the palsy is significantly asymmetrical, it can easily be misdiagnosed as unilateral. The presence of a small esotropia in the primary position with a large V-pattern on down-gaze strongly suggests a bilateral rather than a unilateral palsy.

Dysthyroid eye disease with inferior rectus muscle contracture

A-pattern is frequently seen in dysthyroid eye disease, especially following orbital decompression.
• An A-pattern exotropia is a recognized complication in patients with dysthyroid eye disease who have undergone liberal inferior rectus recession to free one or both tight inferior rectus muscles (Roper-Hall & Burde 1987). The A-pattern may be explained in part by loss of adduction by the recessed muscles. An A-pattern exotropia can result in diplopia on down-gaze, making reading uncomfortable. This condition is difficult to treat successfully, therefore precautions should be taken to avoid it. The risk can be reduced by combining inferior rectus recession with medial transposition of the muscle by up to one muscle's width: this procedure can be used with adjustable sutures.
• A significant incidence of A-pattern has been reported following orbital decompression by either a transantral or an ethmoidal approach (Roper-Hall & Burde 1987). Fells (1987) found A-pattern esotropia to be more common than A-pattern exotropia after anterior ethmoidal decompression. He attributed the A-pattern to postdecompression retroplacement of the globe, which resulted in tightening of the superior oblique tendon and consequent overaction of this muscle. Scott and Thalacker (1981) suggested that the

anatomical course of the medial rectus muscle was changed by decompression and that this accounted for the A-pattern.

• A characteristic type of A-pattern esotropia has occasionally followed bilateral two-wall orbital decompression on our unit (Kranemann *et al.* 1997). The features are no significant decrease in size of the esotropia until the eyes are approximately 15–20° in down-gaze; there is then a progressive reduction in the esotropia to orthotropia or control to a small esophoria. This A-pattern esotropia is certainly mechanical in origin and responds to recession of the medial rectus muscle alone.

• An A-pattern esotropia only on up-gaze is occasionally seen in thyroid eye disease associated with limited elevation of both eyes. A 'convergence retraction' type movement of the eyes in an attempt to elevate against the mechanical resistance of the contracted inferior rectus muscles is seen. A similar pattern of movement occurs in the congenital fibrosis syndrome (see Chapter 21).

Investigation of V- and A-patterns

Aims

The aims of investigation are:
• to detect and measure the V- and A-pattern;
• to determine the reason for the pattern if possible;
• to assess its significance in the management of the strabismus.

Observation of the patient

Significant information can be obtained from simply observing the patient.

• Abnormal head posture. Elevation or depression of the chin can be used to place the eyes in the position of least deviation to obtain binocular single vision; for example, a patient with an A-pattern esotropia may elevate his chin. In children, the head posture may be adopted only intermittently, probably because it is uncomfortable to maintain. The examiner should watch the child at play and the parents should be asked to observe his head position at home. Examination of unposed photographs may be helpful. An abnormal head posture is a favourable prognostic sign but it can

easily be lost in childhood, and early surgical treatment may be indicated to preserve and extend the field of binocular single vision.

• Palpebral fissures. Mongoloid and antimongoloid fissures are strongly indicative of the presence of V- and A-pattern, respectively.

Clinical investigation

Cover test

The cover test is the best method of detecting V- and A-patterns. It should be performed in the primary position and on up-gaze and down-gaze, for both distance and near fixation. Accommodation must be controlled by:

• testing with the patient wearing his refractive correction, especially if he is hypermetropic; the test may need to be repeated without the correction as the spectacle frames may restrict fixation on up-gaze and down-gaze;

• using an accommodative target for fixation, ensuring that it is seen clearly.

We recommend testing all patients at distance fixation, where accommodation is least active.

Ocular movements

The observer should look particularly for underaction and overaction of the vertically acting muscles. A unilateral underaction must be differentiated from an asymmetrical bilateral condition. An alternate cover test should be used to compare the degree of deviation in the relevant positions of gaze.

When testing elevation and depression the eye may be seen to diverge or converge significantly only in the extreme positions. This is often the case where there is a mechanical cause and in some patients with oblique dysfunction, in particular when overaction of the superior oblique results in an A-pattern. The position at which the alphabet pattern occurs should be recorded, and its significance in the management of the strabismus assessed.

Measurement of the deviation

Measurement in the primary position and on elevation and depression can be made using the prism cover test or the major amblyoscope. Prism cover test measurements on up-gaze and down-gaze are easier to standardize if they are made with the patient's chin depressed or raised as far as possible compatible with fixation on the target, rather than by moving the target into the required gaze position. It is important to repeat the measurements with a lesser degree of chin depression and elevation to distinguish alphabet patterns that are present only at the extremes of gaze from those which show a progressive change in the horizontal deviation. This method can be used both for near and distance measurements, although we prefer to use distance fixation.

Alternatively the major amblyoscope can be used; this method has the advantage of being repeatable under the same conditions, but does not always reveal the full difference in the angle of deviation due to difficulty in measuring the angle more than 20° from the primary position. It is, however, useful in measuring the V-pattern in bilateral superior oblique muscle palsies, as it can record excyclotropia on up-gaze and down-gaze. We find the prism and cover test and the major amblyoscope complementary and recommend that patients should be measured using both techniques.

Investigation of binocular function

Knowledge of the patient's binocular function is crucial to the management of a constant strabismus, determining whether a functional result is possible. Nondissociative methods should be used for preference (see Chapter 7). It may be revealing to use Bagolini's striated glasses or a stereotest in the position of least deviation, starting from the primary position and moving the test slowly into the relevant position of gaze, comparing the patient's responses.

Hess chart

Lack of normal binocular vision prevents the use of the Hess screen in many patients with primary esotropia or exotropia, but a chart can often be plotted in those with vertical muscle palsies or mechanically restricted movement, who are more likely to have retained binocular single vision. The Hess chart is particularly useful in patients with bilateral superior oblique palsies and in those with dysthyroid eye disease who may have an A-pattern. The V- and A-pattern is revealed by the inward or outward slope of the two fields (Figs 17.1–17.4). The chart is useful in confirming the diagnosis and providing a record for subsequent comparison.

Field of binocular single vision

This should be plotted if binocular single vision is present in any position of gaze and the patient can appreciate diplopia. The field is useful as a guide to the choice of surgical treatment and as a means of documenting the response to treatment.

Significance of V- and A-patterns

V- and A-patterns can influence the diagnosis, prognosis and management of strabismus.

Differential diagnosis

Certain alphabet patterns have diagnostic significance.
• A large V-pattern is strongly suggestive of a bilateral rather than unilateral fourth nerve palsy.
• An A-pattern in infantile esotropia suggests dissociated vertical deviation (DVD) rather than bilateral inferior oblique muscle overaction.
• A V-pattern in an apparent Brown's syndrome confirms the diagnosis and rules out an isolated inferior oblique palsy.

Prognosis

A V- and A-pattern may allow binocular single vision to develop or to be maintained in up-gaze or down-gaze, indicating a good prognosis.

Management

Alphabet patterns influence the choice and extent of strabismus surgery, whether it is planned to restore binocular single vision or to improve alignment (see below).

Management of alphabet patterns

Most alphabet patterns do not require treatment. Those requiring surgery usually show at least 15 Δ difference in angle from up-gaze to down-gaze, making the pattern cosmetically unsightly. The exceptions are patients with symptoms, including an uncomfortable head posture. The aims of surgery are to achieve concomitance on up-gaze and down-gaze and restore or improve binocular single vision without the need for an uncomfortable head posture or to achieve better ocular alignment for cosmetic purposes. When there is no potential for binocular single vision the upper eyelids mask an increase in angle on up-gaze, and although an obvious strabismus in this gaze position may be cosmetically poor in childhood, it is likely to be less noticeable in adult life. If other members of the family are above average height and the child is tall for his age, the deviation on up-gaze is less likely to remain a cosmetic problem.

Alphabet patterns should be taken into consideration when performing horizontal muscle surgery, otherwise poor or unpredictable results may occur. This particularly applies to esotropia, when an ignored V-pattern may lead to a postoperative consecutive exotropia on up-gaze which progressively increases with time. A V- or A-pattern may also cause the surgeon to modify the amount of horizontal muscle surgery performed. For example, patients with A-pattern esotropia are particularly at risk of consecutive exotropia and should therefore be treated more conservatively.

Surgical procedures to correct V- and A-patterns

The general principles of surgical management are outlined below.
• Identify alphabet patterns that will respond to treatment directed at the underlying horizontal or vertical strabismus. These include mechanical conditions such as the late A-pattern esotropia on down-gaze in thyroid eye disease, and the A- or V-pattern in Duane's retraction syndrome.
• Correct oblique muscle dysfunction if present. Surgery is aimed at correcting overaction of the inferior oblique muscles in V-pattern, and of the superior oblique muscles in A-pattern. Large alphabet patterns may not respond fully to oblique muscle surgery unless the latter is combined with surgery on the horizontal or vertical rectus muscles. V-esotropia on down-gaze is a feature of acquired bilateral superior oblique palsy, and the choice of surgery is influenced by the amount of cyclotorsion present.
• In the absence of significant oblique muscle dysfunction, horizontal muscle surgery for the underlying strabismus can be adjusted to correct the alphabet pattern.

Surgery is usually performed on both eyes and comprises one or more of the following procedures.

Oblique muscle surgery
• Weakening procedures:
   1 myectomy or recession of the inferior obliques;
   2 tenotomy or tenectomy of the superior obliques.
• Strengthening procedures:
   1 tuck of the superior obliques;
   2 Harada–Ito transposition procedure on the superior obliques.
Strengthening procedures are mainly used to correct the superior oblique underaction, the V-pattern and the resulting excyclotropia, which occurs particularly in acquired bilateral superior oblique palsy. Strengthening procedures are rarely performed on the inferior oblique muscles.
• Transposition of the inferior or superior oblique by anteropositioning (desagittalization).

Horizontal muscle surgery
• Upward or downward transposition of the horizontal rectus muscles, which is almost invariably combined with recession or less commonly with resection. Vertical transposition of a rectus muscle weakens its horizontal action in that direction at the expense of strengthening the vertical component of its action. An *aide-mémoire* is that recessed muscles are shifted in the direction of maximum deviation and resected muscles are shifted in the direction of least deviation. For example, in A-pattern esotropia the recessed medial recti would be transposed upwards or the resected lateral recti would be transposed downwards.

Vertical muscle surgery
• Weakening procedures:
   1 recession of the superior or inferior rectus muscles;
   2 lateral transposition of the superior or inferior recti to weaken adduction.
• Strengthening procedures:
   1 resection of the superior or inferior rectus muscles;

2 medial transposition of the superior or inferior recti to strengthen adduction.

Application to V- and A-patterns

V-pattern

With overaction of the inferior oblique muscles
Weakening of both inferior obliques is an effective means of treating V-pattern and is the operation of choice in many cases.

• V-esotropia. Recession or myectomy can be combined with either recession of both medial rectus muscles or with recession of the medial rectus and resection of the lateral rectus of the squinting eye. The surgeon may wish to take into account the loss of abduction which may result from inferior oblique weakening when deciding on the amount of horizontal muscle surgery, but this is often negligible. Anteropositioning of both inferior obliques (desagittalization) combined with recession of both medial recti is favoured by Gobin (1964); however, we prefer to reserve this procedure only for the treatment of DVD with V-pattern.

When the V-pattern is due to acquired bilateral superior oblique palsy the maximum change in the horizontal angle occurs on down-gaze. Surgery to correct the associated excyclotropia by a tuck or by a Harada–Ito procedure (see Chapter 9) on both superior oblique muscles will result in improvement to the V-pattern.

• V-exotropia. When there is significantly more exotropia in the distance, weakening of the inferior obliques can be combined with recession of both lateral rectus muscles. If the near and distance angles of deviation are approximately equal, inferior oblique weakening can be combined with resection of the medial rectus and recession of the lateral rectus in the squinting eye.

Patients with pseudo inferior oblique overaction should be distinguished from those with true overaction of the muscles and managed as described below.

Without overaction of the inferior oblique muscles
The operation of choice in most cases is a symmetrical vertical transposition of the horizontal rectus muscles by up to one muscle width; this amount is usually required if the procedure is to be effective. An asymmetrical transposition of both muscles in one eye can be performed, for example moving the recessed lateral rectus up and the resected medial rectus down; this is less effective than symmetrical surgery.

• V-esotropia. The recessed medial rectus muscles are displaced downwards with symmetrical surgery. The recessed medial rectus is displaced downwards and the resected lateral rectus upwards with asymmetrical surgery.

• V-exotropia. The recessed lateral rectus muscles are displaced upwards with symmetrical surgery. The recessed lateral rectus is displaced upwards and the resected medial rectus displaced downwards with asymmetrical surgery.

An alternative transposition procedure is to slope the reinsertion of a recessed or resected horizontal rectus muscle, usually in both eyes. In V-pattern esotropia, the lower border of the medial rectus is recessed more than the upper border. In V-pattern exotropia, the upper border of the lateral rectus is recessed more than the lower border. The effect of sloped recessions is usually slight and we do not recommend this approach.

A-pattern

With overaction of the superior oblique muscles
Most A-pattern strabismus is associated with overaction of the superior oblique muscles, with the greater change in horizontal alignment occurring from the primary position to down-gaze. In A-esotropia there may be underaction of the inferior obliques, and in A-exotropia there is usually underaction of the inferior rectus muscles. Weakening the overacting superior oblique muscles, usually with a posterior tenotomy, is effective in most patients. A silicon superior oblique tendon expander is occasionally required in markedly asymmetrical inferior rectus underaction with superior oblique overaction.

• A-esotropia: posterior tenotomy of both superior oblique muscles.

• A-exotropia: posterior tenotomy of both superior oblique muscles. Consecutive exotropia is commonly associated with an A-pattern and asymmetrical overaction of both superior oblique muscles, greater on the side of the deviating eye. We recommend correction of A-patterns measuring 20 PD or more to prevent recurrence of the exotropia.

Table 17.1 Surgical correction of V- and A-patterns.

Condition	Transposing horizontal recti	Weakening vertical muscles	Strengthening vertical muscles	Anteropositioning	Transposing vertical recti
A-esodeviation	Recession MR, displaced up Resection LR, displaced down	SO	IO	SO	SR lateral
A-exodeviation	Resection MR, displaced up Recession LR, displaced down	SO	IR	SO	IR medial
V-esodeviation	Recession MR, displaced down Resection LR, displaced up	IO	SO	IO	IR lateral
V-exodeviation	Recession LR, displaced up Resection MR, displaced down	IO	SR	IO	SR medial

Key: IO = inferior oblique; IR = inferior rectus; LR = lateral rectus; MR = medial rectus; SO = superior oblique; SR = superior rectus.

An A-pattern may follow the liberal recession of both inferior rectus muscles in thyroid eye disease; medial transposition of both muscles at the time of the recession can reduce this risk.

It should be remembered that A-pattern strabismus with underaction of the inferior rectus muscles may be due to myasthenia gravis, and, if acquired, requires further investigation.

Without overaction of the superior oblique muscles
• A-esotropia. An underaction of the inferior oblique muscles with overaction of the superior rectus muscles is usually present. Resection of the inferior obliques is not practical and recession of the superior rectus muscle is rarely performed in these cases. Transposition of the vertical rectus muscles medially or laterally is relatively ineffective. A simpler and more predictable approach is to recess both medial rectus muscles and transpose the insertions upwards. Asymmetrical horizontal muscle surgery is an alternative approach; the medial rectus muscle can be recessed and transposed upwards and the lateral rectus muscle resected and transposed downwards. This procedure can give good results and overcome the need for chin elevation.
• A-exotropia. This is almost invariably associated with underaction of one or both inferior rectus muscles with overaction of the superior oblique muscles.

We recommend vertical transposition of the horizontal rectus muscles in the rare cases without superior oblique overaction. A symmetrical recession of both lateral recti is combined with downward displacement of the insertions; alternatively, an asymmetrical recession of one lateral rectus with downward displacement of its insertion is combined with a resection of the medial rectus and upward displacement of the insertion.

The surgical possibilities in V- and A-patterns are shown in Table 17.1.

Outcome of surgery for V- and A-patterns

Surgery aims to leave an alphabet pattern slightly undercorrected in most cases as residual patterns are better tolerated than overcorrections; the exception is V-esotropia in bilateral superior oblique palsy, where residual esotropia on down-gaze is often symptom-producing. The expected effects of surgery on the alphabet pattern are shown in Table 17.2.

Postoperative management

Reoperation may be required for patients with surgical undercorrection or overcorrection of the alphabet pattern. Any improvement following surgery may be delayed, especially in patients with binocular potential.

Procedure	Expected change in alphabet pattern
Oblique muscle surgery	
Bilateral inferior oblique weakening	20 Δ
Bilateral superior oblique posterior tenotomies	25 Δ
Bilateral superior oblique complete tenotomies	35 Δ
Bilateral superior oblique tucks	15 Δ
Vertical transposition surgery	
Symmetrical bilateral medial or lateral recti	20 Δ
Asymmetrical unilateral medial and lateral recti	15 Δ
Combined oblique and horizontal muscle surgery	
Inferior oblique weakening and horizontal transposition	30 Δ
Superior oblique weakening and horizontal transposition	45 Δ

Table 17.2 Effect of surgery on the alphabet pattern.

It is important therefore to allow time for the patient to adjust to the postoperative alignment before further intervention is planned.

• Undercorrection may not require further treatment if the alphabet pattern measures less than 20 PD and the patient is symptom free. Further surgery in the absence of oblique muscle dysfunction involves vertical transposition of the horizontal recti or horizontal transposition of the vertical recti.

• Overcorrection may result in the reversal of the alphabet pattern, for example either an A-pattern changing to a V-pattern, symptom-producing cyclotorsion or both conditions. Overcorrection is less common than undercorrection but may complicate weakening of the superior oblique muscles. A bilateral complete superior oblique tenotomy risks the development of insuperable excyclotorsion, especially if performed on the nasal side of the superior rectus muscle. We therefore recommend the posterior tenotomy as the procedure of choice for weakening this muscle for alphabet patterns. Cyclotorsion may also complicate a weakening procedure on oblique muscles that are only mildly overacting: we have seen insuperable incyclotorsion following a bilateral inferior oblique muscle recession in a patient with residual superior oblique muscle palsy, which later required correction by horizontal transposition of the vertical rectus muscles. A tuck of the superior oblique tendon for A-esotropia can result in incyclotorsion,

Brown's syndrome or an induced vertical deviation. If the problem persists, the tuck may need to be revised.

References

Clark, R.A., Miller, J.M. & Demer, J.L. (1997) Location and stability of rectus muscle pulleys inferred from muscle paths. *Investigative Ophthalmology and Visual Science* **38**, 227–240.

Fells, P. (1975) The superior oblique, its actions and anomalies. *British Orthoptic Journal* **32**, 43–53.

Fells, P. (1987) Orbital decompression for severe dysthyroid eye disease. *British Journal of Ophthalmology* **71**, 101–111.

Gobin, M.H. (1964) Anteroposition of the inferior oblique muscle in V-esotropia. *Ophthalmologica* **148**, 325–341.

Gobin, M.H. (1968) Sagittalisation of the oblique muscles as a possible cause for the A, V and X phenomena. *British Journal of Ophthalmology* **52**, 13–18.

Guyton, D.L. & Weingarten, P.E. (1994) Sensory torsion as the cause of primary oblique muscle overaction/underaction and A- and V-pattern strabismus. *Binocular Vision and Eye Muscle Surgery Quarterly* **9** (Suppl.), 209–236.

Jampolsky, A. (1984) Unusual eye movements in alert humans with attached and detached eye muscles. In: *Transactions of the Fifth International Orthoptic Congress, Cannes* (eds A.P. Ravault & M. Lenk), pp. 245–248. LIPS, Lyon.

Kranemann, C., Ansons, A.M., Denning, A. & Spencer, A.L. (1997) The features of A-pattern esotropia in thyroid eye disease. In: *Transactions of the 24th Meeting of the European Strabismological Association, Vilamoura,*

Portugal (ed. M. Spiritus), pp. 214–219. Aeolus Press, The Netherlands.

Kushner, B.J. (1991) Pseudo inferior oblique overaction associated with Y and V patterns. *Ophthalmology* **98**, 1500–1505.

Lang, J. (1968) Squint dating from birth or with early onset. In: *Transactions of the First International Congress of Orthoptics, London*, pp. 231–237. Kimpton, London.

Mein, J. (1968) Clinical features of the retraction syndrome. In: *Transactions of the First International Congress of Orthoptics, London*, pp. 165–177. Kimpton, London.

Mein, J. & Johnson, F. (1981) Dissociated vertical divergence and its association with nystagmus. In: *Orthoptics, Research and Practice. Transactions of the Fourth International Orthoptic Congress, Berne* (eds J. Mein & S. Moore), pp. 14–16. Kimpton, London.

Roper-Hall, G. & Burde, R.M. (1987) Management of A pattern exotropia as a complication of thyroid ophthalmopathy. In: *Orthoptic Horizons. Transactions of the Sixth International Orthoptic Congress, Harrogate* (eds M. Lenk-Schafer, C. Calcutt, M. Doyle & S. Moore), pp. 361–364. British Orthoptic Society, London.

Scott, W.E. & Thalacker, J.A. (1981) Diagnosis and treatment of thyroid myopathy. *Ophthalmology* **88**, 493–498.

Urist, M.J. (1958) The etiology of the so-called A and V syndromes. *American Journal of Ophthalmology* **46**, 835–844.

Urrets-Zavalia, A., Solares-Zamora, J. & Olmos, H.R. (1961) Anthropological studies on the nature of cyclovertical squint. *British Journal of Ophthalmology* **45**, 578–596.

18

Introduction to Paralytic Strabismus

Paralytic or incomitant strabismus occurs when there is limitation of ocular movement, which can be congenital or acquired. The main features of incomitance are:

• The angle of deviation increases as the eyes are turned in the direction of limitation of movement, and decreases when they are turned in the opposite direction, with the exception of some palsies due to mechanical factors, when movement may be limited in opposing directions.

• The secondary deviation—the angle measured with the affected eye fixating—exceeds the primary deviation—the angle measured with the unaffected eye fixating. The development of secondary comitance in long-standing cases can result in equality of the primary and secondary deviation.

Classification

Incomitant strabismus can be classified according to the underlying cause of the limitation of movement as:

• neurogenic
• myogenic
• mechanical.

Incomitant strabismus is loosely referred to as 'paralytic strabismus' and the following terms are used:

• paralysis, when no movement is possible;
• paresis, when some movement is possible;
• palsy, an older term that includes both paralysis and paresis and is generally used in the text.

Characteristics of paralytic strabismus

Both congenital and acquired conditions may be wholly or partially compensated, principally by an abnormal head posture but also by the patient's fusional amplitude, resulting in the development and maintenance of binocular single vision.

In others, the palsy may be decompensated, giving rise to a manifest strabismus and/or to symptoms. A symptom-free manifest strabismus is more likely to occur in children, and symptoms are more usual in adults.

Muscle sequelae

Limitation of movement affecting one muscle or occurring in one direction of gaze is followed by the development of muscle sequelae, determined by Hering's and Sherrington's laws governing ocular movement (see Chapter 6). The pattern of development is:

• overaction of the contralateral synergist (Hering's law of equal innervation);
• contracture of the ipsilateral antagonist (Sherrington's law of reciprocal innervation);
• secondary inhibition of the contralateral antagonist (Hering's law), which occurs because the contracted antagonist in the affected eye requires less innervation.

The characteristics of palsies, which vary considerably in individuals, are largely determined by the extent of the development of muscle sequelae. Factors influencing the characteristics are:

• Duration of the palsy. An overaction of the contralateral synergist occurs at the onset of the palsy, but the remaining muscle sequelae take time to develop.
• Degree of defective movement, which may range from a slight limitation to complete paralysis. Contracture of the direct antagonist is greater when there is marked limitation.
• The fixing eye. Usually the patient fixates with the unaffected eye but other factors, principally a difference in visual acuity between the two eyes, may result in a preference for the paretic eye. Contracture of the ipsilateral antagonist should not develop to the same extent if the paretic eye fixates. Fixation with the paretic eye may occasionally serve to separate the patient's diplopia.

Abnormal head posture

The purposes of the abnormal head posture in paralytic strabismus are:

• to place the eyes in the position of least deviation so that binocular single vision can develop or be maintained;
• to centralize the field of binocular single vision;
• to obtain foveal fixation when movement is grossly restricted;
• to avoid looking in a direction of gaze in which there is discomfort or pain.

Occasionally an atypical head posture may be adopted in order to separate the diplopic images as widely as possible.

Components

The components of an abnormal head posture comprise a head tilt, face turn and chin elevation or depression.

Head tilt

The head is tilted in incomitant strabismus for two reasons: cyclotropia and vertical deviation.

CYCLOTROPIA

If the head is tilted to the right shoulder in a normal subject the right eye will intort and the left eye will extort. If the left eye is already extorted, as it can be in acquired left fourth nerve palsy, the head is tilted to the right and the left extorsion is compensated. Cyclotropia is mainly a function of the oblique muscles. In a superior rectus palsy the head is tilted to the affected side; this is incorrect for any extorsion produced but correct for the vertical element which is the greater of the two in this instance.

VERTICAL DEVIATION

The head is tilted to the side of the lower eye to level up the diplopic images and allow fusion. A head tilt for the vertical deviation is more common in palsies of the vertical rectus muscles and is usually much less than that seen in oblique palsies.

Face turn

This is adopted to place the eyes away from the direction of underaction and into the position of least deviation.

CHIN ELEVATION OR DEPRESSION

The chin is moved up or down for two reasons:

• to place the eyes in the position of least deviation;
• to avoid discomfort; for example, the chin is often elevated in patients with thyroid eye disease who can find it uncomfortable to look up.

Modification of the head posture

Modification of the head posture to a less extreme position can occur if there is:

- improvement in ocular movement;
- extension of the fusion amplitude;
- sensory adaptation, for example, suppression of one image;
- development of concomitance: for example, if the muscle sequelae become fully developed in a superior oblique palsy, there is no longer a need for chin depression.

The head posture is also modified if it is too uncomfortable to maintain. If, for example, there is a head tilt to one side and a face turn to the opposite side, as in an inferior rectus palsy, the patient may obtain binocular single vision by exaggerating one component and abandoning the other.

Investigation of paralytic strabismus

Aims

The aims of investigation are to:
- establish the type of limitation of ocular movement and to differentiate neurogenic palsies from those due to myogenic or mechanical causes;
- diagnose which muscles are underacting and overacting;
- differentiate congenital or long-standing conditions from those of more recent onset;
- find and treat the cause of the palsy if this is unknown and treatment is possible;
- provide a permanent and repeatable record of the condition so that progress can be assessed.

Reasons for presentation

The reasons for presentation vary depending on whether the palsy is congenital or acquired and on whether the patient is an adult or a child.

Congenital palsies
Adults

Patients with congenital palsies most commonly present because of decompensation of the palsy, resulting in symptoms, mainly intermittent diplopia and asthenopia. Occasionally a symptom-free palsy is discovered by chance, for example in a routine sight test. Vertical muscle palsy is most likely to decompensate.

Decompensation can occur at any age and common causes include:
- poor health;
- change in occupation;
- loss of visual acuity in one eye;
- head injury—even quite minor trauma can cause decompensation.

Children

Patients may present because of:
- the parents noticing an anomaly of ocular movement or a head posture;
- a manifest strabismus: young children may develop a horizontal strabismus, usually esotropia, secondary to a palsy affecting a horizontally or vertically acting muscle.

Acquired palsies
Adults

Patients usually present with symptoms, commonly diplopia, which may be constant or intermittent. A few, particularly the elderly, may complain of less obviously related problems, including having to close one eye, blurred vision or simply not seeing as well.

Children

Patients may complain of symptoms or may attend with a manifest strabismus. Those with sixth nerve palsy commonly present with an esotropia that may persist after recovery of nerve function.

History

A full ophthalmic and medical history should be recorded, as described in Chapter 1. Particular attention should be paid to the patient's symptoms, noting:
- the nature of the symptoms;
- when they occur;
- whether the onset was sudden or gradual;
- any change since the onset.

Questions directed specifically to the patient's diplopia are:
- The type of diplopia—horizontal, vertical or torsional. Patients with vertically separated diplopia should be asked about image tilt since information on this aspect is rarely volunteered.

• Any associated symptoms, either preceding or following the onset of diplopia, such as pain around the eye or on ocular movement.

• Whether the diplopia is constant or intermittent; those with intermittent diplopia should be asked when it occurs.

• Whether the diplopia varies during the day, as it does with thyroid eye disease or myasthenia gravis.

• Any change since the onset—reports of improvement may be misleading as the patient may be ignoring one image or have become more tolerant of the diplopia; worsening of diplopia suggests a progressive disease.

• Any previous episodes of diplopia, which mainly occur in cases of diabetes or multiple sclerosis. The diplopia in each episode may be different in character. Details of its progress can be useful in assessing the prognosis.

• Whether and how the diplopia can be overcome. The principal means are:

  1 abnormal head posture;

  2 fusion of the images, e.g. by blinking;

  3 tilting of spectacle frames to induce a prismatic effect in vertical muscle palsies;

  4 closing one eye.

• The effect of the diplopia on the patient's work.

Symptoms suggestive of more widespread disease include:

• disequilibrium, dysphagia and dysarthria, which are features of brainstem involvement;

• peripheral motor or sensory neuropathy;

• new headache, temporal tenderness, jaw claudication and general malaise, which are all symptoms of giant cell arteritis;

• diplopia with sensory loss in the distribution of the trigeminal nerve, which could be due to a cavernous sinus or superior orbital fissure syndrome.

Observation of the patient

While taking the history the examiner should note:

• an abnormal head posture;

• facial asymmetry or signs of facial injury;

• an obvious deviation of the visual axes;

• difference in pupil size;

• ptosis or lid retraction;

• apparent enophthalmos or exophthalmos;

• any difficulty in speech, hearing or locomotion.

Clinical investigation

An ophthalmic and orthoptic examination should be carried out. Ophthalmic examination is described in detail in Chapter 2. Routine examination of the ocular movement disorder can be summarized as follows:

• Visual acuity for near and distance.

• Cover test for near and distance with and without an abnormal head posture. The observer should record the degree of deviation, the distance and position of gaze in which it is maximum, the presence of diplopia and recovery to binocular single vision.

• Version, duction and vergence movements, noting any anomaly of eyelid and globe position.

• Measurement of the angle of deviation for near and distance and in the most relevant gaze positions (e.g. on lateroversion in suspected sixth nerve palsy), usually by prism cover test. Cyclotropia and the nine positions of gaze measurements are often performed using the major amblyoscope, as described in Chapter 5.

• Hess chart and field of binocular single vision to provide a repeatable record (see Chapters 5 and 6).

The examination is modified according to the nature of the disorder and the patient's general condition, reducing investigation to a minimum if this is poor. If the patient is bed-ridden or very infirm, a diplopia chart can be plotted, recording image separation in at least the most relevant gaze positions.

Medical investigation

Medical examination is essential in most acquired nontraumatic palsies and is tailored to the patient and based on an understanding of the palsy's likely aetiology. Factors to consider before arranging further investigations are:

• A sudden onset of complete third nerve palsy with pupil involvement is due to an intracranial aneurysm until proven otherwise. It is a potential neurosurgical emergency and neuro-imaging should be arranged immediately in collaboration with the neurosurgeons.

• Signs that may indicate a serious underlying cause. Patients with known neurological or systemic disease, those presenting with multiple cranial nerve palsies or signs of generalized central nervous system disease require further evaluation. A palsy which progressively worsens, fails to recover or goes on to involve other parts of the nervous system is a warning sign of a progressively expanding lesion and needs further investigation. Likewise, third nerve palsies that present with or develop aberrant regeneration should undergo neuro-imaging.

• A history of significant head trauma is suggested by a skull fracture or subdural haematoma, loss of consciousness, post-traumatic memory loss or other neurological injury, and no further investigation is required. Patients frequently attribute the cause of a palsy to a 'bang on the head'; further questioning reveals that the head injury was minor and unlikely to be an aetiological factor. It is important to remember that an ocular motor nerve already compromised by a tumour or aneurysm may deteriorate further after minor degrees of head trauma and there may be a history of intermittent diplopia prior to the trauma.

• Patients with congenital or long-standing fourth nerve palsy frequently first present in adult life: differentiation from an acquired palsy is usually easy and the main features are summarized in Table 18.1, p. 348. No further investigation is necessary.

• The diagnosis of myasthenia gravis. A typical presentation is a variable and fatiguable palsy frequently involving the inferior rectus, medial rectus or inferior oblique muscles, often with an upper eyelid ptosis and facial muscle weakness. A changing pattern of muscle involvement is observed on follow-up. See Chapter 20 for further details.

• A presumed microvascular aetiology secondary to atheromatous disease is a common cause of an isolated palsy in the over-45 years age group. The diagnosis should always be provisional, if the examination and investigation fail to reveal other causes and spontaneous recovery occurs; the diagnosis should be questioned if recovery does not occur or if other neurological signs develop. Atheromatous risk factors include diabetes mellitus, hypertension, hyperlipidaemia, or a family history of the condition, and smoking. A microvascular event may also cause a palsy in younger patients, especially those who have existing atheromatous risk factors, in particular diabetes. Investigations should be directed at identifying microvascular risk factors and neuro-imaging is not usually required initially.

• Demyelinating disease in patients aged between 20 and 40 years. The sixth cranial nerve is most frequently affected as it has the longest fascicular course of the ocular motor nerves. Spontaneous recovery is the rule and neuro-imaging is not usually required in typical cases.

Routine investigation

All patients should have their blood pressure and urine checked. The following haematological investigations aimed at identifying atheromatous risk factors also serve as a general screen for patients when the diagnosis is uncertain:

• Full blood count.

• Erythrocyte sedimentation rate (ESR). Occult giant-cell arteritis and other forms of vasculitis as well as chronic systemic disease and malignancy may have an elevated ESR.

• Blood sugar. Blood sugar should be measured as a fasting specimen. If the result suggests diabetes, it cannot be assumed that this is necessarily the cause of the palsy.

• Serum lipids.

Serological investigation for syphilis should be performed, as early treatment can halt further neurological damage. The acetylcholine receptor antibody level is helpful if the aetiology of the palsy remains uncertain: a raised antibody level strongly supports a diagnosis of myasthenia gravis. We recommend that patients over the age of 45 years should have a routine chest X-ray. An electrocardiogram is indicated if there are symptoms of cardiac disease.

Further investigation into systemic and neurological disease or suspected malignancy usually requires collaboration with other specialties.

Neuroradiological examination

Neuro-imaging is indicated for a suspected intracranial lesion on the basis of the patient's mode of presentation, the findings on examination and investigation, and the behaviour of the palsy on follow-up.

Bull and Zilkha (1968) found routine skull X-rays unhelpful in the majority of patients presenting with neurological symptoms and recommended that plain radiographs should be confined to a lateral view. Gawler *et al.* (1974) reported a normal skull X-ray in 50% of patients subsequently diagnosed as having intracranial tumours by CT (computed tomography) scan, lending force to the neuro-ophthalmologists' argument that a CT scan should be obtained and the plain skull X-ray abandoned. The results of a CT scan must also be interpreted with caution, since lesions of the posterior fossa and base of the skull can be missed. Magnetic resonance imaging (MRI) greatly increases diagnostic accuracy. However, the results of neuro-imaging performed at an outside clinic should be re-examined with local neuroradiological colleagues before accepting the reported findings. We have frequently encountered reports of 'normal examination' only to find on reviewing the films that the lesion had been missed. If earlier scans have been reported as normal in a patient with a probable intracranial lesion, it is advisable to repeat the neuro-imaging: either the lesion could have been missed or it may have been too small to be apparent at the time.

It is helpful to the neuroradiologist if a detailed referral letter indicates the type of palsy, the affected side and the presence of any other neurological signs. If there is clinical evidence that the lesion lies, for example, in the orbit, superior orbital fissure, cavernous sinus or the brainstem, this information should also be included.

Differential diagnosis of congenital and acquired palsies

The differential diagnosis of congenital or very long-standing palsies and more recently acquired palsies is important for the following reasons:
• If the palsy is acquired and of unknown origin, further investigation must be carried out to find and treat the cause.
• Time must be allowed for spontaneous recovery in acquired palsies, whereas treatment can be carried out immediately if it is certain that the condition is congenital.
• The surgeon should aim to undercorrect the deviation in patients with congenital palsies, especially

those affecting the vertically acting muscles, partly because the patient is accustomed to exercising his extended vertical fusional amplitude and also because a head tilt in an adult patient may persist postoperatively. This does not apply if there is a simple face turn.

Patients with acquired palsies require full and accurate correction of the deviation in order to resume comfortable binocular single vision.

The features that differentiate congenital and acquired palsies are shown in Table 18.1.

Principles of management

Congenital palsies

Children
Surgery is indicated if:
• there is an unsightly abnormal head posture, particularly one involving a head tilt;
• a manifest strabismus is present with evidence of sensory and motor fusion, indicating that binocular single vision could be restored;
• the deviation is decompensating or is considered likely to decompensate in the future.

Aims
Surgery aims:
• to restore and stabilize binocular single vision and prevent symptoms;
• to remove the need for an abnormal head posture before it becomes established and skeletal changes occur.

Age for surgery
Accurate preoperative assessment is advisable so that the correct choice of surgery can be made. Operation should therefore be delayed if possible until the child is 4 or 5 years old; cooperation should then be sufficient for preoperative assessment and surgery can be carried out before the child starts school. Earlier surgery is indicated if decompensation is occurring or if the palsy is very marked.

Adults
Patients can be treated conservatively using relieving prisms or surgery can be carried out. Treatment is indicated only if symptoms are present.

Differential diagnosis of congenital and acquired palsies.

Diagnostic feature	Congenital	Acquired
History	Patients present because of appearance or chance discovery or symptoms. The duration is usually uncertain and often put earlier at subsequent visits. Diplopia is intermittent and the patient is not very inconvenienced by it	Patients present with diplopia in nearly every case. The exact time of onset is known and the patient is very inconvenienced by it. There may be other associated symptoms
Head posture	The patient and his family are often unaware of the head posture or attribute it to other causes. The posture may be slight when related to the degree of limitation of movement. Scoliosis may be present when there is a head tilt. Facial asymmetry is common. The palsy may be so comitant that chin elevation or depression is not advantageous	The patient is aware of the head posture. It is frequently uncomfortable and for this reason he may adopt it intermittently. It may be quite marked in even slight degrees of palsy. A chin elevation or depression is an obvious feature of vertical muscle palsies
Ocular movement/ concomitance	Although there are many exceptions, muscle sequelae may be fully developed leading to relative concomitance. The primary and secondary deviations will be equal and two virtually equal-sized fields will be seen on the Hess chart. Diagnosis of the primarily affected muscle is sometimes difficult	Overaction of the contralateral synergist will be present but other muscle sequelae will not have developed. The secondary deviation will be larger than the primary deviation. The Hess chart of the affected eye will be obviously smaller than that of the normal eye
Fusion amplitude	Patients with congenital vertical palsies usually have a large vertical fusion amplitude of 10 Δ or more. The field of binocular single vision is consequently quite large	Most patients with acquired vertical palsies have a normal vertical fusion amplitude of only 2–3 Δ Exceptions are patients with a gradual onset or long duration, particularly those with thyroid eye disease
Suppression	This is often present to some extent in congenital palsies. In some, binocular vision may have been lost, but in most the suppression is intermittent. A history of intermittent diplopia implies either suppression or the ability to fuse the images	Suppression occurs in young children with acquired palsies unless it can be prevented, but it is rare in adults with the exception of elderly patients, particularly those with other visual problems resulting in poor vision
Torsion	This is extremely rare even in congenital oblique palsies	Torsion is usual in acquired superior oblique palsies
Ptosis	Congenital superior rectus palsies without ptosis may be seen	If there is an acquired superior rectus palsy, ptosis will also be present
Past-pointing	Absent	Present in very recently acquired palsies but so quickly lost that it is of little diagnostic importance

Acquired palsies

Management comprises:

• The investigation and treatment of the cause if this is unknown.

• A period of observation to allow time for spontaneous recovery and treatment for the underlying condition. A period of 9–12 months is necessary in neurogenic palsies. The patient must be medically stable before surgery is performed and the ocular movements must have been static for at least 3 months. A longer observation period is required in most patients with thyroid eye disease. Early surgical intervention is indicated in some cases of mechanically restricted movement.

• The information recorded at each visit should include:

 1 the patient's opinion of any change in his condition;

 2 cover test and assessment of ocular movement;

 3 Hess chart, always including the outer fields where change is first seen;

 4 field of binocular single vision;

 5 measurement of the deviation, at least in the primary position;

 6 a prism cover test can be used to measure the horizontal and vertical deviation for near and distance, and torsion can be measured on the major amblyoscope or by one of the methods described in Chapter 5.

• Relief of symptoms: binocular single vision should be maintained if possible by means of a head posture and/or temporary prisms. Prisms can prevent the development of suppression and amblyopia in children. Occlusion should be avoided if possible but may be useful in the early stages of an acquired palsy or if the angle is too large to compensate. Botulinum toxin A injection is widely used to prevent contracture occurring, particularly in acquired sixth nerve palsy, and can result in binocular single vision (see Chapter 8).

• Further treatment can be considered if recovery does not take place. Recovery is not always full but patients with residual diplopia on extremes of gaze quickly learn to move their heads to maintain binocular single vision. A full record must be made before the patient is discharged to serve as a comparison if there is a recurrence of symptoms.

Neurogenic palsies and mechanical restriction

The differential diagnosis of neurogenic palsies and limited movement due to mechanical restriction is important because of the basic differences in investigation and treatment. Differentiating features are shown in Table 18.2.

Treatment of symptom-producing palsies

Treatment may be conservative or surgical.

Conservative treatment

Treatment using prisms incorporated into the patient's spectacles (or in spectacle frames if he is emmetropic) is indicated in:

• elderly patients who are loath to undergo surgery;

• patients who are unfit for surgery;

• those with small vertical deviations which might be overcorrected surgically.

Other patients may prefer prisms. Prescription is always preceded by a trial prism for at least 4–6 weeks in order to ensure that the patient is comfortable. The methods of assessment are described in Chapter 5.

Surgical treatment

General principles
The aim of surgery in both congenital and acquired conditions is:

• to overcome symptoms;

• to restore concomitance as far as possible;

• to enlarge the field of binocular single vision, which should be centrally positioned, extending into the lower field;

• to overcome or reduce the need for an abnormal head posture;

• to obtain a less noticeable deviation.

Factors influencing the choice of surgery
The choice of surgery must depend mainly on the nature of the limitation of movement. Other factors influencing the choice are:

• The size of the deviation in the primary position.

• The result of the preoperative forced duction test.

Table 18.2 Differential diagnosis of unilateral neurogenic and mechanical paralytic strabismus.

Diagnostic feature	Neurogenic	Mechanical
Deviation	Depending on the extent of the palsy, the deviation in the primary position can be marked	In many cases with mechanical restriction there is little deviation in the primary position, e.g. Duane's syndrome, orbital floor fracture
Diplopia	Except for third cranial nerve palsy, the nature of the diplopia remains the same in different gaze positions, e.g. right image remains above left	Diplopia may reverse, e.g. between up-gaze and down-gaze
Head posture	A head tilt is usual in vertical muscle palsies	Chin elevation or depression compensates vertical deviations of a mechanical type: head tilt is rare
Ocular movements	The amount of movement elicited is often greater on duction than on version. Movement ceases gradually in the direction of limitation. Maximal limitation is in the position of main action of the affected muscle	Duction and version movements are equally limited. Movement ceases suddenly when the mechanical factor intervenes. Movement is usually limited on, e.g., depression rather than on laevodepression
Hess chart	Although the field of the affected eye will be smaller, there is proportional spacing between the inner and outer fields. Both fields are displaced according to the deviation	The outer field of the chart will be very close to the inner field in the direction of maximum limitation of movement. The field of the affected eye may be very narrow, either horizontally or vertically. Typically the field is limited in, e.g., up-gaze rather than dextro-elevation (with the exception of Brown's syndrome). There is no contracture of ipsilateral antagonists
Retraction of the globe	None	The globe often retracts when turned in the direction opposite to the site of the mechanical lesion
Pain on movement	None	Found in acquired lesions and in some cases of Brown's syndrome
Forced duction	Full passive movement unless secondary muscle contracture has occurred over a long period	Limited passive movement, generally in the direction opposite to the site of the lesion, sometimes in the same direction or in both directions
Intraocular pressure	Remains unchanged in different gaze positions	Will be raised when looking away from the site of the mechanical lesion; a difference of more than 6 mmHg between two opposite directions of gaze is significant

- Whether a muscle is paralysed or has some function. Resections can strengthen a muscle that has some residual function: in the absence of any function, a transposition of adjacent muscles is indicated (see Chapter 9).
- The extent of the development of muscle sequelae. Muscle contracture is particularly important as it will not resolve spontaneously and will adversely affect the results of surgery on other muscles if it is left untreated.
- The presence of both horizontal and vertical components of the deviation.
- Cyclotropia. If this is sufficient to prevent fusion of the images, for example after any vertical deviation has been neutralized with prisms, surgical treatment will be needed to reduce it.
- The presence of a large A- or V-pattern which could limit the field of binocular single vision unless recognized and treated.

Factors influencing the extent of surgery
- Whether the condition is congenital or acquired. Less correction is required in congenital palsies.
- The fusion amplitude. Those with an expanded vertical fusion amplitude require less surgery.
- The duration of a head tilt, which will determine if it will resolve postoperatively. If the tilt has been present for many years, undercorrection is advisable.

References

Bull, J.W.D. & Zilkha, K.J. (1968) Rationalising requests for X-ray films in neurology. *British Medical Journal* **IV**, 569–570.

Gawler, J., de Boulay, G.H., Bull, J.W.D. & Marshall, J. (1974) Computer-assisted tomography (EMI scanned). Its place in the investigation of suspected intracranial tumours. *Lancet* ii, 419–423.

19

Neurogenic Palsies

Neurogenic strabismus can be congenital or acquired. The aetiology of congenital palsies is often unknown and some may be the result of non-neurogenic causes, such as anatomical variations in the origin or insertion of the extraocular muscles or even absence of the muscle or tendon. However, because they resemble acquired neurogenic palsies, and must be differentiated from them, they are included in this section. Palsies of the third (oculomotor), fourth (trochlear) and sixth (abducens) cranial nerves are discussed.

Classification

Acquired
- third nerve palsy
- fourth nerve palsy
- sixth nerve palsy
- ocular neuromyotonia

Congenital
- third nerve palsy
- fourth nerve palsy

- sixth nerve palsy
- double elevator palsy
- double depressor palsy
- Möbius' syndrome

Incidence

Neurogenic strabismus can be:
- unilateral or bilateral, with unilateral palsies being more common;
- isolated or involve multiple ocular motor nerves;
- present in the setting of an underlying systemic disease, for example leukaemia;
- present in the setting of more generalized neurological disease, for example multiple sclerosis.

Rucker (1958, 1966), reporting on two large series of neurogenic strabismus confined to acquired infranuclear palsies, found an incidence of:
- 41–52% sixth nerve palsies;
- 27–34% third nerve palsies;
- 7–8% fourth nerve palsies;
- 13–19% multiple palsies.

The series included cases due to trauma, those referred by neurologists with associated serious illness, and others in which the ocular motor disorder was the only presenting symptom. Congenital disorders were specifically excluded. The cause of the paresis was undetermined in 28% and 22% in each series, respectively.

Rush and Younge (1981) reviewed a comparable series of 1000 cases with identical selection criteria and found a similar distribution of the incidence of cranial nerve palsies. They noted that, despite the development of more sophisticated diagnostic techniques, the percentage of palsies in which no cause could be identified remained surprisingly high. There was a 51% chance of spontaneous recovery in the group with no known cause as opposed to an overall recovery rate of 48%.

Other authors have reported a much higher incidence of fourth nerve palsies. Much depends on whether a series of patients includes congenital as well as acquired palsies, whether the patients reviewed include children as well as adults, and whether the study has been conducted in a general ophthalmology department or a neuro-ophthalmology unit.

Tiffin *et al.* (1996) reported on a series of 165 acquired third, fourth and sixth cranial nerve palsies who were seen in the orthoptic department and found an incidence of:
- 57% sixth nerve palsies;
- 21% fourth nerve palsies;
- 17% third nerve palsies;
- 5% multiple palsies.

Acquired palsies

Aetiology

The main causes of neurogenic palsies are:
- Trauma.
- Space-occupying lesion:
  1 tumour;
  2 vascular: aneurysm; carotid cavernous fistula; subdural haematoma.
- Microvascular: diabetes, hypertension.
- Inflammatory:
  1 Tolosa–Hunt syndrome;
  2 postviral: herpes zoster; meningitis/encephalitis.
- Vasculitis.
- Demyelination.
- Ophthalmoplegic migraine.
- Miller Fisher/Guillain–Barré.
- Acquired immunodeficiency syndrome.

Trauma

Closed head trauma is a major cause of both fourth and sixth nerve palsies, and it often results in bilateral palsies. It is important to note that a patient may relate his symptoms to a past fall or collision, but on further questioning it becomes clear that either the injury did not involve direct head trauma or the symptoms predated it or arose long after the injury. It should be remembered that neurological disease can result in imbalance and an increased propensity to fall. A fall may therefore be the first indication of an underlying neurological condition.
- The sixth nerve passes up the petrous-temporal bone to its upper border, where it makes a right-angle bend under the petrosphenoid ligament. Classically it is taught that this point is where the nerve is particularly prone to damage, either through traction caused by a shift in the brainstem or directly through a fracture of the base of the skull (Wolff 1928).
- The fourth nerve nucleus lies in the dorsal midbrain; the nerve leaves the brainstem as a number

of fine rootlets, which pass posteriorly to cross those emerging from the opposite nucleus. The rootlets join to sweep forwards round the midbrain to enter the cavernous sinus. Closed head injury probably results in tearing of the rootlets as they exit from the dorsal surface of the midbrain. Quite trivial head injury can cause a unilateral palsy, while severe head injury can result in a bilateral palsy.

• Severe head injury is one of the most frequent causes of complete or partial third nerve palsy. Distal fascicular damage or partial rootlet avulsion are important mechanisms of the injury (Balcer *et al.* 1996). Coincidental damage to the anterior visual pathway and other neurological sites is common (Elston 1984).

• Head trauma is a recognized cause of a central disruption of both motor and sensory fusion. Thus the potential for binocular single vision should be investigated prior to undertaking strabismus surgery.

Space-occupying lesions

Tumours

Either primary or secondary intracranial tumours are a common cause of ocular motor palsies in both adults and children. The reported incidence of tumours varies between series and probably reflects the source of patients. Rush and Younge (1981) identified tumour as the cause of the palsy in:

• 15% of sixth nerve palsies;
• 13% of third nerve palsies;
• 4% of fourth nerve palsies.

Rucker (1966) found a higher incidence of tumour (26%) in sixth nerve palsies, and Moster *et al.* (1984) reported a 29% incidence of tumour in a highly selected series of young adults with isolated sixth nerve palsy. Diplopia may be the first presenting symptom. The sixth nerve is the most commonly affected by direct or indirect damage, and children not infrequently present with a symptomatic esotropia. The third nerve is rather less often involved. It is rare for an isolated fourth nerve palsy to be caused by a tumour except for acquired nontraumatic bilateral palsies.

Primary tumours most likely to cause direct damage are:

• meningioma
• pituitary tumour
• craniopharyngioma
• glioma
• chordoma
• lymphoma and leukaemia
• nasopharyngeal carcinoma.

Pituitary tumours usually affect the third nerve before involving the other ocular motor nerves, but Rucker (1966) reported cases in which the sixth nerve was primarily affected. Lymphomas may be a feature of more widespread malignant disease of the lymphatics. Nasopharyngeal carcinomas can be difficult to detect clinically, and may require multiple biopsies of the nasopharynx before the diagnosis can be made.

Secondary (metastatic) tumours are more common than primary tumours as a cause of ocular motor nerve palsies. The most frequent primary sites are carcinoma of the lung in men and carcinoma of the breast in women.

The pattern of neurological dysfunction can have important localizing value for the site of the tumour.

Well-recognized syndromes include:

• The cavernous sinus and superior orbital fissure syndrome: all three ocular motor nerves can be involved; in addition involvement of the ophthalmic division of the trigeminal nerve can result in pain and/or anaesthesia. Involvement of the sympathetic fibres results in a Horner's syndrome. Lesions situated in the posterior cavernous sinus may affect the maxillary division of the trigeminal nerve.

• The orbital apex syndrome: in addition to the nerves affected by the superior orbital fissure syndrome there are signs of proptosis and a compressive optic neuropathy, with or without optic atrophy.

• Brainstem syndromes: these are discussed in detail under the individual ocular motor nerves.

• Cerebellopontine angle syndrome: the commonest tumour at this site is an acoustic neuroma, which frequently results in damage to the eighth, seventh, sixth and fifth cranial nerves. A characteristic primary positional jerk nystagmus, termed Bruns' nystagmus, is occasionally seen and is discussed in more detail in Chapter 23.

Aneurysm

Aneurysms of the blood vessels forming the circle of Willis are an important cause of ocular motor palsies. The position of the aneurysm dictates the nature of the palsy, but the third cranial nerve is chiefly affected.

The main sites where aneurysms can selectively damage the ocular motor nerves include:
• Posterior communicating artery aneurysms which compress the third cranial nerve as it passes below and lateral to the artery. The characteristics are pain around the eye and headache, both of which precede the palsy, and a sudden and often rapid onset of the palsy with a dilated pupil in nearly all cases. The pupil fibres at this point are believed to lie on the upper temporal aspect of the nerve, making them very vulnerable to damage from external pressure.
• Carotid artery aneurysms can also cause a third nerve palsy but if the sympathetic fibres to the dilator pupillae are affected, the pupil will not be widely dilated, thus differentiating the lesion from a posterior communicating artery aneurysm. The pupillary reaction to light will be impaired. Large carotid artery aneurysms can involve all the ocular motor nerves, resulting in total ophthalmoplegia. The fifth nerve may also be affected.
• Basilar artery aneurysms may cause ocular motor palsies. Lustbader and Miller (1988) reported a case of isolated pupil-sparing third nerve palsy, and we have seen cases of sixth nerve palsy.

It is essential that all patients with sudden onset of a nontraumatic third nerve palsy are urgently evaluated for the possibility of an expanding and possibly leaking aneurysm. If left untreated there is a high risk of a fatal subarachnoid haemorrhage.

Carotid cavernous fistula
Carotid cavernous fistula is an abnormal communication between the internal or external carotid system and the cavernous sinus. It can occur spontaneously, usually from meningeal branches of the carotid artery, and give rise to 'slow flow' fistulas. A more serious 'high flow' fistula can arise, usually post-traumatically, where there is direct communication between the internal carotid artery and the cavernous sinus.

The symptoms and signs are due to the raised pressure from arterialization of the orbital venous system and from ocular hypoxia. They include:
• visual loss;
• proptosis;
• dilatation of the episcleral and conjunctival vessels, giving the appearance of a chronic 'red eye';

• pulsation of the globe can sometimes be observed and a bruit heard in high-flow fistulas;
• palsies of the ocular motor nerves can occur to a variable degree;
• swelling and hypoxia of the extraocular muscles can result in myogenic strabismus;
• the signs are occasionally bilateral.

The symptoms and signs may resolve spontaneously. Persistent carotid cavernous fistula that continues to cause concern can be treated by selective thromboembolization by a neuroradiologist.

Subdural haematoma
Head trauma may result in bleeding into the subdural space. The features are those of an expanding space-occupying lesion.

Microvascular
Diabetes
Occlusive disease of the vasa nervorum, the network of small blood vessels supplying the nerves, is a recognized problem in diabetes. It is probable that poor diabetic control makes the patient more vulnerable to microvascular occlusion. Occlusive disease is more common in diabetes of long duration and usually affects patients over 40 years of age. These patients often have other signs of vascular disease, such as ischaemic autonomic neuropathy.

Acquired sixth or third nerve palsy may be the presenting sign of previously undiagnosed diabetes in the older patient, occurring in 40–50% of patients (Burde & Roper-Hall 1977). The fourth nerve is less often affected.

Goldstein and Cogan (1960) reported the symptoms and signs characteristic of a diabetic third nerve palsy as:
• Palsy accompanied by severe headache.
• Pupil usually spared because the vasa nervorum supplies the inner aspect of the nerve, whereas the pupillary fibres are relatively superficial. The incidence of pupil sparing varies in different series from 62 to 83% (Rucker 1958, 1966; Green *et al.* 1964), and when involved is rarely total.

Diabetic neuropathy tends to recur, sometimes affecting one nerve in one episode and a different nerve on a later occasion. It must be remembered that dual pathology can occur, and the presence of diabetes does not mean that it is the cause of the palsy. Ocular motor palsies due to aneurysm and tumour can occur in patients who are diabetic.

Hypertension and atheroma

Similar occlusive microvascular problems are seen in hypertensive patients, most commonly affecting the sixth nerve. Typically the palsy is painless. Patients may have severe atheromatous blood vessel disease in the absence of hypertension or diabetes. Palsies affecting the sixth, fourth and third nerves together with brainstem neurological signs may be the result of brainstem stroke.

Inflammatory

Tolosa–Hunt syndrome

This syndrome is caused by a nonspecific granulomatous inflammation (pseudotumour) in the anterior part of the cavernous sinus. Tolosa (1954) reported narrowing of the carotid artery in the sinus, a finding subsequently confirmed by Hunt *et al.* (1961).

The condition is characterized by:

- ophthalmoplegia—all three ocular motor nerves can be affected;
- pain;
- loss of sensation over the area of distribution of the first division of the trigeminal nerve;
- Horner's syndrome;
- visual loss if the optic nerve is involved.

The syndrome responds to treatment with systemic steroids but can recur. Tumours at the orbital apex can mimic the Tolosa–Hunt syndrome and may show an initial response to steroids due to a reduction of the surrounding oedema. The appearance of the syndrome on magnetic resonance (MR) scanning and in particular the disappearance of the lesion with steroid treatment helps differentiate it from mass lesions at this site (Thomas *et al.* 1988).

Viral infections

Benign sixth nerve palsy in childhood is most likely viral in origin. However, this diagnosis should only be made after thorough investigation has failed to reveal an alternative cause.

HERPES ZOSTER OPHTHALMICUS (HZO)

The first signs of HZO are a strictly unilateral rash following the distribution of the first division of the trigeminal nerve and severe pain. In a significant number of cases, any one or all of the ipsilateral ocular motor nerves may be affected shortly after the onset of the rash. The sixth and third nerves are more frequently involved than the fourth nerve. Contralateral ocular motor palsies have been described (Kelly & Dulley 1976). Other neurological symptoms may develop, suggesting that the disease is not confined to the trigeminal nerve. The majority of ocular muscle palsies recover spontaneously in 3–12 months, but Kelly and Dulley have shown that there is often a clinically demonstrable residual underaction of the affected muscle or muscles.

Vasculitis

Inflammation affecting the blood vessels can arise from a number of different disease processes. Polyarteritis nodosa and systemic lupus erythematosis can both cause a neuropathy; however, isolated involvement of the ocular motor nerves in the absence of other signs of the disease is unusual, although giant-cell arteritis can cause isolated involvement of the ocular motor nerves.

Giant-cell arteritis (temporal or cranial arteritis)

This condition is an inflammatory disease of the arteries occurring usually in people who are over 60 years of age. It typically presents as an irreversible ischaemic optic neuropathy of sudden onset that affects one eye, but is very often followed by involvement of the other. We have seen giant-cell arteritis present as an isolated fourth and sixth nerve palsy. Patients give a clear history of recent headaches, temporal tenderness, jaw claudication and generalized malaise: the finding of a raised erythrocyte sedimentation rate facilitates an early diagnosis. A temporal artery biopsy shows evidence of inflammation of the vessel wall. The condition should be regarded as a medical emergency, and treated with high-dose systemic steroids to reduce any further risk of sight-threatening complications.

Meningitis/encephalitis

Meningitis and encephalitis can arise from viral and bacterial infections. Involvement of all three ocular motor nerves can occur. Recovery may occur following treatment of the underlying infection.

Demyelinating disease (multiple sclerosis)

Optic neuritis is the most common manifestation of multiple sclerosis, although many patients may present first to the ophthalmologist with a disorder of ocular motility, including:

• internuclear ophthalmoplegia, often bilateral, which is perhaps the most frequently encountered motility disturbance;

• sixth nerve palsy;

• occasionally third nerve palsy;

• rarely fourth nerve palsy since the nerve is less vulnerable due to its short fascicular pathway.

Patients with multiple sclerosis usually first present aged between 16 and 40 years. Diagnosis is based on the occurrence of more than one demyelinating event affecting a different site at a different time, and should be supported by other investigations. These include:

• magnetic resonance imaging scan showing characteristic plaques of demyelination;

• lumbar puncture showing protein changes in the cerebrospinal fluid;

• visual evoked potentials showing delayed latency following even a subclinical episode of optic neuritis.

Ophthalmoplegic migraine

This is a rare disorder. The diagnosis is only made after examination has failed to uncover any other abnormalities and must include normal neuro-imaging. Onset is nearly always in childhood.

The features are:

• sudden onset of nausea and vomiting;

• hemicranial pain;

• ipsilateral third nerve palsy, usually with pupil involvement.

The headache subsides with the onset of the third nerve palsy. Recurrence is the rule, and third nerve function may not completely recover over time. There is often a family history of migraine (Polomeno *et al.* 1981).

Miller Fisher syndrome

This syndrome was first described by Miller Fisher in 1956 (1956), and is often referred to as the bulbar variant of the Guillain–Barré syndrome.

It consists of a demyelinating or axonal neuropathy resulting in:

• Ophthalmoplegia from involvement of the ocular motor nerves. The third cranial nerve is frequently involved resulting in both an external and an internal ophthalmoplegia. Disorders of supranuclear ocular motor pathways with palsy of up-gaze and internuclear ophthalmoplegia have also been reported (Zasorin *et al.* 1985).

• Arreflexia from involvement of the dorsal root ganglia of the spinal cord.

• Ataxia from involvement of the Purkinje cells of the cerebellum.

Most cases are self-limiting; however, it can develop into the Guillain–Barré syndrome, requiring respiratory support.

Acquired immunodeficiency syndrome

The acquired immunodeficiency syndrome puts the patient at increased risk of opportunistic infection. Secondary infection may affect the brainstem or the subarachnoid course of the ocular motor nerves.

Nuclear palsies

Nuclear palsies are rarely isolated due to the extensive size of the causative lesion in most instances. The clinical findings are therefore often complicated by involvement of adjacent supranuclear eye movement control centres.

Third nerve

The third nerve nucleus lies in the floor of the aqueduct of Sylvius at the level of the superior colliculus in the midbrain. Each third nerve nucleus supplies four extraocular muscles and the levator muscle. The levator is supplied by a common single caudal nucleus; the superior rectus by the contralateral nucleus; and the medial rectus, inferior rectus and inferior oblique muscles are supplied from the ipsilateral nucleus. The parasympathetic supply to the pupil and ciliary body comes from the Edinger–Westphal nucleus, which lies just caudal to the third nerve nucleus complex.

The brainstem centres concerned with vertical gaze control are in close proximity to the third nerve nucleus. They include the rostral interstitial nucleus of the medial longitudinal fasciculus and the interstitial nucleus of Cajal.

For a unilateral third nerve palsy to be nuclear in origin there should be bilateral ptosis and bilateral superior rectus paresis. The reason for the bilateral superior rectus paresis is that the axons from the contralateral superior rectus subnucleus pass through the ipsilateral subnucleus before forming the third nerve. Most cases probably also have an associated supranuclear vertical gaze palsy that results in a bilateral failure of voluntary up-gaze. In this setting the bilateral superior rectus weakness can only be confirmed to be of nuclear origin by demonstrating a deficient vestibular input by means of the doll's head manoeuvre, when neither eye will elevate. An intact Bell's phenomenon indicates that the lesion is supranuclear.

Sixth nerve

The sixth nerve nucleus lies close to the mid-line in the tegmental area of the pons. It consists of motor neurones supplying the ipsilateral lateral rectus, and interneurones that pass through the medial longitudinal fasciculus to the contralateral medial rectus. In close proximity to the sixth nerve nucleus is the paramedian pontine reticular formation, the horizontal gaze centre, which inputs to the nucleus. The facial nerve passes around the sixth nerve nucleus and indents the floor of the fourth ventricle.

Isolated lesions involving the sixth nerve nucleus result in an ipsilateral horizontal gaze palsy in addition to a lower ipsilateral motor neurone facial paralysis.

Infranuclear palsies

The majority of acquired palsies are the result of lesions below the level of the nucleus for the corresponding nerve, and these are considered in the following sections.

Acquired third nerve palsies

Summary of aetiology

A third nerve palsy may be caused by:
• Compression by a posterior communicating artery aneurysm, which almost always results in pupil involvement. Those cases without pupil involvement which are due to intracranial aneurysm tend to result in incomplete paresis of the extraocular muscles supplied by the third nerve (Guy & Day 1989).
• Direct damage from adjacent tumours, such as meningiomas, affecting areas of the base of the skull or adjacent to the pituitary fossa and cavernous sinus.

• Closed head trauma, which results in pupillary involvement in most cases.
• Microvascular disease due to diabetes or hypertension, usually sparing the pupil.

The fascicular portion of the third nerve may be damaged in association with other brainstem structures, giving rise to two characteristic syndromes:
• Weber's syndrome, comprising an ipsilateral third nerve palsy and contralateral hemiparesis arising from damage to the cerebral peduncle and third nerve.
• Benedikt's syndrome, which is an ipsilateral third nerve palsy with contralateral hemiparesis and contralateral ataxia with intention tremor. These signs arise from damage to the cerebral peduncle, third nerve and the red nucleus.

It has always been assumed that lesions giving rise to divisional or single muscle palsies must affect the third nerve after its separation into two divisions in the cavernous sinus. However, MR scans have shown that a lesion of the fascicular portion of the nerve within the brainstem can cause a divisional palsy (Guy et al. 1985), as can intracranial aneurysms at the site of the posterior communicating and superior cerebellar arteries. This confirms the view of anatomists, who postulated many years ago that the nerve was organized into a divisional pattern close to its origin in the brainstem.

Features

The features of third nerve palsy (Table 19.1) are:
• Crossed diplopia with a vertical element reflecting the exotropia with slight hypotropia; although the eye may be intorted, torsional diplopia is a rare complaint. Diplopia may not be appreciated when the deviation is large, due to the remote position of the second image. Ptosis covering the visual axis will also prevent the appreciation of diplopia.
• An abnormal head posture may be adopted to maintain binocular single vision if the palsy is partial, particularly if it only involves a single muscle. A head posture may also be used to help separate diplopic images that cannot be joined. A head posture is not required if a ptosis covers the visual axis.
• Ocular movements may be very limited, with no elevation or depression demonstrable. Adduction past the mid-line may not be possible.

Table 19.1 Summary of ocular motility findings in third nerve palsy.

Type	Ocular posture	Abnormal head position	Muscle sequelae
All muscles affected	Exotropia, intorsion hypotropia	Face turn to unaffected side	Overaction contralateral LR, SR, SO and IO
Superior division	Hypotropia with true ptosis and pseudoptosis	Head tilt, face turn to affected side and chin elevation	Overaction contralateral IO, contracture of ipsilateral IR, secondary inhibitional palsy of contralateral SO
Inferior division	Exotropia, intorsion and hypertropia	Head tilt to unaffected side; face turn to unaffected side	Overaction contralateral LR, SR and SO
Medial rectus	Exotropia	Face turn to unaffected side	Overaction contralateral LR, contracture ipsilateral LR, secondary inhibitional palsy of contralateral MR
Superior rectus	Hypotropia	Head tilt, face turn to affected side and chin elevation	Overaction contralateral IO, contracture of ipsilateral IR, secondary inhibitional palsy of contralateral SO
Inferior rectus	Hypertropia	Head tilt to unaffected side, face turn affected side, chin depression	Overaction contralateral SO, contracture ipsilateral SR, secondary inhibitional palsy of contralateral IO
Inferior oblique	Hypertropia, intorsion, slight exotropia	Head tilt to affected side, face turn to unaffected side and chin elevation	Overaction contralateral SR, contracture ipsilateral SO, secondary inhibitional palsy of contralateral IR

Key: IO = inferior oblique muscle; IR = inferior rectus muscle; LR = lateral rectus muscle; MR = medial rectus muscle; SO = superior oblique muscle; SR = superior rectus muscle.

- Pupillary involvement results in a dilated pupil; however, if the sympathetic fibres are affected by the same lesion, the features are of a poorly reactive or atonic-type pupil. Rarely, lesions affecting the third nerve in the cavernous sinus may cause a constricted pupil from an associated Horner's syndrome or as a result of aberrant regeneration.
- Aberrant regeneration is a feature of a compressive or traumatic third nerve palsy. It does not occur in microvascular lesions: its development in a patient without a history of trauma demands neuro-imaging to exclude a space-occupying lesion.

Investigation

A medical and ophthalmic history should be taken and ophthalmic and orthoptic investigation carried out, as outlined in Chapter 18.
- Nontraumatic third nerve palsy involving the pupil should be assumed to be caused by an expanding aneurysm until neuro-imaging has excluded the possibility.
- Nontraumatic third nerve palsy sparing the pupil is unlikely to be caused by an aneurysm; in the rare instance when this is the cause, then pupil involvement is likely to occur within a week or two of the initial symptoms. We therefore recommend that all third nerve palsies where the aetiology is unknown are reviewed every 2–3 days for the first week after presentation, and the patient is also instructed to reattend if he observes a change in the size of the pupil or any new symptoms.
- If the pupil is not widely dilated, particular note should be made of its reaction to light, as an associated Horner's syndrome may result in a relative atonic pupil.
- Confirming the integrity of the fourth nerve can be difficult. The main action of the superior oblique is depression when the eye is adducted. This function cannot be tested properly when adduction is limited.

Instead, the patient should be instructed to abduct the eye and then try to look down, when intorsion should be seen if the fourth nerve is intact. Observation of an iris landmark or a conjunctival vessel can aid detection of intorsion.

• A sixth nerve palsy should be suspected if there is a small degree of exotropia in spite of quite marked limitation of adduction. Even when the eye is very exotropic, it is possible to demonstrate lateral rectus function by observing the saccadic velocity or performing a force generation test.

• Fifth nerve function should be routinely assessed; reduced corneal sensitivity in association with a third nerve palsy requires further investigation.

• Signs of aberrant regeneration in the absence of a history of trauma demand further investigation.

• The potential for binocular single vision should be confirmed prior to undertaking strabismus surgery as some patients may have suffered central disruption of the fusion mechanism.

• The possibility of myasthenia should not be forgotten in any case where the aetiology is unknown.

Classification

A palsy may be unilateral or bilateral, and the pupillary fibres may or may not be involved.

Complete

Complete third nerve palsy is palsy involving both the upper and lower division of the third nerve; the pupil may or may not be involved. Two groups are recognized.

• Total paralysis of all the extraocular muscles involved, in addition to the levator muscle. The sphincter pupillae and ciliary muscle may or may not be affected. The ptosis frequently recovers without recovery of the extraocular muscles.

• Paresis of all the extraocular muscles affected, in addition to the levator muscle. The sphincter pupillae and ciliary muscle may or may not be affected.

Incomplete

Incomplete third nerve palsy can present in various forms and the pupil may or may not be involved.

• Palsy of groups of muscles (divisional palsies) comprising:

　1 palsy of the superior division of the nerve affecting the superior rectus and levator muscles;

　2 palsy of the inferior division, affecting the medial rectus and inferior rectus, the inferior oblique and both the intraocular muscles.

• Single muscle palsy.

Complete third nerve palsy

This may be total or partial and the pupil may or may not be affected. All or some of the characteristics described below will be present.

Features

The features are outlined below.

• The affected eye is exotropic, intorted and a little hypotropic despite the fact that the superior oblique has no significant depressor action with the eye in abduction.

• Muscle sequelae include overaction of the contralateral lateral and superior rectus muscles and the superior and inferior oblique muscles. If a partial ptosis is present and the patient fixes with the affected eye, upper eyelid retraction of the contralateral eye will be apparent.

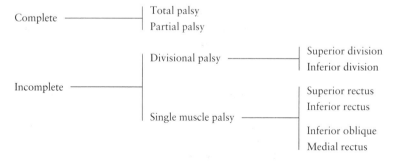

Tree 19.1 Classification of third nerve palsy.

• Aberrant regeneration is seen in association with trauma or space-occupying lesions (see below).

• If the ptosis is partial the patient may complain of diplopia. In some an abnormal head posture, usually a face turn away from the affected eye, will provide a small area of single vision; if so a field of binocular single vision should be plotted

• Diplopia will not be present in total paralysis of the extraocular muscles because the ptosis covers the pupil; there will be no need for an abnormal head posture. The ptosis frequently recovers before the extraocular muscles; it is therefore not uncommon to find a total paralysis of extraocular muscles with no ptosis.

• If the pupil is involved it will be dilated and as the ciliary muscle is also affected there will be an accommodative palsy.

Management

The incidence of spontaneous recovery is low in acquired third nerve palsy unless it is due to microvascular disease. A palsy due to aneurysm or trauma may show some improvement but this is rarely complete and is frequently complicated by aberrant regeneration.

Conservative treatment

Symptoms are only present if the ptosis does not cover the visual axis.

• Prisms are of limited use because the diplopia reverses in different positions of gaze. The deviation may also be too large for the use of prisms and an intorted image may prevent fusion. However, a larger and better-located field of binocular single vision can occasionally be obtained in partial palsies.

• Occlusion may be required in those cases where diplopia is troublesome or there is concern over the appearance.

• Some patients find that they can easily ignore the remote image; in others with long-standing deviations an acquired suppression response appears to develop.

• Photophobia may be a problem in patients with mydriasis from internal ophthalmoplegia. In those patients not helped by tinted glasses, constriction of the pupil can be induced by the instillation of pilocarpine 1% eye drops as required. Some patients are helped by a painted contact lens with a small pupil.

• Ptosis crutches fitted to spectacle frames are useful when bilateral ptosis is present or when the palsy affects the patient's only seeing eye.

• Botulinum toxin has a role in improving alignment and in investigating binocular potential. It is effective in temporarily aligning the visual axes when injected into the lateral rectus or a vertical rectus in a partial palsy. Repeated botulinum toxin injections can offer an alternative to surgical alignment in these cases. Reduction in the deviation can facilitate the investigation of binocular function in some patients when this is in doubt. Botulinum toxin is unlikely to bring about a significant change in alignment in a total palsy.

Surgical treatment

Surgery should not be undertaken until the deviation is stable. The surgical approach depends on whether the palsy is total or partial.

TOTAL PALSY

• The complexity of the ocular muscle imbalance makes the prognosis for establishing even a small field of binocular single vision poor (Fig. 19.1). Surgery should therefore be considered to improve the appearance, or in a patient whose only eye is affected by the palsy, to move the eye into the primary position. In most cases surgery is aimed at treating the exotropia.

• Postoperative diplopia should be anticipated; however, assessing the likely tolerance and adaptation to it is difficult in these patients. As stated above, botulinum toxin in our hands has not been effective in achieving temporary alignment, and the large size of the deviation prevents the successful use of Fresnel prisms. Patients with ptosis that covers the visual axis should be provided with a ptosis prop after surgical alignment of the visual axes to assess their tolerance of diplopia. Surgery for the ptosis should only be considered if diplopia is acceptable to the patient. Interestingly, some patients do not experience postoperative diplopia (Elston 1984), despite improved alignment and absence of fusion, presumably because they have developed an acquired form of suppression.

• A successful surgical outcome consists of good alignment in the primary position, with little to no movement in any field of gaze. The patient needs to understand the need to reduce all eye movement, particularly abduction, to prevent a recurrence of the exotropia.

Field of Left Eye (fixing with right eye) Field of Right Eye (fixing with left eye)

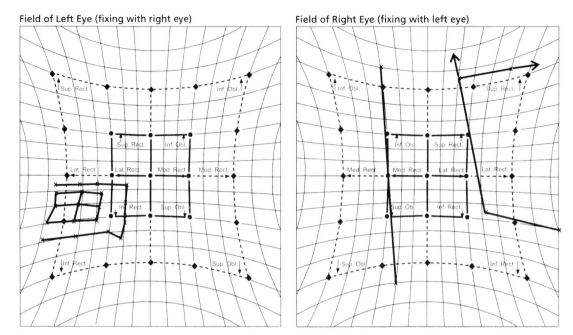

Fig. 19.1 Hess chart of a patient with a complete total left third nerve palsy. The left eye is exotropic and hypotropic with limitation of adduction, elevation and depression.

Horizontal muscle surgery combined with traction sutures

Surgery on the horizontal muscles is the safest, easiest and most predictable of the methods available. Despite the use of an extensive amount of recession and resection, there is still a tendency for the exotropia to recur. The combined use of horizontal rectus surgery and traction sutures to anchor the eye in adduction for a 6-week period postoperatively is therefore recommended (Lee & Gregson 1993). We perform a 12–16 mm recession of the lateral rectus combined with an 8 mm resection of the medial rectus muscle. Ethibond traction sutures are passed under the insertion sites of both vertical recti and brought out through the medial aspect of the upper and lower lids. The sutures are tied over short lengths of rubber bolsters, and this provides the necessary tension to keep the eye anchored in adduction for 6 weeks (see Chapter 9).

Postoperative problems include:
• absence of eye movement, forcing the patient to use extensive head movement;
• overlapping diplopia, preventing the lifting of any ptosis;
• overaction of the contralateral synergist muscles, which can cause a variable and unsightly deviation if the affected eye is used for fixation.

Other procedures have been suggested, including superior oblique mobilization and transposition, and medial transposition of the vertical rectus muscles. In our opinion, there is nothing to be gained by the use of these more complex procedures.

PARTIAL PALSY

In this group of patients there is a better chance for establishing a useful central area of binocular single vision because the extraocular muscles have a degree of residual function.

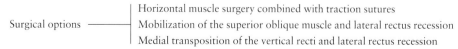

Surgical options —— Horizontal muscle surgery combined with traction sutures
Mobilization of the superior oblique muscle and lateral rectus recession
Medial transposition of the vertical recti and lateral rectus recession

Tree 19.2 Surgical options to correct the exotropia in total third nerve palsy.

The principles of treatment are to:
- investigate the likely postoperative sensory outcome with prisms or botulinum toxin to confirm whether binocular single vision can be achieved;
- optimize the position and range of movement of the affected eye;
- balance the defect by operating on the overacting synergists of the unaffected eye.

The surgical options depend on whether there is a mainly horizontal deviation or a combined horizontal and vertical deviation. In this subgroup, it is assumed that all affected muscles are incompletely paralysed.

Horizontal deviation (Fig. 19.2)
Correction of the exotropia by recession of the lateral rectus and resection of the medial rectus of the affected eye using adjustable sutures is the procedure of choice. The possible persistent incomitance on contralateral gaze, due to residual limitation of adduction of the affected eye, can be improved by recessing the contralateral lateral rectus muscle.

Providing the unaffected eye is used for fixation, aberrant regeneration resulting in upper eyelid elevation on attempted adduction can be improved by combining surgery on the affected eye with a lateral rectus recession on the unaffected eye.

Horizontal and vertical deviation (Fig. 19.3)
The vertical deviation can often be improved by vertical transposition of the horizontal recti after the appropriate amount of recession and resection has been undertaken. Further surgery can be performed on the muscles of the contralateral eye if required. Noonan and O'Connor described a technique by which the vertical deviation and pseudoptosis can be corrected by operating on the vertical recti of the unaffected eye (Noonan & O'Connor 1995).

Incomplete third nerve palsy

Third nerve palsy involving groups of muscles
Superior division palsy
This condition is more likely to be congenital than acquired. Acquired cases may be due to intracranial aneurysms (Guy & Day 1989) and therefore neuro-imaging is recommended when the aetiology is uncertain. Both muscles supplied by the superior division, the superior rectus muscle and the levator muscle, will be affected.

Field of Left Eye (fixing with right eye)

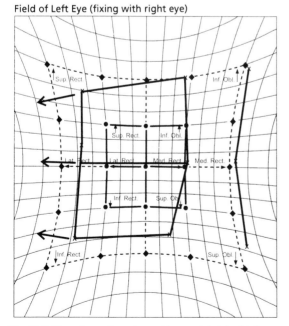

Field of Right Eye (fixing with left eye)

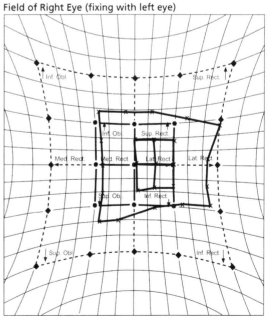

Fig. 19.2 Hess chart of a patient with a partial right third nerve. The right eye is exotropic with no significant vertical deviation due to symmetrical involvement of the elevators and depressors of the right eye.

Field of Left Eye (fixing with right eye)   Field of Right Eye (fixing with left eye)

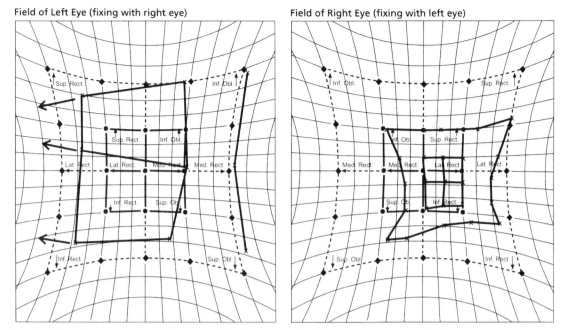

Fig. 19.3 Hess chart of a patient with a partial right third nerve palsy affecting all muscles supplied by the oculomotor nerve.

FEATURES
The features are outlined below.

• The affected eye is hypotropic, giving rise to pseudo-ptosis; the coexisting true ptosis can be assessed with the affected eye fixing in the primary position.

• There is underaction of the superior rectus and ptosis, which is often partial. If the patient fixes with the affected eye the unaffected eye may show apparent upper eyelid retraction.

• There is overaction of the contralateral inferior oblique and contracture of the ipsilateral inferior rectus. Secondary inhibitional palsy of the contralateral superior oblique is also seen.

• A head posture consisting of a chin elevation, with the head tilted and face turned to the affected side, makes best use of the field of binocular single vision, which is displaced down and to the side of the unaffected eye.

MANAGEMENT
Conservative treatment
• No treatment is indicated if the patient is not troubled by diplopia; this is most likely in cases of mild palsies when the field of binocular single vision is reduced only on up-gaze.

• The use of prisms may be effective in long-standing cases in which a spread of concomitance has occurred.

• Sector occlusion to the upper part of the spectacle lens of the affected eye can relieve diplopia on up-gaze and allow binocular single vision to be maintained in other fields of gaze.

Surgical treatment
Strabismus surgery should always be carried out prior to ptosis repair. Surgery is not usually required for diplopia that is only present on up-gaze unless it is interfering with the patient's occupation or leisure activities. Surgery to relieve diplopia on up-gaze may result in it occurring on down-gaze and even in the primary position. The type of surgical procedure depends on the amount of residual superior rectus muscle function and on the type of muscle sequelae that has developed.

Mild superior rectus weakness (Figs 19.4 & 19.5): This can be associated with:

• An incomitant deviation with overaction of the contralateral inferior oblique muscle, which should be weakened in the first instance.

• Concomitance with a significant deviation present in down-gaze and in the contralateral field of gaze: If

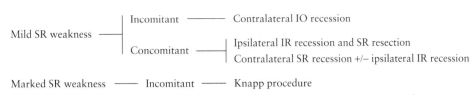

Mild SR weakness ── Incomitant ──── Contralateral IO recession

Concomitant ──── Ipsilateral IR recession and SR resection
Contralateral SR recession +/− ipsilateral IR recession

Marked SR weakness ──── Incomitant ──── Knapp procedure

Tree 19.3 Surgical options to correct the vertical deviation in third nerve palsy involving the superior division.

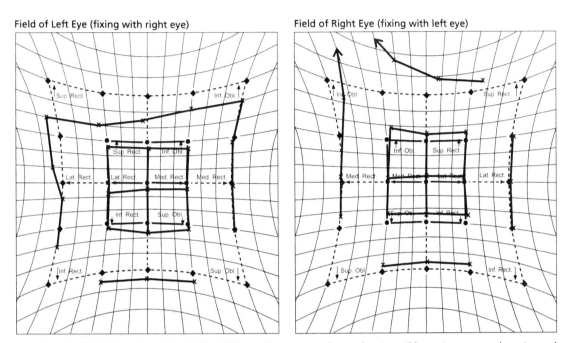

Field of Left Eye (fixing with right eye)

Field of Right Eye (fixing with left eye)

Fig. 19.4 Hess chart of a patient with an isolated left superior rectus weakness, showing mild superior rectus underaction and contralateral inferior oblique overaction.

the deviation is less than 15 Δ in the primary position, we recommend recession of the contralateral superior rectus. If the deviation is greater than 15 Δ, then the ipsilateral inferior rectus should also be recessed. An alternative approach is to perform an ipsilateral inferior rectus recession and superior rectus resection.

Marked superior rectus weakness (Fig. 19.6): In this situation there is significant paresis of the superior rectus muscle. The first procedure should be a forced duction test to confirm that the ipsilateral inferior rectus is not causing mechanical restriction. In the presence of a negative forced duction test we recommend performing an ipsilateral Knapp procedure: a subclinical paresis of the ipsilateral inferior rectus may be uncovered by this procedure resulting in diplopia in down-gaze; the patient should be warned of this risk before proceeding with surgery. If further

improvement in the field of binocular single vision on up-gaze is required following this procedure, surgery to reduce the action of the overacting contralateral inferior oblique or superior rectus can be carried out.

Inferior division palsy (Fig. 19.7)

This condition is very rare. The medial rectus, inferior rectus and inferior oblique muscles are affected in addition to the sphincter pupillae and ciliary muscle.

FEATURES

The features are as follows:
• the affected eye is exotropic, intorted and hypertropic with dilatation of the pupil;
• there is overaction of the contralateral lateral rectus, superior rectus and superior oblique muscles;

Field of Left Eye (fixing with right eye) Field of Right Eye (fixing with left eye)

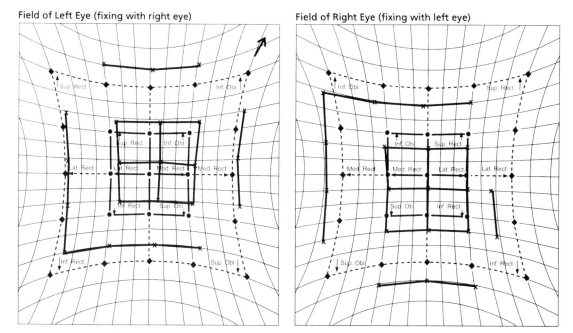

Fig. 19.5 Hess chart of a patient with an isolated right superior rectus weakness. There is a spread of concomitance and the vertical deviation measures approximately equal in all positions of gaze.

Field of Left Eye (fixing with right eye) Field of Right Eye (fixing with left eye)

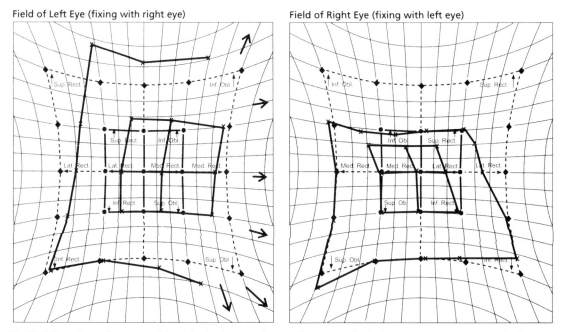

Fig. 19.6 Hess chart of a patient with a right third nerve palsy mainly involving both elevators (superior rectus and inferior oblique) with mild limitation of the inferior rectus and a partial right lateral rectus palsy. There is an A-pattern on attempted up-gaze as a result of aberrant innervation to the right medial rectus muscle.

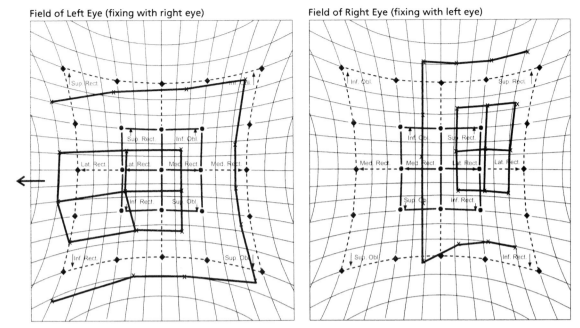

Field of Left Eye (fixing with right eye)   Field of Right Eye (fixing with left eye)

Fig. 19.7 Hess chart of a patient with a right inferior divisional third nerve palsy. The medial and inferior rectus are involved with no apparent involvement of the inferior oblique muscle.

- there is unlikely to be any field of binocular single vision, therefore no need for a head posture;
- accommodation is defective in the affected eye.

MANAGEMENT
The management options are similar to those offered to patients with an incomplete palsy of all the extraocular muscles supplied by the third nerve (see above for further details).

Third nerve palsy affecting single muscles
Acquired palsies affecting single muscles are relatively uncommon; the inferior rectus followed by the superior rectus are those most frequently encountered in our practice. Each can be simulated by other conditions and should be differentiated from them. Treatment is indicated if the condition is symptom-producing or results in a poor appearance. Management can be conservative, using prisms or botulinum toxin, or surgical. Surgical options are discussed below.

Medial rectus muscle
An isolated acquired medial rectus muscle palsy is extremely rare. Most acquired cases in which this is apparent are due either to internuclear ophthalmoplegia, myasthenia gravis or a mechanical condition such as Duane's retraction syndrome or a medial wall blow-out fracture.

FEATURES
The features are given below.
- The affected eye will be exotropic, and the exotropia increases for near fixation. Overaction of the contralateral lateral rectus will be present, and contracture of the ipsilateral lateral rectus and secondary inhibitional palsy of the contralateral medial rectus muscle may be observed (Fig. 19.8).
- There will be a face turn towards the unaffected side if a field of binocular single vision can be achieved.

MANAGEMENT
Further management depends on whether the palsy is total or partial.

Partial palsy
The procedure of choice is a recession of the lateral rectus and a resection of the medial rectus, both in the affected eye.

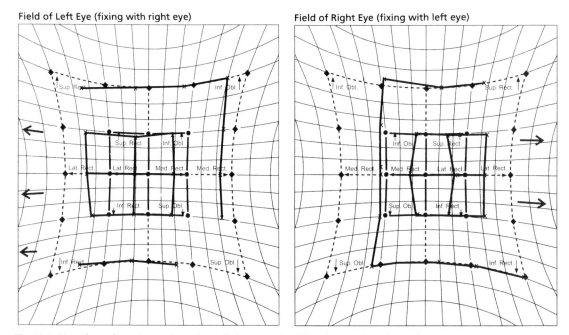

Field of Left Eye (fixing with right eye)   **Field of Right Eye (fixing with left eye)**

Fig. 19.8 Hess chart of a patient with a right medial rectus palsy. There is contralateral lateral rectus overaction.

Total palsy

In this situation a medial transposition of the vertical recti to the insertion site of the paralysed medial rectus combined with a lateral rectus recession or botulinum toxin injection is recommended. The vertical recti need to be resected at the time of transposition to compensate for the slackening that occurs in these muscles.

Inferior rectus muscle

Both congenital and acquired palsies are seen; bilateral involvement is not unusual in congenital cases.

The differential diagnosis in an acquired palsy includes myasthenia gravis, skew deviation and mechanical limitation. Inferior rectus palsy can occur as an isolated acquired phenomenon, possibly related to a vascular insult to the third nerve nucleus or, rarely, from a brainstem tumour (Pusateri *et al.* 1987).

FEATURES

The features are summarized as follows.

• There will be hypertropia and possibly a slight exotropia of the affected eye. An A-pattern suggests bilateral involvement. Full development of muscle sequelae will result in overaction of the contralateral superior oblique, contracture of the ipsilateral superior rectus and secondary inhibitional palsy of the contralateral inferior oblique.

• The chin will be depressed. Few patients show a head tilt (von Noorden & Hansell 1991): if present it is usually to the unaffected side to compensate for the hypertropia or, more rarely, to the affected side to compensate for torsion.

• The Bielschowsky head tilt test should result in the greatest vertical deviation when tilting the head to the unaffected side. However, paradoxical responses are common and the test is unreliable in this disorder, although it can help differentiate an inferior rectus palsy from a contralateral inferior oblique palsy (see Fig. 19.13).

MANAGEMENT

Conservative management with prisms is not always effective due to the incomitant nature of the deviation. However, prisms may prove useful in those cases in which concomitance has spread into the contralateral field of gaze.

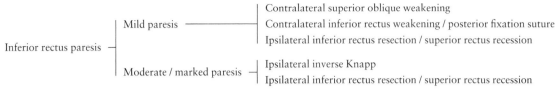

Tree 19.4 Surgical options to correct the vertical deviation in inferior rectus palsy.

The type of surgical procedure depends on the amount of residual inferior rectus muscle function and the types of muscle sequelae that have developed.

General surgical principles

The type of surgical procedure can be categorized according to which eye is operated on:

Surgery on the affected eye:
• Resection of the inferior rectus and recession of the superior rectus muscle (von Noorden & Hansell 1991).
• Augmenting the action of the affected inferior rectus muscle by performing an inverse Knapp procedure.

Surgery on the fellow eye:
• Balancing the defect by:
 1 weakening the contralateral superior oblique;
 2 recession of the contralateral inferior rectus with or without a posterior fixation suture, which is reserved for cases in which concomitance has spread into the contralateral field of gaze.

Surgical treatment

The two main subtypes of inferior rectus palsy seen clinically are:
• inferior rectus muscle underaction associated with only mild muscle paresis;
• moderate to marked inferior rectus palsy.

Inferior rectus muscle underaction with only mild muscle palsy (Fig. 19.9): An inferior rectus underaction is seen in skew deviation without associated inferior rectus paresis.

Surgery on the contralateral eye aiming to balance the defect consists of:
• A weakening procedure of the overacting superior oblique muscle using a posterior tenotomy or performing a complete tenotomy with a tendon spacer. A complete tenotomy carries the risk of postoperative torsional diplopia.
• Occasionally, the deviation on down-gaze appears almost concomitant, with a significant vertical devi-

ation present in the contralateral field of gaze. In these cases surgery on the contralateral inferior rectus muscle is indicated (Saunders 1984).

Surgery on the affected eye involves:
• A resection of the inferior rectus, combined with a superior rectus recession if necessary.

Moderate to marked inferior rectus palsy (Fig. 19.10): This is by far the more common situation in our experience.

Surgery on the affected eye consists of:
• An inverse Knapp procedure: this optimizes both the range of ocular movement and the potential field of binocular single vision. The improvement in the field of binocular single vision can take 3–6 months to become apparent, therefore no further intervention should be planned until at least 6 months have elapsed. If further surgery is required, it can focus on balancing the defect by weakening any overaction of the contralateral superior oblique or inferior rectus muscle.
• Resection of the affected inferior rectus muscle with or without a recession of its ipsilateral antagonist, the superior rectus muscle, is an alternative approach when there is residual inferior rectus function (von Noorden & Hansell 1991).

When the vertical deviation in the primary position is less than 5 Δ, the inverse Knapp procedure runs the risk of reversal of the deviation in both the primary position and in contralateral gaze. It is preferable in this situation to direct surgery at the contralateral eye, aiming to balance the defect.

Superior rectus muscle

Superior rectus underaction, usually bilateral, is a common feature of V-pattern exotropia and is usually congenital in origin. Not infrequently, the superior rectus underaction passes unnoticed until the patient undergoes an eye movement assessment, when diplopia is observed on extreme elevation. We have also seen patients who were required to wear a

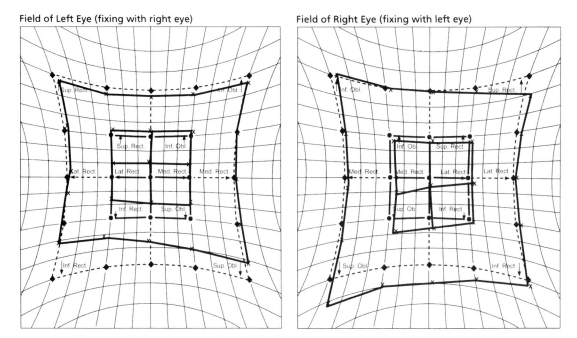

Fig. 19.9 Hess chart of a patient with a mild left inferior rectus palsy. There is contralateral superior oblique overaction.

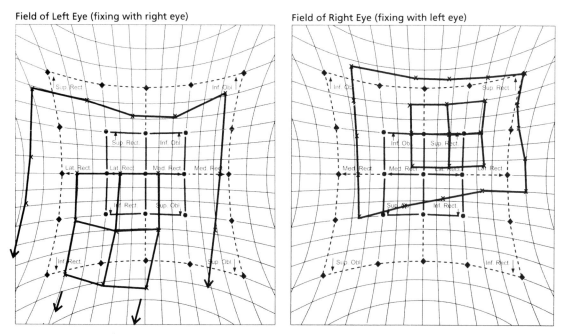

Fig. 19.10 Hess chart of a patient with a marked right inferior rectus palsy. There is a large vertical deviation in the primary position and spread of concomitance into the contralateral lower field.

supporting neck collar following an injury to the cervical spine; the resulting restriction of head movement necessitated more extreme eye movements and made them aware of long-standing superior rectus muscle weakness.

The characteristics and management of superior rectus muscle palsy are the same as those of a superior divisional palsy, as described earlier in this chapter.

DIFFERENTIAL DIAGNOSIS OF SUPERIOR
RECTUS AND CONTRALATERAL SUPERIOR
OBLIQUE PALSY (Fig. 19.11)
The differential diagnosis is based on:
• Comparison of the amount of vertical deviation in extreme positions of gaze by the use of the alternate cover test: this may show that the deviation increases on dextrodepression, indicating a left superior oblique palsy, rather than on dextroelevation as it would in a primary right superior rectus underaction. If the full muscle sequelae have developed, the differential diagnosis of the primary underacting muscle is often difficult and the diagnosis must be based on the preponderance of features outlined below.

• Inspection of the outer fields of the Hess chart.
• The patient's fixation preference: the majority of patients fixate with the unaffected eye.
• Excyclotorsion of the globe: a primary acquired underaction of the superior oblique is more likely to result in excyclotorsion and is the probable diagnosis if this is present. Although extorsion is rarely if ever demonstrable subjectively in congenital superior oblique palsy, it can often be seen objectively by fundus photography.
• Comparison of the near and distance vertical deviation: hypertropia that increases for near fixation suggests a superior oblique palsy. If the muscle sequelae are fully developed, the deviation may be the same for both distances.
• Compensatory head posture: the chin should be elevated in a superior rectus palsy and depressed in a superior oblique palsy, but if concomitance develops due to the muscle sequelae this tends to disappear, leaving only the head tilt and face turn.
• Partial upper-lid ptosis may be present on the affected side in superior rectus palsy.
• Bielschowsky head tilt test: a positive result indicates

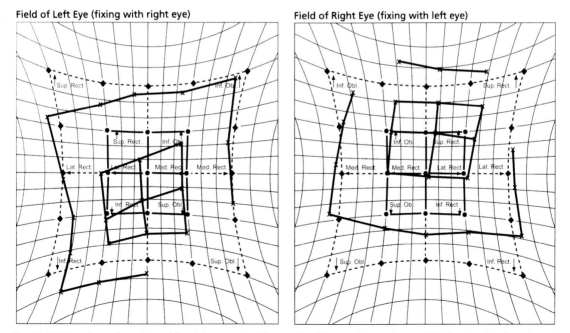

Fig. 19.11 Hess chart of a patient with a right superior oblique palsy. The muscle sequelae are fully developed with ipsilateral inferior oblique overaction, contralateral inferior rectus overaction and superior rectus underaction.

a superior oblique palsy, but a negative result does not always imply a primary superior rectus palsy.

Inferior oblique muscle

An isolated inferior oblique palsy, either congenital or acquired, is very rare. Post-traumatic cases have been reported (Muchnick *et al.* 1985) and we have seen cases due to myasthenia gravis. Congenital underaction affecting one or both muscles is a feature of A-pattern esotropia. Inferior oblique palsy must be differentiated from Brown's syndrome, which is relatively common and must be considered the probable diagnosis until proved otherwise.

FEATURES

The features are summarized as follows.

• The affected eye will be hypotropic, intorted and may be slightly esotropic. An A-pattern is probable in bilateral cases. Overaction of the contralateral superior rectus and contracture of the ipsilateral superior oblique are seen, with secondary inhibitional palsy of the contralateral inferior rectus (Figs 19.12 & 19.13).

• If present, the field of binocular single vision will be displaced down and to the unaffected side: there will be a head tilt to the affected side and face turn to the normal side with chin elevation.

MANAGEMENT

A negative forced duction test at the time of surgery will confirm the diagnosis and exclude Brown's syndrome. Surgery can be undertaken on the unaffected eye to balance the defect or on the ipsilateral antagonist, the superior oblique muscle.

Surgery on the unaffected eye

The contralateral superior rectus is recessed (Pollard 1993). This can be combined with a resection of the contralateral inferior rectus if the primary position deviation is large.

Surgery on the affected eye

The ipsilateral superior oblique can be weakened (Oliver & von Noorden 1982b), ideally using a controlled tenotomy and tendon spacer. It may be possible to restore binocular single vision in the primary

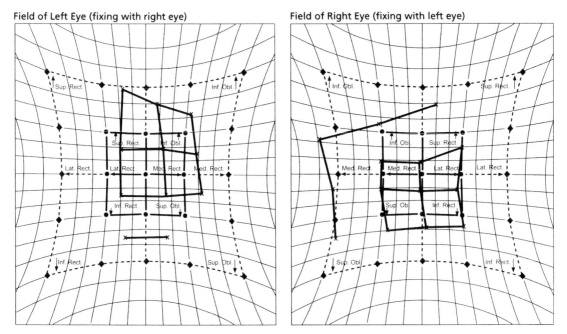

Fig. 19.12 Hess chart of a patient with a right inferior oblique palsy. There is a hypotropia in the primary position and contralateral superior rectus overaction.

Field of Left Eye (fixing with right eye)   Field of Right Eye (fixing with left eye)

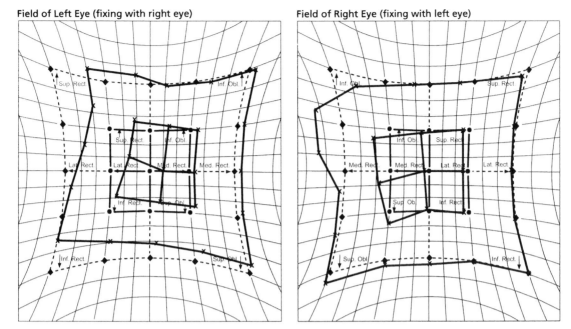

Fig. 19.13 Hess chart of a patient with a left inferior rectus palsy showing contralateral inferior oblique underaction as a result of fully developed muscle sequelae.

position and on down-gaze but elevation in adduction will continue to be limited.

DIFFERENTIAL DIAGNOSIS OF INFERIOR OBLIQUE PALSY AND BROWN'S SYNDROME

The differential diagnosis is based on the following observations.

• A forced duction test, demonstrating that passive movement is normal in inferior oblique palsy and restricted in Brown's syndrome.

• An A-pattern occurs in inferior oblique palsy whereas Brown's syndrome tends to show a V-pattern.

• Incyclotropia is usually present in inferior oblique palsy but not in Brown's syndrome.

• Muscle sequelae should develop as expected in inferior oblique palsy whereas development is confined to overaction of the contralateral superior rectus in Brown's syndrome. This can be seen very clearly on the Hess chart. The field of the affected eye will be displaced down in inferior oblique palsy but that of a patient with Brown's syndrome will show little or no abnormality in the primary position or in the lower field. Brown's syndrome is discussed in Chapter 21.

Aberrant regeneration (misdirection syndrome)

Aberrant regeneration is a condition in which neurological signals destined to supply one group of muscles are redirected to supply a different group.

Aetiology

Aberrant regeneration occurs as a result of injury to the nerve after it has left the brainstem. Lesions more proximal to the nucleus have been reported but are very rare. It can only occur if there is structural damage to the nerve's supporting framework as well as its axons. In one theory the axons distal to the site of injury degenerate while those proximal to the injury site grow forwards and enter the wrong myelin tubes to supply inappropriate muscles, hence the synonym of misdirection syndrome. Other mechanisms have been suggested, including reorganization of the third nerve structure at the level of the nucleus.

Incidence

Aberrant regeneration occurs in a few congenital third nerve palsies but is more common in acquired palsies due to trauma or space-occupying lesions. It may rarely be the presenting sign of a slow-growing intracranial tumour or aneurysm (Schatz *et al.* 1977; Cox *et al.* 1979), and is termed primary aberrant regeneration when there is no evidence of a preceding third nerve palsy. It does not occur when the cause is microvascular, presumably because the structural framework of the nerve remains intact in this condition.

Aberrant regeneration can take place as early as 6 weeks after the onset of the palsy but more commonly develops after 8–12 weeks have elapsed. Infants who have sustained birth trauma resulting in an oculomotor palsy will show aberrant regeneration in 4–6 weeks.

Aberrant regeneration is relatively common and is important because it both complicates the surgical management and is often sufficiently unsightly to distress the patient. Sudden eyelid elevation is invariably the main cosmetic problem, made more bizarre by a residual ptosis when the eye is in the primary position.

Features

The features are summarized as:
• elevation of the upper eyelid on down-gaze (the pseudo-von Graefe phenomenon), which usually increases on down-gaze in adduction;
• adduction of the eye on attempted up-gaze and in some cases on attempted down-gaze;
• retraction of the globe on up-gaze and/or down-gaze;
• constriction of the pupil on attempting adduction.

Management

Aberrant regeneration resulting in elevation of the upper eyelid on attempted adduction often results in temporary improvement in the appearance of a partial ptosis. If surgery is required for an associated exotropia then operating on the horizontal recti of the contralateral eye will result in an increased stimulus to the lateral rectus of this eye and its synergist, the medial rectus of the affected eye. This should result in an improvement in the ptosis and the abnormal lid movement.

Acquired and congenital fourth nerve palsies

Fourth nerve palsy results in underaction of the superior oblique muscle. Both congenital and acquired palsies are common.

Summary of aetiology

The nerve has no anatomical associations that lead to typical presentations and help to identify and localize the lesion, and the aetiology of a number of fourth nerve palsies remains unknown.

Known causes of acquired palsies include:
• closed head injury, which accounts for most acquired bilateral palsies and many unilateral palsies;
• diabetes;
• intracranial tumours;
• myasthenia gravis.

Béchac *et al.* (1984) reported four cases of bilateral fourth nerve palsy due to lesions sited close to the aqueduct of Sylvius.

There is increasing evidence that some congenital cases are due to an anatomical anomaly of the superior oblique tendon, resulting in a complete absence, an abnormal insertion or an excessively lax tendon (Plager 1990). An autosomal dominant form of inheritance of congenital superior oblique palsy has also been reported (Botelho & Giangiacomo 1996).

Features

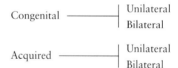

Tree 19.5 Classification of fourth nerve palsy.

Congenital fourth nerve palsies

Unilateral

Unilateral palsies may show the following features:
• The patient frequently presents with an abnormal head posture in childhood. A number of children have undergone unnecessary investigation and, in some cases, actual orthopaedic treatment for a head posture that later turns out to be due to a superior oblique palsy. All children with an abnormal head posture should initially have a full ophthalmic examination to exclude an ocular cause.
• Facial asymmetry, which is common and consists of a reduction in the distance between the lateral canthus and the corner of the mouth on the side of the head posture.

- Intermittent diplopia that can occur later in childhood or in adult life as the first symptom of decompensating congenital palsy. An abnormal head posture is common and can often be observed on old photographs, although the patient is usually unaware of it.
- A large hyperphoria, sometimes exceeding 20 Δ, with the abnormal head posture. A manifest vertical deviation is often present with the head straight. Diplopia may be appreciated; however, nonspecific symptoms are also common when the deviation is manifest; suppression may also occur. The vertical deviation will increase on near fixation.
- The horizontal deviation may be convergent or divergent.
- Absence of symptomatic excyclotorsion; objective excyclotorsion can be observed on fundus examination.
- A positive response to the Bielschowsky head tilt test is present when the head is tilted to the affected side.

Bilateral

Bilateral palsies may show the following features:
- A constant V-pattern esotropia, with hypertropia of the nonfixing eye (Hermann 1981). Any compensatory head posture is likely to be a chin depression. These patients often have associated inferior oblique muscle overaction and are not infrequently misdiagnosed as childhood primary esotropia. The presence of a positive Bielschowsky head tilt test to either side confirms a bilateral superior oblique palsy and helps in the differentiation of these patients from primary esotropia with associated inferior oblique overaction.
- Absence of symptomatic excyclotorsion, although it may be demonstrated objectively by fundus photography.
- A positive response to the Bielschowsky head tilt test, with reversal of the hypertropia on right and left tilt.

Acquired fourth nerve palsies

Most acquired fourth nerve palsies have:
- a recent onset of symptoms, principally diplopia;
- no evidence of enlarged vertical fusion reserves;
- subjective awareness of any head posture present;
- a history of significant head trauma.

Unilateral

Patients with unilateral palsies are occasionally aware of cyclotorsion, but this rarely approaches the magnitude seen in bilateral palsies. The response to the Bielschowsky head tilt test is the same as for congenital palsies.

Bilateral

Torsional diplopia is often the main symptom in symmetrical cases, invariably preventing fusion. The typical head posture in these cases is a marked and obvious chin depression, which is the only means of avoiding diplopia.

Acquired bilateral palsies show:
- Reversal of hypertropia on right and left gaze and on dextro- and laevodepression, which is diagnostic: occasionally this may be evident only on dextroelevation and laevoelevation as a result of overaction of the inferior oblique muscles. The response to the Bielschowsky head tilt is positive to either side.
- A V-pattern and symptomatic excyclotorsion, often measuring greater than 10° in the primary position (Sydnor *et al.* 1982).

Compensatory head posture

Unilateral palsy
- Head tilt to the unaffected eye.
- Face turn to the unaffected eye.
- Chin depression.
  The head tilt is adopted to overcome vertical diplopia rather than cyclotropia.

Bilateral palsy
- Chin depression which is often marked and difficult to maintain.
- Head tilt and face turn to less-affected side in asymmetrical cases, usually with some chin depression.

Investigations

Investigating cyclotorsion
- It is important to question the patient about image tilt during binocular viewing; this will only be appreciated in the fields of gaze where diplopia is present. A subjective measurement of any cyclotorsion should be made in the cardinal positions of gaze. We prefer to use the major amblyoscope for this purpose, as it is easy to combine measurement of cyclotorsion with measurement of the horizontal and vertical

deviation. The double Maddox rod provides a reliable alternative.

• Patients with congenital palsies rarely report image tilt, although we have found subjective torsion in a few patients when specifically questioned. Cyclotorsion increases on down-gaze and is least on up-gaze.

• Cyclotorsion is a barrier to fusion and its effect on the potential for binocular single vision should be assessed in the cardinal positions of gaze. To do this the horizontal and vertical components of the deviation must be neutralized, either using prisms or the major amblyoscope: the latter has the advantage of also neutralizing cyclotorsion, making it easier to confirm the patient's fusional ability. Most patients with acquired palsies should be able to fuse 6–8° of unilateral cyclotorsion. Insuperable cyclotorsion will require surgical correction to re-establish fusion. Central disruption of fusion occasionally follows a post-traumatic fourth nerve palsy: surgery is unlikely to relieve diplopia in these cases, although Pratt-Johnson and Tillson (1987) reported that the outcome was not always totally unfavourable.

Medical investigation

This is discussed in detail in Chapter 18.

Differential diagnosis

Differential diagnosis of congenital and acquired fourth nerve palsies

The differences between congenital and acquired palsies are set out in Chapter 18. Points of particular relevance to superior oblique palsy are:

• facial asymmetry is common in congenital palsy;
• old photographs may demonstrate a head posture;
• subjective cyclotropia, which is not a complaint in congenital palsy, but can usually be demonstrated in acquired palsy;
• the vertical fusion amplitude in congenital palsies with binocular single vision is usually well in excess of the normal 2–4 Δ, which is the usual finding in acquired palsies.

Differential diagnosis of unilateral and bilateral fourth nerve palsies

The differential diagnosis of unilateral and bilateral fourth nerve palsies is important in planning surgical treatment. Very asymmetrical bilateral fourth nerve palsy can mimic a unilateral palsy, especially when traumatic in origin. The bilateral nature of the defect is only revealed after surgery has been performed to correct the more obvious defect: it is therefore good practice to view every case of superior oblique palsy as potentially bilateral until proven otherwise. It is our practice to warn all patients with apparently unilateral traumatic superior oblique palsy that there is a 10% chance of a masked bilateral palsy, which will probably require further treatment.

The differential diagnosis is based on:

• Reversal of hypertropia. It is essential to perform an alternate cover test on extremes of right and left gaze, especially on dextro- and laevodepression: occasionally this may be evident only on dextroelevation and laevoelevation in some patients as a result of overaction of the inferior oblique muscles. The outer fields of the Hess screen correspond to 30° of eccentric gaze; very asymmetrical bilateral palsies may only show the characteristic reversal of hypertropia beyond this point, and it is therefore not apparent on the Hess chart.

• Degree of hypertropia. A small hypertropia in the primary position, in spite of obvious limitation of depression in adduction on one side, strongly suggests a bilateral palsy.

• The degree of excyclotropia. Scott and Kraft (1986a) considered that excyclotropia in excess of 10° in the primary position was diagnostic of bilateral palsy, while other authors have suggested the threshold for diagnosis should be 12 or 15° (Ellis & Helveston 1976; von Noorden et al. 1986). Better differentiation between a unilateral and a bilateral superior oblique palsy can be obtained from comparing the measurement of cyclotorsion in down-gaze and in the primary position; excyclotorsion of 20° or more on down-gaze has a 90% probability that the superior oblique palsy is bilateral (Kraft et al. 1993). It should be possible to detect and measure left excyclotropia when fixing with the right eye, and right excyclotropia when fixing with the left eye in bilateral palsies. However, patients with unilateral palsies can report the same type of excyclotropia in each eye if the paretic eye is consistently used for fixation, for example a right excyclotropia fixing with right and left eyes (Oliver & von Noorden 1982a). Diplopia should be assessed fixing with each eye, using a linear target, preferably held horizontally, to elicit image tilt. If the main complaint is torsional diplopia a bilateral palsy is probable. Sensory and/or motor adaptation to cyclotropia may take place with time, resulting in a decrease in subjective measurements.

• V-pattern. A large V-pattern or a Y-pattern is typical of a bilateral palsy.

• Head posture. A chin depression without head tilt suggests a bilateral palsy.

• Bielschowsky head tilt test. A bilaterally positive head tilt test with right hypertropia on right tilt and left hypertropia on left tilt confirms that the palsy is bilateral.

Classification of superior oblique palsy

The classification of superior oblique palsy is based on the degree and type of muscle sequelae (see Chapter 9 for further details).

If fully developed there will be:

• Overaction (contracture) of the ipsilateral inferior oblique, which is often the most obvious feature of a congenital palsy, and was seen in 98% of 63 patients in one series (Robb 1990).

• Overaction of the contralateral inferior rectus.

• Secondary inhibitional palsy of the contralateral superior rectus, resulting in a more concomitant vertical deviation. This sometimes makes it difficult to differentiate a primary superior oblique palsy from a primary superior rectus palsy (see above).

Management

With the exception of some traumatic palsies, there is a 90% probability that patients with isolated acquired unilateral palsies and no neurological disease will improve spontaneously within 6 months. Recovery after 12 months have elapsed is rare. Bilateral palsies rarely recover fully.

Conservative treatment

Some patients adopt an abnormal head posture to obtain a comfortable area of binocular single vision. Others either find any head posture uncomfortable or are simply unable to achieve a field of single vision. Prisms may be helpful, especially in cases in which a spread of concomitance has developed.

Surgical treatment

Surgical intervention for patients with acquired palsies should be delayed until no further recovery is seen to be taking place, which usually means that observation should be continued for 9–12 months.

Surgical management largely depends on the degree of residual superior oblique muscle paresis and the types of muscle sequelae that have developed.

Factors that have an important bearing on surgical management include:

• Whether the palsy is unilateral or bilateral: acquired bilateral palsies frequently have a V-pattern and significant cyclotorsion, requiring surgery to both eyes.

• The degree and types of muscle sequelae, which influence:

1 the amount of vertical deviation in the cardinal positions of gaze;

2 whether recession of an overacting inferior oblique will be sufficient or if surgery on other muscles will be required.

• The degree of vertical deviation, which is largely influenced by the extent of the superior oblique underaction. Up to 15–20 Δ of hypertropia can often be corrected by recession of the ipsilateral inferior oblique. A deviation exceeding 20 Δ will require in addition a reces-sion of the ipsilateral superior rectus or contralateral inferior rectus, depending on the nature of the muscle sequelae.

• The extent of superior oblique limitation: if this exceeds –2, a strengthening procedure on this muscle is generally indicated, particularly if there is a V-pattern with esotropia on down-gaze.

• Insuperable cyclotorsion will require strengthening of both or one superior oblique muscle.

• The degree of horizontal deviation:

1 if an esodeviation exceeds 10 Δ in the primary position, surgery on the cyclovertical muscles is unlikely to be sufficient to correct it and recession of the medial rectus muscles may be required;

2 a V-pattern with exotropia on up-gaze, usually associated with bilateral inferior oblique overaction, can be treated by recession of these muscles;

3 a V-pattern with esotropia on down-gaze, usually associated with significant superior oblique underaction, will require a strengthening operation on the affected muscle, or on both superior obliques

Field of Left Eye (fixing with right eye)   Field of Right Eye (fixing with left eye)

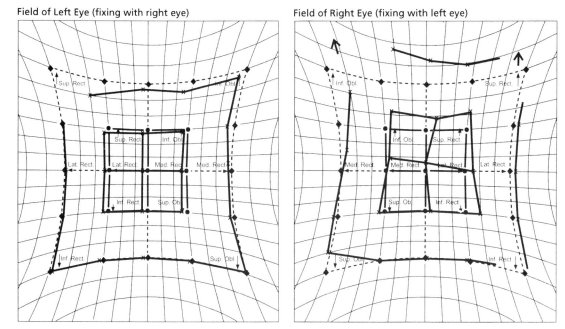

Fig. 19.14 Hess chart of a patient with a right superior oblique palsy. The muscle sequelae are limited to ipsilateral inferior oblique overaction, with minimal remaining limitation of the superior oblique.

in bilateral palsies. Alternatively the medial rectus muscles can be inferoplaced.

• The vertical fusion amplitude: most adult patients with decompensating congenital superior oblique palsy are more comfortable if surgically undercorrected, partly because of the large vertical fusion amplitude commonly found in these cases and also because an abnormal head posture is unlikely to resolve completely after successful surgery.

An excellent management plan for both unilateral and bilateral superior oblique palsies was proposed by Scott and Kraft (1986a,b) based on Knapp's original classification (Knapp 1978): we favour the surgical options proposed by these authors. Eight main categories of unilateral superior oblique palsy and five categories of bilateral palsies are described, and several subcategories are included. As a number of these subcategories are uncommon, we will concentrate on those most frequently seen in clinical practice. We include one category not described by Scott and Kraft.

The classification of unilateral superior oblique palsy is based on the known muscle sequelae that follow superior oblique paresis. The first three classes

show the greatest deviation in the field of action of either the affected superior oblique or its ipsilateral antagonist, or an equal deviation in each field. The other classes show the variable spread of concomitance that can occur in the opposite field of gaze.

Surgical treatment of unilateral superior oblique palsy

Overaction of the ipsilateral antagonist (inferior oblique) (Scott class 1)

FEATURES (Fig. 19.14)

The features are:

• no significant residual limitation or underaction of the superior oblique following recovery of function;

• ipsilateral inferior oblique overaction of +2 or more;

• a deviation in the primary position of less than 15 Δ;

• no significant deviation in the field of gaze away from affected superior oblique.

TREATMENT

The treatment of choice is a recession of the over-acting ipsilateral inferior oblique. This operation is a self-calibrating procedure, with the surgical effect increasing proportionately with the magnitude of the overaction (Dyer 1962); it is therefore effective for a wide range of inferior oblique overaction. There is little risk of reversal of the deviation following this procedure.

Overaction of the ipsilateral antagonist (inferior oblique) and contralateral synergist (inferior rectus) (Scott class 2)

FEATURES (Fig. 19.15)
The features are:
• a mild residual superior oblique underaction remaining of −1 or −2 with overaction of the contralateral inferior rectus;
• an ipsilateral inferior oblique overaction of +3 or more;
• deviation in the primary position of less than 15 Δ;
• no significant deviation in the field of gaze away from the affected superior oblique.

TREATMENT
Recession of the overacting ipsilateral inferior oblique is recommended in the first instance and is generally effective providing superior oblique function is well

preserved. If a vertical deviation persists in the field of action of the superior oblique, either a recession of the contralateral inferior rectus or a superior oblique tuck is indicated. Some young children with congenital superior oblique palsy requiring early surgery probably have an excessively lax superior oblique tendon. Because of their age, these patients are difficult to assess fully preoperatively and significant underaction of the superior oblique can be overlooked. This may be the reason why inferior oblique weakening is sometimes inadequate (Reynolds *et al*. 1984). Patients who present later probably have milder forms of tendon laxity or else the laxity plays a much less significant part.

Overaction of the contralateral synergist (inferior rectus) (Scott class 3)

FEATURES
Two subgroups exist, depending on the amount of residual weakness of the affected superior oblique.
• Mild superior oblique weakness remains as a −1 to −2 limitation.
• Moderate to marked superior oblique weakness persists with a −3 to −4 limitation. There is frequently

Field of Left Eye (fixing with right eye)

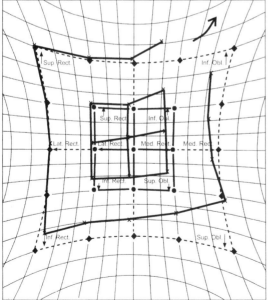

Field of Right Eye (fixing with left eye)

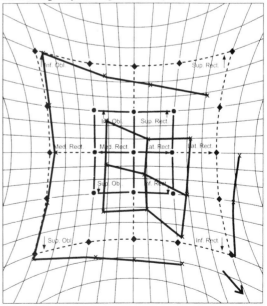

Fig. 19.15 Hess chart of a patient with a left superior oblique palsy. The muscle sequelae are fully developed with left inferior oblique overaction, contralateral inferior rectus overaction and superior rectus underaction.

Field of Left Eye (fixing with right eye)   Field of Right Eye (fixing with left eye)

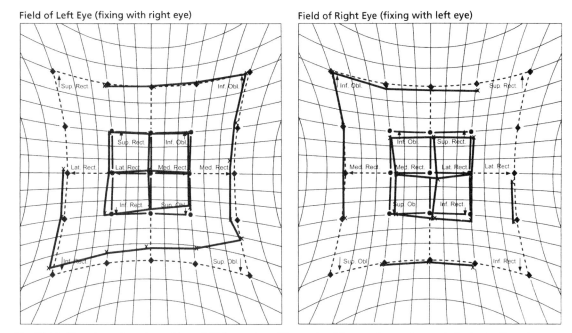

Fig. 19.16 Hess chart of a patient with a mild left superior oblique palsy. The muscle sequelae are limited to ipsilateral superior oblique underaction and contralateral inferior rectus overaction.

an associated esodeviation and V-pattern on down-gaze in addition to significant cyclotorsion.

TREATMENT

Mild superior oblique weakness (Fig. 19.16)

A recession of the overacting contralateral inferior rectus would appear to be the operation of choice. However, this can easily result in reversal of the vertical deviation in the primary position and/or on down-gaze. Three prism dioptres of vertical correction in the primary position is achieved for each millimetre recessed, increasing to 5 Δ mm^{-1} on down-gaze; therefore, even a small recession can result in an under-action and increased incomitance. We have found that if the hypertropia in the primary position exceeds 10 Δ, the risk of reversal following an inferior rectus recession of 3–4 mm is slight.

We recommend the following:

• If the deviation in the primary position is greater than 10 Δ, a recession of the contralateral inferior rectus on adjustable sutures should result in an improvement in the superior oblique underaction without significant risk of reversal.

• If the deviation in the primary position is less then 10 Δ, recession of the contralateral inferior rectus can be combined with a recession of the superior rectus in the same eye, both on adjustable sutures. The superior rectus recession reduces the risk of reversal of the deviation in the primary position (Pratt-Johnson & Tillson 1994). An alternative approach is to perform an ipsilateral superior oblique tuck.

Moderate to marked superior oblique weakness (Fig. 19.17)

This is frequently associated with an esodeviation and cyclotorsion on down-gaze; we recommend a strengthening procedure on the affected superior oblique muscle. A Harada–Ito procedure is effective in correcting the torsional component and results in some improvement in the deviation in the field of action of the affected superior oblique muscle, but it has no real effect on the vertical deviation in the primary position nor on a V-esotropia on down-gaze (Ohtsuki *et al.* 1994). The Harada–Ito procedure can be combined with a recession of the contralateral inferior rectus muscle to obtain a greater correction of the vertical

Field of Left Eye (fixing with right eye)   Field of Right Eye (fixing with left eye)

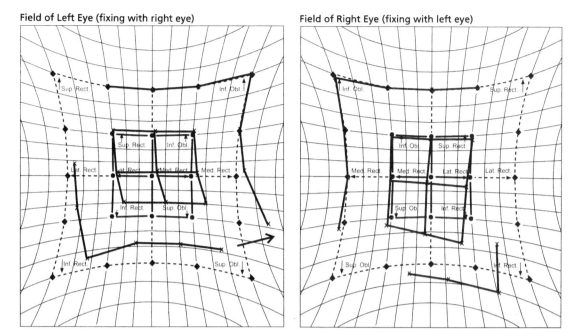

Fig. 19.17 Hess chart of a patient with a marked left superior oblique palsy. There is a V-pattern on down-gaze.

deviation (Younis *et al.* 1995). A superior oblique tuck will correct up to 10 Δ of hypertropia in the primary position and may also be more effective in correcting both the cyclotropia and the vertical deviation on down-gaze; it can, however, cause an iatrogenic Brown's syndrome (Morris *et al.* 1992). If the hypertropia in the primary position exceeds 12 Δ, a superior oblique tuck can be combined with recession of the contralateral inferior rectus muscle.

Overaction of the ipsilateral antagonist (inferior oblique) and contralateral synergist (inferior rectus) with spread of concomitance on up-gaze (Scott class 4)

FEATURES (Fig. 19.18)
The features are:
• a mild superior oblique weakness of −1 or −2 remains with an overaction of the contralateral inferior rectus;
• ipsilateral inferior oblique overaction is +2 or more;
• the vertical deviation in the primary position exceeds 15 Δ;
• a significant vertical deviation is present in the field of gaze away from the affected superior oblique, in particular in up-gaze.

TREATMENT
A recession of the overacting ipsilateral inferior oblique is not sufficient to correct the vertical deviation in the opposite field of gaze, and should therefore be combined with a recession of the ipsilateral superior rectus on adjustable sutures (Khawam *et al.* 1967). Caution is required when weakening both elevators as it is easy to cause a significant postoperative limitation of up-gaze, and it may be safer to weaken the superior rectus first, especially if the inferior oblique overaction does not exceed +2.

Overaction of the ipsilateral antagonist (inferior oblique) and contralateral synergist (inferior rectus) with spread of concomitance on down-gaze (Scott class 5)

FEATURES (Fig. 19.19)
The features are:
• a moderate residual superior oblique weakness of −2 to −3;
• ipsilateral inferior oblique overaction of +1 to +2;
• deviation in the primary position greater than 15 Δ;
• a significant deviation present in the field of gaze away from the affected superior oblique, particularly in down-gaze.

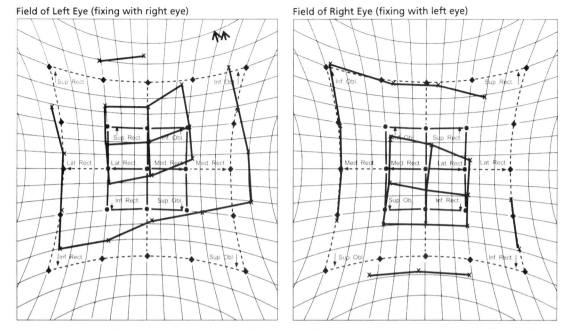

Fig. 19.18 Hess chart of a patient with a left superior oblique palsy with spread of concomitance on up-gaze. There is a large vertical deviation in the primary position and a significant deviation in the ipsilateral field of gaze.

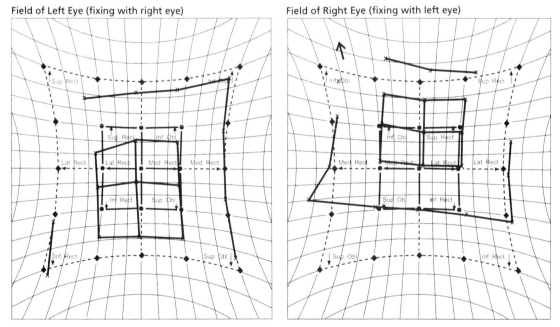

Fig. 19.19 Hess chart of a patient with a right superior oblique palsy with spread of concomitance on down-gaze. There is a large hypertropia in the primary position and a significant deviation in the ipsilateral lower field of gaze.

This group differs from the previous group in that the residual superior oblique weakness outweighs the inferior oblique overaction, resulting in a larger deviation in down-gaze. In some of these patients contracture of the ipsilateral superior rectus may be demonstrable on forced duction test, indicating a mechanical restriction of down-gaze (Jampolsky 1995).

TREATMENT

A forced duction test on down-gaze will indicate whether significant ipsilateral superior rectus contracture is present; it should be suspected if there is an overaction of the contralateral superior oblique muscle. If contraction is demonstrated, both the superior rectus and the ipsilateral inferior oblique should be recessed.

If the forced duction test is negative, Scott and Kraft (1986a) recommend a recession of the overacting ipsilateral inferior oblique combined with a recession of the overacting contralateral inferior rectus. If there is a –3 limitation in the field of action of the affected superior oblique, which may be associated with an esodeviation on down-gaze and cyclotorsion, we would recommend that the affected superior oblique muscle is strengthened with a tuck if the tendon is found to be lax at operation, or by a Harada–Ito procedure if no laxity if present. A tuck should correct up to 10 Δ of vertical deviation in the primary position. The significant deviation in the field of gaze away from the affected superior oblique will not improve with surgery on the superior oblique alone, and a recession of the contralateral inferior rectus muscle on adjustable sutures is also indicated.

Concomitant vertical deviation (Scott class 7)

FEATURES (Fig. 19.20)

Long-standing superior oblique palsies not infrequently show a considerable spread of concomitance, resulting in little variation in the vertical deviation in the different fields of gaze.

The features are:

• no significant limitation of the affected superior oblique;

• overaction of the ipsilateral inferior oblique up to +2.

TREATMENT

The treatment options depend on the amount of vertical deviation in the primary position.

Field of Left Eye (fixing with right eye)

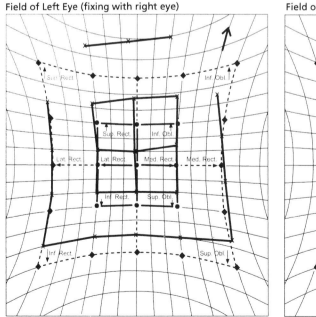

Field of Right Eye (fixing with left eye)

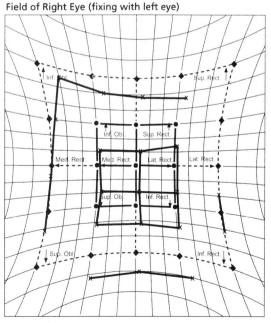

Fig.19.20 Hess chart of a patient with a left superior oblique palsy with spread of concomitance on up-gaze and down-gaze.

• If the deviation is 15 Δ or less, a recession of the ipsilateral superior rectus on adjustable sutures is indicated.

• If it is greater than 15 Δ, a recession of the ipsilateral superior rectus should be combined with a recession of the contralateral inferior rectus. We prefer to put the superior rectus on an adjustable suture and use a fixed suture for the inferior rectus.

Mild amounts of preoperative ipsilateral inferior oblique overaction usually remain unchanged or may even reduce following the recommended surgery.

Surgical treatment of bilateral superior oblique palsy

Successful management can be difficult, especially if the palsy is asymmetrical. The aims of surgery should be to achieve binocular single vision in the primary position and in down-gaze.

A strengthening procedure on both the superior oblique muscles is required to correct excyclotorsion. Factors influencing the choice between a superior oblique tuck and the Harada–Ito procedure are summarized in Table 19.2.

The Harada–Ito procedure is as effective as the tuck in correcting excyclotorsion and there is little risk of a significant Brown's syndrome developing following this procedure. It will correct small amounts of vertical deviation in the field of action of the superior oblique, but if a large vertical deviation is present a tuck is the preferred choice. Treatment of the V-esotropia on down-gaze requires either a tuck or a Harada–Ito.

Bilateral superior oblique palsy can be congenital or acquired. Congenital bilateral palsies can present as a constant esotropia with a V-pattern. Surgery on the horizontal muscles is required for the esotropia, and if the inferior oblique muscles are overacting these should be weakened or, if not overacting, the medial recti can be inferoplaced to improve the V-pattern.

Bilateral acquired superior oblique palsy is categorized into symmetrical or asymmetrical for the purpose of treatment.

Symmetrical palsies

These are categorized on the features of the V-pattern, showing an exodeviation on moving from the primary position to up-gaze, an esodeviation from the primary position to down-gaze or a combination of both findings. A further group of patients have insuperable cyclotorsion without a significant horizontal or vertical deviation in the primary position.

V-PATTERN EXODEVIATION ON UP-GAZE

This is an uncommon situation, the features are the same as for a unilateral palsy associated with overaction of the ipsilateral antagonist (Scott's class 1).

Features (Fig. 19.21)
The features are:
• no significant cyclotorsion;
• bilateral inferior oblique overaction with V-pattern exodeviation on up-gaze;
• no significant residual limitation or underaction of the superior oblique following recovery of function.

	Superior oblique tuck	Harada–Ito
Vertical deviation corrected (in the field of action of superior oblique)	15 Δ (0–40 Δ)	5 Δ
Iatrogenic Brown's	16%	Insignificant
Cyclotorsion (primary position)	10 degrees	10 degrees
V-esotropia	15 Δ	12 Δ

Table 19.2 Effect of alternative bilateral strengthening procedures on the superior oblique muscle.

Field of Left Eye (fixing with right eye)　　　　Field of Right Eye (fixing with left eye)

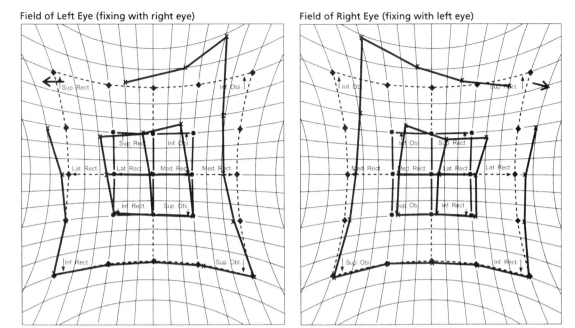

Fig. 19.21 Hess chart of a patient with symmetrical bilateral superior oblique palsy. There is a V-pattern exotropia on up-gaze and the muscle sequelae are limited to bilateral inferior oblique overaction with full recovery of superior oblique function.

Treatment

Treatment consists of bilateral inferior oblique recession.

V-PATTERN ESODEVIATION ON DOWN-GAZE

The features are the same as for a unilateral palsy associated with overaction of the contralateral synergist and moderate to marked limitation in the field of action of the superior oblique (Scott's class 3).

Features (Fig. 19.22)

The features are:

• significant excyclotorsion, greatest on depression of gaze;

• V-pattern with esotropia on down-gaze.

Treatment

The treatment of choice is bilateral superior oblique strengthening. A superior oblique tuck will help correct the V-esotropia on down-gaze, which is less likely to respond to a Harada–Ito procedure. Postoperatively a residual V-pattern esotropia frequently persists

on down-gaze; this can be treated by bilateral inferior placement of the medial rectus muscles.

V-PATTERN EXODEVIATION ON UP-GAZE AND
V-PATTERN ESODEVIATION ON DOWN-GAZE

This subgroup combines the features of the two categories described above.

Features (Fig. 19.23)

The features are:

• significant excyclotorsion, greatest on down-gaze;

• V-pattern esotropia on down-gaze;

• bilateral inferior oblique overaction with V-pattern exotropia on up-gaze.

Treatment

The treatment is bilateral inferior oblique recession combined with a bilateral superior oblique strengthening procedure, preferably using a tuck.

CYCLOTORSION

A significant amount of excyclotorsion is present,

Field of Left Eye (fixing with right eye)   Field of Right Eye (fixing with left eye)

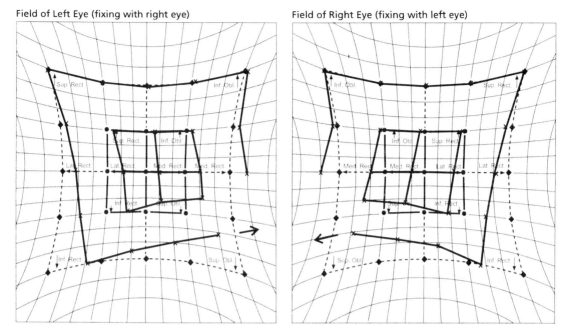

Fig. 19.22 Hess chart of a patient with symmetrical bilateral superior oblique palsy. There is a V-pattern esotropia on down-gaze associated with bilateral superior oblique underaction.

Field of Left Eye (fixing with right eye)   Field of Right Eye (fixing with left eye)

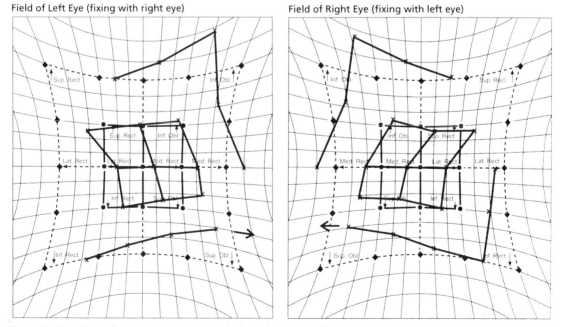

Fig. 19.23 Hess chart of a patient with symmetrical bilateral superior oblique palsy. There is a V-pattern esotropia on down-gaze with bilateral superior oblique underaction and a V-pattern exotropia on up-gaze with bilateral inferior oblique overaction.

preventing fusion. There is often no significant vertical or horizontal deviation in any position of gaze.

Features (Figs 19.24 & 19.25)
The features are:
• significant excyclotorsion, greatest in down-gaze;
• no V-pattern or superior oblique underaction.

Treatment
The treatment of choice is a bilateral Harada–Ito procedure that will correct the excyclotorsion without influencing the vertical and horizontal deviation.

Asymmetrical palsies

These are asymmetrical forms of the above first three categories (Fig. 19.26). Management is especially difficult and is generally based on performing symmetrical bilateral inferior oblique recessions in the presence of asymmetrical bilateral inferior oblique overaction. If there is also asymmetrical bilateral superior oblique limitation a superior oblique tuck is performed on the eye with the greater involvement, using a Harada–Ito procedure on the less involved eye. Further surgery is frequently required.

Masked bilateral palsy

The term 'masked bilateral superior oblique palsy' should be reserved for cases which show evidence of superior oblique dysfunction in the contralateral eye following surgery for an apparently unilateral palsy (Fig. 19.27). This condition was first described by Jampolsky (1971). The dysfunction may take the form of superior oblique underaction, inferior oblique overaction, excyclotorsion or a positive Bielschowsky head tilt test: more than one feature may be present. The unmasking may be evident within a few weeks of the initial surgery or may take some months to develop. The pathophysiology remains unknown. This condition must be distinguished from overcorrection of a unilateral palsy.

The reported incidence of masked bilateral superior oblique palsy varies according to the population studies; it is generally higher in traumatic palsies. Price *et al.* (1987), reviewing their series of acquired bilateral superior oblique palsy, concluded that about 38% were initially masked; in contrast, 3% of masked palsies were found in a series of idiopathic bilateral palsies in children (Robb 1990).

TREATMENT
Treatment is required if the palsy is symptom producing or causing cosmetic concern. Conservative management involves:
• reassurance, which is often necessary when explaining the situation, especially if diplopia is present;
• reinforcement of the use of a small compensatory head posture;
• prisms;
• surgical treatment, which is the same as for a unilateral palsy.

Atypical situations associated with superior oblique palsy

Atypical situations are occasionally seen in association with superior oblique palsy. These include:
• Underaction of the ipsilateral inferior oblique muscle: Spencer and Harcourt (1984) reported a delayed onset of ipsilateral inferior oblique weakness in approximately 9% of consecutive cases of acquired fourth nerve palsy. The underaction became apparent some weeks or months after the onset of the palsy and coincided with some recovery of superior oblique function. Although the condition resembled Brown's syndrome, some cases were nontraumatic, and in others there was no evidence of periorbital trauma. The authors postulated that there was perhaps more widespread cranial nerve damage which remained masked until recovery of the fourth nerve palsy began.
• Overaction of the contralateral superior oblique: von Noorden (1986) reported this finding in 19% of patients with unilateral superior oblique palsy; this was attributed to contracture of the ipsilateral superior rectus.
• Excyclotropia of the nonparetic eye in unilateral palsy: patients with unilateral superior oblique palsy who habitually fixate with the nonparetic eye may show subjective excyclotropia of this eye. It is believed that this phenomenon is due to a monocular sensorial adaptation to the cyclodeviation (Oliver & von Noorden 1982a).
• Congenital absence of the superior oblique tendon: absence of the superior oblique tendon should be anticipated in patients with congenital or long-standing superior oblique palsy when planning surgery. Two surgical strategies should be available, the first to be used if the tendon is found and the second if the tendon is absent. Previous studies indicate that

Field of Left Eye (fixing with right eye)

Field of Right Eye (fixing with left eye)

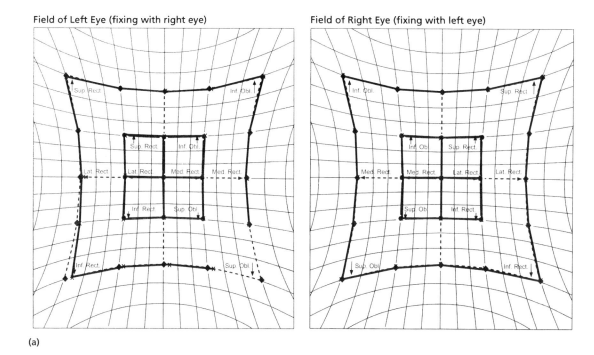

(a)

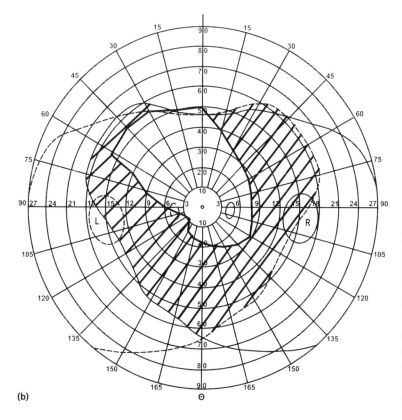

(b)

Fig. 19.24 (a) Hess chart of a patient with bilateral superior oblique palsy without a significant vertical or horizontal deviation. The major amblyoscope measurements (Fig. 19.25) show the high level of excyclotorsion. (b) Field of binocular single vision of the same patient showing diplopia in all down-gaze positions due to insuperable excyclotorsion.

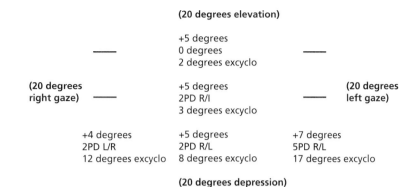

(20 degrees elevation)

	+5 degrees	
——	0 degrees	——
	2 degrees excyclo	

(20 degrees right gaze) —— +5 degrees / 2PD R/I / 3 degrees excyclo —— (20 degrees left gaze)

Fig. 19.25 Major amblyoscope measurements for same patient as Fig. 19.24.

+4 degrees	+5 degrees	+7 degrees
2PD L/R	2PD R/L	5PD R/L
12 degrees excyclo	8 degrees excyclo	17 degrees excyclo

(20 degrees depression)

congenital absence of the tendon should be suspected if there is:

1 a superior oblique palsy with an associated horizontal deviation;

2 an unusually large vertical deviation, with spread of concomitance and evidence of overaction of the contralateral superior oblique muscle;

3 amblyopia;

4 persistent underaction of the superior oblique muscle and a marked head tilt after ipsilateral inferior oblique recession.

Surgical treatment of the vertical deviation depends on the spread of concomitance and on the results of preoperative forced duction testing. It can include weakening of the ipsilateral inferior oblique, the ipsilateral superior rectus and the contralateral inferior rectus muscles (Wallace & von Noorden 1994).

Postoperative management
Undercorrections
A change in the alignment often continues for several months following an inferior oblique recession.

Field of Left Eye (fixing with right eye)　　　Field of Right Eye (fixing with left eye)

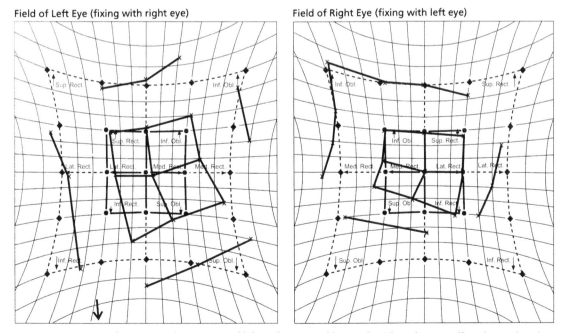

Fig. 19.26 Hess chart of a patient with asymmetrical bilateral superior oblique palsy. The right eye is affected more than the left and there is a V-pattern esotropia on down-gaze.

Field of Left Eye (fixing with right eye)   Field of Right Eye (fixing with left eye)

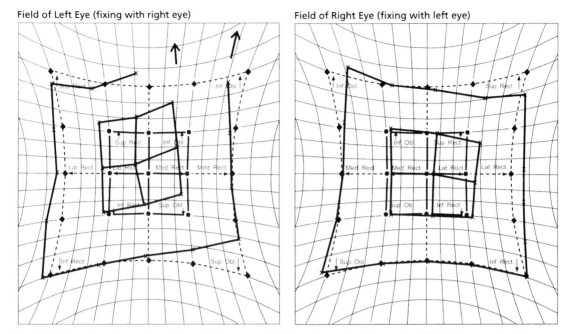

Fig. 19.27 Hess chart of a patient with marked asymmetrical bilateral superior oblique palsy. Slight right superior oblique underaction and inferior oblique overaction are evident in the outer field.

Occasionally, little improvement is seen on the first postoperative day but a few weeks later all evidence of inferior oblique overaction has disappeared. Similarly, in Scott's class 2 with inferior oblique overaction and superior oblique underaction, postoperative improvement in superior oblique action after an inferior oblique recession can take a month or two to become apparent.

The further management of undercorrection depends on the type of deviation present and may be conservative or surgical. Time should be allowed for these possible changes.

Overcorrection

Overcorrection may occur in the primary position or on eccentric gaze. The risk of developing an overcorrection and its type are related to the underlying muscle imbalance, the muscles operated on and the amount of surgery performed. The following general points can be made.

• Overcorrection following a unilateral inferior oblique recession is only likely to occur when there is a masked bilateral palsy. An inferior oblique recession is therefore a safe procedure with little risk of worsening the condition.

• A Brown's syndrome may follow a superior oblique tuck, with reduction or reversal of the vertical deviation on elevation in adduction. All patients should be warned that this is often a 'trade-off', with any gain in single vision on down-gaze at the cost of loss of single vision on up-gaze.

• An inferior rectus recession probably carries the greatest risk of overcorrection, both in the primary position and on down-gaze. Details of how best to avoid this are discussed earlier.

• Simultaneous inferior oblique and contralateral inferior rectus weakening procedures carry a significant risk of overcorrection, with 25% reported by Robb (1990).

• A combined ipsilateral inferior oblique and superior rectus weakening procedure can occasionally result in compromised up-gaze with reversal of the deviation.

Acquired sixth nerve palsy

Sixth nerve palsy results in underaction of the lateral

rectus muscle. Acquired palsies are common, congenital palsies are rare.

Summary of aetiology

Lesions can affect any part of the nerve pathway. Localization is based on the presence of other neurological signs.

Fascicular

Demyelination, vascular disease and metastatic tumours are likely causes of fascicular damage. The sixth nerve is closely related to the seventh nerve and pyramidal tracts.

Lesions in this region result in:

• Foville's syndrome with damage to the pontine tegmentum, resulting in partial sixth nerve palsy, ipsilateral facial weakness, loss of taste of the anterior two-thirds of tongue, ipsilateral Horner's syndrome, ipsilateral facial sensory loss and ipsilateral peripheral deafness.

• Millard–Gubler syndrome with damage to the ventral pons, resulting in sixth nerve palsy and contralateral hemiplegia, with or without ipsilateral facial paralysis.

Peripheral

Causes of peripheral nerve damage are:

• Closed head injury.

• Localized compression of the nerve by a primary pituitary tumour, craniopharyngioma or meningioma in the base of the skull or close to the pituitary fossa or cavernous sinus. Aneurysms involving the basilar artery can also result in an isolated sixth nerve palsy, as can metastatic tumours. Each can present as an isolated sixth nerve palsy.

• Bacterial infection of the middle ear. This can spread to the petrous temporal bone, involving the sixth and fifth nerves, presenting as a sixth nerve palsy with ipsilateral facial pain (Gradenigo's syndrome). Antibiotic therapy has made this syndrome a rarity.

The false localizing sign

The sixth nerve is peculiarly vulnerable to damage caused by raised intracranial pressure, most likely as it passes over the apex of the petrous temporal bone. A lesion remote from the nerve, for example an occipital lobe tumour, can raise pressure. One or both sixth nerves are then subjected to traction as the rise in pressure causes a downward displacement of the brainstem. Sixth nerve palsy due to raised intracranial pressure is described as a false localizing sign because it provides no information as to the site of the lesion.

Features

The features of unilateral sixth nerve palsy are:

• An esodeviation which increases in the distance. There may be binocular single vision for near in mild cases.

• A face turn towards the affected side, more marked when looking in the distance. The head posture may be normal for near fixation. The field of binocular single vision will be displaced to the unaffected side. If abduction is absent or very restricted and the patient fixes with the affected eye there is likely to be a face turn to the affected side to allow foveal fixation.

• Patients with a mild degree of palsy can sometimes maintain binocular single vision with a chin depression.

• Secondary changes in the other horizontal rectus muscles if the muscle sequelae have fully developed, comprising:

1 overaction of the contralateral medial rectus;
2 contracture of the ipsilateral medial rectus;
3 secondary inhibitional palsy of the contralateral lateral rectus.

The features of bilateral sixth nerve palsy are:

• Usually a marked esotropia, greater for distance fixation initially but often equally marked for near in long-standing palsies.

• A face turn to the side of the fixing eye to allow foveal fixation.

• Contracture of the medial rectus muscles, often preventing abduction to the mid-line in total palsy.

Medical investigation

This is discussed in detail in Chapter 18.

Differential diagnosis

MECHANICAL DISORDERS

• Duane's syndrome is the likely diagnosis in a suspected congenital sixth nerve palsy. Careful examination should show a retraction of the globe. There is often only a small esotropia in spite of obvious limitation of abduction.

• High myopia can lead to a progressive loss of abduction; these patients may not be aware of diplopia.

• Thyroid eye disease, which nearly always shows the characteristic exophthalmos and eyelid signs.

• Orbital trauma involving a blow-out fracture of the medial orbital wall, which can usually be differentiated by the history and CT scan.

OTHERS

• Infantile esotropia not infrequently has pseudo-abduction weakness, but abduction can usually be improved after spinning the child around or occluding the contralateral eye for a few hours. In cases where abduction fails to improve, a forced duction test under ketamine anaesthesia can differentiate limitation of abduction due to medial rectus contracture from lateral rectus palsy.

• Symptom-producing esophoria of the divergence weakness type can easily be differentiated from sixth nerve palsy by the absence of lateral incomitance and by normal saccadic velocities.

• Myasthenia gravis can mimic a neurogenic palsy and should always be considered.

Differentiating between a total and a partial sixth nerve palsy

Identifying whether the lateral rectus muscle is totally paralysed or has residual function is important in planning surgical treatment. Important factors to consider include:

• the presence of abduction past the mid-line, which indicates residual lateral rectus function and identifies a partial palsy;

• failure to abduct past the mid-line can be the result of a total palsy or can be caused by mechanical restriction due to contracture of the ipsilateral medial rectus.

The identification of residual lateral rectus function in this situation depends on:

• The forced generation test: a local anaesthetic is instilled and the conjunctiva is grasped at the nasal limbus with the eye adducted. The patient is instructed to abduct the eye: if there is residual lateral rectus function, the examiner can feel a tug on the forceps (Scott 1971). The test can also be performed in a less invasive fashion by placing a cotton tip bud on the temporal limbus and instructing the patient to abduct the eye.

• Botulinum toxin injection: botulinum toxin injected into a contracted medial rectus will reduce the contracture in most instances: abduction beyond the mid-line should then be possible in a partial palsy. In long-standing cases of sixth nerve palsy with marked medial rectus contracture residual lateral rectus function may only become apparent after the injection (Riordan-Eva & Lee 1992).

• Saccadic velocity analysis: saccadic velocity assessment within the available field of movement can help differentiate between a total and a partial palsy of the lateral rectus muscle.

• Electromyography: the action potentials within the lateral rectus muscle can be recorded using electromyography; an increased signal in the muscle as the eye attempts to abduct indicates residual lateral rectus function.

Differentiating between a unilateral and a bilateral sixth nerve palsy

Differentiation is based on:

• an incomitant esotropia increasing on both right and left gaze, which suggests a bilateral palsy;

• full development of muscle sequelae in a long-standing unilateral palsy, which results in inhibition of the lateral rectus in the unaffected eye, simulating an asymmetrical bilateral palsy;

• bilateral contracture of the medial rectus muscles, which develops in long-standing total bilateral palsies;

• slow peak saccadic velocity on abduction, which can easily be assessed clinically and provides a reliable indicator of unilateral or bilateral palsy;

• a V-pattern esotropia, which is more likely in the presence of a bilateral palsy.

Classification and management

Sixth nerve palsy can be unilateral or bilateral, total or partial. Management can be conservative or surgical.

Conservative treatment

Conservative treatment is indicated in the early period following the onset of the palsy, but may also be useful later once the condition has stabilized. Acquired palsies should be managed conservatively for the first 9–12 months, or until stabilization has occurred.

Early-stage treatment

This is aimed at the relief of diplopia and an uncomfortable head posture. The problem of medial rectus contracture complicating future surgical management should be considered; the role of botulinum toxin in its prevention is discussed below.

RELIEF OF SYMPTOMS

The options available include prisms, occlusion and botulinum toxin.

• Prisms are effective in mild palsies or when the development of muscle sequelae has resulted in a more concomitant deviation. Fresnel prisms are the most convenient, dividing the strength between the two eyes if necessary. Higher-powered prisms may in some instances have more of an occluding effect rather than promoting binocular single vision in some patients. If diplopia is only present in the distance, Fresnel prisms can be attached to the upper half of spectacles.

• Occlusion may occasionally be the only way of relieving the symptoms, in addition to hiding the esotropia. Sector occlusion of the nasal part of the spectacle lens can relieve diplopia on lateral gaze and allow binocular single vision in other gaze directions. Different grades of occluder are available in the form of Bangerter foils.

BOTULINUM TOXIN

The roles of botulinum toxin in patients with a sixth nerve palsy include the following.

• Short-term re-establishment of binocular single vision in adults and children. The use of botulinum toxin early in the course of a sixth nerve palsy is effective in re-establishing binocular single vision and relieving symptoms in a significant proportion of patients (Lee *et al.* 1994). The esotropia associated with sixth nerve palsy may result in amblyopia in children. Binocular single vision can be restored and amblyopia prevented by the early use of botulinum toxin. Caution is required when using botulinum toxin during this stage as it can interfere with monitoring recovery in lateral rectus function. Occasionally the effects of the botulinum toxin spill over to affect the superior oblique or inferior rectus muscles,

further complicating observation of change. In view of this we routinely perform neuro-imaging on all patients in whom the cause is unknown when botulinum toxin injection is planned.

• Possible prevention of irreversible medial rectus contracture. There is good evidence that the longer the duration of the lateral rectus palsy the greater the contraction of the medial rectus muscle (Lee *et al.* 1984). However, it remains controversial as to whether botulinum toxin can prevent its occurrence. We have observed cases of total lateral rectus palsy of 6 months duration which went on to complete spontaneous recovery, suggesting that in some patients at least, significant medial rectus contracture was not established at this stage. We routinely inject botulinum toxin into the ipsilateral medial rectus in an effort to prevent contracture in patients with no evidence of recovery after 6 months duration.

• Achievement of long-term cure. The use of botulinum toxin in patients with a relatively concomitant esotropia after good recovery of lateral rectus function can result in good alignment which is maintained long after the effects of the toxin have worn off: the patient apparently 'locks-on' to binocular single vision.

• As an adjunct to surgery. The ipsilateral medial rectus muscle can be weakened with botulinum toxin, and this can be combined with horizontal transposition of the vertical rectus muscles for total lateral rectus palsy (see 'Surgical treatment' below).

• Manipulation of acute surgical overcorrections (see 'Postoperative management' below).

Late-stage treatment

The conservative management options in patients with chronic sixth nerve palsy are:
• maintenance of an abnormal head posture;
• the use of Fresnel prisms or of prisms incorporated in the spectacles;
• repeat injections of botulinum toxin.

Surgical treatment

Important factors that influence the surgical management include:
• whether the palsy is unilateral or bilateral;
• if it is total or partial;
• the presence or absence of demonstrable binocular single vision.

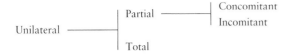

Tree 19.6 Factors influencing the choice of surgery in sixth nerve palsy.

The differences between partial and total palsies and unilateral and bilateral palsies were discussed earlier in this section.

Unilateral lateral rectus palsy

A unilateral palsy may be partial or total, when no abduction is possible. If partial it may remain incomitant or develop concomitance with time.

PARTIAL LATERAL RECTUS PALSY

The muscle sequelae may be:
• incomplete, with overaction of the contralateral medial rectus muscle resulting in an incomitant hori-

zontal deviation maximum in the direction of the lateral rectus palsy (Fig. 19.28);
• fully developed, with overaction of the contralateral medial rectus, contraction of the ipsilateral medial rectus and underaction of the contralateral lateral rectus resulting in a concomitant horizontal deviation (Fig. 19.29).

Factors determining surgical treatment

Important factors to consider include:
• The choice of surgery, which is influenced by whether the deviation is concomitant or incomitant.
• The amount of surgery, which is governed by the amount of residual lateral rectus function and the size of the deviation for near and distance. In general, larger deviations associated with little residual lateral rectus function require the greatest amount of surgery (Scott 1971).
• The forced duction test: a positive forced duction test on abduction identifies significant contracture of the medial rectus. Caution is required in this situation as significant recovery in lateral rectus function may have occurred but is masked by the mechanical

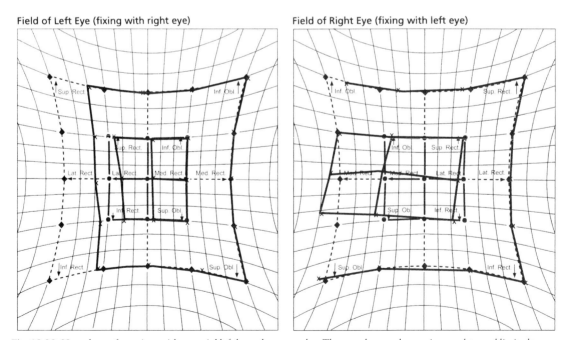

Field of Left Eye (fixing with right eye)   Field of Right Eye (fixing with left eye)

Fig. 19.28 Hess chart of a patient with a partial left lateral rectus palsy. The muscle sequelae are incomplete and limited to right medial rectus overaction.

Field of Left Eye (fixing with right eye)　　　　　　Field of Right Eye (fixing with left eye)

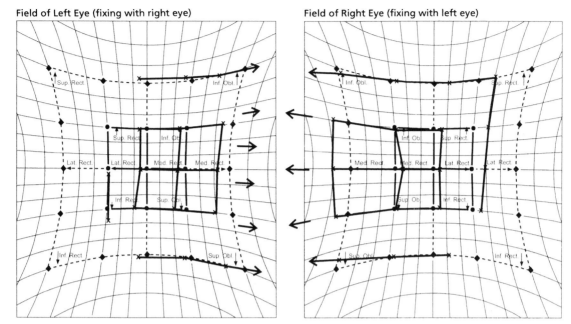

Fig. 19.29 Hess chart of a patient with a partial left lateral rectus palsy. The muscle sequelae are fully developed, with overaction of the contralateral medial rectus, contraction of the ipsilateral medial rectus and underaction of the contralateral lateral rectus resulting in a concomitant horizontal deviation.

restriction of abduction. Unless this is taken into account surgery may result in a greater than expected response.

Choice of surgery

The surgical options include the following.

• A recession of the medial rectus and resection of the lateral rectus of the affected eye. This is the recommended procedure when the deviation is relatively concomitant and measures 30 Δ or less. If the esotropia is larger than 30 Δ then consideration should be given to operating on three or more horizontal muscles.

• A recession of the medial rectus and resection of the lateral rectus of the affected eye, combined with a posterior fixation suture to the contralateral medial rectus. This is the recommended procedure when there is a significant and relatively incomitant deviation in the primary position. The addition of the posterior fixation suture serves to reduce the lateral incomitance by balancing the defect. Occasionally, medial rectus contracture will be the main reason for lateral incomitance; in this situation a recession of the contracted muscle will promote a more concomitant situation.

• A contralateral medial rectus posterior fixation suture: lateral rectus palsy can result in an esotropia on abduction with no significant deviation in the primary position or on contralateral gaze. Conventional horizontal muscle surgery could lead to overcorrection in the primary position, whereas a posterior fixation suture on the contralateral medial rectus should balance the defect on lateral gaze without altering the angle in the primary position.

Other procedures have been described, including a recession of the contralateral medial rectus and a resection of the affected lateral rectus for incomitant cases. However, a resection should not be performed on the affected lateral rectus without also relieving any contracture present in the ipsilateral medial rectus.

Outcome

Important issues to consider following surgical treatment of partial unilateral lateral rectus palsy are:

• A central area of binocular single vision, extending to down-gaze, can be established in most cases.

Field of Left Eye (fixing with right eye) **Field of Right Eye (fixing with left eye)**

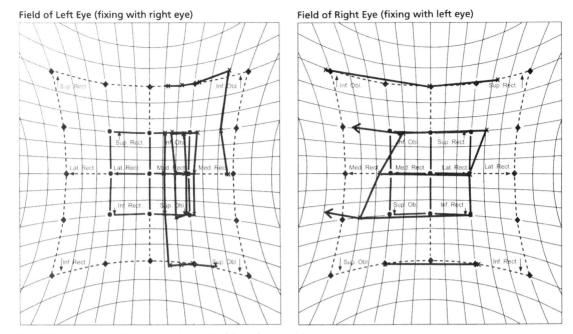

Fig. 19.30 Hess chart of a patient with a total left lateral rectus palsy.

Options
- Full-width lateral transposition of vertical rectus muscles
- Hummelsheim's operation
- Jensen's operation
- Preservation of the anterior ciliary vasculature
- Horizontal muscle surgery

Tree 19.7 Surgical options in total lateral rectus palsy.

• Resection of the lateral rectus by 4–5 mm can result in significant mechanical restriction of adduction, because the affected lateral rectus muscle fibres are frequently replaced by noncontractile fibrous tissue. The restriction will be further aggravated if the ipsilateral medial rectus is recessed at the same time, resulting in significant loss of binocular single vision on contralateral gaze.

As a precaution, we use adjustable sutures whenever possible and routinely use an adjustable suture on both the recessed and resected muscle in this group of patients.

TOTAL LATERAL RECTUS PALSY (Fig. 19.30)
In patients with no sign of recovery of lateral rectus function, surgical options are influenced by the relative risk of anterior segment ischaemia. These risk factors include:

• increasing age, with more likelihood of atheromatous risk factors such as hypertension and diabetes;
• haematological abnormalities such as sickle-cell anaemia;
• the presence of high myopia, previous retinal detachment surgery and previous strabismus surgery.

Choice of surgery
Our preferred option is a full-width lateral transposition of the vertical rectus muscles combined with a medial rectus recession.

In patients under 20 years of age we routinely recess the ipsilateral medial rectus 6 mm. In patients older than this, who may be at greater risk of developing anterior segment ischaemia, we use botulinum toxin to weaken the ipsilateral medial rectus (Fitzsimons *et al.* 1988; Rosenbaum *et al.* 1989). The muscle is injected with botulinum toxin one week before the transposition procedure to ensure that the toxin has been effective, and allow documentation of any side-effects, such as 'spill over' involving other muscles: surgery may have to be delayed if this is significant.

Procedures that attempt to preserve the vascular supply to the anterior segment are usually combined with a necessary medial rectus recession. These include:
• Hummelsheim's operation: lateral transposition of part of the vertical recti.
• Jensen's operation: postinsertion union of the vertical recti to the lateral rectus.
• Dissection of anterior ciliary vessels from the vertical recti prior to transposition (McKeown *et al.* 1989).
• Horizontal muscle surgery: a 12 mm recession of the ipsilateral medial rectus and a 12 mm resection of the affected lateral rectus combined with a traction suture to hold the eye in a position of abduction. This procedure tends to result in a relatively fixed position of the eye and a poor field of binocular single vision. It may be indicated in situations when there is no binocular potential.

Outcome

Important issues following surgical treatment of a total unilateral lateral rectus palsy are given below.
• The Hummelsheim and Jensen operations involve extensive surgical dissection which results in post-operative fibrosis and adhesions, making any reoperation difficult. We prefer to use the simpler full-width transposition procedure, which can be combined with a recession of the medial rectus muscle or with the use of botulinum toxin in patients at risk of anterior segment ischaemia.
• A central area of binocular single vision can be established, with a degree of abduction beyond the mid-line. The pre-existing contralateral field of single vision is compromised, as the operated eye often shows a −1 to −2 limitation of adduction.
• An initial postoperative exodeviation of 15–20 Δ appears to be the most favourable outcome, leading to long-term alignment.
• A postoperative vertical deviation may result from:
 1 the surgical technique: to reduce the risk of a hypertropia of the operated eye we laterally transpose the superior rectus less than the inferior rectus;
 2 a side-effect from the botulinum toxin;

3 failure to identify the presence of an associated fourth nerve palsy.

Bilateral palsy
CHOICE OF SURGERY

In general, bilateral palsies are more difficult to manage successfully than unilateral palsies. The basic surgical approach is the same as for unilateral palsies. Surgery can be performed simultaneously on both eyes, or staggered, operating first on the eye with the more marked palsy. Occasionally an operation on one eye only is successful in treating a bilateral palsy, therefore staged surgery is our preferred option in these patients.

Bilateral palsies are considered as:
• Bilateral total palsy: we recommend staggering the surgery with an initial full-width unilateral lateral transposition of the vertical recti combined with unilateral medial rectus recession (surgical or using botulinum toxin). The fellow eye is operated on in a similar way if necessary.
• Bilateral partial palsy: we recommend an initial medial rectus recession and lateral rectus resection to the eye with the greatest palsy. The fellow eye is treated in a similar way if necessary (Fig. 19.31).
• Bilateral mixed palsy (a total palsy on one side and a partial palsy on the other): the eye with the total palsy should have a full-width lateral transposition of the vertical recti combined with medial rectus recession; the eye with the partial palsy can be treated with a medial rectus recession and a lateral rectus resection if necessary. Surgery should be performed sequentially.

Postoperative management
Undercorrections

Undercorrections require treatment only if symptomatic. Further treatment may comprise the following.
• Conservative measures, using prisms if binocular single vision can be restored, or occlusion if it cannot be achieved. Botulinum toxin in our hands has proved useful in this situation.
• Further surgery may be required. If a unilateral procedure was performed on the affected eye, further surgery can often be carried out on the contralateral eye. When a unilateral transposition procedure has been combined with botulinum toxin to the ipsilateral medial rectus, some degree of contracture may remain,

Field of Left Eye (fixing with right eye) Field of Right Eye (fixing with left eye)

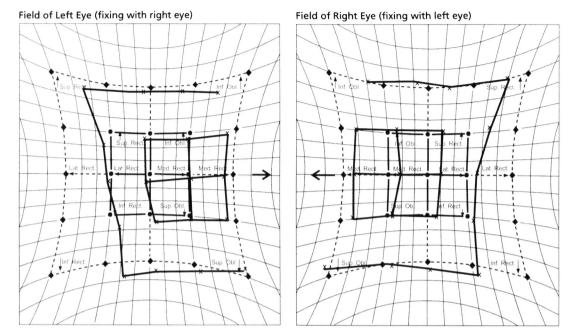

Fig. 19.31 Hess chart of a patient with a partial bilateral lateral rectus palsy. A V-pattern esotropia is present.

especially if the palsy is long-standing. A medial rectus recession should be considered; there appears to be less risk of anterior segment ischaemia developing if this is performed 4–6 months after the transposition procedure.

• In situations where persisting lateral incomitance in the direction of the affected lateral rectus persists, a posterior fixation suture to the contralateral medial rectus may be indicated.

• A transposition procedure may require revision if the eye is still unable to reach the primary position.

Overcorrections

The deviation may be overcorrected in the primary position or on eccentric gaze. Treatment is required only if the condition is symptomatic. The following general points apply.

• Some can be managed conservatively with prisms.

• An overcorrection following a medial rectus recession and lateral rectus resection which fails to respond to prisms should be treated with botulinum toxin to the resected lateral rectus muscle. This has been effective in our hands in producing a long-term correction

of the exodeviation if carried out within 2 months of the initial surgery.

• Those failing to benefit from conservative treatment will require further surgery.

Sixth nerve palsy in the absence of potential for binocular single vision

The surgical aim is to achieve an acceptable appearance. In our experience, it has proved very difficult to obtain a stable alignment when there is total lateral rectus palsy. There is often an early recurrence of esotropia, requiring further treatment.

Below are two examples of patients showing an early return of esotropia.

• A child who underwent bilateral lateral transposition of the vertical recti combined with medial rectus recession of 6 mm showed an early return of the esotropia. A further recession of both medial rectus muscles on 3 mm loops has resulted in a stable small-angle esotropia.

• An adult who underwent a unilateral lateral transposition of the vertical recti with recession of the medial rectus showed an early return of the esotropia. This patient has subsequently been treated with long-term botulinum toxin injections into the recessed medial rectus muscles.

Ocular neuromyotonia

Description
Ocular neuromyotonia is a rare disorder resulting in transient, involuntary spasm of an extraocular muscle leading to intermittent strabismus and diplopia.

Aetiology

In most of the reported cases of neuromyotonia there is a history of radiotherapy treatment to a parachiasmal tumour months or years previously, in others there are no abnormal findings from the history, examination or investigation. It is thought that damage to the ocular motor nerve in the cavernous sinus results in demyelination, and ephaptic transmission (axon to axon) leads to the neural signal spreading to adjacent axons causing a self-perpetuating reverberating circuit and the sustained muscle contraction. A similar mechanism has been proposed for hemifacial spasm and aberrant regeneration in third nerve palsy. Other explanations include reorganization of neurones in the brainstem secondary to retrograde degeneration and ephaptic transmission in the nuclei.

Features

• Intermittent diplopia occurs lasting from seconds to a few minutes.
• A history of radiotherapy to the region of the optic chiasm is present in the majority of cases.
• Sustained eccentric gaze induces muscle spasm resulting in strabismus that persists after the eyes return to the primary position. Eccentric gaze may need to be maintained for several minutes to induce the neuromyotonia and the spasm persists for several seconds or minutes. The spasm usually develops in the agonist muscles that move the eyes into the eccentric position.
• The condition is nearly always unilateral and involvement of all the extraocular muscles except the inferior oblique has been described. The levator muscle and iris sphincter can also be affected.

Differential diagnosis

Other causes of intermittent diplopia include:
• decompensating heterophoria;
• neurogenic strabismus;
• myogenic strabismus, in particular myasthenia gravis;
• mechanical strabismus;
• superior oblique myokymia;
• cyclical third nerve palsy, in which periods of muscle spasm alternate with muscle palsy;
• internuclear ophthalmoplegia;
• convergence spasm, which also involves the pupil and the ciliary muscles.
    Ocular neuromyotonia can readily be distinguished from other causes of transient diplopia by its characteristic features.

Management
Neuro-imaging should be performed on all patients to exclude a recurrence of the original tumour in those with a previous history of radiotherapy or a compressive cause in those without such a history.

Treatment
Spontaneous resolution of diplopia is rare. If the diplopia occurs frequently and is disabling then carbamazepine is effective in abating or reducing the frequency of attacks.

Congenital palsies

Aetiology

Congenital palsies include those which are either present at birth or develop within the first 6 months of life. The aetiology often remains unknown; however, some are caused by neurogenic or myogenic factors, while others are related to anatomical defects, such as the congenital absence of a muscle.
    A palsy can arise as:
• an isolated defect, such as congenital fourth nerve palsies;
• a complication of intracranial disease, such as a hydrocephalus or brainstem glioma;
• part of a craniofacial anomaly, for example a superior oblique palsy in Crouzon's disease and plagiocephaly;
• a familial trait;

- a genetic defect in association with other signs;
- a rare cyclic oculomotor palsy.

It should be recognized that the palsy can be associated with certain conditions: the possibility that the muscle may be absent is particularly important when planning surgical intervention.

Congenital third nerve and sixth nerve palsies are discussed in this section. Congenital fourth nerve palsies have been discussed in more detail above in the section 'Acquired and congenital palsies of the fourth nerve' and is only briefly covered in this section.

Congenital third nerve palsy and third nerve palsy acquired in childhood

Subtypes
Subtypes of congenital third nerve palsy that differ from acquired palsies either in their clinical appearance or in their management are discussed below. Other congenital subtypes of third nerve palsy are discussed alongside their acquired counterparts.

Complete palsy affecting all extraocular muscles
A congenital third nerve palsy is usually isolated. Typically there is some degree of ptosis which usually does not cover the visual axis, and a variable degree of paresis of all the extraocular muscles supplied by the third nerve, often with evidence of aberrant regeneration. Unilateral cases are more common but bilateral cases occur. Despite most reports supporting the isolated nature of congenital third nerve palsy, some cases may have associated nonprogressive neurological abnormalities (Hamed 1991).

Aetiology
In most cases the aetiology remains unknown. As aberrant regeneration is common, the causative lesion is likely to be infranuclear. A history of birth trauma or forceps delivery is often recorded; whether this is coincidental or is the cause has yet to be established.

Features
The clinical features are outlined below.
- Signs of third nerve palsy, which are often reported to evolve over the few months after birth.

- The affected eye is exotropic and intorted with a possible small hypodeviation.
- Muscle sequelae comprise overaction of the contralateral lateral rectus, the superior rectus and the superior and inferior oblique muscles.
- Ptosis, which will cover the visual axis in total palsy but is more usually partial.
- Pupil involvement is common, usually as dilation but with constriction occurring in some cases with aberrant regeneration.
- Amblyopia.

Management
All cases should be assessed by a paediatrician to confirm that the defect is isolated; we believe that the paediatrician should also be involved in planning further investigations, including neuro-imaging.

The ophthalmological management of these cases should follow the same basic principles that are applied to all cases of childhood strabismus. With parental cooperation we have been successful in reversing most cases of amblyopia, and later going on to achieve an improved cosmetic appearance.

CORRECTION OF REFRACTION ERROR
Significant refractive errors should be corrected, with special attention to anisometropia.

Spectacle correction may not adequately neutralize the refractive error because the eye is viewing eccentrically through the lens.

RESTORATION OF VISUAL ACUITY
Amblyopia develops rapidly in both complete and partial palsies and is mainly strabismic. Rarely, amblyopia can develop in the uninvolved eye if the affected eye is used for fixation in a unilateral palsy.

Mechanisms for the development of amblyopia in congenital third nerve palsy are:
- stimulus deprivation from complete ptosis;
- strabismic from the exotropia and cyclovertical deviation;
- anisometropia: the affected eye may be myopic as it is recognized that there is a connection between early deprivation of the visual stimulus and the axial length of the globe; visual deprivation usually but not invariably results in myopia rather than hypermetropia (von Noorden & Lewis 1987).

Part-time total occlusion of the fixing eye or the eye with better visual acuity is the mainstay of amblyopia treatment. If the exotropia is marked, occlusion treatment may be poorly tolerated, although we have not usually found this to be the case. Some amount of maintenance occlusion is required in nearly all cases. Patients with partial ptosis may adopt a chin elevation when occluded and should be encouraged to do so.

Botulinum toxin may be useful in facilitating amblyopia management. We have had limited success with injection into the lateral rectus of the affected eye in cases of total third nerve palsy. It seems logical to attempt to centralize the affected eye to facilitate occlusion, especially in ambulant children who also wear spectacles for anisometropia and who will not otherwise tolerate occlusion. The need for repeat injections and the use of general anaesthesia needs to be made clear to the family before starting this form of therapy.

Binocular single vision is not a realistic goal in total palsies.

SURGICAL TREATMENT

Patients with ptosis covering the visual axis will require ptosis surgery to prevent stimulus-deprivation amblyopia. A frontalis sling is the procedure of choice.

The surgical options available to correct the strabismus are discussed above in the section 'Acquired third nerve palsies'. Because traction sutures are needed to ensure a stable cosmetic alignment in a total complete palsy, surgical intervention may have to be deferred until there is sufficient cooperation to facilitate postoperative management.

Acquired third nerve palsy in early childhood

This is a rare disorder. However, we have seen cases caused by infection (meningitis) and trauma. As recovery can occur, it is important to guard against the loss of binocular single vision and the development of amblyopia.

In one instance, we were able to maintain horizontal binocular alignment in an infant aged 8 months who developed an asymmetrical bilateral third nerve palsy with moderate exotropia after contracting meningitis. Some recovery of third nerve function followed two courses of botulinum toxin injected into both lateral rectus muscles over a 6-month period. Subsequent surgical correction of the exotropia has resulted in stable binocular alignment despite persisting vertical incomitance.

Double elevator palsy

Double elevator palsy is characterized by limitation of up-gaze in both adduction and abduction. It can affect one or both eyes and is considered to be congenital. Acquired palsy of up-gaze has been reported in dorsal midbrain lesions as one of several neurological signs (Jampel & Fells 1968; Lessel 1975).

Aetiology

The presence of Bell's phenomenon and full passive movement strongly suggest that the lesion is supranuclear, but secondary contracture of the inferior rectus can result in an added mechanical restriction. Absence of a Bell's phenomenon could be the result of an upper division of third nerve palsy in which a spread of concomitance has resulted in equal limitation of up-gaze in both adduction and abduction.

Features

The features are:
- ptosis, with a pseudo-component due to hypotropia;
- either binocular single vision or hypotropia in the primary position;
- an intact Bell's phenomenon in some cases;
- an abnormal chin elevation, adopted to maintain binocular single vision or to maintain fixation if the palsy is bilateral;
- a minor degree of passive restriction of up-gaze detected with the forced duction test.

Differential diagnosis

The differential diagnosis includes:
- Congenital fibrosis of the inferior rectus muscle.
- Blow-out fracture of the orbital floor.
- Thyroid eye disease.
- Brown's syndrome, which can show a spread of limitation of elevation into the field of abduction. In these cases, the forced duction test will indicate that the major part of the limitation of up-gaze can be accounted for by mechanical restriction.

• Congenital absence of the superior rectus muscle (Mather & Saunders 1987).
• Upper division of third nerve palsy in which a spread of concomitance has resulted in equal limitation of up-gaze in both adduction and abduction.

In a study of 15 patients with uniocular limitation of elevation, Metz (1979) reported that those without hypotropia in the primary position showed no evidence of elevator palsy on saccadic velocity analysis and the limitation of elevation was the result of contracture of the inferior rectus. In contrast, saccadic velocity analysis of patients with hypotropia in the primary position showed that an elevator palsy was present in 50%.

Management

Conservative treatment
Treatment may not be required if binocular single vision can be maintained without the need for a cosmetically poor or uncomfortable chin elevation.

In the majority of cases surgery is indicated for:
• a hypotropia and pseudoptosis in the primary position;
• a marked compensatory head posture;
• ptosis which interferes with fixation in the primary position or is cosmetically poor.

Surgical treatment
In general, strabismus surgery must be carried out before surgery for ptosis. We have undertaken surgery for the hypotropia combined with a frontalis sling in one patient with a marked hypotropia and no demonstrable levator function in order to avoid postoperative occlusion of the visual axis by the ptosis.

A minor degree of passive restriction of up-gaze with the forced duction test is common; however, this restriction only accounts for part of the overall limitation of up-gaze. This is in contrast to situations in which the primary cause is mechanical, when the forced duction test will indicate that all the limitation of up-gaze can be accounted for in this way.

The surgical treatment of double elevator palsy is a vertical transposition of the horizontal recti (Knapp procedure; Knapp 1969). If a positive forced duction test indicates secondary contracture of the inferior rectus, this muscle is recessed at the same sitting: this has been the case in most of our patients.

Postoperative management
UNDERCORRECTIONS
Undercorrection may arise from:
• Recession of the inferior rectus as the sole procedure. Even if there is only a minor restriction of up-gaze on the forced duction test, recessing the inferior rectus will not be effective and the muscle will eventually re-contract. In this situation early intervention is required, using a Knapp procedure with further recession of the inferior rectus if necessary. Botulinum toxin can be used as an alternative if the inferior rectus has already been maximally recessed.
• Performing only a Knapp procedure. If a significant hypotropia persists in the primary position we have been able to improve alignment by recessing the ipsilateral inferior rectus 5–6 mm, performed within a month or two of the original surgery.

Double depressor palsy

This is a rare congenital anomaly and probably represents either an inferior rectus palsy or a congenital absence of that muscle in which the spread of concomitance has resulted in limitation of down-gaze in both adduction and abduction. The forced duction test on down-gaze may indicate mechanical restriction from secondary contracture of the ipsilateral superior rectus muscle.

Surgical management consists of inferior transposition of the horizontal rectus muscles (inverse Knapp procedure) combined with a recession of the ipsilateral superior rectus muscle if the forced duction test indicates mechanical restriction on down-gaze.

Cyclic oculomotor palsy

This very rare condition is characterized by short spasms of overaction of the muscles supplied by the third nerve, followed by longer episodes of third nerve palsy. Most cases present in the first two years of life and nearly all are unilateral (Fells & Collin 1979).

Aetiology
Loewenfeld and Thompson (1975) suggested that the disorder resulted from damage to the third nerve in infancy, with some nerve fibres remaining intact and still able to function. The damaged portion allowed

abnormal projections to develop from the immature supranuclear centres. They postulated that these abnormal connections permitted subthreshold stimuli to reach the third nerve nucleus, resulting in the spastic phase. The cyclic nature of the overactivity is similar in some ways to the active phase of superior oblique myokymia, but this condition usually lacks a paretic phase and occurs in adults rather than children.

Features

The features are:
• A variable degree of paresis, with ptosis, exotropia and mydriasis during the paretic phase.
• The spasmodic phase occurs every few minutes and usually lasts for up to 30 s. Upper eyelid twitching precedes lid elevation, the eye becomes straight or even esotropic, and miosis occurs. This phase may be precipitated by attempted adduction or by emotional disturbance.

The cycle may continue at a reduced rate during sleep.

There is no known effective treatment for cyclic oculomotor palsy.

Congenital sixth nerve palsy and sixth nerve palsy acquired in infancy

Congenital sixth nerve palsy is very rare, and when it occurs as an isolated finding in the first weeks of life it usually resolves spontaneously (Reisner *et al.* 1971).

Most cases of suspected congenital sixth nerve palsy represent one of the following conditions:
• Duane's retraction syndrome;
• infantile esotropia;
• nystagmus blockage syndrome.
All of these show true or apparent limitation of abduction.

Sixth nerve palsy acquired in childhood

This may be caused by tumour (leukaemia), infection (meningitis), trauma, hydrocephalus or may follow an apparently benign viral illness. A paediatrician should assess all patients. As most cases of acquired sixth nerve palsy in childhood either recover spontaneously or respond well to treatment, it is important that binocular single vision is not lost and amblyopia is prevented whilst monitoring for recovery.

Loss of binocular single vision can be prevented in most cases by:
• encouraging the adoption of a head posture;
• Fresnel prisms;
• botulinum toxin injection into the medial rectus muscle;
• occlusion treatment alternating between the eyes to prevent amblyopia.

The surgical management of persistent childhood sixth nerve palsy is discussed in the earlier section on acquired sixth nerve palsies.

Möbius' syndrome

This syndrome is a congenital disorder that can have a varying spectrum of clinical features, and probably results from either a developmental defect or a hypoxic or traumatic insult to the developing brain. The features are usually bilateral, but may be asymmetrical. The sixth, seventh, ninth and twelfth nerves are usually involved; an associated horizontal gaze palsy is often present. Most cases are sporadic.

Features

The features are:
• Facial palsy: the lack of facial expression may affect bonding between parent and child: poor or occasionally absent lid closure may lead to corneal exposure. The mouth is often kept open.
• Sixth nerve palsy: marked limitation of abduction is present. Some patients show a horizontal gaze palsy with no deviation in primary position, others have a marked esotropia which leads to contraction of the medial rectus muscles and a positive forced duction test. A face turn may be adopted to allow foveal fixation with the preferred eye. Vertical gaze is intact and the presence of Bell's phenomenon serves to protect the cornea and prevent exposure keratitis in most cases.
• Bulbar palsy (ninth and twelfth cranial nerves): swallowing difficulties may make feeding difficult; speech development is often delayed. The tongue is often atrophic.
• Other associations: deafness, pectoral muscle hypoplasia, syndactyly and mental retardation.

Differential diagnosis

The differential diagnosis includes:

• lack of facial expression, which can also be seen in infantile muscular dystrophy and facioscapulo-humeral dystrophy;

• the ocular movement disorder may be confused with Duane's syndrome, infantile esotropia, ocular motor apraxia and horizontal gaze palsy.

Management

A multidisciplinary approach to these patients is important, and families should have access to genetic advice.

Close supervision of the child's development is of utmost importance.

• Correction of refractive errors. Significant refractive errors should be corrected, with special attention to any significant anisometropia.

• Restoration of visual acuity. Binocular single vision is absent: strabismic amblyopia should be managed with occlusion therapy.

• Ocular treatment. Lagophthalmos can result in exposure keratitis that may require the use of ocular lubricants and taping of the eyelids at night. Strabismus surgery is indicated to improve the appearance of an unsightly esotropia. Large medial rectus recessions can often improve the deviation in the primary position, at the expense of adduction and convergence.

Congenital unilateral superior oblique palsies in children

Congenital superior oblique palsy can present in childhood with:

• an abnormal head posture;

• symptoms due to decompensation;

• a manifest vertical strabismus.

Early surgery is indicated to overcome a severe compensatory head posture before structural changes in the neck muscles take place and to prevent decompensation and possible loss of binocular single vision. The features and management of this group are discussed in the earlier section on superior oblique palsy. Most are probably due to a congenital anomaly of the superior oblique tendon resulting in excessive laxity. Helveston described the different types of congenital abnormalities of the superior oblique muscle (Helveston *et al.* 1992):

• a loose floppy tendon;

• nasal insertion site of the tendon;

• absent scleral insertion site of tendon, with tendon inserting into Tenon's capsule;

• absence of the reflected tendon.

In addition to the abnormalities described by Helveston, the superior oblique muscle and tendon may be completely absent. Superior oblique palsy that decompensates in early childhood is probably the result of severe tendon laxity or absence of the tendon or muscle. Most patients that we have treated at this age have manifest deviations in the primary position and the largest angle in the field of action of the affected superior oblique muscle; weakening the ipsilateral inferior oblique muscle in this situation is unlikely to be effective (Reynolds *et al.* 1984) and a superior oblique tuck is our preferred choice.

References

Balcer, L.J., Galetta, S.L., Bagley, L.J. & Pakola, S.J. (1996) Localisation of traumatic oculomotor nerve palsy to the midbrain exit site by magnetic resonance imaging. *American Journal of Ophthalmology* **122**, 437–439.

Béchac, G., Bec, P., Delfour, N., Jeanrot, N. & Marion, B. (1984) Bilateral fourth nerve palsy. Excyclovergence, as a warning of peri-aqueduct stenosis. In: *Transactions of the Fifth International Orthoptic Congress, Cannes* (eds A. Ravault & M. Lenk), pp. 135–142. LIPS, Lyon.

Botelho, P.J. & Giangiacomo, J.G. (1996) Autosomal-dominant inheritance of congenital superior oblique palsy. *Ophthalmology* **103**, 1508–1511.

Burde, R.M. & Roper-Hall, G. (1977) Diabetic ophthalmoplegia. *American Orthoptic Journal* **27**, 48–52.

Cox, T.A., Wurster, J.B. & Godfrey, W.A. (1979) Primary aberrant oculomotor regeneration due to intracranial aneurysm. *Archives of Neurology* **36**, 570–571.

Dyer, J.A. (1962) Tenotomy of the inferior oblique muscle at its scleral insertion. *Archives of Ophthalmology* **68**, 176–181.

Ellis, F.D. & Helveston, E.M. (1976) Superior oblique diagnosis and classification. In: *Strabismus Surgery*, pp. 127–135. Little, Brown, & Co., Boston.

Elston, J.S. (1984) Traumatic third nerve palsy. *British Journal of Ophthalmology* **68**, 538–543.

Fells, P. & Collin, J.R.O. (1979) Cyclic oculomotor palsy. *Transactions of the Ophthalmological Society of the United Kingdom* 99, 192–196.

Fisher, C.M. (1956) Unusual variant of acute idiopathic polyneuritis (syndrome of ophthalmoplegia ataxia and areflexia). *New England Journal of Medicine* 255, 57–65.

Fitzsimons, R., Lee, J.P. & Elston, J. (1988) Treatment of sixth nerve palsy in adults with combined botulinum toxin chemodenervation and surgery. *Ophthalmology* 95, 1535–1542.

Goldstein, J.E. & Cogan, D.G. (1960) Diabetic ophthalmoplegia with special reference to the pupil. *Archives of Ophthalmology* 64, 592–600.

Green, W.R., Hacket, E.R. & Schlezinger, N.S. (1964) Neuro-ophthalmologic evaluation of oculomotor paralysis. *Archives of Ophthalmology* 72, 154–167.

Guy, J.R. & Day, A.L. (1989) Intracranial aneurysms with superior division paresis of the oculomotor nerve. *Ophthalmology* 96, 1071–1076.

Guy, J., Savino, P.J. & Schatz, N.J. (1985) Superior division paresis of the oculomotor nerve. *Ophthalmology* 92, 777–784.

Hamed, L.M. (1991) Associated neurologic and ophthalmologic findings in congenital oculomotor nerve palsy. *Ophthalmology* 98, 708–714.

Helveston, E.M., Krach, D., Plager, D.A. & Ellis, F.D. (1992) A new classification of superior oblique palsy based on congenital variations in the tendon. *Ophthalmology* 99, 1609–1615.

Hermann, J.S. (1981) Masked bilateral superior oblique paresis. *Journal of Pediatric Ophthalmology and Strabismus* 18, 43–48.

Hunt, W.E., Meagher, J.N., Lefever, H.E. & Zeman, W. (1961) Painful ophthalmoplegia: its relationship to indolent inflammation of the cavernous sinus. *Neurology* 11, 56–62.

Jampel, R.S. & Fells, P. (1968) Monocular elevation paresis caused by a central nervous system lesion. *Archives of Ophthalmology* 80, 45–57.

Jampolsky, A. (1971) Vertical strabismus surgery. In: *Symposium Strabismus. Transactions of the New Orleans Academy of Ophthalmology*, pp. 366–385. C.V. Mosby, St Louis.

Jampolsky, A. (1995) The superior rectus contracture syndrome. In: *Update on Strabismus and Pediatric Ophthalmology. Proceedings of the Joint ISA and AAPOS & S Meeting, Vancouver* (ed. G. Lennerstrand), pp. 279–282. CRC Press, Boca Raton.

Kelly, V. & Dulley, B. (1976) Ocular motor defects associated with herpes zoster ophthalmicus. In: *Transactions of the Third International Orthoptic Congress, Boston* (eds J. Mein, S. Moore & L. Stockbridge), pp. 367–377. Symposia Specialists, Miami.

Khawam, E., Scott, A.B. & Jampolsky, A. (1967) Acquired superior oblique palsy. Diagnosis and management. *Archives of Ophthalmology* 77, 761–768.

Knapp, P. (1969) The surgical treatment of double elevator palsy. *Transactions of the American Ophthalmological Society* 67, 304–321.

Knapp, P. (1978) Paretic squints. In: *Symposium on Strabismus. Transactions of the New Orleans Academy of Ophthalmology* (ed. J. Allen), pp. 350–357. Mosby, St Louis.

Kraft, S.P., O'Reilly, C., Quigley, P.L., Allan, K. & Eustis, H.S. (1993) Cyclotorsion in unilateral and bilateral superior oblique paresis. *Journal of Pediatric Ophthalmology and Strabismus* 30, 361–367.

Lee, D.A., Dyer, J.A., O'Brien, P.C. & Taylor, J.Z. (1984) Surgical treatment of lateral rectus muscle palsy. *American Journal of Ophthalmology* 97, 511–518.

Lee, J.P. & Gregson, R.M.C. (1993) Traction sutures in the management of fixed divergent strabismus. In: *Transactions of the 21st ESA Meeting, Salzburg* (ed. H. Kaufmann), pp. 397–399.

Lee, J., Harris, S., Cohen, J., Cooper, K., MacEwan, C. & Jones, S. (1994) Results of a prospective randomised trial of botulinum toxin therapy in acute unilateral sixth nerve palsy. *Journal of Pediatric Ophthalmology and Strabismus* 31, 283–286.

Lessel, S. (1975) Supranuclear paralysis of monocular elevation. *Neurology* 25, 1134–1136.

Loewenfeld, I.E. & Thompson, S.H. (1975) Oculomotor paresis with cyclic spasms: a critical review of the literature and a new case. *Survey of Ophthalmology* 20, 81–124.

Lustbader, J.M. & Miller, N.R. (1988) Painless, pupil-sparing but otherwise complete oculomotor nerve paresis caused by basilar artery aneurysm. *Archives of Ophthalmology* 106, 583–584.

Mather, T.R. & Saunders, R.A. (1987) Congenital absence of the superior rectus muscle: a case report. *Journal of Pediatric Ophthalmology and Strabismus* 24, 291–295.

McKeown, C.A., Lambert, H.M. & Shore, J.W. (1989) Preservation of the anterior ciliary vessels during extraocular muscle surgery. *Ophthalmology* 96, 498–506.

Metz, H.S. (1979) Double elevator palsy. *Archives of Ophthalmology* 97, 901–903.

Morris, R.J., Scott, W.E. & Keech, R.V. (1992) Superior oblique tuck surgery in the management of superior oblique palsies. *Journal of Pediatric Ophthalmology and Strabismus* 29, 337–346.

Moster, M.L., Savino, P.J., Sergott, R.C., Bosley, T.M. & Schatz, N.J. (1984) Isolated sixth nerve palsies in younger adults. *Archives of Ophthalmology* **102**, 1328–1330.

Muchnick, R.S., Stoj, M. & Hornblass, A. (1985) Traumatic inferior oblique muscle paresis. *Journal of Pediatric Ophthalmology and Strabismus* **22**, 143–146.

Noonan, C.P. & O'Connor, M. (1995) Surgical management of third nerve palsy. *British Journal of Ophthalmology* **79**, 431–434.

von Noorden, G.K. & Hansell, R. (1991) Clinical characteristics and treatment of isolated inferior rectus paralysis. *Ophthalmology* **98**, 253–257.

von Noorden, G.K. & Lewis, R.A. (1987) Axial length in unilateral congenital cataracts and blepharoptosis. *Investigative Ophthalmology and Visual Science* **28**, 750–752.

von Noorden, G.K., Murray, E. & Wong, S.Y. (1986) Superior oblique paralysis, a review of 270 cases. *Archives of Ophthalmology* **104**, 1771–1776.

Ohtsuki, H., Hasebe, S., Hanabusa, K., Fujimoto, Y. & Furuse, T. (1994) Intraoperative adjustable suture surgery for bilateral superior oblique palsy. *Ophthalmology* **101**, 188–193.

Oliver, P. & von Noorden, G.K. (1982a) Excyclotropia of the nonparetic eye in unilateral superior oblique paralysis. *American Journal of Ophthalmology* **93**, 30–33.

Oliver, P. & von Noorden, G.K. (1982b) Results of superior oblique tenectomy in inferior oblique paresis. *Archives of Ophthalmology* **100**, 581–584.

Plager, D.A. (1990) Traction testing in superior oblique palsy. *Journal of Pediatric Ophthalmology and Strabismus* **27**, 136–140.

Pollard, Z.F. (1993) Diagnosis and treatment of inferior oblique palsy. *Journal of Pediatric Ophthalmology and Strabismus* **30**, 15–18.

Polomeno, R.C., Waters, G.V., Andermann, F., Kirkham, T.H., Bekhor, S. & Little, J.M. (1981) Ophthalmoplegic migraine of childhood and adolescence: A disorder of the 3rd, 4th and 6th cranial nerves. In: *Orthoptics, Research and Practice. Transactions of the 4th International Orthoptic Congress, Berne* (eds J. Mein & S. Moore), pp. 101–107. Henry Kimpton, London.

Pratt-Johnson, J.A. & Tillson, G. (1987) The investigation and management of torsion preventing fusion in bilateral superior oblique palsies. *Journal of Pediatric Ophthalmology and Strabismus* **24**, 145–150.

Pratt-Johnson, J.A. & Tillson, G. (1994) *Management of Strabismus and Amblyopia. A Practical Guide.* Thieme Medical Publishers, New York.

Price, N.C., Vickers, S., Lee, J.P. & Fells, P. (1987) The diagnosis and surgical management of acquired bilateral superior oblique palsy. *Eye* **1**, 78–85.

Pusateri, T.J., Sedwick, L.A. & Margo, C.E. (1987) Isolated inferior rectus muscle palsy from a solitary metastasis to the oculomotor nucleus. *Archives of Ophthalmology* **105**, 675–677.

Reisner, S.H., Perlman, M., Ben-Tovim, N. & Dubrawski, C. (1971) Transient lateral rectus muscle paresis in the newborn infant. *Journal of Pediatrics* **78**, 461–465.

Reynolds, J.D., Biglan, A.W. & Hiles, D.A. (1984) Congenital superior oblique palsy in infants. *Archives of Ophthalmology* **102**, 1503–1505.

Riordan-Eva, P. & Lee, J.P. (1992) Management of VIth nerve palsy – Avoiding unnecessary surgery. *Eye* **6**, 386–390.

Robb, R.M. (1990) Idiopathic superior oblique palsies in children. *Journal of Pediatric Ophthalmology and Strabismus* **27**, 66–69.

Rosenbaum, A.L., Kushner, B.J. & Kirschen, D. (1989) Vertical rectus muscle transposition and botulinum toxin (Oculinum) to medial rectus for abducens palsy. *Archives of Ophthalmology* **107**, 820–823.

Rucker, C.W. (1958) Paralysis of the third, fourth and sixth cranial nerves. *American Journal of Ophthalmology* **46**, 787–794.

Rucker, C.W. (1966) The causes of paralysis of the third, fourth and sixth cranial nerves. *American Journal of Ophthalmology* **61**, 1293–1298.

Rush, J.A. & Younge, B.R. (1981) Paralysis of cranial nerves III, IV and VI. Cause and prognosis in 1000 cases. *Archives of Ophthalmology* **99**, 76–80.

Saunders, R.A. (1984) Incomitant vertical strabismus. *Archives of Ophthalmology* **102**, 1174–1177.

Schatz, N.J., Savino, P.J. & Corbett, J.J. (1977) Primary aberrant oculomotor regeneration: a sign of intracavernous meningioma. *Archives of Neurology* **34**, 29–32.

Scott, A.B. (1971) Active force tests in lateral rectus palsy. *Archives of Ophthalmology* **85**, 397–404.

Scott, W.E. & Kraft, S.P. (1986a) Classification and surgical management of superior oblique palsies: I. Unilateral superior oblique palsies. In: *Pediatric Ophthalmology and Strabismus: Transactions of the New Orleans Academy of Ophthalmology*, pp. 15–38. Raven Press, New York.

Scott, W.E. & Kraft, S.P. (1986b) Classification and surgical management of superior oblique palsies: II. Bilateral superior oblique palsies. In: *Pediatric Ophthalmology and Strabismus: Transactions of the New Orleans Academy of Ophthalmology.* pp. 265–291. Raven Press New York.

Spencer, F. & Harcourt, R.B. (1984) A paradoxical pattern of ocular movement associated with acquired superior oblique dysfunction. In: *Transactions of the Fifth International Orthoptic Congress, Cannes* (eds A. Ravault & M. Lenk), pp. 261–266. LIPS, Lyon.

Sydnor, C.F., Seaber, J.H. & Buckley, E.G. (1982) Traumatic superior oblique palsies. *Ophthalmology* **89**, 134–138.

Thomas, D.J.B., Charlesworth, M.C., Afshar, F. & Galton, D.J. (1988) Computerised axial tomography and magnetic resonance scanning in the Tolosa–Hunt syndrome. *British Journal of Ophthalmology* **72**, 299–302.

Tiffin, P.A.C., MacEwen, C.J., Craig, E.A. & Clayton, G. (1996) Acquired palsy of the oculomotor, trochlear and abducens nerves. *Eye* **10**, 377–384.

Tolosa, E.J. (1954) Peri-arteritic lesions of the carotid siphon with clinical features of carotid infraclinoid aneurysms. *Journal of Neurology, Neurosurgery and Psychiatry* **17**, 300–302.

Wallace, D.K. & von Noorden, G.K. (1994) Clinical characteristics and surgical management of congenital absence of the superior oblique tendon. *American Journal of Ophthalmology.* **118**, 63–69.

Wolff, E. (1928) A bend in the 6th cranial nerve – and its probable significance. *British Journal of Ophthalmology* **12**, 22–24.

Younis, M.H., Vivian, A. & Lee, J.P. (1995) Unilateral modified Harada–Ito procedure for excyclotorsion secondary to unilateral superior oblique palsy. In: *Update on Strabismus and Pediatric Ophthalmology. Proceedings of the Joint ISA and AAPOS & S Meeting, Vancouver* (ed. G. Lennerstrand), pp. 313–316. CRC Press, Boca Raton.

Zasorin, N.L., Yee, R.D. & Baloh, R.W. (1985) Eye-movement abnormalities in ophthalmoplegia, ataxia and areflexia (Fisher's syndrome). *Archives of Ophthalmology* **103**, 55–58.

20
Myogenic Palsies

A myogenic palsy is a form of paralytic strabismus in which the weakness of ocular movement is due to a primary problem affecting the muscle itself rather than one disrupting the nerve supply or causing mechanical restriction.

Classification

The following conditions are included and discussed under myogenic palsies:
- myasthenia gravis;
- Lambert–Eaton–Rooke syndrome;
- chronic progressive external ophthalmoplegia;
- orbital myositis;
- rhabdomyosarcoma.

Thyroid eye disease principally involves the extraocular muscles; however, the features of the disease are mechanical and not paretic. It is therefore discussed in Chapter 21.

Myasthenia gravis

Thomas Willis first described this condition in 1683. The term myasthenia is derived from Greek, and means 'weak muscle', while gravis is from Latin and means 'heavy', which may be interpreted as severe. The term 'myasthenia' is used subsequently in this chapter.

Aetiology and pathology

Myasthenia is an autoimmune disorder. Normally acetylcholine (the neurotransmitter) is released from the terminal portion of the motor axon at the synaptic gap. Acetylcholine binds to the receptor sites at the motor end-plate causing a depolarizing wave to spread along the excitable membrane of the muscle, which results in muscle contraction.

Patients who develop myasthenia form antibodies to these receptor sites at the muscle end-plate (acetylcholine receptor site antibodies). These antibodies prevent acetylcholine from binding, and so reduce the effectiveness of the neurotransmitter. Acetylcholine continues to be released in an attempt to maintain muscle contracture until stores are exhausted, hence the characteristic early muscle fatigue. Structural changes follow, with loss of receptor sites on the post-synaptic membrane, reaching a stage when even if adequate quantities of acetylcholine were available,

Tree 20.1 Summary of the symptoms and signs in myasthenia gravis.

Symptoms and signs ——— Ptosis
Diplopia
Orbicularis weakness
Limb girdle weakness
Bulbar and respiratory muscle weakness

the muscle would no longer be in a position to bind it and contract. Receptor site antibodies can be detected in the serum of around 80–90% of patients with generalized myasthenia but only in 50–60% of patients with ocular myasthenia.

Extraocular muscles may be preferentially involved for one of three possible reasons:
• their higher firing rate, with a dense concentration of receptors resulting in early expression of any weakness;
• a increased sensitivity of the neuromuscular junction in extraocular muscle;
• different circulating antibodies preferentially directed at specific sites on the extraocular muscles.

Features

The essential features of myasthenia are summarized below.
• It is a disorder of neuromuscular transmission due to a reduction of acetylcholine receptor sites at the motor end-plate of skeletal muscles.
• It is characterized by excessive fatiguability of striated muscle, which may be general, affecting all striated muscles, or surprisingly selective.
• The order of frequency of affected muscle groups is: extraocular, facial, bulbar, neck, limb girdle, distal limb and trunk muscles.
• Extraocular muscles are commonly affected in all types of myasthenia. Diplopia and ptosis mark the onset of the disease in about 70% of cases, and with time they will be seen in 90% of cases, some of which later progress to more generalized muscle involvement (Osserman 1967).
• When the respiratory muscles are severely affected the illness can prove fatal, and is termed a 'crisis'.
• Other autoimmune diseases may be associated, such as diabetes, thyroid eye disease, pernicious anaemia and rheumatoid arthritis.

Symptoms and signs

Symptoms and signs of myasthenia can be ocular or systemic. They have a diurnal variation, being least in the morning and becoming worse as the day progresses. Symptoms are usually exacerbated by intercurrent illness.

Ocular symptoms and signs

The ocular symptoms and signs are the same whether the disease is confined to the eye muscles or if the eye involvement is one aspect of systemic disease. It is unusual to see a patient with myasthenia who does not show either ptosis, diplopia or evidence of orbicularis weakness.

PTOSIS
This is often the presenting sign of myasthenia, and is present in most patients to some degree. The ptosis occurring in myasthenia has the following significant characteristics:
• It is usually bilateral and often asymmetrical, unlike the more symmetrical ptosis seen in chronic progressive external ophthalmoplegia.
• The degree of ptosis increases during the day, and may vary from day to day. Ptosis affecting different sides at different times is diagnostic of myasthenia.
• Frontalis overaction is seen as the patient tries to increase lid elevation, and in rare instances there will be upper eyelid retraction rather than ptosis. The upper eyelid fold may be reduced or absent.

The assessment of patients with ptosis is discussed in Chapter 2. Important points in the evaluation of patients with myasthenic ptosis include:
• Variability in the ptosis, which can be assessed by asking the patient to stop blinking while maintaining fixation on a target in the primary position. The ptosis slowly increases after a few seconds in most myasthenic patients. A similar increase can be observed by

asking the patient to sustain up-gaze for a minute or two.

• Cogan's lid twitch sign (Cogan 1965), which can be demonstrated by first asking the patient to look down for 15 s, then instructing him to make a fast refixation movement to the primary position. Lid movement follows eye movement on down-gaze, but when the eye returns to the primary position the lid momentarily moves above its previous level (the lid twitch) before returning to its ptotic position. Approximately 50% of Cogan's series of patients with myasthenic ptosis demonstrated this sign, although it is not specific for myasthenia, and can occur, for example, in patients with third nerve palsy associated with aberrant regeneration, as well as in other conditions.

• Anomalous eyelid movements: 'flutter-like' upper eyelid movements are seen, often associated with repeated blinking. These probably represent multiple lid twitches.

• Enhanced ptosis: if the examiner holds up the eyelid on the more affected side in asymmetric ptosis, the innervational drive to both upper eyelids is reduced and the ptosis on the less affected side is seen to increase (Gorelick et al. 1981).

DIPLOPIA

Variable diplopia, often vertical, is the classic symptom of myasthenia. Separation of the images increases and the diplopia becomes more difficult to control as the day progresses or after a period of prolonged reading or driving.

Myasthenia may cause any type of ocular muscle palsy, but more typically results in one or more of the following:

• pseudo-internuclear ophthalmoplegia (Fig. 20.1a,b)
• isolated inferior rectus palsy (which is otherwise rare);
• pseudo-gaze palsy;
• pseudo-isolated third, fourth or sixth nerve palsy;
• gaze-paretic nystagmus.

Features suggestive of myasthenia on ocular movement assessment include:

• variability of measurements, both during the examination and between assessments;
• increase in the amount of limitation of movement on sustained gaze;

• normal saccadic velocities in the presence of a moderate amount of limitation of eye movement can help differentiate myasthenia from other causes of ophthalmoplegia (Yee et al. 1987).

Saccadic eye movement recording may demonstrate either higher than normal peak saccadic velocities or, less commonly, intrasaccadic fatigue.

ORBICULARIS WEAKNESS

Most patients with myasthenia can adequately close their eyelids. However, a sizeable number are unable to 'bury' their eyelashes or cannot prevent the examiner opening the eyelids with only gentle pressure. It is unusual to see lagophthalmos or exposure keratitis. Osher and Griggs (1979) reported that 12% of myasthenic patients showed the 'peek' sign, in which the lid margins separated after momentary opposition to gentle sustained lid closure, resulting in widening of the palpebral fissure and scleral exposure. The patient thus appeared to 'peek' at the examiner (Osher & Griggs 1979).

Systemic symptoms and signs

The symptoms in generalized myasthenia depend on which muscle groups are affected. A feeling of fatigue and a lack of energy is a common complaint.

• Limb girdle muscle: this may cause difficulty in rising from a seated position, and in climbing stairs or performing tasks which require the arms to be kept above the head for any length of time.

• Facial muscles: a lack of facial expression due to weakness of the facial muscles may be noted by the patient or by relatives and friends.

• Jaw muscles: difficulty with chewing and dysphagia (difficulty in swallowing) as the meal progresses, occasionally associated with nasal regurgitation of fluids.

• Bulbar muscles: dysarthria (difficulty of speech) which becomes more pronounced as the conversation progresses. Dysphagia may also occur.

• Respiratory muscles: breathlessness on exertion, which may rapidly deteriorate with an intercurrent infection or surgical trauma. The introduction of systemic steroid therapy can result in some patients rapidly going into respiratory crisis.

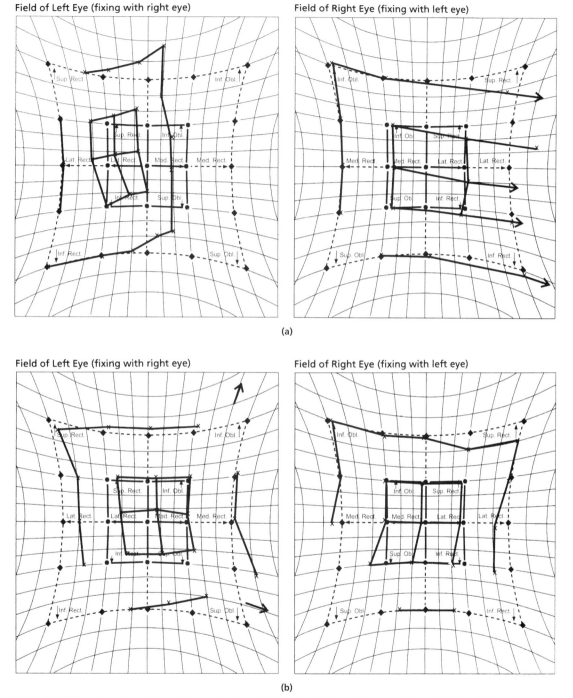

Fig. 20.1 (a) Hess chart of a patient with myasthenia gravis showing a left pseudo-internuclear ophthalmoplegia and superior oblique palsy. (b) Hess chart of same patient following treatment with pyridostigmine.

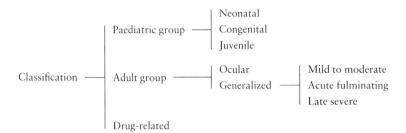

Tree 20.2 Classification of myasthenia gravis.

Classification of myasthenia gravis

Paediatric group

• Neonatal myasthenia: rarely a baby born to a myasthenic mother may exhibit signs of myasthenia, probably due to transplacental antibody transfer. The disease in this instance is usually self-limiting, with recovery expected in 6 weeks.

• Congenital myasthenia: this occurs in infants of nonmyasthenic mothers, and tends not to be antibody mediated. Ocular involvement is common, with some cases responding to systemic anticholinesterases.

• Juvenile myasthenia: the juvenile form may develop any time from birth to puberty and is similar to the adult form of the disease, but tends to progress slower with a higher proportion of spontaneous remissions (Morris 1982).

Adult group

Adult myasthenia is divided into four main types, depending on which muscle groups are affected and on the severity of the disease.

• Ocular myasthenia: the disease is limited to the eye muscles, which appear to be particularly susceptible to myasthenic changes. If the disease does not progress to involve other muscle groups within 2 years of onset, the condition usually but not invariably remains ocular (Osserman 1967).

• Mild to moderate generalized myasthenia: the onset of the disease is gradual, the extraocular muscles are often affected before the disease spreads to affect skeletal and bulbar muscles. The respiratory muscles are spared in this group, therefore mortality is low.

• Acute fulminating myasthenia: the onset is rapid with early involvement of the respiratory muscles and a significant mortality.

• Late severe myasthenia: severe myasthenia develops in the ocular or mild generalized group at least 2 years after the first signs of muscle weakness.

Drug related

The condition of D-penicillamine-induced myasthenia was described by Bucknall *et al.* (1975, 1979) after Osserman had prepared his original classification of myasthenia. D-penicillamine is a drug used in the treatment of certain autoimmune disorders, such as rheumatoid arthritis or systemic lupus erythematosus. Some patients on this drug develop myasthenic symptoms, which resolve when the penicillamine is stopped. A case of D-penicillamine-induced ocular myasthenia has been reported (Katz *et al.* 1989). D-penicillamine is also used to treat other conditions which do not have an autoimmune basis, and in this group D-penicillamine-induced myasthenia is a rarity, implying that susceptible patients must have an underlying abnormality of the immune system to develop this response. Antibiotics such as streptomycin have also been reported as inducing myasthenic symptoms.

Investigations

Tensilon test

Edrophonium (Tensilon) is a short-acting anticholinesterase that is injected intravenously. It improves the function of myasthenic muscles within 1 min following injection and is effective for approximately 5 min. The test is useful for assessing the function of any group of muscles; however, eyelid muscles and extraocular muscles provide an opportunity to make a quantifiable assessment of the effects of injection. Some patients may show a hypersensitivity reaction to the drug, although the risks of this are reduced by the prior test dose (see below), and serious reactions can

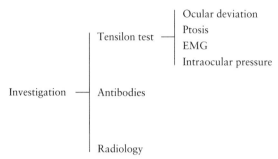

Tree 20.3 Investigations in myasthenia gravis.

occur, including respiratory depression and brady-cardia. The test should be performed in a hospital setting where resuscitation facilities are available. Patients should be warned that they may experience salivation and lacrimation following the injection.

Method

An indwelling needle is inserted into an accessible vein. Three syringes are prepared:

- A 1 mL syringe containing 10 mg (1 mL) of Tensilon.
- A 1 mL syringe containing 0.6 mg of atropine sulphate (see below).
- A 2 mL syringe containing 2 mL of normal saline.

A test dose of 2 mg (0.2 mL) of Tensilon is administered and flushed through with a small amount of saline and the patient is observed for any improvement in muscle function over a period of 3 min.

- A small group of patients will show a significant response to this test dose, permitting a diagnosis of a positive test to be made.
- Some patients will show a hypersensitivity reaction to this dose, exhibiting features of excessive parasympathetic stimulation such as abdominal cramps and bradycardia. These adverse effects can be reversed with the use of atropine. Patients showing such a hypersensitivity to this amount of Tensilon should not proceed further with the test.

If there is no untoward systemic reaction to the test dose and no evidence of a positive response, then the remaining 8 mg (0.8 mL) of Tensilon is administered and flushed through with a small amount of saline.

Assessment of results

The effect of Tensilon is assessed by comparing muscle function before and after the injection. The use of an objective and quantifiable assessment method is preferred.

- Hess chart. Because of the short effect of Tensilon the patient should be seated at the screen at the time of the injection. A Hess chart should be plotted immediately before the test dose is administered then repeated twice during the 3 min that the test dose is effective. If no effect is noted, then the remaining 8 mg is injected and the Hess chart is plotted twice again. It should be possible for all the serial Hess charts to be plotted by one orthoptist. A chart plotted 10 min after the last injection should be comparable with the chart plotted before the injection. The test is said to be positive when a change of 3 Δ or more in the vertical deviation or 5 Δ or more in the horizontal deviation occurs after an intravenous injection of Tensilon (Retzlaff *et al.* 1969). In practice, any change in the deviation greater than 5 Δ (half a small square on the Hess chart) should be recorded as a positive response (Fig. 20.2a,b).
- Observation of ptosis. The patient should be seated in a chair that can be easily reclined in case of an adverse reaction to the Tensilon. Two observers should be present, and the patient should be instructed to assume comfortable gaze on a distant object; the presence of frontalis overaction should be minimized. Both observers should note any improvement in the ptosis, in addition to measuring any change. In patients suspected of malingering or where subjective interpretation is difficult, a placebo injection of normal saline is given and the response compared.
- Electromyography (EMG). This can be used to measure the action potentials of contracting muscle fibres before and after injecting Tensilon. In myasthenia, the EMG shows fatigue of single fibre response following repetitive stimulation and an enhanced response after Tensilon. The technique of EMG is described in Chapter 6.

Other techniques include the measurement of intraocular pressure before and after the Tensilon test. A positive response is a rise of more than 5 mmHg and is due to increased compression of the globe by improved muscle tone.

Interpretation of response to Tensilon

- Although a positive response nearly always indicates a diagnosis of myasthenia, there are reports of positive responses in the presence of other intracranial

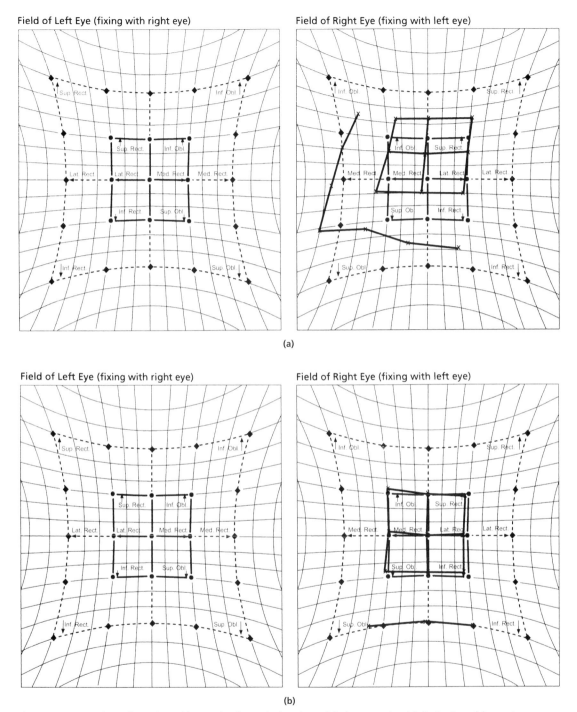

Fig. 20.2 (a) Hess chart of a patient with myasthenia gravis showing a right hypertropia with limitation of depression.
(b) Hess chart of same patient following Tensilon injection demonstrating a positive response with complete recovery of depression.

disease. The diagnosis of myasthenia based solely on the response to Tensilon should not detract from continuing to monitor all patients and, in the presence of other neurological signs, or when the natural history of the condition suggests a progressive course, then appropriate neuro-imaging should be arranged.

• A negative response to Tensilon does not exclude the diagnosis of myasthenia, as some myasthenic patients do not respond well to anticholinesterases. Muscles that have been chronically affected also become permanently weakened and do not respond either to Tensilon or to the longer-acting anticholinesterases.

• A negative response may occasionally follow the administration of only the main dose (8 mg) of Tensilon. If a patient is extremely sensitive to the drug, the muscles can change rapidly from a myasthenic state to a cholinergic state, and no improvement in muscle function is observed. It is therefore important to observe the response to the initial test dose (2 mg) of Tensilon before proceeding further with the test.

Anti-acetylcholine receptor site antibodies

In myasthenia, antibodies are directed to the postsynaptic muscle end-plate and their presence can be measured in the serum. Patients with generalized myasthenia are more likely to have demonstrable antibodies (80–90%) compared with those with ocular myasthenia (40–50%). The presence of such antibodies makes a diagnosis of myasthenia highly probable, but absence does not exclude it.

Radiology

The thymus can be become enlarged in myasthenia. A CT scan of the thoracic inlet should be performed on all patients diagnosed with myasthenia.

Management

In general, patients with evidence of generalized myasthenia are treated more aggressively that those with the ocular form.

Generalized myasthenia
Enhancing neuromuscular transmission

Initial treatment should be with anticholinesterases such as pyridostigmine (Mestinon) given orally, at an initial dose of 60 mg three time a day. This treatment is frequently effective in relieving symptoms in patients in the early stages of the disease with mild muscle involvement.

Suppression of the immune system

Patients with evidence on CT scan of thymus gland enlargement (due to a thymoma or thymic hyperplasia) should be considered for thymectomy. Following thymectomy, two-thirds of patients enter a complete remission or respond to lower levels of medical treatment. One of the mechanisms by which thymectomy works may be by the removal of reserves of the B-cells responsible for the production of the acetylcholine receptor antibody.

Systemic steroids are often effective in the treatment of myasthenia, and initially patients should be started on 10 mg of prednisolone, which can then be slowly increased if necessary. Steroid side-effects may prevent the optimum level of systemic steroids being maintained. Azathioprine is a useful agent that has an additive effect to any systemic steroids, allowing the steroid dose to be reduced. Close monitoring of all patients on systemic immunosuppression treatment is essential. Steroids are probably effective by their action in reducing antibody production and decreasing receptor activity.

Plasmaphoresis to reduce the level of circulating antibodies has been used (Seybold *et al.* 1982), along with human immunoglobulin.

Providing rehabilitative support

It is important that all patients with ocular symptoms who are on medical treatment are seen by an orthoptist. The use of Fresnel prisms in conjunction with medical treatment can result in a lower maintenance level of treatment and as a result fewer systemic side-effects occur.

Tree 20.4 Summary of management options in myasthenia gravis.

Management ──┬── Enhance neuromuscular transmission
             │   Suppression of the immune system ──┬── Medical
             │   Rehabilitation   └── Surgical

Ocular myasthenia

Myasthenia that remains confined to the ocular muscles for longer than 2 years is unlikely to progress to generalized myasthenia. Ocular myasthenia is not life threatening, therefore consideration needs to be given to the potential side-effects of any treatment. Thymectomy is at present not indicated in ocular myasthenia. Ptosis props can be used to support the upper eyelid on flexible loops of wire mounted on the spectacle frame. Prisms are often ineffective due to the variability of the deviation. Occlusion of one eye may be preferred in some cases rather than risk the systemic side-effects of medical treatment.

Botulinum toxin

Botulinum toxin has a role in confirming binocular potential in patients prior to embarking on surgical treatment.

Strabismus surgery

Surgery is contraindicated in the active stage of the disease because of the variability of the deviation. However, once the condition is quiescent, patients may benefit from strabismus surgery (Acheson *et al.* 1991; Davidson *et al.* 1993). Surgery performed under general anaesthesia has a risk of causing a myasthenic crisis; intensive care support must therefore be available prior to embarking on surgery under general anaesthesia. We prefer to operate on adult patients under local anaesthesia, using adjustable sutures where possible.

Lambert–Eaton–Rooke syndrome (LERS)

This is a disorder of neuromuscular transmission which differs from myasthenia in that the transmission defect is presynaptic rather than postsynaptic (Vincent 1988).

Aetiology

There is a strong association between LERS and malignancy, predominantly small-cell carcinoma of the lung. In a review of 50 cases O'Neill *et al.* (1988) showed an incidence of 62% of this typical carcinoma. LERS may predate the diagnosis. However, if the syndrome has been present for more than 2 years without evidence of malignancy the risk of its subsequent development declines sharply.

Features

Extraocular muscle involvement is unusual in this syndrome. The features tend to be:
• limb girdle and axial weakness;
• autonomic symptoms are common, particularly a dry mouth;
• ptosis occurs less frequently than in myasthenia; O'Neill *et al.* reported a 52% incidence.

The resting muscle action potential is reduced but unlike the response in myasthenia, it increases progressively after repetitive nerve stimulation, or following a short period of voluntary contracture (facilitation).

There is a variable response to Tensilon injection. Dell'Osso *et al.* (1983), using an electro-oculographic technique, found a positive response in two out of five patients.

An assay is now available to identify circulating antibodies.

The management of patients with LERS is limited to excluding underlying malignancy.

Chronic progressive external ophthalmoplegia (CPEO)

A number of muscle disorders are caused by or associated with defects in mitochondrial function. CPEO is the most frequently encountered disorder of this type found in clinical practice. Since nearly all mitochondrial DNA is maternally transmitted, almost all cases of CPEO arise in this way.

It seems likely that CPEO represents a number of different conditions that have in common the presence of a progressive external ophthalmoplegia. Petty *et al.* (1986) reviewed the clinical features of 66 patients with histologically defined mitochondrial myopathy. They found a variety of clinical presentations, but 55% showed progressive ophthalmoplegia and 36% of the total group had a pigmentary retinopathy. However, 27% of the patients with the typical mitochondrial changes found on muscle biopsy (ragged red fibres) had primary neurological signs such as ataxia and seizures.

Features

CPEO is characterized by progressive symmetrical loss of ocular motility accompanied by ptosis and orbicularis weakness. Smooth muscle is not affected and pupillary reactions and accommodation remain normal. In the late stages of the disease, the eyes are virtually immobile and secondary fibrotic changes occur, introducing a marked mechanical element, which can be identified by forced duction testing. The symmetrical involvement of both eyes and the slow progressive nature of the condition mean that most patients are not aware of diplopia and usually present with advanced limitation of ocular movement. However, not all patients have equal restriction in the early stages, so that diplopia may be the presenting symptom in a minority of cases. Some groups of patients have no evidence of ptosis. Saccadic velocities are always reduced (Metz & Meshel 1974).

Clinical syndromes associated with CPEO

CPEO may occur alone or in association with a variety of systemic disorders. The term 'ophthalmoplegia-plus' has been used to describe these various syndromes. The best known of them is described below, but it should be noted that the collection of physical signs into syndromes is not supported by laboratory findings.

Kearns–Sayre–Daroff syndrome

This is characterized by:
• CPEO, usually starting in childhood;
• fine pigmentary retinopathy;
• heart conduction block.

All the above features should occur before 20 years of age to fulfil the standard criteria for the diagnosis. Many other less commonly associated conditions have been described, including ataxia, dementia, raised CSF protein and short stature, but the presence of these findings is variable.

Differential diagnosis

A progressive external ophthalmoplegia may be caused by a number of different conditions; these need to be excluded before making the diagnosis of CPEO. Conditions that may cause a progressive external ophthalmoplegia include:

• Myasthenia: the presence of a positive response to Tensilon, anti-acetylcholine receptor antibodies, or normal saccadic velocities strongly supports the diagnosis of myasthenia.
• Mechanical disorders such as thyroid eye disease: most patients will show the characteristic ocular features of thyroid eye disease. However, 10% of patients with myasthenia gravis will also have thyroid eye disease. Some will show a variable ptosis or strabismus, including the presence of a divergent strabismus in the setting of thyroid eye disease (see Chapter 21).
• Supranuclear gaze palsy: supranuclear disorders should show improvement in movement on doll's head testing, whereas CPEO will remain unchanged.
• Multiple cranial nerve palsies: an asymmetrical disorder of eye movement similar to CPEO can be seen with brainstem demyelination and the Miller Fisher syndrome. Other neurological symptoms and signs suggestive of primary brainstem disease are often present.

Management

All patients should have an ECG and fundus examination to identify those with the Kearns–Sayre–Daroff syndrome. The ECG must be repeated yearly in those patients with no evidence of heart conduction defects.

The progress of the disease can be recorded, but the bilateral nature of the disorder reduces the value of the Hess chart as an indicator of change. Fields of uniocular fixation may be useful.

The disorder may be somewhat asymmetrical in the early stages, giving rise to diplopia, which may be relieved by prisms. The eyes are relatively immobile in the later stages and prisms are then of little benefit. Should the eye become anchored in a grossly eccentric position, then muscle surgery to straighten it may be justified. However, the potential anaesthetic dangers of heart block or pharyngeal muscle weakness may contraindicate intervention. Usually surgery is not required. Ptosis props may help the ptosis. Ptosis surgery runs the risk of causing serious exposure keratitis due to the associated poor orbicularis function and absent Bell's phenomenon.

Orbital myositis (orbital pseudotumour)

This condition is characterized by an inflammatory swelling of one or more of the extraocular muscles. It may be:

• unilateral or bilateral;
• acute or chronic.

In some cases there is a previous history of an upper respiratory tract infection (Purcell & Taulbee 1981). In a group of eight patients seen by us, three patients showed evidence of a raised influenza antibody titre, and one patient a raised antistreptolysin (ASO) titre (unpublished data). Four out of the 12 patients reported by Weinstein *et al.* (1983) gave a history of ocular or systemic autoimmune disease.

Features

When only one muscle is affected, the typical limitation of movement is:

• paretic in the direction of the involved muscle's action;
• mechanical in the opposite direction, because the inflammatory process prevents adequate muscle relaxation.

   The Hess chart, saccadic velocity measurements and forced duction testing (see Chapter 5) can confirm these signs. The patient often complains of pain, made worse by ocular movement. Computed tomography (CT) shows marked swelling of the affected muscles.

   Other signs of orbital inflammatory disease will be present to a variable degree. In severe cases there may be:

• lid swelling
• chemosis
• proptosis.

Differential diagnosis

Orbital myositis should be distinguished from the following conditions.

• Thyroid eye disease: ocular myositis can resemble thyroid eye disease in presentation. The two conditions can usually be differentiated by:

   1 lid retraction and lid-lag, which are typical of thyroid eye disease but are absent in orbital myositis;

   2 thyroid function, which should be normal in myositis, with absence of thyroid autoantibodies;

   3 the onset is usually gradual in thyroid eye disease and more acute in myositis;

   4 thyroid eye disease is usually bilateral, with evidence of multiple muscle involvement on CT imaging;

   5 in myositis there is CT scan evidence of involvement of the extraocular muscle tendon, which is usually spared in thyroid eye disease.

• Orbital pseudotumour: orbital myositis probably represents a subgroup of idiopathic orbital pseudotumour. With pseudotumour there is usually enhancement of the orbital fat on CT imaging without evidence of muscle enlargement.

• Orbital cellulitis: this is an infective disease associated with systemic symptoms. Most cases arise secondary to adjacent sinus infection.

• Orbital rhabdomyosarcoma: this tumour usually occurs in childhood, when it is rare for orbital myositis to occur.

Management

Orbital myositis may occasionally be self-limiting. However, in some cases of acute orbital myositis the condition can become chronic. The early use of systemic steroids may reduce the risk of acute orbital myositis recurring and possibly becoming chronic (Weinstein *et al.* 1983).

Conservative treatment of strabismus

Mild restriction of ocular motility only requires treatment if it is symptom producing. Some patients can be managed with prisms.

Botulinum toxin

Botulinum toxin has been used successfully in a group of patients reported by Bessant and Lee (1995), and we would support their view that botulinum toxin should be the first line of treatment in those patients failing to respond to conservative management.

Strabismus surgery

Strabismus following orbital myositis is usually mechanical. Surgery should be delayed until the condition has stabilized, and the patient is off systemic treatment. Even then, the patient should be warned about the risk of further attacks.

Rhabdomyosarcoma

This is a highly malignant tumour of striated muscle and usually presents in childhood; there are isolated case reports of the tumour occurring in later life. The affected patient may present with a squint and show restriction of ocular movement, or the tumour growth may be so rapid that there is acute proptosis and orbital signs suggesting orbital cellulitis. Prompt diagnosis is essential. Prognosis has improved following advances in radiotherapy and chemotherapy.

References

Acheson, J.F., Elston, J.S., Lee, J.P. & Fells, P. (1991) Extraocular muscle surgery in myasthenia gravis. *British Journal of Ophthalmology* 75, 232–235.

Bessant, D.A.R. & Lee, J.P. (1995) Management of strabismus due to orbital myositis. *Eye* 9, 558–563.

Bucknall, R.C., Dickson, A.StJ., Glick, E.N., Woodland, J. & Zutchi, D.W. (1975) Myasthenia gravis associated with penicillamine treatment for rheumatoid arthritis. *British Medical Journal* 5958 (i), 600–602.

Bucknall, R.C., Ballint, G. & Dorkins, R.L. (1979) Myasthenia associated with D-penicillamine therapy in rheumatoid arthritis. *Scandinavian Journal of Rheumatology* 28, 91–93.

Cogan, D.G. (1965) Myasthenia gravis. *Archives of Ophthalmology* 74, 217–221.

Davidson, J.L., Rosenbaum, A.L. & McCall, L.C. (1993) Strabismus surgery in patients with myasthenia. *Journal of Pediatric Ophthalmology and Strabismus* 30, 292–295.

Dell'Osso, L.F., Ayyah, D.R., Daroff, R.B. & Abel, L.A. (1983) Edrophonium test in the Eaton–Lambert syndrome: quantitative oculography. *Neurology* 33, 1152–1163.

Gorelick, P.B., Rosenberg, M. & Pagano, R.J. (1981) Enhanced ptosis in myasthenia gravis. *Archives of Neurology* 38, 531.

Katz, L.J., Lesser, R.L., Merikangas, J.R. & Silverman, J.P. (1989) Ocular myasthenia after D-penicillamine administration. *British Journal of Ophthalmology* 73, 1015–1018.

Metz, H.S. & Meshel, L. (1974) Ocular saccades in progressive external ophthalmoplegia. *Annals of Ophthalmology* 6, 623–628.

Morris, J.E. (1982) Ocular presentation of juvenile myasthenia gravis. *American Orthoptic Journal* 32, 51–55.

O'Neill, J.H., Murray, N.M. & Newsome-Davis, J. (1988) The Lambert–Eaton syndrome; review of 50 cases. *Brain* 111, 577–596.

Osher, R.H. & Griggs, R.C. (1979) Orbicularis fatigue. The 'Peek' sign of myasthenia gravis. *Archives of Ophthalmology* 97, 677–679.

Osserman, K.E. (1967) Ocular myasthenia gravis. *Investigative Ophthalmology* 6, 277–287.

Petty, R.K.H., Harding, A.E. & Morgan-Hughes, J.A. (1986) The clinical features of mitochondrial myopathy. *Brain* 109, 915–938.

Purcell, J. & Taulbee, W.A. (1981) Orbital myositis after upper respiratory tract infection. *Archives of Ophthalmology* 99, 437–438.

Retzlaff, J.A., Kearns, T.P., Howard, F.M. & Cronin, M.L. (1969) Lancaster red-green test in evaluation of edrophonium effects in myasthenia gravis. *American Journal of Ophthalmology* 67, 13–21.

Seybold, M., Tsoukas, C., Lindstrom, J., Fong, S. & Vaughan, J. (1982) Leukoplasmapheresis for myasthenia gravis. *Neurology* 39, 433–435.

Vincent, A. (1988) Disorders of neuromuscular transmission. *Current Opinion in Neurology and Neurosurgery* 1, 793–799.

Weinstein, G.S., Dresner, S.C., Slamovits, T.L. & Kennerdell, J.S. (1983) Acute and subacute orbital myositis. *American Journal of Ophthalmology* 96, 209–217.

Yee, R.D., Whitcup, S.M., Williams, I.M., Baloh, R.W. & Honrubia, V. (1987) Saccadic eye movements in myasthenia gravis. *Ophthalmology* 94, 219–225.

21
Mechanical Disorders of Ocular Motility

Mechanical restriction of ocular movement is caused by elements within the orbit which either interfere with muscle contraction and relaxation or otherwise prevent free movement of the globe. Physical restraint that interferes with normal muscle function is sometimes referred to as a leash or tether.

A leash may be direct or indirect:

• Direct: for example, a tight or shortened muscle or tendon, tightened overlying conjunctiva or surrounding connective tissue. These factors have the effect of limiting movement when gaze is directed away from the leash.

• Indirect: for example, a large retinal explant, a sinus mucocele or adhesions between the conjunctiva and orbit following trauma may limit eye movement when gaze is directed towards the leash.

Direct leashes are far more common in clinical practice.

Classification

This classification of mechanical disorders of ocular movement that follows is based on the clinical features of each condition. In some, it is possible to have both a mechanical and a paralytic component, for example in orbital blow-out fracture. In these cases, all aspects of the management are considered in this chapter. In others in which there is a primary myogenic, neurogenic or concomitant disorder with subsequent development of a mechanical component, management is discussed in the relevant chapter.

Mechanically caused conditions that result in a predictable pattern of restricted ocular movement can be divided into two groups, depending on the age of onset:
- Group 1: congenital or with onset in early childhood:
  1. Duane's retraction syndrome;
  2. Brown's syndrome;
  3. congenital fibrosis syndrome;
  4. adherence syndromes.
- Group 2: acquired later in childhood or in adult life:
  1. thyroid eye disease;
  2. orbital injuries;
  3. restriction following retinal detachment and cataract surgery;
  4. orbital inflammation;
  5. orbital tumours;
  6. secondary Brown's syndrome.

This list is not comprehensive. Mechanical restriction can also result from other causes, including strabismus surgery and ionizing radiation within the orbit, with unpredictable ocular movement patterns.

Characteristics of mechanically limited ocular movement

Important characteristics of mechanically limited ocular movement are listed below.
- A positive forced duction test, which is the essential feature of mechanical restriction.

- Normal saccadic velocity until the point of mechanical restriction is reached: this feature can differentiate a mechanical restriction from a neurogenic palsy.
- Retraction of the globe, which strongly suggests mechanical limitation: it occurs when gaze is directed away from the site of the leash and is best seen by viewing the affected eye from the side or by comparison of the two eyes by observing ocular movement from above the patient.
- Equal limitation of duction and version: although this is commonly seen with mechanical disorders it is not uncommon to find that with effort the duction movement can be made to exceed the version movement, although the increased movement is not easily sustained by the patient. In contrast, the increased duction movement seen in neurogenic palsies is both larger and better sustained.
- Reversal of the deviation in opposite directions of horizontal and vertical gaze, which is usually indicative of a mechanical factor.
- Limited development of muscle sequelae, often confined to overaction of the contralateral synergist in the unaffected eye.
- Abnormal patterns of movement, particularly the up-shoot and/or down-shoot resulting from a tight lateral rectus muscle in some cases of Duane's syndrome.
- Torsional movements of the globe which are frequently seen, especially when horizontal gaze reaches the point of mechanical restriction. These movements should not be interpreted as torsional nystagmus.

General principles of management

Treatment is directed to ensuring that the patient is comfortable and has a satisfactory appearance. In many cases these criteria are already met and treatment is not required. When indicated, treatment is usually surgical, with the following aims:
- To centralize and if possible enlarge the field of binocular single vision, reducing the need for an abnormal head posture.
- To reduce or eliminate anomalous ocular movements caused by mechanical restriction, for example, an up-shoot or down-shoot on attempted adduction. It is not always possible to increase the range of ocular movement.

• To correct the cosmetic defect, which may be caused by a strabismus or by other factors such as enophthalmos or eyelid anomalies.

The results of surgery are neither as consistent nor as permanent as they are in other forms of strabismus. Despite this limitation, great benefit can still be obtained by appropriately timed and selected surgical intervention.

Duane's retraction syndrome

This syndrome was first described by Stilling (1887) and Türk (1896) and is also known as the Stilling–Türk–Duane's syndrome. Duane (1905) discussed the disorder in more detail and it became generally known as Duane's retraction syndrome. The retraction syndrome is a congenital disorder and has been reported in a neonate aged just 1 day (Archer *et al.* 1989). Despite its congenital origin it is rarely recognized until later in childhood, when defective eye movement or an obvious compensatory head posture brings it to attention. Occasionally the problem remains unnoticed or unreported into adult life. The syndrome is thought to be unilateral in approximately 80% of cases, but since bilateral Duane's syndrome is usually markedly asymmetrical, it is possible that more subtle anomalies are missed and the incidence of bilateral involvement is higher. The left eye is affected more than twice as frequently as the right eye. Females show a slightly higher incidence than males, and a hereditary basis has been reported (Kirkham 1970).

Aetiology

Evidence has been presented which strongly suggests that the findings in Duane's retraction syndrome are due to innervation of the lateral rectus by extra branches of the third nerve in place of absent or deficient sixth nerve fibres. Hotchkiss *et al.* (1980) reported on the autopsy findings of two patients with documented Duane's syndrome. The sixth nerve and nucleus were absent in both cases. The inferior division of the third nerve was seen to bifurcate, giving off several small branches that entered the lateral rectus. The innervated portion of the muscle appeared healthy, in contrast to the fibrotic denervated portion.

Hoyt and Nachtigaller (1965) had earlier reported on the literature, describing several instances of similar third nerve misdirection to the lateral rectus. Huber (1984) reported examining a patient undergoing neurosurgery for removal of an acoustic neuroma: only two thin atrophic sixth nerve fibres were seen. Huber suggested that in Duane's syndrome the lateral rectus could have three parts:
• a normally innervated portion;
• a portion innervated by the third nerve;
• a denervated and therefore fibrotic portion.

If this is the case both biopsy and electromyography of the lateral rectus could have misleading results. The presence of a normally innervated portion would explain the variable limitation of abduction seen in Duane's syndrome; those patients capable of a significant amount of abduction would have a larger innervated portion of the muscle, whereas those lacking all abduction would lack all normal innervation.

Disruption of embryological development at the second stage is probably responsible for the cranial nerve abnormalities reported. A higher than normal incidence of skeletal and other congenital anomalies supports this view. The causes of this disruption are largely unknown, although Papst and Esslen (1960) reported on the high incidence of Duane's syndrome and other ocular motility disorders resulting from the use of the drug thalidomide during pregnancy. The high incidence of ocular motor disorders was confirmed by Miller (1992) in a review of 86 patients with thalidomide embryopathy, 31 had classic Duane's syndrome. Precise information was available about the timing of drug use and this was compared with the known sensitive periods for development. In cases where the drug was taken from day 20 to day 23, horizontal gaze palsies resulted, and between day 24 and day 35 classic Duane's syndrome occurred.

Misdirection of third nerve fibres to the lateral rectus results in a common nerve supply to the antagonistic horizontally acting muscles; in consequence co-contraction of the medial and lateral rectus muscles occurs on attempting adduction, limiting the amount of excursion. Abduction is limited because the lateral rectus is not adequately innervated by the sixth nerve and receives its maximal innervation by the third nerve when the eye is adducted. Co-contraction can also explain retraction of the globe and the up-shoot and down-shoot on adduction commonly seen.

Features

The main features of Duane's syndrome are described below, and illustrated in Figs 21.1–21.3.

• Limitation of horizontal eye movement, usually comprising a moderate or marked limitation of abduction. In most cases there is little or no limitation of adduction; in others adduction is restricted but to a lesser extent than abduction. Less commonly, the limitation of adduction exceeds the limitation of abduction. One or, more rarely, both eyes can be affected: the pattern of defective movement can differ in each eye in bilateral cases and is commonly very asymmetrical, with the movement of one eye restricted far more than the other.

• Compensatory head posture, which is mainly adopted to centralize the often narrow field of binocular single vision. Occasionally the head posture is used to facilitate foveal fixation if the patient's preferred eye has marked limitation of movement. The head posture is determined by the deviation in the primary position and by the pattern of ocular movement. Most patients are esotropic, with an increased deviation for distance, therefore the common head posture is a face turn to the affected side, more marked for distance fixation and reduced or not required for near. Patients with greater limitation of adduction have exotropia, which increases for near fixation and is compensated by a face turn to the unaffected side, particularly for near. Some patients can abduct better with the eyes in an elevated position, giving rise to a V-pattern and to a chin depression to minimize the esotropia. The opposite also occurs, with improved abduction on depression of gaze, an A-pattern and chin elevation. A V- or A-pattern is also seen when there is an up-shoot or down-shoot on adduction. Chin elevation or depression may be combined with a face turn. Patients with very asymmetrical bilateral Duane's syndrome adopt similar head postures, dictated by the defective movement in the more affected eye. When both eyes are affected to a marked extent, the patient is more likely to present with a manifest strabismus and may need to adopt a face turn to

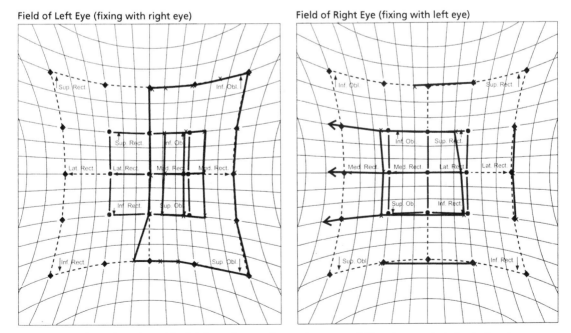

Fig. 21.1 Hess chart of a patient with a left Duane's retraction syndrome, type I. There is an esodeviation in the primary position with marked limitation of left abduction and overaction of the contralateral medial rectus muscle.

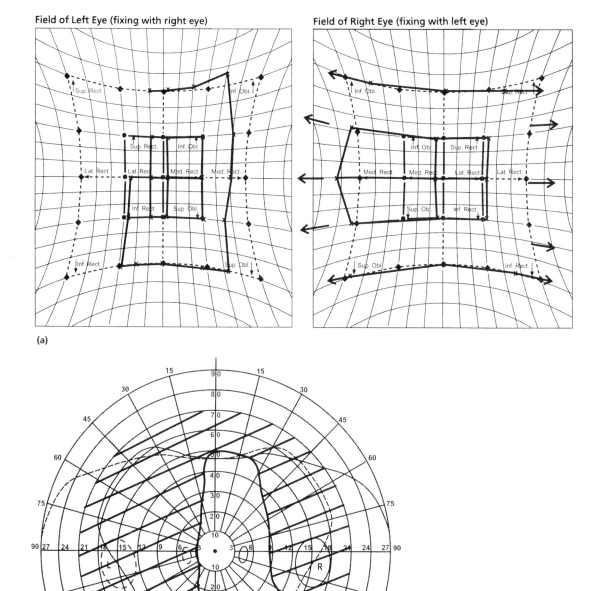

(a)

(b)

Fig. 21.2 (a) Hess chart of a patient with a left Duane's retraction syndrome, type III, without significant deviation in the primary position. (b) Uniocular field of fixation of the same patient. There is marked restriction of abduction and moderate restriction of adduction of the left eye.

Field of Left Eye (fixing with right eye)   **Field of Right Eye (fixing with left eye)**

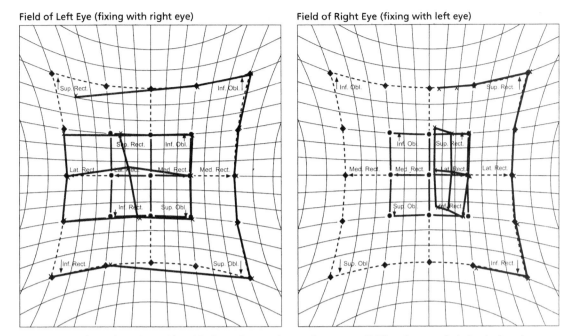

Fig. 21.3 Hess chart of a patient with a right Duane's retraction syndrome, type II. There is an exodeviation in the primary position with marked limitation of right adduction and overaction of the contralateral lateral rectus muscle.

maintain fixation. Patients who maintain binocular single vision can be seen to use head tracking rather than eye tracking. The obvious head movement is an important diagnostic sign, and is necessitated by the restricted field of binocular single vision.

• Manifest strabismus, usually esotropia, when the head is straight. Exotropia mainly occurs when adduction is more limited than abduction. The strabismus is markedly incomitant in unilateral cases and in asymmetrical bilateral cases, with a marked increase in the deviation when the patient is made to fix with the more affected eye.

• Retraction of the globe on adduction, with narrowing of the palpebral fissure. Both globe retraction and limitation of adduction are caused by co-contraction of the horizontal rectus muscles: narrowing of the palpebral fissure is the direct result of globe retraction. The magnitude of the co-contraction is closely related to the amount of retraction, the extent of limitation of adduction and the presence of up-shoot and down-shoot of adduction. In general the greater the co-contraction, the greater the retraction and limitation of movement. In a few cases retraction of

the globe can cause displaced orbital fat to bulge through the septum orbitale and a swelling can be seen below the eye as it attempts adduction. Widening of the palpebral fissure on attempted abduction is also observed but is probably of no significance since it also occurs in cases of acquired sixth nerve palsy.

• Up-shoot and/or down-shoot on adduction. An up-shoot of the eye on attempted adduction is commonly seen, usually more apparent when the eye is adducted above the mid-line; a down-shoot frequently occurs in the same eye when adducted below the mid-line. Co-contraction of the horizontal recti on attempted adduction causes the globe to slip up or down behind the tight lateral rectus muscle, allowing the medial rectus to act as an elevator when the eye is above the mid-line and as a depressor when it is below the mid-line. The greater the co-contraction the more marked the up-shoot and down-shoot. A tight lateral rectus can also contribute to the restriction of adduction. Depression or elevation on abduction, which is much less common, can be explained in a similar way, when a tight medial rectus causes slippage of the globe and the lateral rectus acts to bring about upward or downward movement. An up-drift or down-drift is seen in the abducting eye when there is inferior or superior oblique muscle overaction in the contralateral eye and this eye maintains fixation.

• Absence of diplopia. Patients may rarely complain of diplopia, although some are aware of crossed diplopia on contralateral version. Diplopia is sometimes elicited using red and green goggles and a spotlight, making it possible to plot the field of binocular single vision.

• Poor convergence. Convergence deficiency is sometimes present when there is significant limitation of adduction, and may trouble an older child or adult, although this is uncommon.

• Associated ocular abnormalities, which are well documented and include colobomata, heterochromic iridis, lens opacities, microphthalmos and persistent pupillary membrane. The underlying refractive error in patients with the retraction syndrome does not differ significantly from that found in a normal population (Tredici & von Noorden 1985; Raab 1986).

• Skeletal and facial abnormalities and evidence of abnormal neural development which have been reported include Goldenhar's and Klippel–Feil syndromes, abnormal ear formation, deafness, syndactyly, cleft palate and spinal meningocele (Pfaffenbach *et al.* 1972).

Specific features of the condition

Abnormal head posture

An abnormal head posture is mainly adopted to centralize the field of binocular single vision. Occasionally it is used to place the fixing eye in an optimum position. This can occur if the syndrome is bilateral, or if the affected eye is preferred for fixation.

The head posture is determined by the deviation in the primary position. Most patients are esotropic, with an increased deviation for distance. Therefore, the head posture is commonly a face turn to the affected side, more marked for distance fixation and reduced or not required for near.

If there is an exotropia, the face is turned to the unaffected side to compensate for the limitation of adduction that will be more troublesome for near fixation. If an A- or V-pattern is present the chin may

be elevated or depressed to make use of the position of minimum deviation.

Globe retraction and up-shoot and down-shoot on adduction

The magnitude of the co-contraction of the horizontal recti on adduction is closely related to the retraction of the globe, the limitation of adduction and the presence of up-shoot or down-shoot. Marked up-shoot and down-shoot tends to be observed in the presence of marked limitation of adduction and severe globe retraction. The mechanism for the up- and down-shoot has been shown to be due to slippage of the globe around a tight lateral rectus muscle. The latter can result in mechanical restriction of adduction and is a contributory factor in some cases. Depression or elevation of the eye on attempting abduction, which is much less common, may be explained in a similar way, with the lateral rectus acting to bring about upward or downward movement. Rarely up-shoots and down-shoots may arise from co-innervation of the vertical and lateral rectus muscles; in this situation a moderate hypertropia is frequently present in the primary position and a gradual up-drift or down-drift of the eye occurs.

Not all the diagnostic features of the retraction syndrome may be apparent in the very young child, making the diagnosis in those below the age of 1 year difficult (Caputo *et al.* 1996).

Useful diagnostic clues in Duane's retraction syndrome are:

• a significant face turn;

• obvious head tracking: because the field of binocular single vision is so restricted the child turns his face to follow or fixate an object to either side;

• the small size of an esotropia despite marked limitation of abduction.

Although abduction is very obviously limited, in a few patients the defect is slight with no evidence of globe retraction on adduction, so that the diagnosis can be missed. The retraction syndrome has been diagnosed only after surgery for an esotropia (Elsas 1991). We have observed this in a patient with esotropia associated with slight limitation of abduction without retraction on adduction. Following horizontal muscle surgery, features of Duane's syndrome became apparent, with limitation of adduction and associated retraction of the globe. Further surgery was later required.

Classification

Both Brown (1950) and Huber (1974) have classified Duane's syndrome according to the characteristics of the limitation of movement.

BROWN'S CLASSIFICATION

Type A: with limited abduction and less-marked limitation of adduction, as described by Duane.
Type B: showing limited abduction but normal adduction.
Type C: in which the limitation of adduction exceeds the limitation of abduction. There is an exotropic deviation and a face turn to compensate the loss of adduction.

HUBER'S CLASSIFICATION

This classification takes account of the electromyographic evidence of differing aetiology.
Duane (type) I: characterized by marked limitation of abduction, explained by maximal innervation reaching the lateral rectus when the eye is adducted.
Duane (type) II: characterized by limitation of adduction, explained by co-contraction of the horizontal recti on attempted adduction.
Duane (type) III: characterized by limitation of both abduction and adduction, explained by co-contraction of the horizontal recti, as in type II, but also demonstrating loss of innervation to the lateral rectus on attempted abduction.

Huber's subtyping adequately describes the disordered horizontal motility seen in Duane's syndrome and is supported by electromyographic findings. However, many patients do not fit neatly into this classification; in particular, types I and III probably represent a continuum rather than being separate entities, likewise type II and the condition known as synergistic divergence (described below).

VARIANTS OF DUANE'S SYNDROME

• Congenital adduction deficiency with synergistic divergence. This is a rare disorder of ocular motility characterized by an exotropia with marked limitation of adduction. On attempted adduction, the affected eye moves further into the field of abduction increasing the size of the exotropia. This condition is also known colloquially as the 'the splits' and using electromyography it has been shown that the limitation of adduction results from anomalous and excessive innervation of the antagonist lateral rectus muscle.
• Co-innervation with other branches of the third nerve. In some patients co-innervation of the lateral rectus muscle and vertically acting muscles supplied by the third nerve can occur, leading to up-drift and down-drift on horizontal gaze.

Diagnosis

The aims of diagnosis are summarized as follows:
• accurate recording of the various features of the condition;
• differentiation of unilateral and bilateral Duane's syndrome;
• assessment of the extent to which the syndrome is compensated;
• evaluation of the cosmetic effect of the compensatory head posture, globe retraction and up-shoot or down-shoot on adduction.

Methods

• The cover test is performed routinely with and without any abnormal head posture for near and distance.
• Ocular movements should be tested, noting any difference in the amount of horizontal movement elicited when tested above and below the mid-line and observing any up-shoot or down-shoot on adduction or abduction. The presence of an A- or V-pattern should be noted. The observer should look carefully for signs of bilateral involvement. The near point of convergence should be measured.
• Changes in lid and globe position on horizontal gaze should be carefully assessed. Change in the depth of the palpebral fissure can be quantified as a percentage of the normal, for example a 50% reduction on adduction. Unless obvious retraction of the globe is seen, the patient should be observed from either side at eye level as each eye is adducted, or from above, when it is easier to see the comparative position of the globes.

• The deviation should be measured fixing with each eye for near and distance with the head straight. Quite marked incomitance is often present in the primary position and is best measured using the prism cover test.

• Confirmation of binocular single vision should be obtained whenever it is in doubt, using a base-out prism, a stereo-test, Bagolini glasses or the Worth four dot test, depending on age and cooperation. Most patients maintain binocular single vision with an abnormal head posture.

• It is usually possible to plot a Hess chart but particular care must be taken to stabilize the patient's head. Head movement is natural to a patient with this condition and a very small change in position can significantly alter the chart.

• The presence or absence of diplopia should be investigated. If diplopia can be elicited, using a spotlight and red and green glasses if necessary, it should be possible to obtain a field of binocular single vision. Again, it is imperative that the patient's head should be kept straight and static.

• The innervation pattern of the horizontal rectus muscles can be recorded using electromyography, as demonstrated first by Breinin (1957) and later by Huber (1974). Electromyography is rarely necessary to make a diagnosis but we have occasionally found it useful in investigating adult patients who initially present with features of Duane's syndrome which they relate to a recent event, usually trauma.

Differential diagnosis

Acquired simulated Duane's retraction syndrome

Disorders simulating Duane's syndrome can result from:

• Trauma to the eye or localized inflammation inhibiting the action of the lateral rectus. This can result in restriction of both abduction and adduction and in retraction of the globe on attempting adduction. Spontaneous recovery may occur depending on the cause and on the extent of damage to the lateral rectus muscle.

• Liberal resection of the lateral rectus has the same effect as trauma.

In both instances there will be limitation of passive horizontal movement. Ocular movement may be painful if inflammation is the cause of the limitation. These conditions differ from true Duane's syndrome in that innervation to the muscles follows a normal pattern. Restriction of ocular movement is purely mechanical.

Möbius' syndrome

Möbius' syndrome is a congenital and usually sporadic disorder of ocular movement characterized by bilateral facial weakness and loss of abduction, often symmetrical. It can superficially resemble bilateral Duane's syndrome. Distinguishing features are the lack of facial expression due to facial nerve palsy and absence of retraction of the globe and narrowing of the palpebral fissures (see Chapter 19).

Congenital sixth nerve palsy

Congenital sixth nerve palsy is very rare. Features which suggest this diagnosis include an esotropia, often of large angle, with limited abduction but no evidence of limited adduction nor the associated globe retraction and the up-shoot and or down-shoot which are typical of Duane's syndrome. Despite these differences, the differential diagnosis can still present problems (Souza-Dias 1992). The presence of other neurological deficits, especially papilloedema, demands further investigation.

Infantile esotropia

Infantile esotropia, often alternating, may present with apparent limitation of abduction affecting both eyes; abduction can usually be demonstrated, either by occluding the contralateral eye for a period, or by rotating a young child to induce vestibular nystagmus, thus demonstrating movement past the mid-line. No other characteristics of Duane's syndrome will be present.

Management

The majority of patients with Duane's syndrome maintain comfortable binocular single vision and remain compensated, usually with a comparatively slight face turn. Symptoms are uncommon and often the patient's friends are unaware of the abnormality because he moves his head rather than eyes. Surgical treatment is therefore required in only a few cases.

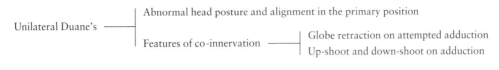

Unilateral Duane's ———┤ Abnormal head posture and alignment in the primary position

Features of co-innervation ———┤ Globe retraction on attempted adduction
Up-shoot and down-shoot on adduction

Bilateral Duane's

Tree 21.1 Factors influencing surgery in Duane's syndrome.

Surgery is indicated for the following reasons:
• decompensation, giving rise to manifest strabismus in childhood or resulting in symptoms at a later stage;
• a cosmetically poor compensatory head posture;
• a cosmetically poor manifest strabismus, most often seen when both eyes are affected;
• severe globe retraction with or without up-shoot and down-shoot.

Surgical treatment

The aims of surgery are:
• to correct a manifest strabismus;
• to centralize the field of binocular single vision, enlarging it if possible;
• to overcome or reduce the need for a large compensatory head posture;
• to reduce the consequences of co-innervation of the medial and lateral recti on attempted adduction.

Improvement of horizontal ocular movement is very unlikely to be achieved and is not the purpose of surgery. This should be clearly understood by the patient or his parents before surgery is undertaken.

Kraft (1993) suggested that surgical treatment of Duane's syndrome should be based on features of the condition that are likely to influence the type and amount of any surgery rather than on Huber's classification. The surgeon should consider:
• whether the condition is unilateral or bilateral;
• the presence of an abnormal head posture and the size of the deviation in the primary position; in most cases surgery should be delayed until 5–6 years of age;
• characteristics related to co-innervation of the medial and lateral recti on adduction, namely globe retraction with narrowing of the palpebral fissure and the presence of up-shoot and down-shoot.

With a few modifications, we have adopted a similar approach in our surgical treatment of the condition.

Unilateral Duane's syndrome

ABNORMAL HEAD POSTURE AND THE
DEVIATION IN THE PRIMARY POSITION

The most common reason for operating on patients with Duane's syndrome is to correct a head posture. The direction and size of the head posture is determined by the type of deviation in the primary position and by which eye is affected by the syndrome. Duane's syndrome may present with esotropia and exotropia.

Duane's syndrome with esotropia

This is the commonest form seen in our practice; most patients have type I Duane's. The size of the esotropia in the primary position is important when deciding on the amount and type of surgery. Surgery should include a recession of the ipsilateral medial rectus muscle.

Amount of surgery:
• Esotropia not greater than 15 Δ: ipsilateral medial rectus recession 5 mm.
• Esotropia between 15 and 25 Δ: ipsilateral medial rectus recession 5 mm; contralateral medial rectus recession 3 mm.
• Esotropia 25 Δ or greater: bilateral medial rectus recession 5 mm.

Other surgical options include adding a posterior fixation suture to the contralateral medial rectus muscle in an attempt further to balance the defect of restricted abduction and enlarge the field of binocular single vision.

Fells and McCarry (1987) described their experience using horizontal transposition of the vertical rectus muscles in patients with Duane's syndrome. Although their results were good, we recommend that the effective and simpler recession of the medial rectus muscle should be the procedure of first choice.

Duane's syndrome with exotropia

Duane's syndrome with exotropia is comparatively rare; most patients that we have seen show type II or type III Duane's. Adduction is limited with marked globe retraction on attempted adduction: in addition, there is often marked up-shoot and down-shoot. In type III Duane's the head posture is often relatively slight, and the main concern is the obvious globe retraction. Patients with type II Duane's, on the other hand, may show marked face turn to the side of the unaffected eye.

Surgery comprises a recession of the lateral rectus muscle. The amount and type of surgery depends on:
• the size of the exotropia in the primary position;
• the degree of mechanical restriction of adduction;
• the magnitude of the globe retraction and any up-shoot and down-shoot on attempted adduction.

RETRACTION OF THE GLOBE ON ADDUCTION
Co-innervation of the medial and lateral rectus muscles is responsible for most cases of globe retraction, although a tight lateral rectus muscle can be a contributory factor in some. The most severe globe retraction is found in Duane's type II and III. Surgical treatment comprises recession of the lateral rectus muscle in the affected eye; it is usually required only if there is at least a 50% narrowing of the palpebral fissure on adduction.

Important factors influencing the type and amount of surgery include:
• The presence of a contributory mechanical component to the limitation of adduction. A forced duction test greater than +1 limitation of adduction indicates a tight lateral rectus, which should be recessed 8–10 mm. A forced duction test of 0 or +1 limitation of adduction rules out muscle tightness, a larger lateral recession of 12–16 mm is required to achieve a satisfactory result.
• The presence of an abnormal head posture and the size of any deviation, discussed above.
• Up-shoot and down-shoot on adduction, discussed below.

UP-SHOOT AND/OR DOWN-SHOOT ON ATTEMPTED ADDUCTION
The magnitude of the co-contraction of the horizontal rectus muscles on adduction is closely related to the amount of retraction of the globe, the degree of limitation of adduction and the presence of up-shoot or down-shoot, which can be effectively managed by preventing the globe slipping over the ipsilateral lateral

rectus muscle on attempted adduction. This can be achieved by the following procedures:
• a large recession of the lateral rectus muscle;
• a lateral rectus muscle posterior fixation suture;
• a Y-splitting of the lateral rectus muscle (Jampolsky 1984; Rogers & Bremer 1984).

Most cases of up-shoot and down-shoot are associated with significant retraction of the globe on adduction and we usually combine a large recession of the ipsilateral lateral rectus muscle with a Y-splitting procedure.

Bilateral Duane's syndrome
Cases of bilateral Duane's syndrome may be more common than previously thought, in particular asymmetrical forms with only minimal involvement of the fellow eye. Different forms of Duane's syndrome may be present in the same patient, further complicating any surgical management. Surgical management is based on the same principles as for unilateral Duane's syndrome, with most cases requiring treatment for an abnormal head posture. Binocular potential is less common in this subgroup, particularly when both eyes are equally affected, with most patients requiring cosmetic surgery to correct an unsightly strabismus. Botulinum toxin has been effective in achieving stable long-term cosmetic alignment in a case of bilateral symmetrical type I Duane's that we have treated.

Postoperative management
Most cases of Duane's syndrome show considerable improvement following surgery. Less successful results occur due to an undercorrection or overcorrection.

Undercorrection
An undercorrection of a head posture or primary position alignment of the visual axes will require further surgery, preferably on the muscles of the fellow eye. Following an ipsilateral medial rectus muscle recession for a Duane's type I, a contralateral medial rectus muscle recession, combined with a posterior fixation suture if necessary, will often be effective.

Overcorrection
Overcorrection following surgery for Duane's syndrome is rare, but has been reported in association with severe limitation of adduction following a large ipsilateral medial rectus recession (Nelson 1986).

When there is significant retraction of the globe on adduction due to horizontal rectus muscle co-contraction, weakening the medial rectus muscle could result in increased co-contraction, leading to severe limitation of adduction. We recommend that the ipsilateral lateral rectus muscle is also recessed in these cases.

Mechanical restriction of the superior oblique tendon

Brown (1950) reported on a patient with limited elevation of the eye in adduction and a positive forced duction test in whom a tight superior oblique anterior tendon sheath was found at surgery. Division of the sheath resulted in immediate free passive movement and in improvement in elevation in adduction. This condition was assumed to be congenital and has become known as Brown's syndrome (or the superior oblique tendon sheath syndrome). An essential diagnostic feature of the syndrome is restricted elevation in adduction but normal depression in adduction. It is now believed that most cases of Brown's syndrome develop in infancy and that few, if any, are congenital.

The syndrome can be acquired later in childhood or in adult life through inflammation or trauma affecting the trochlear region, which can trap the superior oblique tendon. However, not all patients with this type of lesion show the characteristics of a classical Brown's syndrome; in some patients, particularly those with trochlear injury, it results in defective depression in adduction as well as defective elevation. We prefer not to apply the term 'Brown's syndrome' to this condition. The management of classical Brown's syndrome, whether acquired in infancy or later life, differs from that of patients with restricted elevation and depression, and the two groups are therefore considered separately. It should be noted that this classification depends on the clinical findings rather than the aetiology.

Brown's syndrome

Brown's syndrome is usually unilateral with less than 10% of bilateral cases; there is no preference for the right or left eye. Females are affected with the same frequency as males, and there does not appear to be any genetic basis for the disorder. Most patients maintain binocular single vision, although

the anomaly can be associated with esotropia or exotropia.

Patients with Brown's syndrome show all or some of the following characteristics:
• Limitation of elevation in adduction. If the restriction of movement is severe, there may also be some limitation of direct elevation and even of elevation in abduction.
• Down-drift of the affected eye on contralateral version, sometimes accompanied by widening of the palpebral fissure.
• Overaction of the contralateral superior rectus muscle. Other muscle sequelae do not develop, therefore there is no overaction of the superior oblique on the affected side.
• An A- or V-pattern. Fells (1975) reported a significant incidence of A-pattern in esotropic patients with Brown's syndrome, but in our experience a V-pattern is predominant whether or not there is an associated horizontal strabismus (Mein 1971).
• A very typical Hess chart, showing the limitation of elevation and no or minimal abnormality in the lower field (Figs 21.4 & 21.5).
• Discomfort on attempting elevation in adduction, which can range from reluctance to assume that position of gaze to actual pain.
• Improvement in elevation in adduction on repeated testing in that direction of gaze, sometimes accompanied by a 'click' (the so-called 'click syndrome'), followed in some cases by overaction of the ipsilateral inferior oblique with evidence of restricted movement on down-gaze. The development of a 'click' may be a good prognostic sign indicating that the condition may spontaneously resolve.
• Absence of cyclotropia.
• An abnormal head posture, comprising a head tilt to the affected side, a face turn to the contralateral side and chin elevation. The head posture is confined to chin elevation if the syndrome is bilateral and symmetrical. Many patients with Brown's syndrome can maintain comfortable binocular single vision without an abnormal head posture.
• A positive forced duction test.

Aetiology

The abnormality in most cases of Brown's syndrome involves the superior oblique tendon and/or

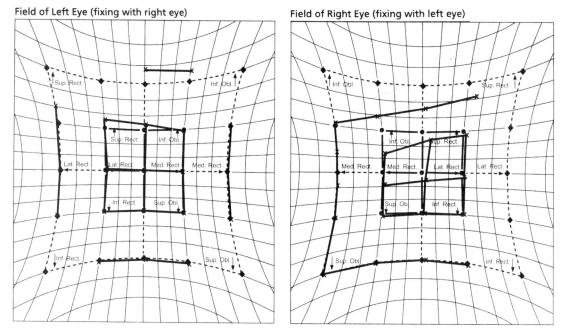

Fig. 21.4 Hess chart of a patient with a mild right Brown's syndrome.

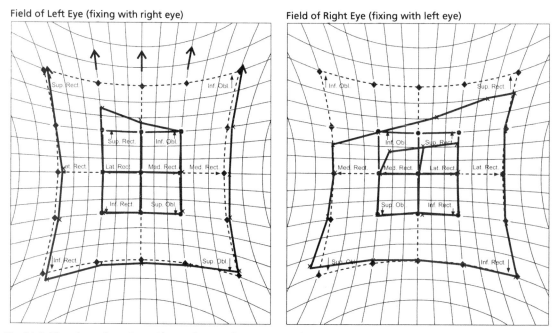

Fig. 21.5 Hess chart of a patient with a moderate right Brown's syndrome associated with mild ipsilateral superior oblique weakness but with no deviation in the primary position.

the trochlear complex. Its aetiology remains uncertain and may vary from one patient to another. Several theories have been proposed, and the main ones are described below.

DEVELOPMENTAL ANOMALY

One theory is that the condition arises due to a developmental anomaly affecting the trochlear/superior oblique complex. Sevel studied the embryological development of this region (Sevel 1981) and noted that the superior oblique tendon and the trochlea were connected during embryological development by thick trabeculae which gradually remodelled, leaving behind fine remnants which persisted after birth. He postulated that failure of the embryological trabeculae to remodel could explain some cases of Brown's syndrome.

Helveston et al. (1982) made a number of observations following a study of the anatomy and physiology of the trochlea and intratrochlear superior oblique tendon. These included:

1 A bursa-like structure separating the tendon and trochlea, the distension of which could result in an acquired Brown's syndrome, with or without a click.

2 The intratrochlear superior oblique tendon is normally enveloped in a vascular sheath, which may be important for maintaining the smooth passage of the tendon through the trochlea. The vascular sheath may help maintain the relatively high metabolic demands of the region and help dissipate the heat and repair the 'wear and tear' generated through the normal movement of the tendon through the trochlea. Similar vascular sheaths can be found surrounding other tendons, and the condition trigger finger has been likened to acquired Brown's syndrome (Sandford-Smith 1973), attributed to thickening of the sheath surrounding the tendon of the digits of the hand.

3 The superior oblique tendon itself is made up of fibres that span the whole length of the tendon with little in the way of connections between adjacent fibres. Movement of the tendon through the trochlea is believed to be achieved by differential movement of individual fibres; those situated centrally move more extensively than the more peripheral fibres during periods of contraction and relaxation of the superior oblique muscle. The tendon therefore does not move like a cord through a pulley, but rather behaves like a telescope with the component parts of the tendon sliding over each other. Disruption of the telescopic action by either developmental or acquired connections between the individual superior oblique fibres may be responsible for some cases of Brown's syndrome.

INELASTIC SUPERIOR OBLIQUE TENDON (Parks 1977)

A relatively inelastic tendon would result in a positive forced duction test but cannot be proved unless the posterior tendon is explored. However, an iatrogenic Brown's syndrome is usually observed after plication (tucking) of the tendon as a stage in the surgical treatment of fourth cranial nerve palsy. The inferior oblique is then prevented from elevating the eye in adduction as the superior oblique fails to relax, which gives some support to Park's view.

NODULE OR SWELLING ON THE TENDON

The concept of a nodule or swelling on the tendon just posterior to the trochlea, preventing free passage through it, was first proposed by Sandford-Smith (1969). If the swelling could be forced through the trochlea, a click could be felt or even heard and elevation in adduction improved. Sandford-Smith pointed out the similarity between Brown's syndrome and stenosing tenovaginitis (trigger finger), which is also acquired in early childhood. A number of disease processes can cause an inflammatory response and result in swelling on the tendon. These include rheumatoid arthritis, scleritis and systemic lupus erythematosus (Trimble et al. 1984). Some patients with Brown's syndrome respond to retrotrochlear injection of local steroids, supporting the view that an inflammatory process is responsible. Booth-Mason et al. (1985) have reported a patient with carcinoma of the prostate who developed a secondary deposit in the trochlear area. Trauma affecting the trochlea usually results in restriction of elevation and depression and is discussed below.

OTHER POSSIBLE CAUSES

Other possible causes of Brown's syndrome which have been reported are fibrous attachments between the superior rectus and the underlying superior oblique tendon, abnormality of the superior oblique insertion and paradoxical innervation of the inferior oblique and the superior oblique (Feric-Seiwerth & Celic

1972), similar to that found in Duane's retraction syndrome but without supporting anatomical evidence.

Natural history

Spontaneous improvement over a long period of time undoubtedly occurs in a significant number of patients with early-onset Brown's syndrome (Adler 1959; Costenbader & Albert 1959; Mein 1971; Waddell 1982). Whether the presence of a click signifies that spontaneous improvement is likely to occur remains uncertain. However, we have found that cases of Brown's syndrome which show a click are usually intermittent and therefore carry with them a better long-term prognosis.

Investigation

The aims of the investigation are:
• to record the findings;
• to assess the degree of compensation;
• to differentiate a click syndrome.

Once an initial examination of ocular movements has been made, a Hess chart should be plotted. If this test is deferred until later in the examination the full extent of limited elevation in adduction may not be shown. Serial charts can be used to record change. A field of binocular single vision should be plotted if diplopia can be elicited. The deviation in the primary position should be measured by prism cover test and the strength of binocular single vision assessed using stereotests, positioned in the lower field if necessary. Binocular function should be investigated if a manifest strabismus is present.

If a click is suspected, it can best be detected by placing a finger over the trochlea and asking the patient to look up and in. If a click occurs the examiner can feel the sudden movement of the tendon through the trochlea. It is advisable to repeat this procedure on the other side, placing a finger over the opposite trochlea. A bilateral click can sometimes be felt in patients whose symptoms are related only to one side.

Differential diagnosis

Brown's syndrome should be differentiated from the following conditions.

• Isolated inferior oblique palsy. This is a very rare condition, and is perhaps more frequently seen following orbital trauma or in association with myasthenia gravis.
• Double elevator palsy. This condition can be readily differentiated from Brown's syndrome by comparable limitation of up-gaze on both adduction and abduction and by the presence of a ptosis. Bell's phenomenon may be intact, confirming the absence of any mechanical restriction of elevation.
• Orbital blow-out fracture. Blow-out fracture of the orbit typically results in limitation of elevation, which is usually greatest in abduction with retraction of the globe on attempted up-gaze. Enophthalmos and infraorbital nerve anaesthesia may also be present.
• Congenital ocular muscle fibrosis syndrome. Fibrosis of the inferior rectus will result in limitation of up-gaze. The limitation will be greatest in abduction with retraction of the globe on attempted up-gaze; bilateral cases often show a convergent retraction movement. In some cases intraoperative forced duction testing will be required to differentiate the two conditions.
• Adherence syndrome. Inferior oblique muscle surgery which is complicated by rupture of the tendon's capsule, haemorrhage and anterior orbital fat prolapse may lead to the development of a progressive hypotropia of the operated eye. This arises from the development of inflammatory adhesions between the orbital connective tissue septae, the extraocular muscles and the sclera, resulting in mechanical restriction of elevation which is greatest in abduction.

Management

Conservative treatment

The majority of patients with Brown's syndrome of early onset maintain symptom-free binocular single vision with a relatively slight head posture. The field of binocular single vision is usually adequate and in the optimum position on depression of gaze. These patients are well compensated and do not require treatment. Children should be kept under observation. The parents should be told that the syndrome may improve with time but if it does not, up-gaze will be used less as the child grows in height and the anomaly will become less noticeable.

Retrotrochlear steroid injection

The use of local steroids in the management of Brown's syndrome was first proposed by Roper-Hall and Roper-Hall (1972), who used this treatment in late-onset Brown's syndrome, either to reduce an inflammatory reaction or to prevent the development of fibrous tissue secondary to trauma. The technique also appears to be effective in improving elevation in the short term in early-onset Brown's syndrome (Trimble *et al.* 1984; Trimble 1988). Accurate placing of the injection is essential. Treatment does not have a sustained effect in all cases and is indicated only in patients who would otherwise require surgery.

Surgical treatment

Surgical intervention in Brown's syndrome is not predictable; the results may range from no change in elevation in adduction to a superior oblique palsy, and operation should be avoided if possible, particularly in view of the possible spontaneous improvement. In cases in which binocular single vision is only maintained at the expense of a marked head posture or in those that are decompensating, surgery still has a role to play. A weakening procedure on the superior oblique tendon should be performed: partial tenotomy and recession procedures are not effective in improving the restriction of elevation in adduction and a tenotomy of the superior oblique tendon is the operation of choice. Exploration of the posterior tendon should not be attempted as it could lead to serious fibrosis and would limit the passage of the tendon through the trochlea in both directions.

Choice of surgery

Tenotomy with preservation of the intermuscular connective tissue septum

We advise this procedure. Division of the anterior tendon on the nasal side of the superior rectus muscle should improve elevation in adduction whether the underlying defect was a shortened tendon or a lesion preventing free passage of the tendon through the trochlea. Care is taken to preserve the intermuscular connective tissue septum. Fine connections between the intermuscular septum and the tendon can allow the muscle to continue to function normally despite a free tenotomy, and their presence explains why a superior oblique palsy does not necessarily develop.

The result is however, unpredictable. Parks (1977) has reported a success rate of around 50%. Elevation in adduction does not necessarily improve in all cases, while in some tenotomy can lead to total loss of superior oblique action, necessitating treatment for a superior oblique palsy. In spite of its poor predictability, tenotomy has the best chance of success.

Tenotomy with removal of the intermuscular connective tissue septum

A 2–4 mm portion of the superior oblique tendon can be excised together with the intermuscular connective tissue septum to reduce the incidence of recurrent Brown's syndrome and to manage patients when a previous tenotomy has failed to correct the defect. Theoretically, the likelihood of reattachment of the tendon to the globe is lessened. The incidence of superior oblique palsy may be comparatively higher using this procedure rather than a tenotomy (Parks 1978).

Superior oblique tendon expander

Wright (1991) described the use of a silicon spacer to effectively lengthen the tendon and produce a graded amount of superior oblique weakness in an attempt to overcome the unpredictable outcome following superior oblique tenotomy. However, more experience is required, especially longer periods of follow-up, before the silicon expander can be recommended for routine use.

Other procedures

Other surgical procedures that might be considered but are less commonly used include:

• Recession of the contralateral superior rectus muscle, which would probably be used only if earlier surgery had been insufficient, or if the patient preferred to fixate with the affected eye, making the overaction more obvious.

• Taking down the superior oblique tendon tuck which has resulted in a marked iatrogenic Brown's syndrome in a primary superior oblique palsy.

If there is a manifest horizontal strabismus, surgery may be indicated for functional or cosmetic reasons. Surgery for Brown's syndrome will be needed if the prognosis for binocular single vision is good but should only be considered in cosmetic cases if the restriction is marked and unsightly. The horizontal angle can be corrected using conventional techniques.

Postoperative management

The response to superior oblique tenotomy may be delayed by days or in some cases several weeks. During the postoperative period, all patients should be instructed to carry out ductional exercises, occluding the non-operated eye and forcing the operated eye to look in the field of elevation in adduction.

Trapped superior oblique tendon

This condition is virtually always acquired and is mainly caused by trauma in the trochlear region from industrial injuries or road traffic accidents, often involving windscreen glass. Inflammation around the trochlea is a less common cause.

Features

The main features are:
• Limitation of both elevation and depression of gaze, more marked when the eye is adducted. Elevation or depression can be asymmetrically affected depending on the manner in which movement of the tendon is impeded. There will be hypotropia of the affected eye on up-gaze and hypertropia on down-gaze. The limitation of elevation may increase with time.
• Vertical and torsional diplopia will be present, which will reverse as gaze changes from the upper to the lower fields. If the right eye is affected the right image will be higher and intorted on up-gaze and lower and extorted on down-gaze.
• Cyclotropia may be present in the primary position and can prevent fusion of the images.
• An abnormal head posture involving a face turn to the sound side is likely; the head tilt and chin position are influenced by the nature of the cyclotropia and by whether up-gaze or down-gaze is more restricted.

Management

Conservative treatment

The patient may achieve a useful field of binocular single vision with an abnormal head posture and will not require treatment. Prisms are of limited value in patients with trapped superior oblique tendon because of the changes which occur in the vertical deviation and significant cyclotropia.

Local steroid injection

Injection of local steroids into the trochlear region may have a place in reducing the degree of subsequent fibrosis.

Surgical treatment

Removal of scar tissue

A considerable amount of scar tissue may form after trauma in the trochlear area. Surgery directed at freeing the tendon from this tissue is at best disappointing and may exacerbate the problem by increasing fibrosis. It should therefore be avoided.

Superior oblique tenectomy

Tenectomy is the only procedure of value in cases of severe tendon trapping. The operation is designed to excise the anterior tendon and its intermuscular septum so that the eye can move freely. The inevitable loss of superior oblique function that results from this procedure can be compensated to some degree by surgery at a later date on either the ipsilateral inferior oblique and/or the contralateral inferior rectus, depending on the findings. Tenectomy should correct any incyclotropia present but by an unpredictable amount, possibly resulting in overcorrection. However, the deviation may be sufficiently reduced to allow the use of prisms to give useful binocular single vision.

Congenital ocular fibrosis syndrome

The term congenital ocular fibrosis syndrome encompasses a spectrum of conditions in which the primary abnormality is fibrosis of the extraocular muscles and adjacent tissues. It is a stationary disorder which is present at birth. Harley *et al.* (1978) have subclassified the congenital ocular fibrosis syndrome into:
• generalized fibrosis;
• fibrosis of the inferior rectus with ptosis;
• congenital unilateral fibrosis;
• vertical retraction syndrome;
• strabismus fixus.

Although they are rare, it is important to recognize that these disorders exist so as to avoid unnecessary investigation and to provide optimum treatment.

Generalized fibrosis syndrome

This is the commonest and most severe form of the condition; the term generalized fibrosis syndrome was first used by Brown, who described three cases (Brown 1950).

Pathogenesis and aetiology

The congenital ocular fibrosis syndrome has been reported in association with other generalized and ocular abnormalities. In most cases these appear to have been coincidental; however, Khawam *et al.* (1987) reported on a family with the condition in which all members had optic nerve coloboma. Perhaps of more significance is the reported association of the congenital ocular fibrosis syndrome and neural misdirection conditions. Brodsky *et al.* (1989) and Traboulsi *et al.* (1993) have all described the Marcus Gunn jaw winking syndrome in these patients, Brodsky's case also had the synergistic divergent form of Duane's retraction syndrome. This association with neural misdirection questions the basis for the classification of the congenital ocular fibrosis syndrome as a primary ocular myopathy and gives credence to the view that it may arise secondarily to a congenital lack of innervation. It is also possible, however, that the defect responsible for the congenital ocular fibrosis syndrome may affect both the muscles and their innervational process (Traboulsi *et al.* 1993).

Features

Laughlin (1956) described the characteristic features of the condition as:
- fibrosis of all extraocular muscles;
- fibrosis of Tenon's capsule;
- adhesions between muscles, Tenon's capsule and the globe;
- inelasticity and fragility of the conjunctiva;
- no elevation or depression of either eye;
- little or no horizontal movement;
- both eyes fixed in a position of downward gaze 20–30° below the horizontal;
- bilateral ptosis;

- backward head tilt with chin elevated;
- the condition is present at birth.

Additional features reported later by Letson (1980) are:
- an autosomal dominant inheritance pattern in most cases;
- a manifest strabismus, either exotropia or esotropia;
- a high incidence of amblyopia;
- reduced visual acuity resulting from the difficulty in providing satisfactory optical correction of significant refractive errors.

The subgroups of the congenital ocular fibrosis syndrome known as fibrosis of the inferior rectus with ptosis (Crawford 1970), congenital unilateral fibrosis (Leone & Weinstein 1972) and the vertical retraction syndrome (Khodadoust & von Noorden 1967) probably all represent localized forms of the generalized syndrome with unilateral or bilateral involvement of a single muscle or muscle groups. They differ from each other in terms of the muscles involved and by their mode of inheritance. The condition of progressive exaggerated A-pattern strabismus described by Fells *et al.* (1982) is another localized form of the disorder.

The strabismus seen in the congenital ocular fibrosis syndrome may not always be the result of extraocular muscle fibrosis: this is especially true for any horizontal strabismus that may be present (Hill *et al.* 1996).

Strabismus fixus

This is a rare disorder in which there is a marked esotropia, associated with extreme tightness of the medial rectus muscles (Duke-Elder & Wybar 1973). The eyes are firmly fixed in adduction and neither active nor passive horizontal movement is possible. Vertical movement is preserved.

Differential diagnosis of the congenital ocular fibrosis syndrome

The differential diagnosis includes neurogenic, mechanical and myogenic disorders. These comprise:
- partial or complete third cranial nerve palsy;
- double elevator palsy;
- Möbius' syndrome;
- Brown's syndrome;

- orbital floor fracture;
- thyroid eye disease;
- chronic progressive external ophthalmoplegia;
- myasthenia gravis.

In most cases, forms of the congenital ocular fibrosis syndrome can be readily differentiated from these conditions on the basis of the mode of presentation, clinical signs, results of investigation and the forced duction test.

Management

The initial management should include the correction of any significant refractive error and an attempt to improve visual acuity by treating any strabismic, anisometropic or deprivational amblyopia. Most patients adopt a chin elevation, which results in eccentric viewing through the spectacle lens and less than optimum optical correction: this may explain why visual acuity rarely reaches 6/6 in bilateral cases with significant refractive errors. Hiatt and Halle (1983) have stressed the importance of repeat refractions in these patients because of the frequent change in refractive status and its potential contribution towards amblyopia. In particular, significant changes in refractive error have been observed following extraocular muscle surgery (Hertle *et al.* 1992), which may cause a change in the magnitude and direction of the force exerted by the rectus muscle on the globe.

Surgical treatment

Not all patients with the congenital ocular fibrosis syndrome require surgery; those without a significant head posture or strabismus can simply be kept under observation.

The aims of surgery are:
- treatment of ptosis covering the visual axis;
- improvement of abnormal head posture;
- alignment of the visual axes in the primary position.

Treatment for the ptosis should be delayed until surgery on the extraocular muscles has been completed whenever possible. Ptosis surgery frequently results in lagophthalmos and risks the development of exposure keratitis.

Amblyopia should be treated before considering extraocular muscle surgery, which we rarely perform before the age of 4–5 years. Successful amblyopia management may be hindered by the presence of a marked hypotropia in unilateral cases; in this instance, early surgery for the hypotropia is indicated to facilitate amblyopia treatment. Surgery should always be preceded by a forced duction test as not all components of the strabismus are necessarily mechanical. Any vertical component to the strabismus should be managed before dealing with the horizontal deviation. Most cases require a recession to one or both inferior rectus muscles to achieve a satisfactory alignment in the primary position and improve the head posture. A recession exceeding 5 mm is frequently required; however, this will compromise down-gaze and cause an A-pattern exotropia in most patients. Lower lid retraction is frequently observed following this amount of surgery on the inferior rectus. In some cases, a satisfactory alignment in the primary position cannot be achieved by recessing the fibrosed inferior recti alone and surgery to other muscles is required. A resection of the ipsilateral superior rectus muscle has been proposed in these cases, although we prefer to use an ipsilateral Knapp procedure, especially if surgery to the horizontal recti is also required, as this can be carried out at the same time as the vertical transposition procedure (Hill *et al.* 1996).

Although normalization of ocular movement is not possible, most patients with the congenital ocular fibrosis syndrome benefit from surgery to improve their head posture and alignment in the primary position.

Adherence syndromes

Adherence syndromes can be congenital or acquired.

Congenital

Johnson (1950) described two varieties of developmental anomaly in the ocular muscles and their fascial sheaths.

1 Abnormal fascial connections between the lateral rectus and inferior oblique muscles, causing mechanical limitation of abduction of the eye.

2 Adherence between the superior rectus muscle and the superior oblique tendon, causing mechanical limitation of elevation.

These anomalies are more rare than was originally predicted, but should be considered as a differential diagnosis in patients with otherwise unexplained limitation of movement. They can be identified at surgery and should be divided if present.

Acquired

Acquired adherence syndromes are much more common and are usually the consequence of strabismus or retinal detachment surgery. Trauma and occasionally orbital infection are also causes. Parks (1972) used the term to describe a complication of inferior oblique myectomy he believed was due to proliferation of fibrofatty tissue and reattachment of the proximal end of the inferior oblique muscle to Tenon's capsule. This results in a hypotropia with mechanical restriction of elevation. Parks described this complication in 26% of disinsertions and 13% of myectomies of the inferior oblique. On the other hand, von Noorden reported seeing this complication after inferior oblique myectomy only twice over a 35-year period (von Noorden 1996). We have seen this complication on two occasions and found the combined use of botulinum toxin to the inferior rectus muscle of the affected eye and an anchoring suture effective in restoring alignment in the primary position (McElvanney *et al.* 1996).

Thyroid eye disease

Description

Thyroid eye disease (TED) is characterized by a constellation of signs which are commonly seen in patients with a past or current history of thyroid dysfunction, usually hyperthyroidism. The main signs are upper eyelid retraction and lid-lag, mechanical restriction of ocular motility, exophthalmos and compressive optic neuropathy. The main symptoms are discomfort, mainly from corneal exposure, diplopia and loss of vision. One or both eyes may be affected. When only one eye appears to be involved, it is likely that the other eye will become affected at a later stage.

Thyroid dysfunction comprises either overaction of the thyroid gland, resulting in thyrotoxicosis, or underaction of the gland, reducing thyroid secretion and causing myxoedema. The most common form of thyroid dysfunction is known as Graves' disease, and consists of hyperthyroidism with the common features of TED in association with systemic abnormalities such as autoimmune thyroid disease, pretibial myxoedema and acropachy (finger clubbing). Not all patients with hyperthyroidism develop TED: in approximately 20% of those who do so, it develops in the 6-month period preceding the diagnosis of the thyroid disorder, in 20% it occurs concurrently with the diagnosis and in 20% it develops in the 6-month period following the diagnosis. In the remaining 40%, the features of TED develop more than 6 months after the onset of hyperthyroidism (Bartley *et al.* 1996). Although most patients with TED are hyperthyroid or have a history of treatment for the condition, 4% are hypothyroid and 6% remain euthyroid. As 10% of patients with TED do not develop thyrotoxicosis some investigators have questioned the link between TED and hyperthyroidism. However, Salvi *et al.* (1990) have shown thyroid abnormalities to be present in nearly all patients.

Analysis of a group of 50 patients with TED studied by us revealed that 84% were hyperthyroid, 4% had primary hypothyroidism and 14% were euthyroid. With a longer follow-up period it is likely that at least some of the euthyroid patients will develop thyroid dysfunction.

Pathology and natural history

Thyroid eye disease is to some extent self-limiting and has two identifiable phases, an acute or subacute inflammatory phase and a cicatricial phase. Some patients may not go through the acute or subacute phase, but present instead with a restrictive myopathy. Most of the characteristic features of the disease are due to the inflammatory process affecting the extraocular muscles and eyelids. The extraocular muscles become enlarged early in the disease process, as shown on computer axial tomography and ultrasound scans (Kennerdell *et al.* 1981; Feldon & Weiner 1982). Biopsy specimens show a round cell infiltrate: these findings are compatible with an inflammatory myopathy, and investigation into its cause have pointed towards an autoimmune aetiology. The primary target cell in the orbit for the immune process appears to be the fibroblast.

There are several hypotheses about the pathophysiology of TED.

• The TSH receptor could be the shared thyroid-orbital antigen (Heufelder & Bahn 1992). While antibodies towards TSH receptor have been found in thyroid patients, the titre does not appear to be increased in patients with TED.

• A 64 kDa antigen shared with the thyroid gland and eye muscle could be responsible (Hiromatsu *et al.* 1988). This antigen can be found in tissue other than the thyroid and orbit and only a minimal correlation exists between the antigen titre and TED status (Ross *et al.* 1994).

• As the major component of the inflammation in TED occurs in the perimysial compartment between individual muscle cells, the orbital fibroblasts are believed to be central to this process. Fibroblast activity may be modulated by cytokines, which are inflammatory mediators derived from T-cells (Bahn 1995).

Environmental factors are important in the development of autoimmune disease and may play a part in influencing its severity. Hagg and Asplund (1987) first identified the association between severe TED and smoking, which was later confirmed by Shine *et al.* (1990). Smoking is known to affect the immune system, either by altering the function of the T-cell, thus changing the balance of the immune chain, or by the products of the cigarette smoke having a direct immunological effect.

The acute and subacute inflammatory phase

Sympathetic overactivity during this phase can result in overaction of Müller's muscle, leading to upper eyelid retraction and lid-lag on down-gaze.

Extraocular muscle oedema due to round cell (lymphocyte) infiltration and the deposition of mucopolysaccharides between the muscle fibres can increase the muscle volume by a factor as high as 10. The increased orbital volume causes proptosis of the globe, which may lead to corneal exposure. Some patients have a tight orbital septum, which can restrict the degree of proptosis, but causes the intra-orbital pressure to rise and can embarrass the blood supply to the optic nerve. The swollen muscles become inelastic and give rise to mechanical restriction of ocular movement. During this phase of the disease botulinum toxin injected into the affected muscles in selected cases has been shown to have a long-term effect in reversing the mechanical restriction (Lyons *et al.* 1990).

Only rarely is there evidence of a paralytic component to the myopathy; however, we have observed this in three situations (Spencer *et al.* 1996):

• in the acute phase associated with a systemic proximal myopathy and thyrotoxicosis;

• in patients with severe inflammation and evidence of optic neuropathy;

• as an isolated finding involving the inferior rectus muscle.

The cicatricial phase

In most patients fibrosis and secondary muscle contraction gradually replace the acute inflammatory phase affecting the extraocular muscles. Fibrotic and contracted muscles do not respond well to botulinum toxin, and no long-term benefit is obtained from its use during this phase. As the muscle swelling subsides the proptosis reduces and the patient's appearance improves. The risk of sight-threatening optic neuropathy, which has been shown to be directly related to the size of the extraocular muscles (Barrett *et al.* 1988), is therefore reduced during this phase of the disease. Upper eyelid retraction usually persists, due either to fibrosis of the levator muscle or to increased innervation to the superior rectus muscle to bring about up-gaze. Diplopia, particularly if vertical, may become less troublesome due to one or more of the following factors:

• the development of symmetrical restriction of ocular movement;

• tightening of the superior rectus muscle in a hypotropic eye, which reduces the amount of hypotropia in the primary position at the expense of limited depression of gaze;

• the gradual development of an exceptionally large vertical fusion amplitude;

• reduction in the degree of proptosis, which allows more effective muscle action and may reduce the restriction of movement.

However, in some cases limitation of movement can increase.

Thyroid dysfunction

The reason for the systemic thyroid dysfunction seen in patients with TED remains uncertain. The probable cause in the majority of patients is a disturbance in the immune mechanism. This belief is supported by the presence of thyroid autoantibodies in the patient's serum and by the strong association between disorders of thyroid function and other autoimmune conditions such as myasthenia, diabetes and pernicious anaemia. Autoimmune disorders typically have a higher prevalence in families, and it is not unusual to find two or more such disorders in the same patient. In our group of patients with TED, 16% had a family history of other autoimmune disease and 42% gave a positive family history for thyroid dysfunction.

Systemic features

Patients with systemic thyroid dysfunction may present with evidence of overactivity or underactivity.

Hyperthyroidism

The features of thyroid overactivity include:
- weight loss;
- increased appetite;
- intolerance of heat;
- anxiety state;
- tremor;
- sweating;
- increased heart rate.

Elderly patients may not show these signs but may present instead with heart failure due to atrial fibrillation.

Hypothyroidism

The features of thyroid underactivity include:
- weight gain;
- decreased appetite;
- intolerance of cold;
- lethargy and increased sleeping time;
- hair loss, including the outer third of the eye brows;
- coarsening of the skin and dry and brittle hair;
- slowing of the ankle jerk reflex;
- reduced heart rate.

Laboratory investigation

Biochemical investigation of thyroid dysfunction should include an analysis of:
- Serum thyroxine (T_4).
- Serum triiodothyronine (T_3). The levels of serum T_4 and T_3 are elevated in patients with thyrotoxicosis and reduced in patients with hypothyroidism.

- Serum thyroid-stimulating hormone (TSH). The TSH level is reduced in the hyperthyroid state and elevated in the hypothyroid state.
- Thyroid autoantibodies. The presence of autoantibodies to thyroid tissue may be found in the serum of affected patients and may be the only detectable serum abnormality in some patients.

Systemic treatment of thyroid dysfunction

Before eyelid or strabismus surgery is considered the patient should be euthyroid and stable. The treatment options for the thyroid dysfunction are outlined below.

Hyperthyroidism

Patients with clinical evidence of thyroid overactivity can be managed using:
- drugs to reduce thyroid function;
- radioactive iodine to irradiate the thyroid gland;
- thyroidectomy;
- beta-blockers, for example propanolol, which may be used in the short term to control some of the sympathetic overactivity. These drugs do not affect the levels of thyroid hormone.

There is no convincing proof that any one treatment regime is better than another as far as preventing or reducing the ocular complications is concerned. However, the development of hypothyroidism following treatment appears either to cause or increase the ocular problems. Hypothyroidism is more likely to occur after radioactive iodine therapy. All patients require careful monitoring after treatment and thyroid replacement therapy should be instituted if a hypothyroid state develops.

Hypothyroidism

The management is simply thyroid hormone replacement, usually with thyroxine. Care must be taken initially, as the increased metabolic rate may induce a strain on the cardiovascular system and cause angina or myocardial infarction.

Ocular involvement in thyroid eye disease

For the purpose of investigation and management ocular involvement can be categorized into:
- the eyelids, orbital tissues and the globe (general ocular involvement);

- the optic nerve;
- the extraocular muscles.

General ocular and optic nerve involvement are considered together, while extraocular muscle involvement is considered separately.

General ocular and optic nerve involvement
Features of general ocular involvement
The features include:

- Ocular discomfort, which is a common symptom and can be due to drying of the corneal epithelium from proptosis, upper eyelid retraction, poor blink pattern or reduction in Bell's phenomenon resulting from contraction of the inferior rectus. Clinically punctate erosions affecting the inferior third of the cornea are seen, highlighted by the use of fluorescein dye. This condition is often aggravated by swollen and hyperaemic conjunctiva, especially over the insertion sites of the horizontal rectus muscles. Superior limbal keratoconjunctivitis, an inflammatory condition, is frequently seen in patients with TED.
- Upper eyelid retraction is the most common sign seen in these patients and is caused by sympathetic overactivity in the early phase of the disease, with overaction of Müller's muscle. Fibrotic contracture of the levator muscle occurs in the cicatricial phase. Upper eyelid retraction can also result from increased innervation to the superior rectus and levator muscles in patients with mechanical restriction of elevation due to a tight inferior rectus muscle.
- Upper eyelid lag, which occurs on down-gaze, returning to its previous position relative to the limbus when the eye movement is completed.
- Proptosis, which is axial and usually symmetrical, although it can be markedly asymmetrical in a minority of patients and strictly unilateral in a few. Thyroid eye disease is the commonest cause of unilateral proptosis.
- Periorbital oedema, which indicates raised intraorbital pressure. Localized swelling between the tarsal plates and the orbital margin represents herniation of orbital fat through deficiencies in the orbital septum.

Features of optic nerve involvement
The features include:

- Loss of visual acuity, which may result from corneal exposure with punctate keratitis, refractive changes or compressive optic neuropathy.
- Loss of vision from optic nerve compression, which can be insidious, resulting in failure to present early to the ophthalmologist: it is therefore important to assess optic nerve function regularly in all patients thought to be at risk of optic nerve compression.
- A subjective change in colour vision, which can be the first sign of early optic nerve compression; for example, patients may state that the colours on the television appear washed out.
- There is no relative afferent pupil defect in symmetrical bilateral compressive optic neuropathy.
- Mild or no optic disc swelling. The central retinal vein leaves the intraorbital optic nerve at its midportion, therefore optic disc swelling is not a consistent feature of compressive thyroid optic neuropathy. Optic atrophy develops when treatment for the optic neuropathy is delayed, and represents structural damage to the optic nerve.

Investigation
A general ocular examination should be carried out as outlined in Chapter 2. Special attention should be paid to measuring and recording the eyelid position and function, the degree of proptosis and the state of the cornea.

Investigation of optic nerve function should include:

- The best corrected visual acuity, which should be recorded on each visit. Contrast sensitivity can be quickly assessed using the Pelli–Robson charts.
- Colour vision should also be measured on each visit using Ishihara plates, which provide a rapid, reliable and reproducible measure.
- Automated visual fields, which are important in confirming the presence of optic neuropathy and in monitoring for change. However, it can be difficult to demonstrate the central scotoma associated with reduced visual acuity in compressive optic neuropathy, especially for levels of 6/9–6/12.
- Serial visual evoked potentials, which provide an objective assessment of optic nerve function. It is important to know that the patient is euthyroid before evaluating the result, as hypothyroid patients without optic nerve compression can show a delay in the P100 component of the VEP.

Management of generalized ocular involvement

MEDICAL TREATMENT

Corneal exposure

Management of corneal exposure is governed by the following factors:

• If it is mild it can be controlled by using artificial tear preparations combined with protective side-pieces fitted to the spectacles to reduce tear evaporation.

• If associated with lid retraction and overaction of Müller's muscle: patients occasionally responded to the use of guanethidine eye drops; however, these are no longer available in the UK.

• In association with marked proptosis and eyelid retraction, corneal exposure may be severe and often fails to respond satisfactorily to medical management. These patients occasionally show temporary improvement with the use of botulinum toxin injected either into the levator muscle to directly reduce the upper eyelid retraction or into the tight inferior rectus muscle, which has an indirect effect on the upper eyelid retraction. Systemic steroid treatment to reduce the amount of proptosis can be used as a short-term option in some patients.

Optic nerve compression

The threat to vision is a medical emergency. The only effective nonsurgical treatment is the use of high-dose systemic steroids, which may be administered orally or parenterally. Difficulty may arise in patients who either do not respond to high-dose systemic steroids or who do not tolerate a reduction in their steroids without reactivation of the underlying disease process. Due to the serious complications associated with the long-term use of high-dose systemic steroids, we only recommend their use in patients who are otherwise unsuitable for surgical decompression of the orbit.

SURGICAL TREATMENT

It should be stressed that whenever possible surgery should not be considered until the patient is euthyroid and his medical condition is stable, except in patients with sight-threatening disease.

Eyelid surgery

Eyelid surgery is indicated to protect the cornea when conservative measures are insufficient or have failed and/or for cosmetic reasons when there is marked upper eyelid retraction and lid-lag. The available options are:

• Disinsertion of an overacting Müller's muscle (Henderson's operation).

• Lengthening of a contracted levator muscle by using donor sclera (Collin 1984). This method offers the best protection and gives excellent cosmesis.

• Lateral tarsorrhaphy, which is rarely used since it is cosmetically unsightly and soon stretches: it provides more protection for the lateral conjunctiva than it does for the cornea and is of little benefit in corneal exposure. Of more importance is that it can limit spontaneous proptosis thereby increasing the intraorbital pressure and the risk of optic nerve compression.

Orbital surgery

Orbital decompression is indicated:

• in patients with significant proptosis who fail to respond to medical treatment for corneal exposure;

• as the first line of treatment of patients with compressive optic neuropathy;

• as part of the rehabilitation of patients with unsightly proptosis without corneal exposure.

It is important that consideration is given to the need to perform an orbital decompression before carrying out surgery to the extraocular muscles.

Principle: The principle of orbital decompression is to create space for the prolapse of the orbital contents by removing one or more of the orbital walls, thus relieving pressure on the optic nerve and reducing proptosis.

Methods: The three options available for increasing orbital volume are:

1 removal of the orbital floor;

2 removal of the medial wall of the orbit;

3 removal of the lateral orbital wall and roof of the orbit.

The preferred primary option is decompression of both the medial wall and orbital floor to allow the orbital contents to prolapse into the ethmoidal and maxillary sinuses. Access is usually through a skin incision along the infraorbital margin between the nose and the eye, being careful to avoid damaging the infraorbital nerve lying in the orbital floor, otherwise anaesthesia of the ipsilateral cheek and upper teeth will result. The Caldwell–Luc approach, in which an incision is made into the maxillary antrum above the premolar teeth, is still preferred by some faciomaxillary surgeons.

Complications:

• It should be noted that a strabismus can be made worse or be caused by orbital decompression. Fells (1987), using an antral-ethmoidal approach, reported a significant incidence of A-pattern esotropia, which we have also observed.

• Significant restriction of movement can follow orbital decompression.

For these reasons it is important that orbital decompression should be carried out before extraocular muscle surgery.

RADIOTHERAPY

Radiotherapy can be used to reduce the size of affected extraocular muscles in order to relieve orbital pressure. Fells *et al.* (1989) compared radiotherapy with surgical decompression and concluded that radiotherapy had little or no detrimental effect on ocular motility, whereas significant restrictions followed surgical decompression. However, the effect of radiotherapy is not immediate and steroids must be used in the interim if vision is at risk. At present, we usually reserve radiotherapy for patients who are unfit for surgery or whose surgical decompression has proved inadequate.

Extraocular muscle involvement

TED affects the extraocular muscles in the following ways.

• The muscles become enlarged during the inflammatory phase, restricting ocular movement and raising intraorbital pressure; however, subclinical involvement is common, when enlargement is seen on ultrasound or CT scan without demonstrable loss of function.

• An extraocular muscle paresis is occasionally seen when there is severe congestive myopathy and uncontrolled hyperthyroidism, or as an isolated finding affecting the inferior rectus muscle (Hermann 1982; Spencer *et al.* 1996).

• Mechanical restriction of ocular movement develops in both the acute and cicatricial phases and is often accompanied by pain on looking in the direction of limited movement.

• Retraction of the globe occurs when movement away from the site of the restriction is attempted; this is commonly seen on up-gaze. A convergence-retraction movement may occur when there is bilateral restriction. Harcourt *et al.* (1978) reported retraction of the globe on down-gaze and increased proptosis on up-gaze in some patients: although contracture of the superior rectus muscle could account for these findings, they were seen and measured in patients with relatively mild limitation of movement.

• A wide spectrum of ocular muscle involvement is seen, ranging from a single muscle in one eye to a number of muscles in both eyes. In order of decreasing frequency the muscles involved are: the inferior rectus, the medial rectus, the superior rectus and the lateral rectus, resulting in restricted up-gaze, lateral gaze, down-gaze or medial gaze, although the lateral rectus is often spared even when enlargement is evident on CT scan. The oblique muscles are rarely if ever involved.

• The common ocular posture is hypotropia of the more affected eye, sometimes with associated esotropia.

• Diplopia is common and is often the presenting symptom in TED. It may be vertical, horizontal or a combination of the two, and is typically worse in the morning. Torsional diplopia is much less common.

• An abnormal head posture, commonly chin elevation, is often adopted, with or without a face turn: its purpose is either to avoid an uncomfortable position of gaze, to centralize a field of binocular single vision or, in a few cases, to facilitate fixation when there is marked bilateral restriction of movement.

• An enlarged vertical fusion amplitude often develops, probably due to the insidious onset of the disease, allowing patients to control quite large vertical deviations.

Management

The management options for the ocular motility disorder largely depend on:

• the stability of both the underlying medical condition and the ocular state;

• the need for orbital decompression.

Stability of the medical condition and ocular state: Before undertaking strabismus surgery the patient should be euthyroid as further treatment for

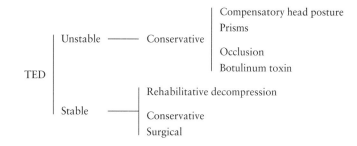

Tree 21.2 Summary of management options for treating the ocular muscle imbalance in thyroid eye disease.

uncontrolled hyperthyroidism may result in instability of the ocular condition; furthermore, uncontrolled hyperthyroidism has a direct effect on the cardiovascular system and may result in the development of dysrhythmias during general and local anaesthesia. Strabismus surgery should be avoided during the acute and subacute inflammatory phase of the disease as ocular alignment is often changing rapidly. Alignment should be stable for at least 3 months before undertaking strabismus surgery.

Orbital decompression: Orbital decompression can be part of the rehabilitation of patients with TED: when indicated it should always precede extraocular muscle surgery for reasons discussed later.

Management options: The management options for the ocular motility disorder depend on the:
• stability of the underlying condition: ocular/general medical;
• requirement for orbital decompression: compressive neuropathy/exposure, rehabilitative.

Despite the apparent variability of muscle involvement in TED, it is possible to categorize the ocular motility disturbances into well-recognized patterns which form the basis for further management.

CONSERVATIVE TREATMENT
The aims of conservative management are:
• to monitor the patient's progress and record and measure change in the condition;
• to overcome symptoms, principally diplopia, and allow comfortable binocular single vision to be maintained.

During the initial period the patient must be kept under frequent observation to assess the rate of change. A Hess chart, field of binocular single vision and field of uniocular vision should be recorded. Many patients can already maintain binocular single vision by means of an abnormal head posture; providing they remain comfortable no further treatment is required.

Prism therapy
The aim of prism therapy is to make the patient comfortable by overcoming diplopia and restoring a useful field of binocular single vision. Although it has been stated that marked incomitance and the likelihood of rapid change in the deviation prevent the use of prisms in patients with TED, this has not been our experience.

In several ways patients with this condition are ideal candidates for prism therapy because:
• the strength of prism required is low in relation to the angle of the deviation because of the increased fusion amplitude;
• the patient must usually wait a considerable time before surgery can be carried out;
• most patients are of an age likely to require spectacles, thus facilitating either the use of Fresnel prisms or prisms incorporated into the refractive prescription.

The majority of patients readily accept prisms in preference to diplopia and find them more tolerable than occlusion. We have not found that frequent change in prism strength is required.

Botulinum toxin
Botulinum toxin has a role during the early stages of the disease process in patients whose diplopia cannot be adequately relieved using prisms. Lyons *et al.* (1990) have shown that during this stage of the disease patients can regain binocular single vision following botulinum toxin treatment and that in 1 out of 6 patients a 'cure' will obviate the need for strabismus surgery. It is also useful in the management of small surgical overcorrection or undercorrection. Despite

the success of botulinum toxin in the early stages of TED, its effect tends to be short-lived: most of the patients we have treated have not returned for further injections, preferring instead simply to ignore the diplopia or resort to occlusion.

Occlusion
Occlusion is used only as a last resort and may be a further handicap to a patient with bilateral limitation of ocular movement.

SURGICAL TREATMENT
The aims of extraocular muscle surgery are to improve the patient's appearance and to establish a field of binocular single vision in the primary position and on down-gaze, extending the area into other fields of gaze if possible, although this is seldom achieved. It is important to ensure that the patient has realistic expectations of the outcome of surgery and understands both its limitations in TED and that the unstable nature of the ocular motility disorder may necessitate further surgery in the future. The patient should be euthyroid and the ocular muscle imbalance should have remained stable for least 3 months before considering surgery.

Important considerations in surgical management are:
• Surgery on patients with TED can be performed under local or general anaesthesia. We find that most patients are suitable for adjustable sutures.
• The forced duction test must first be performed to confirm the presence and extent of mechanical restrictions and later to assess the effectiveness of surgical recession.
• Care should be taken to prevent adjustable sutures from coming into contact with the cornea, which may already be compromised through exposure keratitis. Significant dehydration must be prevented during surgery.
• It is advisable to leave long-standing vertical deviations slightly undercorrected, aiming to align the visual axes just below the primary position. The patient's well-developed vertical fusion amplitude should ensure that comfortable binocular single vision is maintained, whereas patients find it very difficult to adapt the fusion amplitude to control overcorrection.

• Reversal of the deviation can occur if an attempt is made to correct the full vertical deviation with a single inferior rectus recession. A large recession can cause significant underaction on down-gaze.
• When a bilateral inferior rectus recession is required, the risk of developing a postoperative A-pattern can be reduced by medial transposition of both muscles.
• Large bilateral medial rectus recessions, in excess of 10 mm, are on occasions required to achieve satisfactory alignment in the primary position.
• Resection of a muscle can result in worsened mechanical restriction of movement unless great care is taken. This procedure is rarely used in TED.
• Recession of the conjunctiva is often necessary after completion of muscle surgery. The forced duction test is used as a guide to the amount of recession required.

Patterns of ocular muscle imbalance in TED
Despite the apparent variability of muscle involvement in TED, it is possible to categorize the ocular motility disturbances into recognizable patterns on which to base further management.

The pattern of vertical and horizontal ocular muscle involvement in TED can be divided into:
• unilateral or grossly asymmetrical bilateral involvement;
• symmetrical bilateral clinical involvement.

Using this broad classification six patterns can be identified. The features, aetiology and management of each pattern are discussed.
1 Unilateral or grossly asymmetrical restriction of elevation (Fig. 21.6):
• Relatively incomitant, resulting in an increase in the vertical deviation on up-gaze and a reduction on down-gaze, usually with an intact inferior field of BSV.
    Aetiology: a mechanical restriction of the ipsilateral inferior rectus.
    Management: an ipsilateral inferior rectus recession.
• Relatively concomitant (Fig. 21.7), resulting in a vertical deviation that is the same on up-gaze and which decreases minimally or not at all on down-gaze, usually with no field of BSV.
    Aetiology: a mechanical restriction of the ipsilateral inferior rectus and of the contralateral superior rectus.
    Management: if the deviation measures less than 20 Δ in the primary position, an ipsilateral inferior

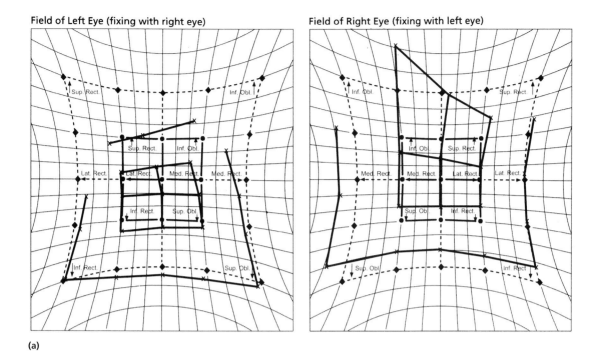

(a)

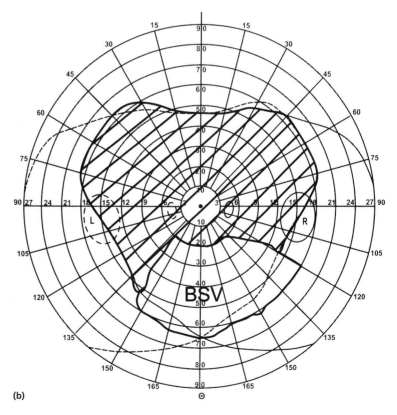

Fig. 21.6 (a) Hess chart of a patient with unilateral thyroid eye disease showing limitation of the left eye on elevation. (b) Field of binocular single vision of the same patient, showing a field of binocular single vision in depression.

(b)

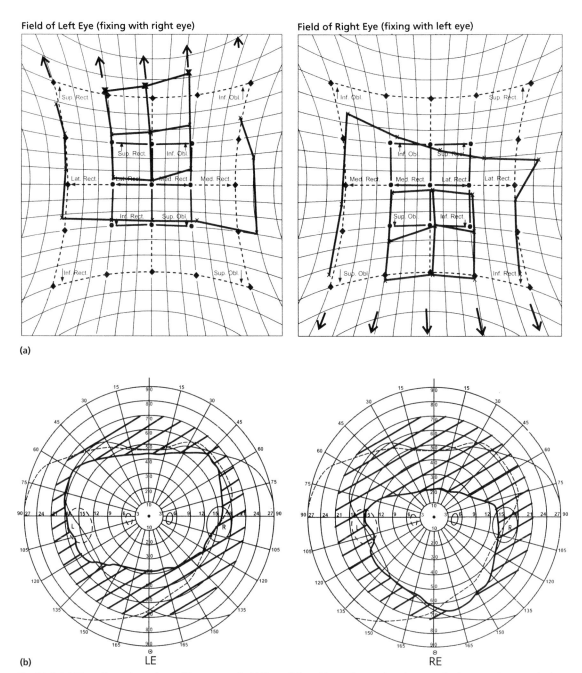

Fig. 21.7 (a) Hess chart of a patient with asymmetrical bilateral thyroid eye disease showing a marked concomitant vertical deviation. (b) Uniocular field of fixation of the same patient. The right eye shows moderate restriction of elevation and the left shows slight restriction of depression.

(c)

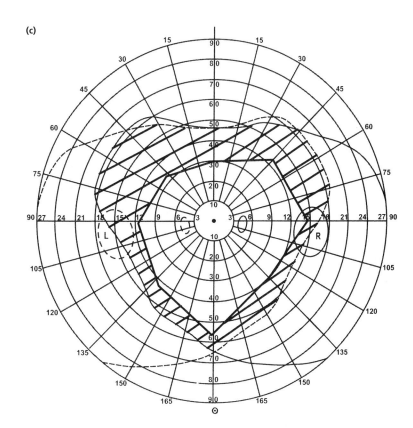

Fig. 21.7 (*Continued*) (c) Field of binocular single vision of the same patient, showing a well-placed central field of binocular single vision.

rectus recession is usually sufficient to restore a useful field of binocular single vision. If the deviation exceeds 20 Δ, the inferior rectus recession should be combined with a recession of the contralateral superior rectus, especially if the forced duction test confirms the presence of a mechanical restriction of the contralateral eye on depression of gaze. Attempting to correct the vertical deviation by operating only on the ipsilateral inferior rectus muscle could lead to significant underaction and reversal of the deviation on down-gaze.

2 Unilateral or grossly asymmetrical bilateral restriction of abduction (Fig. 21.8):

• Relatively incomitant, resulting in an esotropia which increases in the direction of the mechanical restriction and reduces in the opposite field of gaze. There is a face turn way from the side with the mechanical restriction, with an intact field of BSV.

Aetiology: a mechanical restriction of the ipsilateral medial rectus with limitation of abduction. This

pattern of ocular muscle involvement occasionally follows a medial wall decompression procedure.

Management: an ipsilateral medial rectus recession.

• Relatively concomitant (Fig. 21.9), resulting in an esotropia in all horizontal positions of gaze.

Aetiology: bilateral mechanical restriction of both medial rectus muscles is likely.

Management: a unilateral or bilateral medial rectus recession, depending on the size of the deviation.

3 Unilateral or grossly asymmetrical bilateral restriction of both elevation and abduction (Fig. 21.10): The management of this group is the same as for patterns 1 and 2 described above. Surgery should be performed simultaneously on horizontal and vertical muscles if possible. It should be remembered that an ipsilateral recession of both the medial rectus and inferior rectus muscles may worsen any pre-existing exophthalmos and corneal exposure. The need for orbital decompression prior to undertaking strabismus

Field of Left Eye (fixing with right eye)

Field of Right Eye (fixing with left eye)

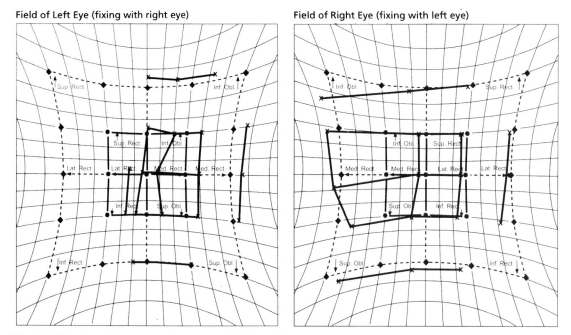

Fig. 21.8 Hess chart of a patient with asymmetrical bilateral thyroid eye disease showing marked restriction of left abduction with overaction of the contralateral medial rectus muscle.

Field of Left Eye (fixing with right eye)

Field of Right Eye (fixing with left eye)

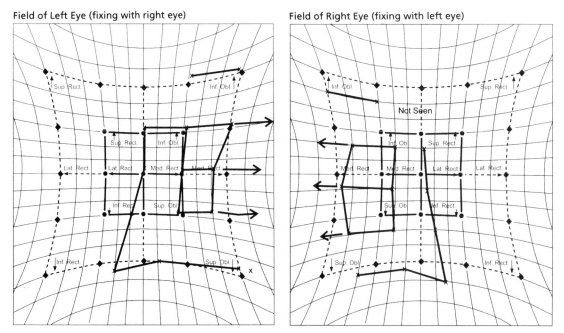

Fig. 21.9 Hess chart of a patient with symmetrical bilateral thyroid eye disease showing a large esodeviation in the primary position and bilateral limitation of abduction.

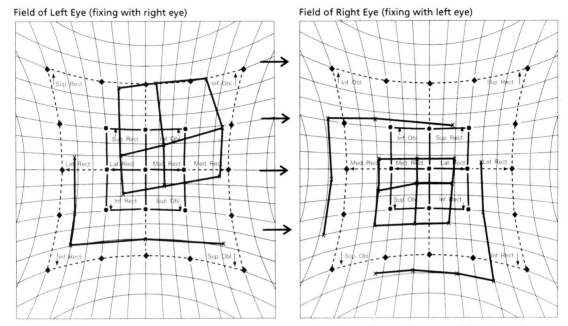

Fig. 21.10 Hess chart of a patient with asymmetrical bilateral thyroid eye disease showing limitation of elevation and abduction of the right eye.

surgery should be considered in patients with significant pre-existing exophthalmos.

4 Bilateral symmetrical restriction of elevation: Significant bilateral inferior rectus muscle involvement is suggested when:

- neither eye is able to maintain fixation in the primary position;
- there is asymmetrical mechanical restriction of elevation, with a −2 to −3 restriction in the more mobile eye;
- an A-pattern esotropia is present on up-gaze, with a convergence retraction movement as the eyes attempt to move into the field of maximum restriction;
- contraction of the superior rectus, if present, will restrict movement on down-gaze.

The Hess chart will not give a true indication of the severity of the extraocular muscle involvement due to the symmetrical nature of the restricted elevation, so the fields of uniocular fixation and BSV should always be examined.

Management: both inferior rectus muscles should be recessed sufficiently to allow the eye to elevate to just above the primary position. The forced duc-

tion test can be used to ensure that the recession is adequate. In cases of asymmetrical inferior rectus involvement, asymmetrical recessions are performed, taking care not to reverse the deviation: reversal can be avoided by aiming for alignment of the eyes just below the primary position.

5 Bilateral restriction of both elevation and abduction: An important finding in this category is an A-pattern esotropia. Factors contributing to an A-pattern in TED include:

- previous orbital decompression;
- mechanical restriction of the inferior rectus muscles;
- underaction or compromised action of both inferior rectus muscles;
- mechanical restriction involving the medial rectus muscles;
- mechanical restriction affecting the superior rectus muscle with limitation of down-gaze and overaction of the superior oblique muscles.

Characteristics of A-pattern esotropia in TED: The A-pattern esotropia seen in TED can be characterized on the basis of the field of gaze in which the maximum change in horizontal deviation occurs.

• A-pattern only apparent on extreme down-gaze. This type of A-pattern esotropia is a frequent complication of bilateral decompression of the medial and inferior orbital walls. The angle of esotropia is maintained until down-gaze of 20–30° is reached, when a relative divergence occurs, resulting in alignment or near alignment of the visual axes.

Aetiology: the cause is presumably related to mechanical factors brought about by the decompression procedure, although we have observed it in patients who have not had prior orbital surgery.

Management: a bilateral medial rectus muscle recession resulted in the disappearance of the A-pattern in five patients we treated in this way.

• A-pattern only apparent on up-gaze. There is a moderate to marked bilateral restriction of elevation. Esotropia increases as the eyes move into the area of mechanical restriction, with the characteristic convergence retraction movement as the patient attempts to sustain up-gaze.

Aetiology: the same phenomena are seen in patients with the congenital ocular fibrosis syndrome in which the inferior rectus muscles are principally involved (Hill *et al.* 1996). It has been suggested that in this condition the A-pattern is the result of convergence as the eyes move into the field of restriction; this may occur because of relative overaction of the superior rectus muscles or from co-innervation of the medial rectus muscles. The variability of the phenomena in patients with TED who have restricted elevation may be analogous to the situation in Brown's syndrome, when an A- or V-pattern may be observed in some patients but not in others.

Management: if the patient can achieve comfortable binocular single vision in the primary position, treatment is not usually required. When up-gaze is severely restricted, an inferior rectus muscle recession should improve elevation and reduce the A-pattern.

• A-pattern occurring from up-gaze to down-gaze. There is a consistent decrease in the amount of esotropia from up-gaze to down-gaze, associated with underaction of both inferior rectus muscles and overaction of the superior oblique muscles.

Aetiology: the A-pattern may develop after recession of the inferior recti or is occasionally seen as a primary phenomenon. It has been reported by Fells (1987) following orbital decompression, and attributed to post-decompression retroplacement of the globe, which resulted in tightening of the superior oblique tendon and consequent overaction of this muscle.

Management: spontaneous improvement will occur in a few patients treated by orbital decompression. A-pattern of this type due to other causes is very difficult to manage successfully. A forced duction test should be performed at the time of surgery to confirm that defective depression of gaze is not due to superior rectus contraction. If surgery is indicated to improve up-gaze, the inferior rectus muscles should be recessed and transposed medially: this procedure should be combined with surgery to weaken both overacting superior oblique muscles, preferably by tenotomy. The esotropia can be corrected by recession of one or both medial rectus muscles, depending on the size of the deviation in the primary position.

6 Mechanical restriction of the superior rectus muscles resulting in limited down-gaze: There is a limitation of depression that is greatest in abduction. A unilateral contracted superior rectus muscle has already been described in pattern 1, it also occurs bilaterally in pattern 4, in which there is bilateral restriction of up-gaze. The presence of superior rectus contraction is confirmed by a forced duction test at the time of surgery (Jampolsky 1995).

Management: recession of the superior rectus muscles, which can be combined with inferior rectus recession if necessary.

Multiple factors are often present in any one patient, resulting in considerable variability of the observed patterns.

Postoperative management

If adjustable sutures are used, we recommend the one-stage procedure under local anaesthesia; early postoperative adjustment is recommended if the two-stage procedure is used: adjustment may be complicated by early adherence of the muscle to the sclera if it is delayed. The use of adjustable sutures on the inferior rectus muscle has been associated with late slippage and a change in the deviation, but we have not found this to be a significant problem. An underaction of the inferior rectus may complicate a large recession of this muscle, resulting in reversal of the deviation on down-gaze in addition to causing lower eyelid retraction.

Some of these patients require Fresnel prisms to maintain a central field of binocular single vision.

Results of surgery in thyroid eye disease

Most patients having strabismus surgery for thyroid eye disease obtain a significant improvement in both the field of binocular single vision and in the extent of the abnormal head posture. Success is usually measured in terms of obtaining a field of binocular single vision in the primary and reading positions with or without the aid of a small prism. Mourits *et al.* (1990), using fixed sutures, reported a success rate of 71% after one procedure and 89% after more than one procedure. Fells and McCarry (1988), comparing fixed and adjustable sutures, obtained success in 66% of patients with fixed sutures compared with 76% of patients using adjustable sutures.

Special forms of strabismus in thyroid eye disease

Cyclotorsion and thyroid eye disease

Patients with mechanical restriction of ocular movement may have cyclotorsion in addition to any vertical or horizontal deviation. Cyclotorsion in patients with TED has been previously reported (Caygill 1972; Trobe 1984), with excyclotropia the more common finding although incyclotorsion has also been described. The incidence in these series was 43% and 66%, respectively, and included two patients with incyclotropia. Its true incidence is difficult to determine as it may remain undetected in patients who do not report a tilted image; moreover, it is rarely a barrier to fusion. The cyclotorsion has been attributed to contraction of the inferior rectus muscles, although we have observed it in patients without significant mechanical restrictions. The mechanism responsible for the concomitant nature of the cyclotorsion is difficult to understand. We have found that the amount of cyclotorsion does not correlate with the degree of limitation of movement, and in a number of our cases the measurement remained the same on up-gaze and down-gaze. The findings imply that although cyclotorsion may be attributed to muscle bulk, it is not related to muscle function. Despite the mechanism

remaining unknown, recession of the rectus muscles can reduce cyclotorsion in addition to improving the range of movement. Where there is gross restriction of ocular movement, correcting the horizontal or vertical component by a recession of the contracted rectus muscle will reduce the amount of cyclotorsion in most cases. Surgery on the superior oblique, in the form of a Harada–Ito procedure, can then be employed in those in which excyclotorsion remains a barrier to fusion. Insuperable excyclotorsion in the absence of significant horizontal or vertical restrictions has been successfully treated by superior oblique surgery as a primary procedure in our hands.

Convergence insufficiency and thyroid eye disease

Convergence insufficiency in TED may occur as a primary event or can develop secondary to a significant ocular muscle imbalance. Primary convergence insufficiency is managed using the standard methods described in Chapter 16, ensuring that spectacles are well centred and tear film deficiencies receive appropriate treatment. The management of secondary convergence insufficiency is more complex, and depends on the type of imbalance found.

Frequently encountered ocular muscle balance defects include:

- large esophoria or esotropia;
- incomitant vertical strabismus;
- A- or V-pattern;
- limitation of adduction following either orbital decompression or strabismus surgery.

Changing varifocal or bifocal lenses to single lens reading glasses allows some patients to adopt a small head posture to achieve comfortable binocular single vision for near. In most patients, management needs to be directed at the underlying defect before any improvement in the symptoms associated with the convergence insufficiency can be obtained.

Myasthenia gravis and thyroid eye disease

Most autoimmune disorders show a familial pattern indicating some genetic predisposition. It is therefore not surprising that patients with one autoimmune disorder are more likely to suffer from a second. Approximately 1 in 500 patients with hyperthyroidism will also have myasthenia gravis, and 1 in 20 patients with myasthenia will have hyperthyroidism. In most cases, the strabismus resulting from one of these two conditions can be readily distinguished from the other.

Important signs suggesting the presence of myasthenia in a patient who otherwise shows evidence of TED include:
• ptosis;
• exotropia;
• fatiguability;
• limitation of movement not supported by a positive forced duction test (Burde 1990).

In these cases further investigation, including a Tensilon test, is mandatory.

Orbital injuries

Orbital injuries usually arise following blunt trauma, either from an object striking the face, for example a fist, or through the patient being thrown against a hard surface, as occurs in road traffic accidents. Limitation of ocular movement and diplopia are common consequences.

Effects of trauma

Trauma to the orbit may result in:
• Soft tissue injury causing oedema and haemorrhage. If there is no fracture of any part of the orbit, limitation of ocular movement should improve spontaneously as the swelling subsides and the haemorrhage absorbs. Palsy of the inferior rectus arising from damage to its nerve supply may persist, resulting in troublesome diplopia on down-gaze.
• Bony injuries may arise from the force of impact causing fractures by direct trauma or indirectly by transmission to the weak orbital plates of the maxillary and ethmoid bones. These are termed 'blow-out' fractures, as it was believed that they were caused by a sudden rise in intraorbital pressure. This is no longer considered to be the predominant mechanism, and trauma to the orbital rim, resulting in a buckling and fracture of the orbital floor, is generally accepted as the more likely cause.

Blow-out fractures may be classified as follows:
• Those in which the orbital rim remains intact: commonly the fracture affects the floor (antral blow-out); much less commonly the medial wall is involved

(ethmoidal blow-out). In a few cases there may be a combined antral and ethmoidal blow-out. These 'pure' blow-out fractures are caused by trauma from an object which is approximately the same size as the orbital aperture, for example a fist, kneecap or cricket or hockey ball, making fights and sports injuries the most usual causes.
• Those in which the orbital rim is fractured in addition to an antral, ethmoidal or combined blow-out. These have been termed 'impure' blow-out fractures. Common causes are road traffic accidents in which the face strikes the steering wheel or dashboard, industrial accidents and falls.

Blow-out fractures cannot occur until the air sinuses have developed. The youngest patient seen by the authors was aged 7 years.

Features

Features to consider are:
• When, where and how the injury occurred, which should always be recorded for medico-legal purposes.
• Diplopia, which is the main symptom of blow-out fractures. Separation of the images is mainly vertical in a fracture of the floor and mainly horizontal in a fracture of the medial wall. Orbital floor fracture frequently results in limitation of both up-gaze and down-gaze, leading to reversal of the diplopia from looking up to looking down. Up-gaze is commonly more restricted than down-gaze, resulting in downward displacement of the small field of binocular single vision which is often present. In medial wall blow-out fracture both adduction and abduction are frequently restricted, so that diplopia is crossed in looking in the direction of the fracture and uncrossed when looking away from it. Although reversal of diplopia is typical of orbital blow-out fracture it is not diagnostic, as similar findings can occur when there is oedema and haemorrhage and no fracture. Koornneef (1979) has described how both horizontal rectus muscles have connective tissue septa which extend to the orbital floor and to the inferior rectus and inferior oblique; therefore the medial and lateral recti are also involved to some extent in fractures of the orbital floor.
• Pain, which occurs when tissue is trapped and is present when the patient looks away from the site of

the lesion, on up-gaze in blow-out fractures of the floor and on abduction in blow-out fractures of the medial wall.

• Loss of vision, which may result from trauma to the eye or the optic nerve: every patient should undergo a complete examination of both the anterior and posterior segments of the eye.

• Limitation of ocular movement, which can be mechanical, neurogenic or myogenic in origin. Mechanical limitation of movement can be due to:

   1 oedema and, to a lesser extent, haemorrhage;

   2 incarceration or entrapment of tissue, especially if the fracture is linear;

   3 herniation of tissue and orbital contents into the maxillary antrum;

   4 displacement of the globe.

It was believed that the inferior rectus and occasionally the inferior oblique became trapped in a linear fracture of the orbital floor or herniated into the antrum when a hole was present, restricting up-gaze. It is now known that connective tissue rather than muscle tissue becomes trapped or herniated. Koornneef (1979) has shown that each muscle has an organized system of connective tissue septa, which becomes trapped or is distorted by the fracture.

• Limitation of movement due to palsy of the inferior rectus muscle, which may be myogenic or neurogenic in origin, resulting in limitation of movement on down-gaze. The reason why there is an increased propensity for the inferior rectus to be affected may be because shortly before the impact to the eye an intact Bell's phenomenon rotates the eye upwards, exposing the muscle to the direct force of the injury. We have observed continuing spontaneous recovery of inferior rectus function 9–12 months after the injury.

• Displacement of the globe, which is commonly backwards (enophthalmos); there may also be downward displacement when there is herniation of fat from the inferior part of the orbit into the antrum. Enophthalmos can progressively worsen over a long period of time. If severe, it can cause serious disfigurement. Proptosis that results from intraorbital haemorrhage is occasionally seen on presentation.

• Retraction of the globe, which occurs when the eye moves away from the site of entrapment, is seen on elevation in a floor blow-out fracture and on abduction in a medial wall blow-out fracture. Fibrosis is another cause of retraction and may account for the few cases in which it is a late sign. The presence of retraction is strongly indicative of entrapment or herniation of tissue into a fracture site. If there is no retraction, the prognosis for spontaneous recovery of ocular movement is better.

• Facial asymmetry, which occurs in 'impure' blow-out fractures, especially those involving a fracture of the zygoma. Facial scarring may also be present, depending on the exact nature of the injury.

• Infraorbital anaesthesia from damage to the infra-orbital nerve, which results in loss of sensation of the ipsilateral cheek and upper teeth.

• A large subconjunctival haemorrhage with no posterior limit, which strongly infers that the bleeding originates from within the orbit and suggests that a fracture may be present.

• Subcutaneous emphysema resulting from air tracking into the subcutaneous tissues, which is seen following fracture of the medial wall. A patient with an orbital blow-out fracture should be instructed not to blow his nose as this can result in the development or worsening of subcutaneous emphysema.

Investigation

Investigations include:

• Visual acuity, which must be recorded for distance and near and regularly monitored since the injury may also have damaged the globe or optic nerve. It is extremely important to assess and record both uncorrected and corrected visual acuity early and certainly before surgery, in view of the possible medico-legal problems which might ensue if it is not certain whether any loss of vision preceded or followed surgical treatment.

• An examination of the ocular media and fundi, noting any signs of trauma, which include hyphaema, angle recession, iris sphincter rupture, lens subluxation, retinal dialysis and choroidal rupture.

• A record of any head posture adopted for near and for distance viewing. If there is limitation of vertical movement, the compensatory head posture is likely to be a chin elevation or depression rather than a head tilt. Patients with medial wall fractures usually adopt a face turn, generally to the affected side, which will be more pronounced for near fixation.

• The ocular movements should be recorded, noting particularly limitation of movement in opposite directions of gaze and retraction of the globe, which is best assessed by viewing both eyes from above. A Hess chart should be plotted, including the outer fields, and a field of binocular single vision should be obtained: this may reveal peripheral areas of diplopia, indicating defective movement which was not apparent on the Hess chart. These tests are essential in monitoring progress.

• The measurement of the position of the globe, both enophthalmos and depression. This is required as a record and should be repeated at regular intervals (see Chapter 2).

• The measurement of the deviation, which should be measured in the primary position for near and distance, fixing with either eye, preferably using a prism cover test. If the patient can cooperate a measurement in the most important gaze positions is useful, for example on up-gaze and down-gaze in cases of orbital floor blow-out fracture.

• Intraocular pressure should be recorded in the position of gaze in which movement is limited and compared with the primary position values.

The forced duction test is uncomfortable to perform in the early period, and cannot differentiate mechanical restriction due to oedema and haemorrhage from that caused by tissue entrapment. In our hands it is not sufficiently sensitive under local anaesthesia to identify mild restrictions. A significant restriction of movement will be associated with retraction of the globe and in such cases the forced duction test will not contribute significantly to the clinical picture.

Radiological examination

The options available in the radiological investigation of an orbital blow-out fracture include:

• Plain radiography: extensive facial fractures causing impure blow-out fractures can be seen using a combination of anteroposterior and lateral plain X-rays of the facial skeleton. 'Pure' blow-out fractures, particularly of the linear type, are rarely visible using this technique but in the presence of an intact orbital rim, a fracture of the orbital floor or medial wall should be suspected if there is blood (fluid level) in the maxillary antrum or ethmoid sinuses, or more rarely, if air is seen in the orbital cavity. A plain radiograph

will not identify all fractures of the orbit and is of little value in patients who show clinical signs suggestive of a fracture.

• Computed tomography (CT) scan: a CT scan is the radiological investigation of choice in patients suspected of a blow-out fracture of the orbit and can accurately identify the site and extent of any fracture. The extraocular muscles and globe are clearly outlined in addition to the orbital skeleton. Scans can be electronically reconstructed in all three planes, so that a complete three-dimensional representation of the effects of the injury on the orbital bones, the eye and the extraocular muscles is possible. An antral blow-out fracture may be seen to affect not only the inferior rectus and inferior oblique, but also the medial rectus, dragging the muscle inferiorly due to involvement of the intermuscular orbital septa in the injury.

• Magnetic resonance imaging (MRI) scan: an MRI scan is not the preferred radiological procedure for imaging the orbit as it does not demonstrate the bony skeleton. It does, however, provide better definition of the soft tissues and may have a role in documenting the extent of any soft tissue injury. Cinematographic MRI scan, demonstrating the relationship of extraocular muscles and soft tissues during movement of the globe, may give a better understanding of the mechanisms involved in the restrictive ocular motility seen in these patients.

Management of pure blow-out fractures

Patients with fractures involving the orbital rim are best treated in collaboration with faciomaxillary surgeons. Prisms may be required postoperatively to overcome any residual diplopia. These so-called 'impure' blow-out fractures are excluded from the discussion which follows.

Most patients are seen shortly after injury and are discussed below under 'Early management'. However, a few are not referred until much later, either because of other serious injury or because the patient did not seek advice; these patients are considered under 'Late management'.

Early management

Limitation of ocular movement in patients with known fractures is likely to be caused partly by mechanical factors comprising fracture, oedema and haemorrhage, and muscle paresis. The roles of the orthoptist and ophthalmologist include:

- identifying the presence of any ocular muscle imbalance;
- monitoring for any change with time;
- identifying the mechanical and paralytic components of the motility disorder;
- conservative management of ocular muscle imbalance:
  1 encouraging the adoption of a head posture to achieve BSV;
  2 the use of Fresnel prisms;
  3 occlusion.

The condition should be monitored mainly by assessment of visual acuity, the Hess chart and field of binocular single vision. The patient should be tested every 3–4 days for the first few weeks after the injury. As the soft tissue oedema and haemorrhage subside, ocular movement may improve and an initial proptosis may change to enophthalmos.

If the motility does not significantly improve, surgery is then considered in the following circumstances:

- Persistent limitation of ocular movement represented by > −2 restriction, on up-gaze in cases of orbital floor fractures and on lateral gaze in medial wall fracture. Limitation of movement on down-gaze is the result of inferior rectus muscle paresis and will not be influenced by surgical repair of the fracture site: initial conservative management of these patients is indicated (Wojno 1987).
- Incarceration or herniation of tissue which is unlikely to regress without surgery. This is visible on radiological investigation and is associated with significant enophthalmos once oedema has subsided. There may be retraction of the globe on attempted movement in the field of restriction and the forced duction test will be positive.
- Cosmetically unacceptable enophthalmos, usually exceeding 3 mm. The use of a CT scan to measure the orbital volume within 20 days of injury may predict the final degree of enophthalmos (Whitehouse *et al.* 1994).

Timing of orbital surgery

The timing of orbital surgery remains controversial. Very early surgery, carried out within 1–3 days of onset, was advocated in the past. More recently, most surgeons consider 14–21 days to be the optimum waiting time to allow for spontaneous improvement, the exception being the presence of significant orbital volume loss through a large fracture site or marked retraction of the globe on attempted up-gaze, which may best be managed by very early surgical invention. There is some evidence that patients under 20 years of age respond less well to treatment (McCarry *et al.* 1984), possibly due to the faster formation of fibrous scar tissue in this age group (Waddell *et al.* 1982). Although successful cases of later surgical intervention have been reported, they are probably exceptions, since the formation of bony callus by that stage is likely to prevent the freeing of trapped tissue. In contrast, Putterman *et al.* (1974) advised observation for a period of 4–6 months: they reported that surgery was not required by most patients in their series at the end of that time and that the few still troubled by diplopia were successfully treated by conventional muscle surgery on the normal eye. This view is supported by a retrospective review by Neufeld *et al.* (1996).

Further discussion of this controversial issue can be found in the excellent articles in which early surgical repair is compared with a more conservative approach (Manson & Iliff 1991; Putterman 1991).

Orbital surgical technique

The aim of surgery is to free incarcerated or prolapsed orbital tissue from the fracture site and so reconstitute as nearly as possible the normal anatomical arrangement of the orbital contents. This is done by approaching the fracture site in the floor or medial wall through a horizontal skin incision overlying the inferior orbital margin, and following a subperiosteal plane of dissection external to the orbital fascia. To prevent re-adhesion of orbital tissue to a linear fracture, or recurrent prolapse through a hole in the fractured bony plate, a suitably shaped silastic plate is placed over the fracture site deep to the periosteum. The subperiosteal space is closed anteriorly along the inferior orbital rim with sutures to stabilize the silastic plate and the skin and muscle incisions are closed in layers. The orbital contents are disturbed as little as possible during surgery to avoid additional scar tissue formation and further mechanical restriction of ocular movement. Attempts to overcome restricted movement by direct surgery on the inferior rectus or medial rectus muscles or by division of supposedly contracted orbital fascial bands should be avoided at this stage.

Late management

Significant enophthalmos will benefit from primary repair of the fracture site, even at a late stage. Patients with persistent diplopia fall into two groups: those who refused initial orbital surgery, and those whose diplopia failed to resolve during follow-up. Putterman *et al.* (1974) recommend extraocular muscle surgery rather than orbital surgery in this group, and we agree with this approach, except where the orbital fracture has not been previously explored or there is significant enophthalmos.

Classification of ocular muscle imbalance in orbital blow-out fractures

The ocular motility features of orbital blow-out fracture are very characteristic and any deviation is almost always incomitant. The features of blow-out fracture of the orbital floor and medial wall are considered separately.

Classification of orbital floor blow-out fractures

Three types of orbital floor blow-out fracture are recognized, based on whether the limitation of ocular movement is mechanical and/or neurogenic in origin.
• Type I. Limited elevation of affected eye because of mechanical restriction.
• Type II. Limited depression of affected eye because of inferior rectus muscle palsy.
• Type III. Combined limited elevation and depression of the affected eye because of mechanical restriction and inferior rectus palsy, respectively.

Type I orbital floor blow-out fractures
FEATURES
• Limitation of ocular movement on up-gaze.
• The forced duction test is positive for mechanical restriction, with the greatest limitation in elevation and abduction.
• The field of binocular single vision is reduced in elevation, resulting in a chin-up compensatory head

posture in some patients. The effect on the patient depends on his needs and requirements; snooker players and mountain climbers, for example, are more likely to be troubled by a loss of binocular single vision in elevation.

Most cases in which elevation is significantly limited can be successfully treated by timely and appropriate intervention with orbital surgery.

MANAGEMENT
Conservative treatment
It is surprising how many patients adapt to a reduced field of binocular single vision in elevation. This fact is highlighted by patients who elect for surgery but later decline it, stating that they are comfortable in spite of unchanging alignment.

Surgical treatment
Surgical principles: The two basic surgical strategies are:
• surgery to increase the range of movement of the affected eye on up-gaze;
• surgery to balance the defect by decreasing the amount of overaction in the muscles of the fellow eye.

Surgical intervention should be avoided if it puts the field of binocular single vision in the primary position and down-gaze at risk.

Categories: The restriction in the range of movement in up-gaze can be categorized into one of three groups, depending on its severity.
• Mild restriction in the movement of the affected eye on up-gaze with overaction of the contralateral inferior oblique muscle (Fig. 21.11). An improvement in the field of binocular single vision can be obtained with a recession of the overacting inferior oblique muscle. However, if mild inferior rectus paresis coexists with up-gaze restriction, this procedure can result in an overaction of the contralateral superior oblique and loss of the field of binocular single vision on down-gaze, and is therefore contraindicated in such cases.
• Moderate restriction in the movement of the affected eye on up-gaze with overaction of the contralateral inferior oblique and superior rectus muscles (Fig. 21.12). The contralateral superior rectus muscle should be weakened: recession can be combined with a posterior fixation suture if necessary. The

Field of Left Eye (fixing with right eye)

Field of Right Eye (fixing with left eye)

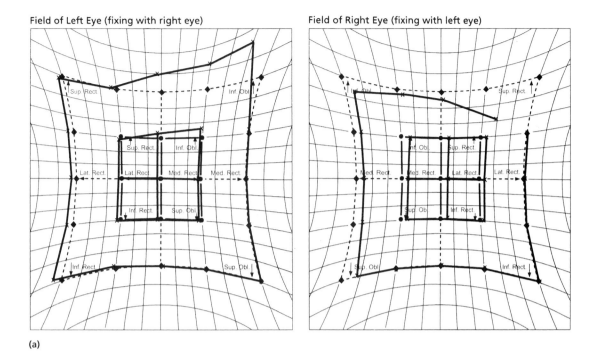

(a)

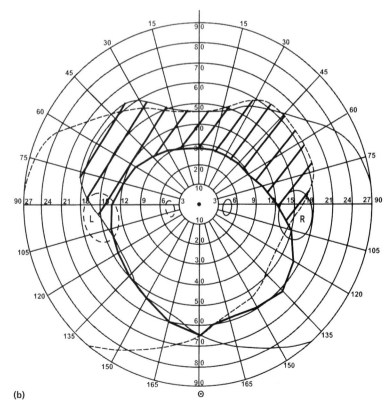

Fig. 21.11 (a) Hess chart of a patient with a type I blow-out fracture of the right orbital floor showing mild limitation of elevation of the right eye. (b) Field of binocular single vision of same patient showing diplopia in elevated positions only. **(b)**

Field of Left Eye (fixing with right eye) Field of Right Eye (fixing with left eye)

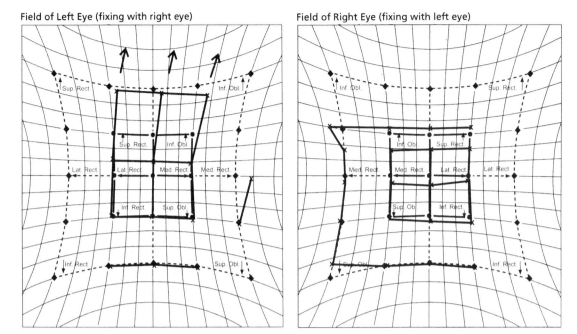

Fig. 21.12 Hess chart of a patient with a type I blow-out fracture of the right orbital floor showing moderate limitation of elevation of the right eye.

simultaneous weakening of both elevators in one eye should be avoided if possible. The use of adjustable sutures can help to prevent reversal of the deviation in the primary position and on down-gaze, and is recommended.

• Marked restriction of movement of the affected eye on up-gaze, preventing fixation in the primary position (Fig. 21.13). These cases present a difficult surgical problem. If the orbital floor has not been adequately explored and all incarcerated tissue freed, surgery should be performed to achieve this. If previous attempts by the orbital surgeon to improve the range of elevation have failed, the strabismus surgeon should re-explore the area around the inferior rectus and inferior oblique complex. All adhesions should be freed. This often results in a temporary improvement in the forced duction test; however, all too often this is not maintained postoperatively, with a recurrence of the original restriction. We have had some success with the combined use of intraoperative botulinum toxin into the inferior rectus muscle and a traction suture to anchor the eye in an elevated position. If the traction suture can be kept in place for

4–6 weeks, we have been able to restore binocular single vision in the primary position without loss of single vision in down-gaze. We do not consider that in this situation any useful improvement in the field of BSV can be obtained by operating on the unaffected eye, in an attempt to match the defect.

A recession of the ipsilateral inferior rectus muscle in an attempt to improve elevation is not recommended in type I orbital blow-out fracture: limitation of depression without improvement in elevation can follow this procedure. The mechanism may be that a subclinical inferior rectus palsy is converted to an overt clinical paresis by the recession, resulting in the limitation of movement on down-gaze.

Type II orbital floor blow-out fractures
FEATURES

• Limitation of ocular movement on down-gaze.

• The forced duction test is negative for mechanical restriction on depression.

• The aetiology is a palsy of the inferior rectus muscle, either because of direct myogenic injury to the muscle or from damage to its nerve supply.

Field of Left Eye (fixing with right eye)

Field of Right Eye (fixing with left eye)

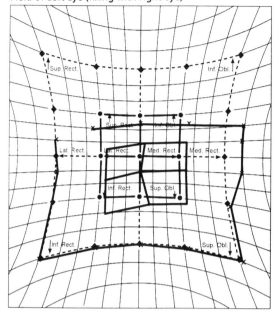 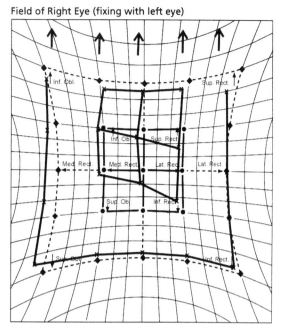

Fig. 21.13 Hess chart of a patient with a type I blow-out fracture of the left orbital floor showing a vertical deviation in the primary position and marked limitation of elevation of the left eye.

• Recovery of inferior rectus function commonly occurs and may continue for 12 months from the time of injury; surgical intervention should be deferred until no further recovery is documented.

MANAGEMENT

Conservative treatment

Conservative management should be continued until there is no further evidence of recovery, usually for 9–12 months. Prisms are usually ineffective as a long-term treatment due to the incomitant nature of the deviation.

Surgical treatment

Surgical principles: The two basic surgical strategies are:

• Surgery to the affected eye to improve ocular movement:

1 a resection of the inferior rectus and recession of the superior rectus muscles;

2 augmenting the action of the involved inferior rectus muscle by an inverse Knapp procedure.

• Surgery to the fellow eye to balance the defect:

1 a recession of the overacting contralateral superior oblique;

2 a recession of the contralateral inferior rectus muscle, with or without a posterior fixation suture.

A resection of the ipsilateral inferior rectus in orbital floor blow-out fracture may cause restriction of elevation or worsen any pre-existing tendency to it; we do not therefore recommend this procedure in these patients.

Categories: The vertical deviation may be associated with an underaction of the inferior rectus muscle, either with preservation of the range of movement or more usually, with limited depression (Fig. 21.14).

• Inferior rectus muscle underaction with a normal range of movement on down-gaze is uncommon. Surgery should be directed at the contralateral eye, aiming to balance the defect with a weakening of the superior oblique muscle using a posterior tenotomy or a tendon spacer. Occasionally the deviation on down-gaze is concomitant, with a significant vertical deviation on both dextro- and laevodepression: a

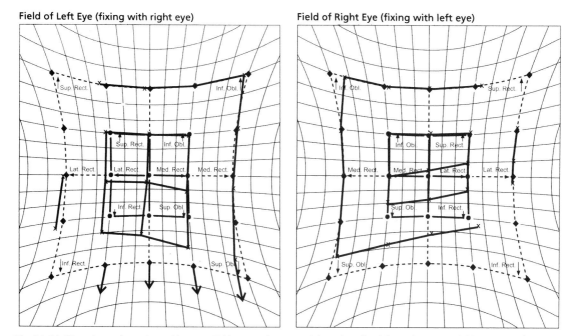

Fig. 21.14 Hess chart of a patient with a type II blow-out fracture of the right orbital floor showing mild limitation of depression of the right eye.

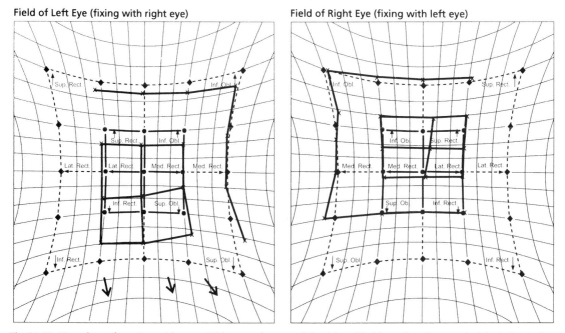

Fig. 21.15 Hess chart of a patient with a type II blow-out fracture of the right orbital floor showing a vertical deviation in the primary position and moderate limitation of depression of the right eye.

recession of the contralateral inferior rectus should be considered. An inverse Knapp procedure should not be used for these cases as reversal of the deviation can occur.

• Inferior rectus underaction with limitation of movement on down-gaze, which is by far the more common finding in our experience (Fig. 21.15). Resection of the inferior rectus muscle could result in restriction of elevation and is not recommended: we prefer instead to improve the range of ocular movement with an inverse Knapp procedure to optimize the field of binocular single vision on down-gaze. The field can continue to improve for 6–9 months postoperatively (Lipton *et al.* 1990). Further intervention should be deferred until this period has elapsed. If necessary the defect should then be matched by operating on either the contralateral superior oblique or the inferior rectus muscles (see Chapter 9).

Type III orbital floor blow-out fractures

FEATURES

Type III combines the features of types I and II (Fig. 21.16).

• Limitation of ocular movement on up-gaze. The forced duction test is positive for mechanical restriction, with the greatest restriction in elevation and abduction.

• Limitation of ocular movement on down-gaze. The forced duction test is negative for mechanical restriction on depression.

• The patient often has a small central island of binocular single vision (Fig. 21.16b), but is considerably handicapped by diplopia on down-gaze.

MANAGEMENT

Conservative treatment

In some cases there may be spontaneous improvement in the range of ocular movement, particularly on depression. Prisms are of no benefit to these patients.

Surgical treatment

It is very difficult to obtain any satisfactory improvement in the field of binocular single vision in this group of patients. If the orbital floor has not been adequately explored and all incarcerated tissue freed, then this should be carried out. There is a risk that surgery to improve the elevation of the eye will result

in further loss of inferior rectus function and cause a vertical deviation in the primary position, with loss of the existing small field of binocular single vision. If the restricted elevation can be improved the patient can then be treated as described for a type II blow-out fracture. It is our experience that most cases unfortunately fail to respond to further orbital surgery at this late stage.

Surgical principles: The surgical strategy is to expand the field of binocular single vision by operating on the unaffected eye, but in our experience most patients are reluctant to consider such treatment.

Surgery can be planned in two stages:

• Stage one: a large recession of the superior and inferior rectus muscle of the unaffected eye. The aim is to balance the limited depression of the affected eye with the large contralateral inferior rectus recession. The superior rectus recession is required to prevent postoperative hypertropia of the operated eye.

• Stage two is carried out if these procedures have been successful in enlarging the field of binocular single vision. A posterior fixation suture to the two recessed muscles can obtain further expansion of the field.

Classification of medial wall orbital blow-out fractures

Medial wall orbital blow-out fracture is more often seen in association with a blow-out fracture of the orbital floor (Figs 21.17 & 21.18) rather than as an isolated condition (Dodick *et al.* 1969). Medial wall fracture has been reported as a complication of ethmoidal sinus surgery with concurrent damage to the medial rectus muscle and occasionally to the optic nerve. In general, medial wall blow-out fracture has a less disabling effect on ocular motility than orbital floor fracture and surgical repair of the fracture frequently results in significant improvement in ocular movement.

Ocular motility imbalance persisting after repair of the medial wall blow-out fracture can be categorized as:

• limitation of abduction arising from mechanical restriction;

• limitation of adduction due either to mechanical restriction or to a neurogenic palsy of the medial rectus.

Field of Left Eye (fixing with right eye) **Field of Right Eye (fixing with left eye)**

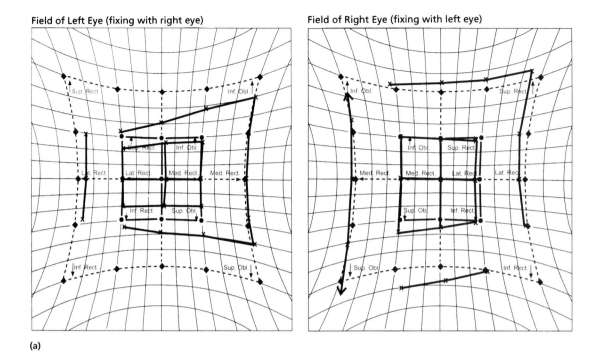

(a)

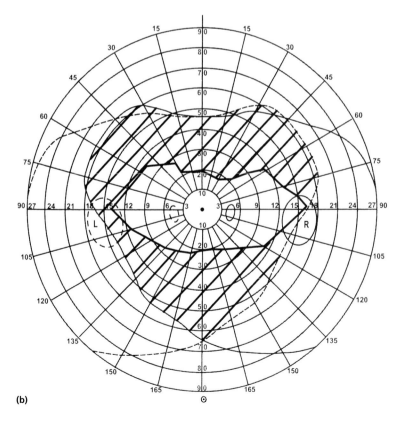

(b)

Fig. 21.16 (a) Hess chart of a patient with a type III blow-out fracture of the left orbital floor showing limitation of elevation and depression of the left eye. (b) Field of binocular single vision of same patient showing a central field of single vision.

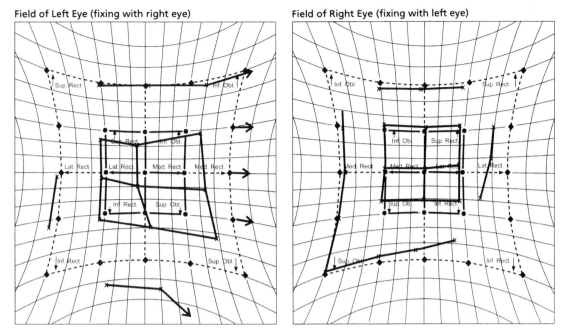

Fig. 21.17 Hess chart of a patient with a blow-out fracture of the right medial wall and orbital floor showing limitation of abduction and depression of the right eye with overaction of the contralateral medial rectus and superior oblique.

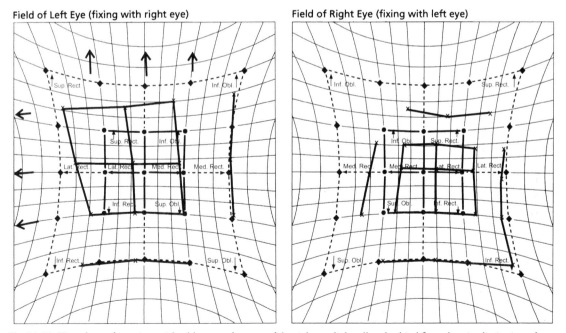

Fig. 21.18 Hess chart of a patient with a blow-out fracture of the right medial wall and orbital floor showing limitation of adduction and elevation of the right eye.

Management

Conservative treatment

There is either spontaneous improvement in ocular movement or a good response to primary surgical repair of the blow-out fracture in most cases: those not improving are kept under observation for 9–12 months before deciding on further management.

Prisms are usually ineffective as a long-term treatment due to the incomitant nature of the deviation.

Surgical treatment

Persistent limitation of adduction is more common than limited abduction and its management is discussed further.

Limitation of adduction from involvement of the medial rectus muscle results in either a mechanical restriction, probably from involvement of the check ligament of the muscle in the fracture site, or a muscle palsy: these conditions may coexist. Further management depends on separating the mechanical and paretic components: we have found the forced duction test, the forced generation test and botulinum toxin to be useful in the differential diagnosis.
• Limitation of adduction due to medial rectus muscle palsy. If this is partial, as is usual, then an ipsilateral medial rectus resection and a lateral rectus recession is the procedure of choice. If the palsy is total, the superior and inferior recti should be transposed medially and the lateral rectus muscle weakened by injection of botulinum toxin (see Chapters 9 and 19 for further details).
• Limitation of adduction due to a mechanical restriction of adduction. The medial wall of the orbit and the medial rectus muscle should be explored and all abnormal adhesions divided. Improvement in the forced duction test at the time of surgery is not always maintained, and further management may be difficult.

Retinal detachment surgery

Disturbance of binocular vision due to motor and sensory factors is not uncommon following vitreoretinal surgery. Over the past 10 years we have seen a change in the surgical management of retinal detachment, which has led to a reduction in the number of cases with troublesome postoperative strabismus. This has been due to the change from large to low-profile explants, less direct interference with the extraocular muscles and the increased use of the vitrectomy and endolaser procedure.

Aetiology

Diplopia can result from mechanical, paralytic, myogenic and secondary strabismus. It can also arise from decompensation of a pre-existing phoria.
• Mechanical restriction of ocular movement is a frequent cause of diplopia after vitreoretinal surgery. It may be the result of:
  1 Oedema involving the orbital connective tissue, conjunctiva and extraocular muscles. Early postoperative inflammation and swelling reduces the elasticity of tissues, leading to restriction of ocular movement. Inflammatory mediators can cause extraocular muscle contracture.
  2 Adhesions forming between the explant, the inferior rectus and the inferior oblique in inferior detachment surgery, and between the explant and the superior rectus in superior detachment surgery. The superior oblique tendon can be trapped by a superiorly placed explant or by an encircling band. Fibrosis is likely to follow and is more common if repeated retinal surgery has been performed.
  3 The explant itself, especially if it has been placed under an extraocular muscle.
• Paralytic strabismus can be the result of a muscle becoming detached during surgery or from damage to its nerve supply.
• Myogenic strabismus results from direct trauma to the extraocular muscle or muscles.
• Sensory factors can degrade binocular single vision and either decompensate a pre-existing phoria or cause a secondary strabismus. Poor image quality or aniseikonia may prevent fusion, even when ocular movement is good. Factors which can disrupt fusion include:
  1 preoperative loss of vision from a macular off retinal detachment or vitreous haemorrhage;
  2 the intraoperative use of expanding intraocular gases, which can prevent fusion for several weeks postoperatively; macular oedema and cataract can also degrade image quality;

Field of Left Eye (fixing with right eye)   **Field of Right Eye (fixing with left eye)**

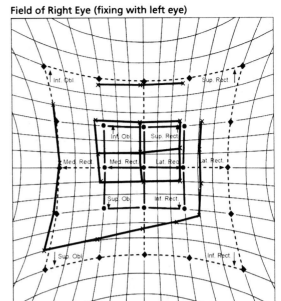

Fig. 21.19 Hess chart of a patient with mechanical restriction of ocular movement following a right retinal detachment repair showing limitation of abduction and depression of the right eye.

3 postoperative metamorphopsia from a macular off detachment and secondary retinal surface membranes can distort vision;

4 a tight encircling band can cause significant myopia and astigmatism may be secondary to retinal explants;

5 marked degrees of anisometropia can result from the use of intraocular oil.

Multiple factors are frequently responsible for the strabismus in any given patient.

Features (Fig. 21.19)

Features of the patient with strabismus after vitreo-retinal surgery include:

• Pain and swelling in the early postoperative period as a result of inflammation, which may recur later due to reactive changes to the explant or to its becoming secondarily infected. The explant can work its way loose, indenting the eyelid, or become extruded through the conjunctiva and require removal.

• Diplopia and pain on eye movement in the field of restricted gaze.

• Horizontal, vertical and occasionally cyclotorsional strabismus.

• Normal visual acuity in the operated eye in some cases.

Management

Conservative management of the strabismus is indicated in the first 3–6 months after vitreoretinal surgery to allow time for spontaneous recovery. Strabismus surgery is indicated only if a detached muscle is suspected or when other methods of dealing with the deviation have failed.

Conservative treatment

The following measures can be considered.

• Correction of anisometropia by contact lenses, which may relieve aniseikonia sufficiently to allow fusion.

• Prisms can be used to overcome diplopia when there is a small angle of deviation unless the image disparity is too great: even if fusion is not obtained in the clinic it is sometimes worthwhile persisting with prisms for a short period to give the patient time to adapt to them.

• Intractable diplopia may be relieved by sector or total occlusion on one spectacle lens.

In our experience the ocular muscle imbalance frequently improves as postoperative inflammation subsides; we therefore delay further treatment, including the use botulinum toxin, until it is apparent that the strabismus will persist.

Botulinum toxin

Botulinum toxin has both a diagnostic and therapeutic role in patients with postretinal detachment strabismus.

• It can be used diagnostically to investigate the patient's binocular potential.

• It can be used therapeutically to treat persistent strabismus, leading to restored fusion or cosmetically improved alignment after one or several injections.

Surgical treatment

Surgery can be considered if conservative measures have failed to restore binocular single vision or improved alignment. In a minority of cases in which the explant is the direct cause of the restricted movement, motor function may be improved by its removal; in most cases this can safely be carried out 3 months after a successful retinal detachment procedure. By this time a firm retinal/choroidal attachment should have been achieved and removal of the explant is associated with only an approximate 10% risk of re-detachment. However, because of additional fibrosis, explant removal does not often solve the problem and further measures will be required.

Aims

The main aim of surgery is to restore binocular single vision in the primary and reading positions in patients with fusion potential. It may not be possible to eliminate diplopia in all gaze directions. The goal in the absence of fusion is to improve ocular alignment without causing intolerable diplopia.

Surgical management depends on the potential for binocular single vision and the magnitude and nature of any restriction of ocular movement.

• Good potential for binocular single vision and mild mechanical restriction of movement. Strabismus

surgery can be performed on the fellow eye, avoiding the need to reoperate on the previously operated eye.

• Good potential for binocular single vision and marked mechanical restriction of movement. Surgery for the strabismus needs to be directed at the restricted eye, aiming to achieve free ocular movement and restore alignment.

• Strabismus due to a muscle palsy. Muscle palsies resulting from damage to the muscle or its nerve supply should be managed in the same manner as neurogenic palsies (see Chapter 19). If a muscle has been lost, attempts to retrieve it are sometimes successful.

• Poor potential for binocular single vision. The risk of postoperative diplopia should be assessed either with prisms or botulinum toxin. Strabismus surgery can be performed on either eye.

After a forced duction test to identify restriction of passive movement, the muscles should be explored and all fibrous tissue meticulously removed. We do not routinely remove explants that are not contributing towards the strabismus. Adhesions between muscle and explant and muscle and sclera should be divided until ductions are normal. It is nearly always necessary to recess affected muscles, using adjustable sutures when possible, and a conjunctival recession should be carried out if there is any evidence of conjunctival contracture.

Cataract surgery

Binocular diplopia is an uncommon complication of cataract surgery and should be differentiated from monocular blurring arising from uncorrected refractive error and media opacity.

Aetiology

Diplopia can result from myogenic, mechanical, paralytic and secondary strabismus.

• Myogenic damage to the inferior rectus can occur when cataract surgery is performed under local anaesthetic. It follows direct injection of the anaesthetic agent into the muscle which can then result in:

  1 Volkmann's ischaemic contracture and fibrosis of the muscle and a mechanical strabismus (Hamed 1991) as a result of the rise in tissue pressure within the muscle's fascial compartment.

2 A direct toxic injury to the muscle fibres by the local anaesthetic agent, resulting in muscle contraction and restriction of ocular movement (Rainin & Carlson 1985).

3 A minor degree of toxic injury that can result in an overaction of a muscle from posterior segmental contracture rather than the contraction and restrictive strabismus seen following the more extensive injury described above (Capo & Guyton 1996).

4 Permanent paresis of vertical recti presumably due to anaesthetic myotoxicity (Esswein & von Noorden 1993).

- Mechanical restriction of ocular movement can follow the placement of a bridle traction suture under the superior rectus muscle. Damage to the global surface of the superior rectus muscle by the suture can result in an adhesion between muscle and globe at this site, creating a posterior fixation suture effect and restricting the upward movement of the eye (Hamed *et al.* 1987).

- Paralytic strabismus is a transient phenomenon in the early postoperative period following peribulbar or retrobulbar local anaesthetic.

- Secondary strabismus is a frequent cause of diplopia and can arise from:

1 Central loss of sensory fusion following surgery on congenital and traumatic unilateral cataract, and when unilateral aphakia is left uncorrected. A characteristic slow oscillating movement, the Heimann–Bielschowsky phenomenon, may be observed in the affected eye and the patient may report oscillopsia.

2 Postoperative anisometropia and high levels of surgically induced astigmatism.

3 The normalization of long-standing anisometropia. The correction of high levels of preoperative anisometropia can result in difficulty in patient adaptation and may result in disruption of fusion from insuperable aniseikonia.

Features

The main features of diplopia arising after cataract surgery are as follows.

- A history of intermittent diplopia or prismatic spectacles strongly suggests decompensation of a pre-existing strabismus as the cause of the diplopia.

- Secondary strabismus arising from high postoperative anisometropia or astigmatism should be readily apparent after refraction.

- Myogenic damage to the inferior rectus can cause:

1 a mechanical strabismus with a hypotropia in the primary position which increases on abduction and elevation; the forced duction test is positive;

2 an overaction of the muscle, with an ipsilateral hypotropia which increases in its field of action;

3 an inferior rectus palsy.

- Damage to the superior rectus can result in a mechanical or paralytic strabismus and apparent overaction of the muscle in the same way as described for the inferior rectus.

Management

The diplopia should initially be managed conservatively to allow time for spontaneous recovery. Diplopia that occurs only on up-gaze is better tolerated than diplopia in other gaze directions and usually does not require further intervention. High levels of postoperative astigmatism may be correctable by suture adjustment. Strabismus and refractive surgery is indicated only when other methods of dealing with the diplopia have failed.

Conservative treatment

The following measures can be considered.

- Single lens spectacles are likely to be better tolerated than bifocal and varifocal lenses when high levels of anisometropia are present. Correction of anisometropia by contact lenses may relieve aniseikonia sufficiently to allow fusion.

- Astigmatism with a plus axis around 90° can be managed by early suture removal, whereas astigmatism with an axis around horizontal cannot be treated in this way. When corrected some patients will be able to tolerate quite large levels of astigmatism, whereas others will need refractive surgery.

- Prisms can be used to overcome diplopia when there is a small angle of deviation unless the image disparity is too great: even if fusion is not obtained in the clinic it is sometimes worthwhile persisting with prisms for a short period to give the patient time to adapt to them.

- Botulinum toxin injection is indicated for a persisting

hypotropia due to inferior rectus contracture that is not correctable by prisms. Contracture of the superior rectus is not readily treated with botulinum toxin injection due to the inevitable ptosis that accompanies toxin injected into the muscle.

• Intractable diplopia may be relieved by occlusion on one spectacle lens.

Surgical treatment

Refractive and strabismus surgery should be delayed until conservative treatment has failed to relieve symptoms.

• Refractive surgery can correct astigmatism and anisometropia that is disrupting fusion. Circumferential corneal incisions are used to relieve astigmatism, and radial or photorefractive keratotomy to correct high levels of myopia responsible for intolerable anisometropia.

• Anisometropia resulting from an incorrect power of intraocular lenses can be treated by surgically exchanging the lens with one of the correct strength.

• Persisting strabismus that is not relieved by prisms is managed on the basis of its aetiology and the nature of the deviation. Decompensation of a pre-existing horizontal phoria is treated by surgery to the medial and lateral rectus muscles. A fourth nerve palsy that has decompensated following cataract surgery should be treated according to the muscle sequelae (see Chapter 19). Vertical strabismus due to inferior rectus contracture should be managed by a recession of the contracted muscle; contracture of the superior rectus is managed in the same way, using adjustable sutures when possible. Vertical deviations greater than 15 Δ may require an additional recession of the contralateral antagonist (Munoz *et al.* 1996). Inferior rectus palsy can be treated with surgery to strengthen the affected muscle or by weakening the overacting muscles in the contralateral eye (see Chapter 19).

Orbital tumours

Orbital tumours may cause a mechanical restriction, either by the tumour mass obstructing movement of the globe or by diffuse infiltration of the periocular tissue.

Mass lesions sited outside the muscle cone, for example lacrimal gland tumours, will cause horizontal or vertical displacement of the globe and usually cause a restriction of movement in the direction of the lesion. Infiltrative tumours are usually metastatic, with the commonest primary sites being breast in women and prostate in men. Secondary deposits in the orbit from breast carcinoma may be of the sclerosing type, resulting in enophthalmos rather than exophthalmos, leading to severe limitation of ocular movement (Trimble 1980).

Occasionally the tumour may cause a very specific restriction of movement: a Brown's syndrome secondary to a discrete prostatic secondary tumour in the region of the trochlea has been reported (Booth-Mason *et al.* 1985). Kivlin and Lundergan (1985) reported an acquired orbital retraction syndrome, with some similarity to Duane's syndrome, also due to a prostatic orbital metastasis. Direct involvement of the muscle fibres is rare, occurring in less than 5% of all cases of orbital metastases. Arnold *et al.* (1989) reported a case of secondary exotropia with restricted adduction due to a metastasis within the belly of the medial rectus following gastric carcinoma.

References

Adler, F.H. (1959) Spontaneous recovery in a case of superior oblique tendon sheath syndrome of Brown. *Archives of Ophthalmology* **61**, 1006.

Archer, S.M., Sondhi, N. & Helveston, E.M. (1989) Strabismus in infancy. *Ophthalmology* **96** (1), 133–137.

Arnold, R.W., Adams, B.A., Camoriano, J.K. & Dyer, J.A. (1989) Acquired divergent strabismus: presumed metastatic gastric carcinoma in the medial rectus muscle. *Journal of Pediatric Ophthalmology and Strabismus* **26**, 50–51.

Bahn, R.S. (1995) The fibroblast is the target cell in the connective tissue manifestations of Graves' disease. *International Archives of Allergy and Immunology* **106**, 213–218.

Barrett, L., Glatt, H.J., Burde, R.M. & Gado, M.H. (1988) Optic nerve dysfunction in thyroid eye disease. *CT Radiology* **167**, 503–507.

Bartley, G.B., Fatourechi, V., Kadrmas, E.F., Jacobsen, S.J., Ilstrup, D.M. & Garrity, J.A. (1996) The chronology of Graves' ophthalmopathy in an incidence cohort. *American Journal of Ophthalmology* **121**, 426–434.

Booth-Mason, S., Kyle, G.M., Rossor, M. & Bradbury, P. (1985) Acquired Brown's syndrome, an unusual case. *British Journal of Ophthalmology* **69**, 791–794.

Breinin, G.M. (1957) Electromyography: a tool in ocular and neurologic diagnosis. II muscle palsies. *Archives of Ophthalmology* 57, 165–175.

Brodsky, M.C., Pollock, S.C. & Buckley, E.G. (1989) Neural misdirection in congenital ocular fibrosis syndrome: implications and pathogenesis. *Journal of Pediatric Ophthalmology and Strabismus* 26, 159–161.

Brown, H.W. (1950) Congenital structural muscle anomalies. In: *Strabismus Ophthalmic Symposium 1* (ed. J.H. Allen), pp. 205–236. Mosby, St Louis.

Burde, R.M. (1990) Graves' ophthalmopathy and the special problem of concomitant ocular myasthenia gravis. *American Orthoptic Journal* 40, 37–50.

Capo, H. & Guyton, D.L. (1996) Ipsilateral hypertropia following cataract surgery. *Ophthalmology* 103, 721–730.

Caputo, A.R., Wagner, R.S., Guo, S. & Santiago, A.P. (1996) Infantile abduction deficit: Duane's retraction syndrome of abducens palsy? A study of 24 cases. *Binocular Vision and Strabismus Quarterly* 11, 213–218.

Caygill, W.M. (1972) Excyclotropia in dysthyroid ophthalmopathy. *American Journal of Ophthalmology* 73, 437–441.

Collin, J.R.O. (1984) *A Manual of Systematic Eyelid Surgery*, p. 70. Churchill Livingstone, Edinburgh.

Costenbader, F.D. & Albert, D.G. (1959) Spontaneous regression of pseudoparalysis of the inferior oblique muscle. *Archives of Ophthalmology* 59, 607–608.

Crawford, J.S. (1970) Congenital fibrosis syndrome. *Canadian Journal of Ophthalmology* 5, 331–336.

Dodick, J.M., Galin, M.A. & Kwitko, M. (1969) Medial wall fracture of the orbit. *Canadian Journal of Ophthalmology* 4, 377–378.

Duane, A. (1905) Congenital deficiency of abduction associated with impairment of adduction, retraction movements, contraction of the palpebral fissure and oblique movements of the eye. *Archives of Ophthalmology (Chicago)* 34, 133–150.

Duke-Elder, S. & Wybar, K. (1973) *Ocular Motility and Strabismus*, Vol. VI, pp. 204–206. Henry Kimpton, London.

Elsas, F.J. (1991) Occult Duane syndrome: Co-contraction revealed following strabismus surgery. *Journal of Pediatric Ophthalmology and Strabismus* 28, 328–332.

Esswein, M.B. & von Noorden, G.K. (1993) Paresis of a vertical rectus muscle after cataract extraction. *American Journal of Ophthalmology* 116, 424–430.

Feldon, S.E. & Weiner, J.M. (1982) Clinical significance of extraocular muscle volumes in Graves' ophthalmopathy. *Archives of Ophthalmology* 100, 1266–1269.

Fells, P. (1975) The superior oblique, its actions and anomalies. *British Orthoptic Journal* 32, 43–53.

Fells, P. (1987) Orbital decompression for severe dysthyroid eye disease. *British Journal of Ophthalmology* 71, 101–111.

Fells, P. & McCarry, B. (1987) Surgical options in Duane's retraction syndrome. In: *Orthoptic Horizons. Transactions of the 6th International Orthoptics Congress, Harrogate* (eds M. Lenk-Schafer, C. Calcott, I.M. Doyle & S. Moore), pp. 438–441. British Orthoptic Society, London.

Fells, P. & McCarry, B. (1988) 'Fixed' versus 'adjustable' sutures in the treatment of dysthyroid ophthalmology. In: *Transactions of the Seventeenth European Strabismological Association, Madrid* (ed. J. Murube), pp. 239–242.

Fells, P., Waddell, E. & Alvares, M. (1982) Progressive exaggerated A-pattern strabismus with presumed fibrosis of extraocular muscles. In: *Strabismus II* (ed. R. Reinecke), pp. 335–343. Grune & Stratton, Orlando.

Fells, P., Rosen, P., Pickard, B. & Plowman, N. (1989) Radiotherapy or surgery for orbital decompression in dysthyroid eye disease? In: *Transactions of the Eighteenth European Strabismological Association, Krakow* (ed. H. Kauffman), pp. 239–242.

Feric-Seiwerth, F. & Celic, M. (1972) Contribution to the knowledge of the superior oblique tendon sheath syndrome (Brown's syndromes). In: *Orthoptics. Transactions of the Second International Orthoptic Congress, Amsterdam* (eds J. Mein, J.J.M. Bierlaagh & T.E.A. Brummelkamp-Dons), pp. 354–359. Excerpta Medica.

Hagg, E. & Asplund, K. (1987) Is endocrine ophthalmopathy related to smoking? *British Medical Journal* 295, 634–635.

Hamed, L.M. (1991) Strabismus presenting after cataract surgery. *Ophthalmology* 98, 247–252.

Hamed, L.M., Helveston, E.M. & Ellis, F.D. (1987) Persistent binocular diplopia after cataract surgery. *American Journal of Ophthalmology* 103, 741–744.

Harcourt, B., Mein, J., Crompton, J. & Johnston, P. (1978) The significance of retraction of the globe on infraduction in certain cases of thyroid eye disease. In: *Strabismus* (ed. R.D. Reinecke), pp. 111–116. Grune & Stratton, New York.

Harley, R.L., Rodrigues, M.M. & Crawford, J.S. (1978) Congenital fibrosis of the extraocular muscles. *Journal of Pediatric Ophthalmology and Strabismus* 15, 346–358.

Helveston, E.M., Merriam, W.W. & Ellis, F.D. (1982) The trochlea: a study of the anatomy and physiology. *Ophthalmology* 89, 124–133.

Hermann, J.S. (1982) Paretic thyroid myopathy. *Ophthalmology* 89, 473–478.

Hertle, R.W., Katowitz, J.A., Young, T.L., Quinn, G.E. & Farber, M.G. (1992) Congenital unilateral fibrosis, blepharoptosis and enophthalmos syndrome. *Ophthalmology* 99, 347–355.

Heufelder, A.E. & Bahn, R.S. (1992) Evidence for the presence of a functional TSH-receptor in retroocular fibroblasts from patients with Graves' ophthalmopathy. *Experimental Clinical Endocrinology* 100, 62–67.

Hiatt, R.L. & Halle, A.A. (1983) General fibrosis syndrome. *Annals of Ophthalmology* 15, 113–119.

Hill, M., Ansons, A., Gray. C. & Spencer, A. (1996) The ocular fibrosis syndrome: the role of vertical transposition of the horizontal rectus muscles in these patients. In: *Trans-actions of the 23rd Meeting of the European Strabismological Association, Nancy* (ed. M. Spiritus), pp. 429–434. Aeolus Press, The Netherlands.

Hiromatsu, Y., Fukazawa, H., Guinard, F., Salvi, M., How, J. & Wall, J.R. (1988) A thyroid cytotoxic antibody that cross-reacts with an eye muscle cell surface antigen may be the cause of thyroid associated ophthalmopathy. *Journal of Clinical Endocrinological Metabolism* 67, 565–570.

Hotchkiss, M.G., Miller, N.R., Clark, A.W. & Green, W.R. (1980) Bilateral Duane's retraction syndrome. A clinicopathologic case report. *Archives of Ophthalmology* 98, 870–874.

Hoyt, W.F. & Nachtigaller, H. (1965) Anomalies of ocular motor nerves. *American Journal of Ophthalmology* 60, 443–448.

Huber, A. (1974) Electrophysiology of the retraction syndrome. *British Journal of Ophthalmology* 58, 293–300.

Huber, A. (1984) Duane's retraction syndrome. Considerations on pathophysiology and aetiology. In: *Transactions of the Fifth International Orthoptic Congress, Cannes* (eds A.P. Ravault & M. Lenk), pp. 119–125. LIPS, Lyon.

Jampolsky, A. (1984) Unusual eye movements in alert humans with attached and detached eye muscles. In: *Transactions of the Fifth International Orthoptic Congress, Cannes* (eds A.P. Ravault & M. Lenk), pp. 245–248. LIPS, Lyon.

Jampolsky, A. (1995) The superior rectus contracture syndrome. *Update on Strabismus and Pediatric Ophthalmology. Proceedings of the Joint ISA and AAPOS & S Meeting, Vancouver* (ed. G. Lennerstrand), pp. 279–282. CRC Press, Boca Raton.

Johnson, L.V. (1950) Adherence syndrome; pseudo-paralysis of the lateral or superior rectus muscles. *Archives of Ophthalmology* 44, 870–878.

Kennerdell, J.S., Rosenbaum, A.E. & El-Hoshy, M.H. (1981) Apical optic nerve compression of dysthyroid optic neuropathy on computed tomography. *Archives of Ophthalmology* 99, 807–809.

Khawam, E., Azar, D., Shami, M. & Hemady, R. (1987) Progressive congenital familial ophthalmoplegia with optic nerve coloboma: report of a family. *Binocular Vision* 2, 223–231.

Khodadoust, A.A. & von Noorden, G.K. (1967) Bilateral vertical retraction syndrome. *Archives of Ophthalmology* 78, 606–612.

Kirkham, T.H. (1970) Inheritance of Duane's syndrome. *British Journal of Ophthalmology* 54, 323.

Kivlin, J.D. & Lundergan, M.K. (1985) Acquired retraction syndrome associated with orbital metastasis. *Journal of Pediatric Ophthalmology and Strabismus* 22, 109–112.

Koornneef, L. (1979) *Sectional Anatomy of the Orbit.* Esculapius, Birmingham, USA.

Kraft, S.P. (1993) Surgery for Duane syndrome. *American Orthoptic Journal* 43, 18–26.

Laughlin, R.C. (1956) Congenital fibrosis of the extraocular muscles. A report of 6 cases. *American Journal of Ophthalmology* 41, 432–438.

Leone, C.R.Jr & Weinstein, G.W. (1972) Orbital fibrosis with enophthalmos. *Ophthalmic Surgery* 3, 71–75.

Letson, R.D. (1980) Surgical management of the ocular congenital fibrosis syndrome. *American Orthoptic Journal* 30, 97–101.

Lipton, J.R., Page, A.B. & Lee, J.P. (1990) Management of diplopia on down-gaze following orbital trauma. *Eye* 4, 535–537.

Lyons, C.J., Vickers, S.F. & Lee, J.P. (1990) Botulinum toxin therapy in dysthyroid strabismus. *Eye* 4, 538–540.

Manson, P.N. & Iliff, N. (1991) Management of blow-out fractures of the orbital floor. II. Early repair for selected injuries. *Survey of Ophthalmology* 35, 280–292.

McCarry, B., Fells, P. & Waddell, E. (1984) Difficulties in the management of orbital blow-out fractures in patients under 20 years old. In: *Transactions of the Fifth International Orthoptic Congress, Cannes* (eds A.P. Ravault & M. Lenk), pp. 283–287. LIPS, Lyon.

McElvanney, A., Ansons, A. & Spencer, A. (1996) The use of 5-fluorouracil, botulinum toxin and traction sutures in the management of the adherence syndrome. In: *Transactions of the 23rd Meeting of the European Strabismological Association, Nancy* (ed. M. Spiritus), pp. 451–456. Aeolus Press, The Netherlands.

Mein, J. (1971) Superior oblique sheath syndrome. *British Orthoptic Journal* 28, 70–76.

Miller, M. (1992) Thalidomide embryopathy. A model for the study of congenital incomitant horizontal strabismus. *Transactions of the American Ophthalmological Society* 89, 634–674.

Mourits, M.P., Koornneef, L., van Mourik-Noordenbos, A.M. *et al.* (1990) Extraocular muscle surgery for Graves' ophthalmopathy: does prior treatment influence surgical outcome? *British Journal of Ophthalmology* 74, 481–483.

Munoz, M., Capo, H. & Siatkowski, R.M. (1996) Results of surgery for vertical strabismus following cataract extraction performed under local anaesthesia. *Binocular Vision and Strabismus Quarterly* 11, 275–280.

Nelson, L.B. (1986) Severe adduction deficiency following a large medial rectus recession in Duane's retraction syndrome. *Archives of Ophthalmology* 104, 859–862.

Neufeld, M., Maurino, V. & Lee, J.P. (1996) Conservative management of diplopia after orbital blow-out fracture. In: *Transactions of the 23rd Meeting of the European Strabismological Association, Nancy* (ed. M. Spiritus), pp. 401–402. Aeolus Press, The Netherlands.

von Noorden, G.K. (1996) *Binocular Vision and Ocular Motility: Theory and Management of Strabismus*, pp. 442–443. Mosby, St Louis.

Papst, W. & Esslen, E. (1960) Zur ätiologie der angerborenen abduzenlahmung. *Klinische Montatsblatte Fur Augenheilkunde* 137, 306–327.

Parks, M.M. (1972) The weakening surgical procedures for eliminating overaction of the inferior oblique muscle. *American Journal of Ophthalmology* 73, 107–122.

Parks, M.M. (1977) The superior oblique tendon. *Transactions of the Ophthalmological Society of the United Kingdom* 97, 288–304.

Parks, M.M. (1978) Surgery for Brown's syndrome. In: *Symposium on Strabismus. Transactions of the New Orleans Academy of Ophthalmology*, pp. 157–177. Mosby, St Louis.

Pfaffenbach, D.D., Cross, H.E. & Kearns, T.P. (1972) Congenital anomalies in Duane's retraction syndrome. *Archives of Ophthalmology* 88, 635–639.

Putterman, A.M. (1991) Management of blow out fractures of the orbital floor. III. The conservative approach. *Survey of Ophthalmology* 35, 292–298.

Putterman, A.M., Stevens, T. & Urist, M.J. (1974) Non-surgical management of blow-out fractures of the orbital floor. *American Journal of Ophthalmology* 77, 232–239.

Raab, E.L. (1986) Clinical features of Duane's syndrome. *Journal of Pediatric Ophthalmology and Strabismus* 23, 64–68.

Rainin, E.A. & Carlson, B.M. (1985) Post-operative diplopia and ptosis: a clinical hypothesis based on the myotoxicity of local anaesthetics. *Archives of Ophthalmology* 103, 1337–1339.

Rogers, G.L. & Bremer, D.L. (1984) Surgical treatment of the upshoot and downshoot in Duane's retraction syndrome. *Ophthalmology* 91, 1380–1383.

Roper-Hall, M.J. & Roper-Hall, G. (1972) The superior oblique 'click' syndrome. In: *Transactions of the Second International Orthoptic Congress, Amsterdam* (eds J. Mein, J.J.M. Bierlaagh & T.E. Brummelkamp-Dons), pp. 360–366. Excerpta Medica.

Ross, P.V., Koenig, R.J., Arscott, P. *et al.* (1993) Tissue specificity and serologic reactivity of an autoantigen associated with autoimmune thyroid disease. *Journal of Clinical Endocrinology and Metabolism* 77, 433–438.

Salvi, M., Zhang, Z.-G., Haegert, D., Woo, M., Liberman, A. & Cadarso, L. (1990) Patients with endocrine ophthalmopathy not associated with overt thyroid disease have multiple thyroid immunologic abnormalities. *Journal of Clinical Endocrinology and Metabolism* 70, 89–94.

Sandford-Smith, J.H. (1969) Intermittent superior oblique tendon sheath syndrome. *British Journal of Ophthalmology* 53, 412–417.

Sandford-Smith, J.H. (1973) Superior oblique tendon sheath syndrome and its relationship to stenosing tenosynovitis. *British Journal of Ophthalmology* 57, 859–865.

Sevel, D. (1981) Brown's syndrome – a possible etiology explained embryologically. *Journal of Pediatric Ophthalmology and Strabismus* 18, 26–31.

Shine, B., Fells, P., Edwards, O.M. & Weetman, A.P. (1990) Association between Graves' ophthalmopathy and smoking. *Lancet* 335, 1261–1263.

Souza-Dias, C. (1992) Congenital VI nerve palsy is Duane's syndrome until disproven. *Binocular Vision Quarterly* 7, 70.

Spencer, A., Ansons, A., Mars, S. & Gray, C. (1996) Myopathic extraocular muscles in thyroid eye disease. A report of 3 cases. In: *Transactions of the 23rd Meeting of the European Strabismological Association, Nancy* (ed. M Spiritus), pp. 350–354. Aeolus Press, The Netherlands.

Stilling, J. (1887) *Untersuchungen uber die entstehung der kurtsichtigheit*. Bergmann, Wiesbaden.

Traboulsi, E.I., Jaafar, M.D., Kattan, H.M. & Parks, M.M. (1993) Congenital fibrosis of the extraocular muscles: Report of 24 cases illustrating the clinical spectrum and surgical management. *American Orthoptic Journal* 43, 45–53.

Tredici, T.D. & von Noorden, G.K. (1985) Are anisometropia and amblyopia common in Duane's syndrome. *Journal of Pediatric Ophthalmology and Strabismus* 22, 23–25.

Trimble, R.B. (1980) Diplopia as a presenting sign of neoplasia. *Transactions of the Ophthalmological Society of the United Kingdom* 100, 498–500.

Trimble, R.B. (1988) An alternative management of Brown's syndrome. In: *Transactions of the Seventeenth Meeting of the European Strabismological Association, Madrid* (ed. J. Murube), pp. 181–185.

Trimble, R.B., Kelly, V. & Mitchell, M. (1984) Acquired Brown's syndrome. In: *Transactions of the Fifth International Orthoptic Congress, Cannes* (eds A.P. Ravault & M. Lenk), pp. 267–272. LIPS, Lyon.

Trobe, J.D. (1984) Cyclodeviation in acquired vertical strabismus. *Archives of Ophthalmology* **102**, 717–720.

Türk, S. (1896) Ueber Retractionsbewegungen der Augen. *Deutsche Medicinische Wochenschrift* **22**, 199–201.

Waddell, E. (1982) Brown's syndrome revisited. *British Orthoptic Journal* **39**, 17–21.

Waddell, E., Fells, P. & Koornneef, L. (1982) The natural and unnatural history of a blow-out fracture. *British Orthoptic Journal* **39**, 29–32.

Whitehouse, R.W., Batterbury, M., Jackson, A. & Noble, J.L. (1994) Prediction of enophthalmos by computed tomography after 'blow-out' orbital fracture. *British Journal of Ophthalmology* **78**, 618–620.

Wojno, T.H. (1987) The incidence of extraocular muscle and cranial nerve palsy in orbital floor blow-out fractures. *Ophthalmology* **94**, 682–685.

Wright, K.W. (1991) Superior oblique silicone expander for Brown's syndrome and superior oblique overaction. *Journal of Ophthalmology and Strabismus* **28**, 101–107.

22

Supranuclear and Internuclear Disorders

Classification

The ocular motor system functions to maintain bifoveal viewing in a variety of situations. There are four basic types of eye movement, each with its own higher centre control system. Fast conjugate refixation movements are generated by the saccadic system, steady viewing and smooth tracking by the pursuit and optokinetic systems, with the vergence system maintaining alignment for objects moving towards or away from the observer. The vestibular ocular system removes the potentially destabilizing effects of head movement by producing eye movements which are equal and opposite to the head movement, providing a stable setting for the other eye movement systems to operate.

Isolated supranuclear motility disorders result in palsies of conjugate movement affecting one or more of the movement systems (so-called 'gaze palsies'). Diplopia is absent as parallelism of the visual axes is maintained.

The lesion responsible for a supranuclear motility disorder is rarely isolated and may affect nuclear and infranuclear structures responsible for eye movement, resulting in mixed disorders of ocular motility in which diplopia may be a symptom.

Anatomical pathways

Horizontal and vertical conjugate eye movements are processed by the brain at two different levels:

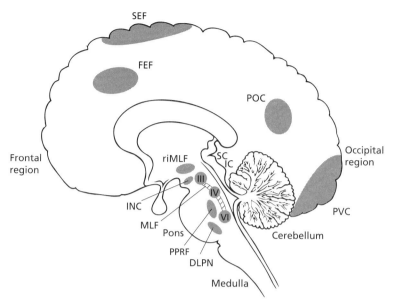

Fig. 22.1 Structures involved in eye movement control. Higher centre control areas for both saccadic and pursuit eye movements include the primary visual cortex (PVC), frontal eye fields (FEF), parieto-occipital cortex (POC) and the cerebellum. The supplementary eye fields (SEF) and the superior colliculus (SC) are specific for saccades. Lower centre control areas include the pontine paramedian reticular formation (PPRF) for horizontal and the rostral interstitial nucleus of the medial longitudinal fasciculus (riMLF) and interstitial nucleus of Cajal (INC) for vertical saccadic eye movements. The dorsolateral pontine nuclei (DLPN) are thought to be involved in pursuit eye movements. III = third nerve nucleus; IV = fourth nerve nucleus; VI = sixth nerve nucleus; MLF = medial longitudinal fasciculus; IC = inferior colliculus.

• The higher centre control areas are involved in the calculation of the amount and type of eye movement in response to a desired change in eye position. Structures involved with saccadic movement are the frontal eye fields, supplementary eye fields, parieto-occipital cortex, superior colliculus and cerebellum. Structures involved with pursuit are the parieto-occipital cortex, frontal eye fields and the cerebellum.

• The lower centre control areas are involved in generating the eye movement signal to the ocular motor neurones. These are the gaze centres and neural integrators in the brainstem. The resulting gaze movement may be a saccade or a smooth pursuit movement (Fig. 22.1).

The higher centre control areas are specific for pursuit and saccadic eye movements and are discussed in their respective sections. The lower centre control area for saccadic movement is discussed below.

Lower centre saccadic control areas

Horizontal gaze centres

These are anatomically ill-defined areas within the pontine paramedian reticular formation (PPRF) on each side of the mid-line at the level of the sixth nerve nuclei. Each centre controls horizontal saccadic movement to the ipsilateral side.

The horizontal gaze centre consists of a collection of neurones responsible for saccadic signal generation. Two important groups are the burst and pause neurones.

• Burst neurones are either short-lead excitatory burst neurones which generate the pulse of neural activity that corresponds to the peak velocity and amplitude of the saccade, or long-lead excitatory burst neurones which show an activity before the onset of the saccade and are believed to be involved in synchronizing the generation of the saccadic pulse.

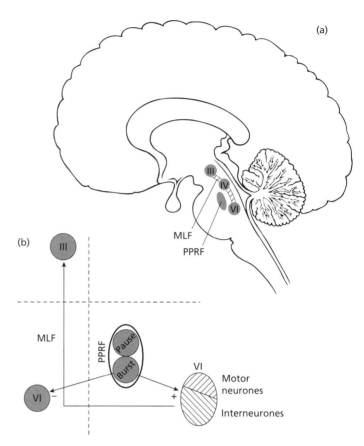

Fig. 22.2 (a,b) Lower centre horizontal saccadic eye movement control areas. Pause cells in the pontine paramedian reticular formation (PPRF) switch off prior to the generation of a horizontal saccade resulting in burst cell activity stimulating the ipsilateral and inhibiting the contralateral sixth nerve nuclei (VI). Sixth nerve motor neurones project to the ipsilateral lateral rectus, and interneurones to the contralateral medial rectus via the medial longitudinal fasciculus (MLF).

• Pause neurones show constant neural activity except just prior to and during a saccade; they are believed to inhibit the burst neurones and prevent unwanted saccadic eye movements being generated.

Fibres from the gaze centre pass to the ipsilateral sixth nerve nucleus. The nucleus contains two different groups of neurones.

• The sixth nerve motor neurones: the axons pass to the ipsilateral lateral rectus muscle and are the axons of the sixth cranial nerve.

• The sixth nerve interneurones: the axons project to the medial rectus subnucleus of the contralateral third nerve via the medial longitudinal fasciculus (MLF) (Fig. 22.2).

A signal is sent from the horizontal gaze centre to the contralateral sixth nerve nucleus that reciprocally inhibits the antagonist muscles. Higher centre input to

the abducens nucleus comes from the saccadic system, pursuit system and the vestibular-optokinetic system to bring about horizontal gaze.

Vertical gaze centres

The centres responsible for the control of vertical conjugate gaze lie in the upper midbrain, and include the rostral interstitial nucleus of the medial longitudinal fasciculus and other neurones in the region of the anterior and posterior commissures. Pathways located in the dorsal and caudal midbrain in the region of the posterior commissure are important in up-gaze. The rostral and ventral region of the midbrain contains the main lower centre control area for vertical eye movement, the rostral interstitial nucleus of the MLF. The uppermost part of this nucleus may be preferentially involved in the generation of signals responsible for down-gaze.

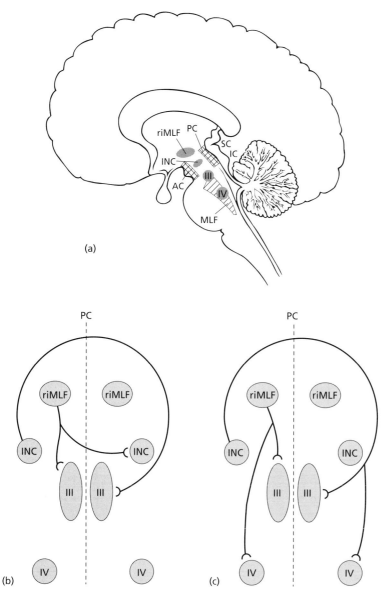

(a)

(b)

(c)

Fig. 22.3 (a–c) Lower centre vertical saccadic eye movement control areas. Structures in the midbrain responsible for vertical gaze include the rostral interstitial nucleus of the medial longitudinal fasciculus (riMLF) and interstitial nucleus of Cajal (INC). Burst neurones in the riMLF send axons to the third nerve nucleus (III) for up-gaze (a), and the third and fourth nerve nuclei (IV) for down-gaze (b). The INC is the vertical neural integrator providing gaze-holding signals which project via the posterior commissure (PC). AC = anterior commissure; MLF = medial longitudinal fasciculus; SC = superior colliculus; IC = inferior colliculus.

The lower centre control areas are supplied bilaterally by the upper centre control areas and act together (Fig. 22.3).

Neural integrators

The brainstem centre responsible for coding eye position is the neural integrator. Eye position signals are coded for saccadic, pursuit and vestibular eye movements. The neural integrator responsible for horizontal gaze involves the cerebellum, the perihypoglossal nuclei in the brainstem and the medial vestibular nucleus. The vertical integration of eye movement probably involves input from the interstitial nucleus of Cajal. For further details see Chapter 23.

Types of gaze movement

Saccadic eye movements

Anatomical pathway

The higher centre control command for voluntary horizontal saccades arises in the frontal eye fields (Brodmann area 8); it then descends via the anterior limb of the internal capsule to the superior colliculus and then on to the brainstem reticular formation in the pons. The pathway decussates at the ponto-mesencephalic junction, hence stimulation of the frontal eye fields results in contralaterally directed saccades. Vertical saccades are generated by signals arising from both frontal eye fields, with the pathway connecting with lower centre control areas in the midbrain (Fig. 22.3). During the saccade visual perception is suspended, therefore the individual is not conscious of the rapid movement of the visual field.

Features

The saccadic system generates the signals for fast conjugate eye movements responsible for voluntary or involuntary movements towards visual, auditory and tactile stimuli. Saccades make up the fast components of optokinetic nystagmus and jerk nystagmus, and random eye movements during sleep.

The saccadic latency is the interval from the appearance of the stimulus to the start of the movement. The interval represents the time it takes the ocular motor system to process the signal before its arrival at the extraocular muscles, and is normally 200 ms. The saccadic eye movement consists of an accelerating phase, with the peak velocity occurring a third of the way into the movement. The amplitude of the saccade has a close relationship with the peak saccadic velocity, with large-amplitude saccades associated with high velocities (Bahill *et al.* 1975). Peak velocities range from 60° s⁻¹ to 600° s⁻¹ for movements of 1–30° in amplitude.

Sequence of events in the generation of a saccade (Figs 22.2 & 22.3)

The sequence of events that takes place in the generation of a voluntary saccade is as follows.

1 The pause cells in the brainstem gaze centres receive an inhibitory stimulus from higher centre con-

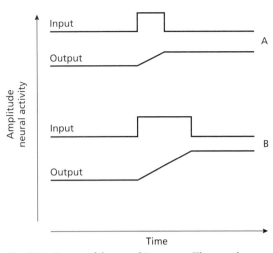

Fig. 22.4 Output of the neural integrator. The neural integrator mathematically processes the pulse signal. In example A the integration of the small input pulse produces a small step increase in output. In example B a large pulse signal, corresponding to a larger velocity and amplitude movement, generates an appropriately large step output.

trol areas such as the frontal eye fields and superior colliculus, indicating that a saccade is planned.

2 The inhibited pause cells allow the burst neurones to generate a burst of neural activity which corresponds to the pulse component of the pulse-step neural signal of the saccade.

3 The pulse signal generated by the burst neurones goes to the ocular motor neurones and is responsible for the rapid acceleration of the eye movement during the saccade. The pulse signal is also directed to the neural integrator, which is located in the cerebellum and the brainstem for horizontal saccades and in the interstitial nucleus of Cajal in the midbrain for vertical saccades.

4 The neural integrator mathematically processes the pulse signal into an eye-position coded output which corresponds to the step signal (Fig. 22.4). The step signal is fed back into the brainstem gaze centre and then on to the ocular motor nerve, and is responsible for maintaining the eye in the new position of gaze.

Inaccurate saccades and corrective movements

A saccade may not always result in the eyes arriving at the desired gaze position. This may be the result of an

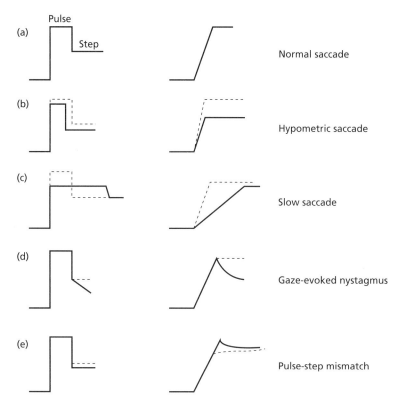

Fig. 22.5 Types of saccadic eye movement inaccuracies. (a) Normal saccade resulting from an appropriately matched pulse and step signal. (b) Hypometric saccade resulting from a deficient pulse-step signal. (c) Slow saccade resulting from a deficient pulse height but normal amplitude with an appropriate pulse–step match. (d) Gaze-evoked nystagmus resulting from a pulse–step mismatch of a normal pulse and a deficient step. (e) Pulse–step mismatch from an excessive pulse and normal step resulting in overshooting the target and a slow drift (glissade) of the eye back to the target.

excessive or deficient pulse-step signal or a mismatch between the pulse and the step components (Fig. 22.5). The cause of the inaccurate saccade may reside in the higher centre control area, the brainstem gaze centre or the neural integrator.

Inaccurate saccades may arise from:
• A deficient pulse-step signal resulting in a hypometric saccade and an undershooting of the target (Fig. 22.5b). A second saccade in the same direction as the first may be generated to allow the eye to reach the target.
• An excessive pulse-step signal resulting in a hypermetric saccade and an overshooting of the target. A second saccade in the reverse direction may be generated to reach the target.
• A deficient pulse height with a normal amplitude and pulse–step match results in a slow saccade (Fig. 22.5c).
• A pulse–step mismatch resulting in a normal pulse and a deficient step (gaze-evoked nystagmus) (Fig. 22.5d). In this situation, the eye reaches the target but

there is a slow drift of the eye back towards the primary position because of the deficient step command.
• A pulse–step mismatch resulting in an excessive or deficient pulse and a normal step leading to either an overshoot or an undershoot of the target, followed by a slow drift of the eye back to the target (glissade) (Fig. 22.5e).

Pursuit eye movements

Anatomical pathway

The higher control areas for pursuit movement lie in the parieto-occipital cortex, with fibres descending to the brainstem for the generation of horizontal pursuit commands; commands also arise from the frontal eye fields (Fig. 22.6a). This descending pathway probably undergoes a double decussation which results in the right cortex generating signals for ipsilateral pursuit movement. The lower centre control area in the brainstem that is responsible for pursuit movement probably involves the dorsolateral pontine nuclei: the

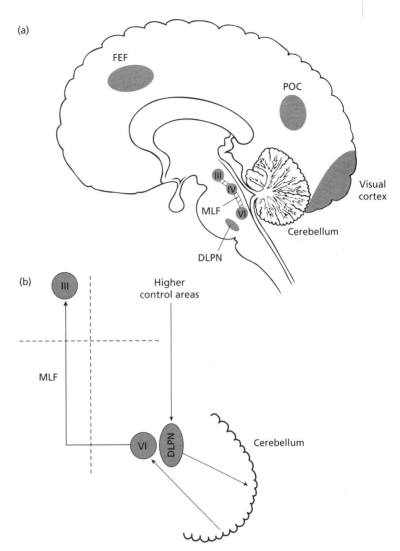

Fig. 22.6 Control areas for pursuit eye movements. (a) Higher centre control of pursuit eye movements involves the visual cortex, parieto-occipital cortex (POC) and the frontal eye fields (FEF). These areas project ipsilaterally to the dorsolateral pontine nuclei (DLPN), which relay in the cerebellum before projecting to the sixth nerve nucleus for horizontal eye movement (VI) (b) and the fourth (IV) and third (III) nerve nuclei in the midbrain for vertical eye movement. MLF = medial longitudinal fasciculus.

projections of these nuclei are poorly understood but are believed not to pass through the PPRF before synapsing at the sixth nerve nucleus for horizontal pursuit. The cerebellum is closely associated with normal pursuit movements, signals being generated during pursuit with the head still and during combined eye-head tracking (cancellation of the vestibular ocular reflex, VOR) (Fig. 22.6a,b).

Features
The pursuit system maintains stable eye tracking or combined eye-head tracking of slowly moving objects.

It counteracts slow movements of the target which may destabilize the retinal image. The normal stimulus for pursuit movements is image movement (retinal slip) in the parafoveal region. Like saccades, pursuit movements have a latency following the stimulus of the order of 100 ms. For target velocities up to 40–50° s^{-1} most eyes are able to track the object accurately, with an eye velocity which is equal to the target velocity (gain = 1). For higher target velocities the eye has increasing difficulties in matching target velocity (gain < 1), either initiating a catch-up saccade or lagging behind the target. Pursuit movements are influenced by the nature of the stimulus, how it is behaving, the attention of the subject and by certain drugs. Combined eye-head tracking of objects requires the normal VOR associated with head movement (eye movement equal and opposite to the head movement) to be suppressed before stable object tracking can take place. This property of the pursuit system to cancel the VOR can be tested clinically, and provides a sensitive measure of the performance of the pursuit system.

Vergence eye movements

Anatomical pathway

The higher control areas responsible for vergence movement are poorly understood. Striate cortex neurones responding to retinal image disparity have been identified in monkeys. Premotor signals are thought to originate in the mesencephalic reticular formation, with separate populations of cells for convergence and divergence. Three subnuclei (a, b and c) have been identified at the level of the medial rectus nucleus, with subnucleus c thought to be involved principally with vergence movements.

Features

The vergence system functions to maintain binocular alignment, permitting stereopsis and avoiding diplopia. It provides the commands for disjugate eye movements. There are two main types of vergence stimuli: retinal blur, which is associated with accommodative vergence, and retinal image disparity, which is associated with fusional vergence. In this respect the vergence system functions differently from the saccadic and pursuit systems which generate conjugate eye movements.

Pure vergence movements have a maximum velocity of approximately $20°$ s^{-1}; however, vergence movements are more often associated with conjugate eye movements, in which case the velocity of the vergence component is increased. The dynamic properties of vergence movements, particularly the relationship between peak vergence velocity and vergence amplitude, are more variable than saccades; they are influenced by the type of stimulus, its size and the conditions of viewing. Convergence is normally associated with accommodation and pupillary miosis, the near triad.

The vestibular ocular reflex and optokinetic system

Anatomical pathway

The vestibular system has two components: peripheral (located in the middle ear) and central (the eighth cranial nerve and the brainstem nuclei in the medulla). The peripheral vestibular apparatus consists of the three semicircular canals and the otolith organs, the saccule and utricle. Each semicircular canal connects centrally by way of a three-neurone arc to a pair of extraocular muscles. The otoliths connect centrally only to the cyclovertical muscles. The vestibular nuclei also play a key role in coding information for gaze-holding and have important connections to the cerebellum.

Features

Both the vestibular and optokinetic systems operate to maintain a stable retinal image during head movement. The head movements may result from the transmitted cardiac pulse, locomotion, or the larger movements associated with whole body rotation. A variety of sensory signals originating from the labyrinthine semicircular canals, otoliths, visual system and peripheral receptors contribute to the generation of compensatory eye movements which serve to counteract the effect of head movement. The semicircular canals respond only to angular acceleration. Translatory head movements (up and down) and static head tilts stimulate the otoliths by virtue of their sensitivity to linear acceleration.

The function of the vestibular and optokinetic systems can be best understood by considering the events taking place during a period of whole body rotation that may occur during a dance routine. As the dancer starts to rotate, the semicircular canals are stimulated. There is a latency of 16 ms before compensatory eye movements are generated; these consist of a slow-phase movement which is opposite to the direction of rotation, and a nystagmus fast phase in the direction of the rotation. When the dancer reaches a constant rotational velocity the signal generated by the semicircular canals declines, the eyes can no longer match the target motion and the retinal image slips across the retina. This retinal slip is the stimulus to the opto-kinetic and pursuit systems, which take over the generation of the compensatory slow eye movement. In humans the otoliths generate counter-rolling of the eyes in response to static head tilt, which compensates for only 10% of the tilt. However, in animals with laterally placed eyes, head tilt stimulates the otoliths principally to generate vertical disjugate eye movement, akin to a skew deviation. It can be seen that in humans the VOR plays a far greater role than the otoliths in generating compensatory eye movements.

Clinical assessment of conjugate gaze movement

A detailed description of the clinical assessment of conjugate gaze movements can be found in Chapter 6.

Supranuclear gaze palsies

The structures involved in horizontal and vertical gaze movements are shown in Fig. 22.1.

Horizontal gaze palsies

Frontal eye field lesions
Unilateral saccadic palsy
AETIOLOGY
The commonest cause is a vascular accident affecting the frontal lobe. Slow-growing frontal lobe tumours cause saccadic paralysis.

FEATURES
Acute pathology affecting the premotor cortex of one cerebral hemisphere may sometimes cause an initial irritative lesion, with tonic deviation of the eyes to the opposite side. This is rapidly followed by the more common signs of failure of function of the damaged premotor cortex, resulting in loss of the ability to generate saccades to the opposite side. In severe cases, particularly if the patient has a reduced level of consciousness, there will be a tonic deviation with gaze directed towards the side of the lesion. This abnormality has been described in the more conscious patient, when there is deviation of Bell's phenomenon towards the side of the lesion on attempted eye closure rather than the usual upward eye movement.

The reduced ability to generate saccades in the direction away from the affected frontal cortex is paralleled by the loss of the fast phase of optokinetic nystagmus. Provided the lesion is isolated and the patient's level of consciousness is satisfactory, smooth pursuit movement can be demonstrated to either side.

VOR stimulation by the doll's head manoeuvre or by caloric testing should show that the horizontal gaze centres in the brainstem remain intact, and results in a full range of movement.

Provided that the lesion is limited to the one frontal cortex, most patients improve with time and are able to make saccades to the opposite side. Saccades may have an increased latency and reduced accuracy, but should regain a normal maximum peak velocity, whereas lesions affecting the PPRF and below slow the velocity. A common finding in affected patients is difficulty in maintaining eccentric gaze away from the affected frontal cortex and the eyes tend to drift back to the mid-line. This induces repeated small corrective saccades in an attempt to maintain the eccentric gaze position (gaze paretic nystagmus).

The relatively transient loss of saccadic function that occurs with isolated frontal cortex lesions may be due to the presence of other systems for saccade generation. When these are also affected, a much more profound and long-lasting saccadic paralysis occurs, for example a combined frontal lobe and superior colliculus lesion. These combined lesions are the result of experimental study and give insight into the nature of eye movement control, but are unlikely to occur in clinical practice.

Posterior hemisphere lesions
Palsy of smooth pursuit
AETIOLOGY
Extensive parieto-occipital lobe damage secondary to vascular accident or tumour is the most likely cortical cause of interruption of smooth pursuit.

FEATURES
An isolated loss of smooth pursuit movement, comparable with a saccadic paralysis, is very rare. When the pursuit system is defective, the patient is able to track a moving target by using a series of small-amplitude saccades in place of the pursuit movement. This is termed saccadic or 'cog wheel' pursuit. Surprisingly, the pursuit system may be normal in pure occipital cortex damage, but is more likely to be impaired if the

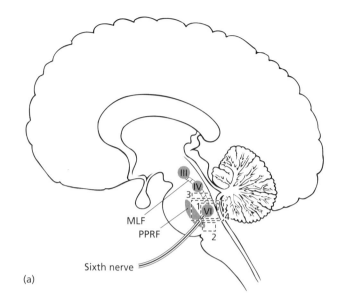

(a)

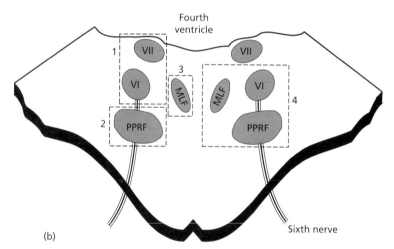

(b)

Fig. 22.7 (a,b) Eye movement control structures involved in pontine lesions. A horizontal gaze palsy can result from (1) a lesion involving the sixth nerve nucleus (VI) or (2) a lesion of the pontine paramedian reticular formation (PPRF). (3) Internuclear ophthalmoplegia results from a lesion of the medial longitudinal fasciculus (MLF). (4) A combination of a PPRF and MLF lesion results in a one-and-a-half syndrome. VII = seventh nerve nucleus.

parietal cortex is also affected. The optokinetic response is similarly impaired when the stripes are rotated in the direction of the lesion, but should be normal when the direction of drum rotation is reversed.

Parieto-occipital lesions cause a contralateral homonymous hemianopia in addition to their motor effects.

Pontine lesion (Fig. 22.7)

Disease processes affecting the pons result in characteristic disturbances of ocular motility through damage to the lower centre eye movement control areas. The two main disorders are:

• unilateral gaze palsy from a lesion involving the PPRF or the sixth nerve nucleus;

• a one-and-a-half syndrome from a lesion involving the PPRF and ipsilateral MLF.

The features of the one-and-a-half syndrome are discussed later.

The proximity of adjacent structures, which are often simultaneously affected, will modify the clinical picture; for example, involvement of the vestibular nuclei may produce a gaze-evoked nystagmus and a deficiency of the VOR.

Unilateral gaze palsy (Fig. 22.7)

AETIOLOGY

A single lesion likely to cause a complete unilateral gaze palsy is most probably located in the pons at the level of the sixth nerve nucleus. The causes include demyelinating disease, vascular occlusions and occasionally tumours. Although intrinsic disease of the brainstem is most likely, compression from an external tumour can also occur.

FEATURES

• Damage to the sixth nerve nucleus and to adjacent structures in the PPRF is always paretic and never irritative. An acute lesion may result in conjugate deviation of the eyes to the opposite side; however, unlike a higher centre lesion, the effect may be longlasting and saccadic velocity remains slow.
• Eye movements are affected on ipsilateral gaze but unaffected on contralateral gaze.
• If damage is mild the gaze palsy may be restricted to slow ipsilateral saccades and a minor degree of limitation of ocular movement with sparing of the pursuit movement. Stimulation of the VOR will demonstrate a full range of eye movement.
• Severe damage leads to a complete palsy of ipsilateral horizontal gaze (both pursuit and saccadic). Large lesions leading to a deficiency of the VOR and the neural integrator with gaze-evoked nystagmus often affect the vestibular nuclei.

A PPRF and sixth nerve nucleus lesion result in a similar deficiency of ipsilateral gaze. The two can be differentiated from each other in that lesions affecting the sixth nerve always affect the VOR and frequently cause a lower motor neurone facial palsy from involvement of the ipsilateral facial nerve. Another important differentiating feature is the nature of saccades generated towards the affected side in the intact field of gaze. In a sixth nerve nucleus lesion these are normal, whereas in PPRF lesions failure to inhibit the contralateral sixth nerve nucleus leads to saccades of small amplitude and low velocity.

Convergence is spared in both sixth nerve nucleus and PPRF lesions.

Ocular motor apraxia

Ocular motor apraxia is a form of saccadic paralysis that can be congenital or acquired.

The congenital form was first documented by Cogan (1952, 1966) and is often referred to as Cogan's ocular motor apraxia. The patient usually presents in infancy because the parents have noticed an apparent lack of visual attention and are concerned that the child may not see. The head thrusts and repetitive blinking that characterize this disorder occur when the child develops head control in the first few months of life. There is an inability to execute voluntary saccades; some patients can generate random saccadic eye movement and the quick phases of the VOR and caloric nystagmus may be intact. Vertical saccades and horizontal and vertical pursuit movements are unaffected. The head thrust is a manoeuvre to change fixation to a new gaze position. The child rapidly turns his head in the desired direction of gaze, usually overshooting the target. Eye movement follows the head movement until the target is fixated on the fovea. Once foveal fixation is achieved, the head is slowly turned back to the mid-line, but the eyes remain fixated on the eccentric target through the activity of the VOR, which prevents the eyes following the return head movement. The rapid blink pattern commonly seen may be a technique to break the fixation at the start of the head thrust manoeuvre. Head thrusting usually reduces as the child matures and learns other ways of overcoming the disability.

Acquired forms of ocular motor apraxia may occur in Huntington's disease, multiple sclerosis and Wilson's disease. The presence of other neurological signs and the involvement of vertical saccadic and pursuit movement can differentiate acquired from congenital forms.

Other congenital gaze palsies

Transient disturbances of supranuclear gaze have been described in healthy neonates (Hoyt *et al.* 1980). Tonic deviation of down-gaze and skew deviation may occur.

Severe disorders of gaze movement are seen in some children with cerebral palsy due to various types of brain damage. These children often show multiple handicaps, including intellectual impairment and generalized motor disabilities. There may be concern that the vision is impaired, as the child does not follow objects. This apparent lack of visual attention may be due simply to the motor difficulties and acuity may be normal. Head thrusting is not usually seen. A head posture, usually a face turn, may be adopted by some children with a unilateral gaze palsy. Some children show improvement of motor function as they grow older. Gaze disorders may also be associated with a variety of types of paralytic or concomitant strabismus.

Vertical gaze palsies

As vertical eye movements are under bilateral upper centre control, vertical gaze palsies due to isolated cerebral lesions do not occur. Lower centre control areas in the midbrain responsible for up-gaze and down-gaze exist. Down-gaze deficits arise from bilateral lower centre lesions; however, up-gaze deficits can arise from a unilateral lesion affecting the fibres and nuclei in the posterior commissure (Fig. 22.3).

Isolated supranuclear vertical gaze palsies are characterized by preservation of vestibular movement. Bell's phenomenon, the VOR and caloric nystagmus will generate eye movements into the affected direction of gaze. Large lesions and progressive disease often also affect the adjacent ocular motor nuclei and infranuclear pathways, leading to loss of vestibular movement.

Dorsal midbrain syndrome (Parinaud's syndrome)
AETIOLOGY
Progressive involvement of the region of the dorsal midbrain is usually due to tumours of the pineal gland (pinealoma); nonprogressive lesions are the result of dorsal midbrain vascular accidents or trauma.

FEATURES
The features are:
• A gaze disorder: the initial sign is a loss of upward saccadic movement in the presence of normal vertical pursuit. If the stripes of an OKN (optokinetic nystagmus) drum are slowly rotated downwards, the absence of a refixating upward movement can be clearly seen. Upward rotation of the drum results in a normal optokinetic nystagmus response due to the preservation of upward pursuit movement. When the

cause is a progressive lesion, loss of upward saccades is followed first by loss of upward pursuit and then by loss of saccadic and pursuit movement in down-gaze.
• Convergence retraction 'nystagmus': a characteristic feature of Parinaud's syndrome is rhythmical convergence of the visual axes and associated retraction of the globes on attempted up-gaze. This is also best demonstrated by testing optokinetic nystagmus, rotating the stripes downwards.
• Pathological upper eyelid retraction (Collier's sign): upper eyelid retraction is usually associated with lid-lag and is best seen on down-gaze. One or both eyes can be affected.
• Pupil abnormalities: the pupils are usually dilated and show a reduction in response to direct and consensual light stimulation. However, pupil constriction is normal on accommodation. This disparity in pupil reaction is known as light/near dissociation.
• Papilloedema: when the cause of Parinaud's syndrome is a space-occupying lesion, usually a pinealoma, there is eventually a rise in intracranial pressure followed by papilloedema. However, this is a late sign.

Progressive supranuclear palsy (Steele–Richardson syndrome)
This disease is due to degeneration of the brainstem reticular formation and may present in the early stages with impairment of vertical saccades. Initially there is a slowing of the vertical saccadic velocity, usually first affecting down-gaze, which is followed in due course by a complete vertical saccadic paralysis. Disorders of horizontal gaze are a late feature; eventually some patients may go on to a complete ophthalmoplegia. Difficulty in voluntarily opening the eyelids may be present (apraxia of lid opening). Other associated neurological signs include axial rigidity and difficulty with speech, swallowing and balance. Patients complain of difficulty in seeing the food on the plate or in walking downstairs. Symptoms are due to the combination of the vertical gaze palsy and axial rigidity limiting neck movement. Progressive dementia develops with death usually occurring 10 years after the clinical onset of the disease.

Parkinson's disease
This is may be associated with impaired up-gaze, but down-gaze is usually unaffected. Saccades may be

hypometric but are of normal velocity. Convergence insufficiency may occur. Paradoxically, prolonged tonic elevation of the eyes (oculogyric crisis) has been described in postencephalitic Parkinsonism.

Tonic downward gaze lesions

The eyes may show a chronic downward deviation associated with a failure of up-gaze in patients with recent bilateral thalamic infarcts. This type of deviation is more commonly seen in children with unrelieved hydrocephalus, when there is often associated upper eyelid retraction (setting-sun sign).

Investigation of supranuclear disorders

As with any paralytic disorder of eye movement, all patients should have a full medical history taken and undergo a full medical examination in addition to the usual ophthalmic and orthoptic assessment.

Particularly relevant tests include:
- qualitative and, if possible, quantitative assessment of saccadic and pursuit movements;
- examination of the VOR and assessment of integrated head and eye movements;
- demonstration of Bell's phenomenon;
- measurement of convergence and accommodation amplitude;
- optokinetic nystagmus to accentuate convergence retraction nystagmus in the dorsal midbrain syndrome and pursuit deficits in patients with parietal lobe lesions;
- qualitative and, if possible, quantitative assessment of nystagmus if present (see Chapter 23 for further details);
- pupil size;
- visual fields.

For further details on the assessment of ocular movements, see Chapter 6.

Internuclear ophthalmoplegia (INO)

Description

Internuclear ophthalmoplegia is a lesion of the medial longitudinal fasciculus resulting in a palsy of the medial rectus muscle and a dissociated gaze-evoked nystagmus, greatest in the abducting eye.

Anatomical pathway

The sixth nerve nucleus acts as the final common pathway for horizontal gaze. Axons from the interneurones, representing the saccadic, pursuit and vestibular-optokinetic systems, travel in the MLF and cross the mid-line to synapse with the contralateral third nerve subnucleus supplying the medial rectus muscle. These are the axons affected in INO (Figs 22.2, 22.6 & 22.7).

Types

The type of INO depends on the precise location of the lesion in the MLF. INO can be unilateral or bilateral, and high or low.

Unilateral

Unilateral lesions appear to affect the interneurones from only one sixth nerve nucleus, resulting in impairment or loss of adduction of the affected medial rectus on attempted conjugate gaze. The saccadic, pursuit and vestibulo-ocular systems are all affected. Milder cases, or those that have partially recovered, may simply show a reduction in the peak saccadic velocity of the affected medial rectus. Limitation of adduction is nearly always associated with abducting nystagmus of the other eye.

If the lesion is discrete and does not affect the medial rectus subnucleus itself or the descending tracts controlling convergence, then the muscle will contract on attempting convergence. Medial rectus contraction in response to a convergence stimulus, but apparent paralysis in response to a conjugate gaze stimulus, is a unique feature of unilateral and bilateral INO and is due to a lesion affecting the lower part of the MLF. If medial rectus contractions in response to both convergence and conjugate gaze are equally affected, the lesion is in the upper part of the MLF close to the third nerve nucleus.

A skew deviation may be seen in unilateral INO, and the hypertropic eye is usually on the same side as the INO.

Bilateral

Lesions that affect the interneurones running in the MLF from both sixth nerve nuclei result in bilateral

INO, with loss of adduction of each eye on attempted contralateral version. Abducting nystagmus is present in each eye on lateral gaze. Provided the lesion is limited to the interneurones, convergence is retained. Bilateral INO is often asymmetric.

Aetiology

The commonest cause of unilateral and often bilateral INO in the younger patient is multiple sclerosis. The ophthalmoplegia may be the presenting feature of the disease. The development of other signs of multiple sclerosis may confirm the diagnosis. However, it is not possible to predict the frequency of severity of subsequent signs and symptoms and great care must be taken in advising patients suspected of having this disorder. Internuclear ophthalmoplegia in the older patient may be due to small blood vessel occlusion; it is usually unilateral owing to the strict mid-line separation of the blood supply to the two halves of the brain stem.

Tumours, intrinsic or metastatic, rarely cause a purely unilateral INO, due to the proximity of the structures relaying in the MLF. Bilateral lesions may be caused by tumour, although the commonest causes are multiple sclerosis and basilar artery branch occlusions.

Features

The principal feature is abducting nystagmus. The reason for this characteristic nystagmus of the abducting eye, which occurs in both unilateral and bilateral INO, is not clear.

Several theories have been suggested, and these are outlined below.

1 An adaptive change to the medial rectus weakness: when the affected eye is used for fixation, innervation to the weak medial rectus results in an undershoot followed by a slow drift towards the target. Central adaptive changes lead to increased innervation to the medial rectus to compensate for the weakness; this results in excessive innervation to the abducting eye, which initially overshoots then slowly drifts back to the target. This pulse–step mismatch results in the dissociated nystagmus. If the affected eye is occluded for a period of a few days then the dissociated nystagmus is abolished, supporting this theory.

2 An increase in the convergence tone: failure of the ipsilateral medial rectus to contract on conjugate gaze leads to inappropriate co-contraction of both medial rectus muscles from an increased convergence tone. Convergence causes the abducting eye to adduct and move off the target; this is followed by a corrective abducting saccade to regain its position. The cycle continues, resulting in the abducting nystagmus (Stroud *et al.* 1974).

3 Interruption of descending pathways: fibres from the contralateral third nerve nucleus to the sixth nerve nucleus descend via the MLF and possibly represent a feedback circuit.

4 A form of gaze-evoked nystagmus: involvement of the neural integrator may result in a dissociated gaze-evoked nystagmus, more apparent in the abducting eye.

5 Preservation of convergence: the older concepts of posterior INO, in which convergence is lost, and anterior INO, in which convergence is retained, are difficult to understand and it is preferable to consider rostral (upper) and caudal (lower) lesions. Rostral lesions are more likely to affect the descending tracts that initiate convergence or the subnucleus of the medial rectus itself, and will result in a loss of response of the affected medial rectus to both gaze and convergence stimuli. Discrete caudal lesions are more likely to spare the subnucleus of the medial rectus and the descending tracts that initiate convergence. Therefore, a convergence movement will be possible in the absence of adduction on contralateral gaze.

6 Preservation of the range of adduction in the presence of a reduced medial rectus saccadic velocity: demyelinating disease has a preferential effect on the high-velocity neural activity normally associated with the pulse signal of a saccade, and less effect on the low-frequency signals seen with pursuit movements.

A form of dissociated nystagmus identical to that seen in internuclear ophthalmoplegia has been reported following surgical paresis of the medial rectus muscle (von Noorden *et al.* 1984).

Diagnosis

Internuclear ophthalmoplegia should always be suspected whenever there is an acquired limitation of adduction.

• There is usually an exophoria or exotropia in the primary position. This will increase on attempted horizontal gaze in the direction of action of the affected medial rectus muscle in cases of unilateral INO.

• Saccadic movements are usually impaired to a greater extent than pursuit movements. Saccadic velocity slowing is a useful diagnostic feature and can differentiate truly unilateral INO from asymmetric bilateral INO. The measurement of saccadic velocity and of the accuracy of the saccades is one of the most useful methods of diagnosing and monitoring the patient's progress.

• Optokinetic nystagmus will be impaired, but the results are difficult to interpret.

A Hess chart can provide a useful record of the progress of the condition.

Differential diagnosis

Internuclear ophthalmoplegia must be differentiated from the following conditions:

• Myasthenia: this can mimic INO very closely. A dissociated nystagmus greatest in the abducting eye is seen in patients with myasthenic medial rectus weakness. Even experienced examiners have mistakenly diagnosed cases of myasthenia as INO. The differential diagnosis of myasthenia is aided by:
  1 variability of the signs;
  2 the presence of Cogan's lid-twitch sign;
  3 involvement of the vertically acting muscles;
  4 a positive response to intravenous edrophonium chloride (Tensilon).

• Orbital trauma: a blow-out fracture of the medial wall can result in a medial rectus underaction; a history of trauma and evidence of mechanical restriction of abduction help with the diagnosis.

• Duane's retraction syndrome: the restriction of abduction and the characteristic changes in the palpebral aperture on horizontal gaze help with the diagnosis.

• Infranuclear medial rectus palsy (partial third nerve palsy): isolated infranuclear medial rectus palsy is extremely rare. The loss of convergence and the absence of abducting nystagmus can differentiate it from an INO.

Management

The natural history depends on the cause; patients with INO due to multiple sclerosis are likely to recover adduction, often very rapidly. However, even when adduction appears full, abducting nystagmus may persist for a much longer period and may continue indefinitely in a few cases, providing evidence to future examiners of a past episode of INO. Those cases due to vascular causes are also likely to show spontaneous recovery. INO secondary to tumour will not recover; progression of the disorder and the development of other neurological signs should give warning of the diagnosis. No specific treatment can be given, except in those few cases due to tumour, when radiotherapy may help. When the cause is vascular disease, attention to any treatable cardiovascular disorder (e.g. hypertension) is advisable.

Diplopia can usually be compensated if necessary by a face turn. Some patients derive benefit from prisms.

One-and-a-half syndrome (paralytic pontine exotropia)

Description

One-and-a-half syndrome consists of a unilateral internuclear ophthalmoplegia and a contralateral horizontal gaze palsy.

Aetiology

An extensive caudal lesion in the pons can affect the horizontal gaze centre and the adjacent MLF, resulting in a palsy of both medial rectus muscles and one lateral rectus (i.e. gaze palsy plus INO) (Fig. 22.7). Causes include demyelination, vascular, tumour and inflammation.

Features

The main clinical and diagnostic features are as follows:

• The only remaining horizontal movement is abduction by the unaffected lateral rectus, which is associated with the typical abducting nystagmus.

- When the patient attempts to fixate with this eye in the primary position, the nystagmus will reduce or cease. There is therefore a palsy of conjugate gaze on one side and an INO on looking to the other side.
- A marked compensatory head posture may be adopted to achieve fixation with the preferred eye.

Although complete 'one-and-a-half' syndromes are rare, partial or incomplete syndromes are more common. They can be diagnosed on clinical assessment.

A Hess chart is useful in monitoring the condition. However, care must be taken in its interpretation, as synergist muscles are affected in patients with lesions involving the horizontal gaze centre as well as the MLF (partial one-and-a-half syndrome). Since the basis of the Hess chart is a comparison of action of synergistic muscles, the test is comparing abnormal with abnormal and, if viewed in isolation, the gaze palsy element may be missed.

Skew deviation

Description

Skew deviation is a vertical strabismus resulting from a disruption of input into the oculomotor and trochlear nuclei. Cyclotorsion is often a feature and other symptoms and signs of central nervous system disease are usually present.

Aetiology

Skew deviation arises from a peripheral or central imbalance of otolith inputs to the oculomotor and trochlear nuclei (Smith *et al.* 1964; Keane 1975).

Structures involved in the pathogenesis of skew deviation include:
- the middle ear and the vestibular nerve;
- the vestibular nuclei in the brainstem;
- the cerebellum;
- the medial longitudinal fasciculus;
- the interstitial nucleus of Cajal in the midbrain.

Features

The features of skew deviation are:
- A vertical strabismus, which can be transient or permanent. Transient deviations are common in unilateral internuclear ophthalmoplegia.

- A deviation, which may be concomitant or incomitant. Incomitant skew deviation must be differentiated from a cyclovertical muscle palsy, and typically resembles a unilateral or bilateral inferior rectus muscle or a unilateral superior rectus underaction.
- Incyclotorsion of the hypertropic eye. This is similar to one-half cycle of see-saw nystagmus and reflects the common occurrence of both disorders with lesions involving the interstitial nucleus of Cajal.
- Other signs of central nervous system disease, usually involving the brainstem and cerebellum.

The strabismus can be monitored using a Hess chart.

Treatment options for supranuclear and internuclear disorders

An isolated supranuclear gaze palsy is uncommon and does not cause diplopia but can result in symptoms because of the restriction of gaze. More common is a supranuclear combined with an internuclear, nuclear or infranuclear palsy in which diplopia is often the presenting symptom. Oscillopsia can result from acquired nystagmus.

Symptoms and corresponding treatments

Patients with supranuclear and internuclear disorders may present complaining of the following symptoms, and should be treated accordingly.

Head posture

The need to adopt an uncomfortable compensatory head posture is more common in vertical compared to horizontal gaze palsies. In the dorsal midbrain syndrome a chin-up head posture may be adopted to move the eyes away from the restricted field of up-gaze or to avoid diplopia or the discomfort associated with convergence retraction nystagmus.

Base-up deviating prisms can treat the chin-elevation. However, ambulatory patients rarely tolerate these. A recession of both inferior rectus muscles can improve the range of up-gaze and help correct the head posture (Buckley & Elston 1997). The use of adjustable sutures can reduce the risk of inducing a vertical deviation, and if large recessions are necessary the inferior rectus tendon should be transposed medially to lessen the incidence of an A-pattern exotropia on down-gaze. Chin-down head postures are a feature of progressive supranuclear gaze palsy, and base-down deviating prisms can help the patient when eating their food.

Diplopia

Double vision can be the result of a lesion affecting the internuclear or infranuclear pathways, the ocular motor nuclei or a skew deviation. The treatment of nuclear and infranuclear disorders is discussed in Chapter 19. Unilateral internuclear ophthalmoplegia rarely causes diplopia in the primary position but can result in symptoms on lateral gaze, and nasal sector occlusion to the spectacle lens of the affected eye can help relieve symptoms.

An exotropia can be associated with bilateral internuclear ophthalmoplegia and the one-and-a-half syndrome, prisms are rarely effective in relieving diplopia and a recession of the lateral recti and a resection of the medial rectus muscles can achieve a central field of binocular single vision.

Skew deviation can result in a concomitant or incomitant vertical deviation. Prisms are often effective in relieving diplopia when the deviation is concomitant. Incomitant skew deviation most often resembles a unilateral or bilateral inferior rectus palsy or a unilateral superior rectus palsy, and is managed in a similar way (see Chapter 19).

Oscillopsia

Image motion on lateral and vertical gaze can result from gaze-evoked, up-beat and down-beat nystagmus, and sector occlusion to spectacle lenses may reduce symptoms. Ocular palatal myoclonus and pendular horizontal nystagmus commonly result in troublesome oscillopsia in the primary position and may respond to medication, botulinum toxin or surgery (see Chapter 23).

Poor cosmesis

A cosmetic concern about the strabismus frequently accompanies other complaints of diplopia and an uncomfortable head posture (Buckley & Elston 1997). Care is needed to ensure that surgery to improve cosmesis does not cause diplopia or worsen it if it pre-exists.

References

Bahill, A.T., Clark, M.R. & Stark, L. (1975) The main sequence: a tool for studying human eye movements. *Mathematical Biosciences* **24**, 191–204.

Buckley, S.A. & Elston, J.S. (1997) Surgical treatment of supranuclear and internuclear ocular motility disorders. *Eye* **11**, 377–380.

Cogan, D.G. (1952) A type of congenital ocular motor apraxia presenting jerky head movements. *Transactions of the American Academy of Ophthalmology and Otolaryngology* **56**, 853–862.

Cogan, D.G. (1966) Congenital ocular motor apraxia. *Canadian Journal of Ophthalmology* **1**, 253–260.

Hoyt, C.S., Mousel, D.K. & Weber, A. (1980) Transient supranuclear disturbances of gaze in healthy neonates. *American Journal of Ophthalmology* **89**, 708–713.

Keane, J.R. (1975) Ocular skew deviation analysis of 100 cases. *Archives of Neurology* **32**, 185–190.

von Noorden, G.K., Tredici, T.D. & Ruttum, M. (1984) Pseudo-internuclear ophthalmoplegia after surgical paresis of the medial rectus muscle. *American Journal of Ophthalmology* **98**, 602–608.

Smith, J.L., David, N.J. & Kintworth, G. (1964) Skew deviation. *Neurology* **14**, 96–105.

Stroud, M.H., Newman, N.M., Keltner, J.L. & Gay, A.J. (1974) Abducting nystagmus in the medial longitudinal fasciculus (MLF) syndrome – internuclear ophthalmoplegia (INO). *Archives of Ophthalmology* **92**, 2–5.

23
Nystagmus and Related Oscillations

Nystagmus is a rhythmical oscillation of the eyes, or less commonly one eye. One component of the oscillation is a slow phase drift away from the assumed position of gaze; this component differentiates nystagmus from nystagmus-like oscillations which comprise only saccadic (fast) elements. Nystagmus can be physiological or pathological: pathological nystagmus is classified depending on whether children or adults are affected. A full classification is given in Table 23.1.

Pathological nystagmus

Description of waveform

Terms describing the waveform characteristics
(Figs 23.1 & 23.2)
TYPE OF WAVEFORM
• Jerk nystagmus. The waveform has two different components: a slow phase or drift away from fixa-

tion, which is the abnormal movement, and a fast corrective movement (saccade) in the opposite direction to regain fixation.
• Pendular nystagmus. The waveform is characterized by equal-velocity slow-phase movements in both directions, similar to the motion of a pendulum.

DIRECTION
Jerk nystagmus is conventionally described by the direction of the fast phase; i.e. if the fast phase is to the right then the nystagmus is described as right-beating. Both jerk and pendular nystagmus can be horizontal, vertical or torsional. In some cases two waveforms are simultaneously present and are superimposed on each other, resulting in other trajectories such as an oblique or elliptical waveform.

Nystagmus can be conjugate or disjugate: the direction of the nystagmus is the same in both eyes in conjugate nystagmus, and is opposite in each eye in disjugate nystagmus.

Table 23.1 Classification of nystagmus and related oscillations.

Pathological nystagmus	Gaze-dependent nystagmus
Childhood nystagmus	Gaze-evoked nystagmus
Congenital forms	Gaze-paretic nystagmus
Congenital nystagmus	Dissociated nystagmus
Sensory	Acquired pendular nystagmus
Idiopathic	Horizontal
Latent/manifest latent	Vertical
Congenital forms of adult nystagmus	Ocular-palatal myoclonus
Acquired forms	Nystagmus associated with monocular visual loss
Spasmus nutans	
Nystagmus associated with intracranial disease	*Physiological nystagmus*
Nystagmus associated with ipsilateral visual loss	Following vestibular stimulation
	Caloric
Adult nystagmus	Rotational
Acquired jerk nystagmus	Following optokinetic and pursuit stimulation
Primary positional	Gaze-dependent
Conjugate	End-point nystagmus
Vestibular nystagmus	
Peripheral	*Nystagmus-like oscillations*
Central	Inappropriate saccades
Periodic alternating nystagmus	Involuntary
Other types of conjugate nystagmus	Saccadic intrusions
Brun's nystagmus	Saccadic oscillations
Disjugate	Superior oblique myokymia
See-saw nystagmus	Voluntary
Convergence retraction nystagmus (really a	Voluntary 'nystagmus'
saccadic abnormality)	Roving eye movements

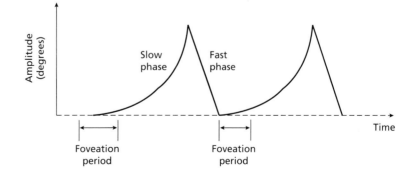

Fig. 23.1 Terms used to describe the waveform characteristics of jerk nystagmus.

AMPLITUDE

The amplitude is measured in degrees and represents the extent of movement between the start of the drift away from fixation and the start of the corrective movement in the opposite direction (Figs 23.1 & 23.2). The amount of movement in both directions should be approximately equal. In the majority of cases the amplitude will increase when the patient looks in the

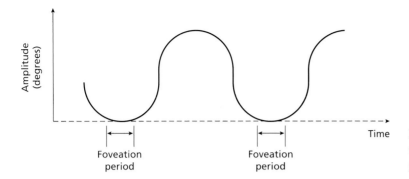

Fig. 23.2 Terms used to describe the waveform characteristics of pendular nystagmus.

direction of the fast phase (Alexander's law). When he looks in the opposite direction, the amplitude will reduce, the oscillations may cease, or the direction of the nystagmus may reverse. There are very few exceptions to this rule, but in some cases of vertical nystagmus the amplitude increases on looking in the direction of the slow phase.

The amplitude is graded as small, medium or large.

FREQUENCY

The number of beats that occur in a given time determines the frequency of the nystagmus. The greater the number of beats the higher the frequency.

The frequency is graded as low, moderate or high.

INTENSITY

The intensity of the nystagmus is the product of the amplitude and frequency. Unidirectional nystagmus is graded as follows:

Grade 1. The nystagmus is present only on looking in the direction of the fast phase.

Grade 2. The nystagmus is present on looking in the direction of the fast phase and in the primary position.

Grade 3. The nystagmus is present on looking in the direction of the fast phase, in the primary position and in the opposite field of gaze.

FOVEATION PERIOD

The foveation period is the area in the waveform where eye velocity is at a minimum and visual acuity is maximal.

NULL REGION

The null region is the field of gaze where the intensity of the nystagmus is minimal, and is therefore the region where visual acuity is usually maximal. The null region usually coincides with the neutral zone, i.e. the eye position where jerk nystagmus changes to a small-amplitude pendular waveform or no nystagmus movement is observed. Some patients may adopt an abnormal head posture to place the eyes in the null region to maximize their visual acuity.

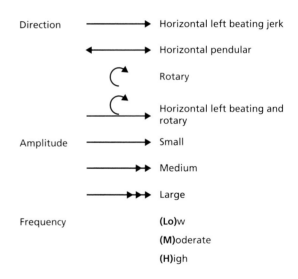

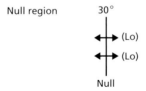

Fig. 23.3 Symbols used for diagrammatic representation of nystagmus characteristics. A null region is depicted at 30° eccentric gaze where the nystagmus has a low-frequency pendular waveform.

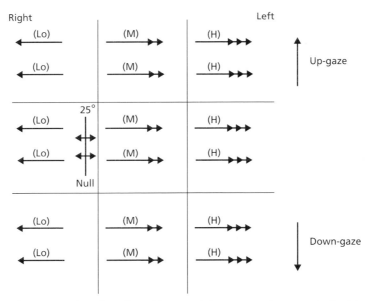

Fig. 23.4 A diagrammatic representation of a patient with congenital nystagmus; the pattern in the right eye is shown above that of the left eye. The nystagmus is symmetrical in both eyes. The nystagmus is horizontal left-beating in the primary position with medium amplitude (size of arrow) and moderate frequency (M). The intensity increases on left gaze (Alexander's law). There is a null region at 25° right gaze where the intensity is least and the waveform pendular. Beyond 25° right-gaze the waveform changes to right-beating with a small amplitude and low frequency. The nystagmus remains the same on up-gaze and down-gaze. When the nystagmus is symmetrical and conjugate, only one eye need be represented in the diagram. If the nystagmus is asymmetrical or disjugate, then the pattern in both eyes should be illustrated.

SYMMETRY

Nystagmus can be unilateral or bilateral. When bilateral the intensity is usually symmetrical but may be asymmetrical between the eyes (dissociated nystagmus); this is a feature of spasmus nutans and the nystagmus seen in internuclear ophthalmoplegia.

Diagrammatic representation of nystagmus characteristics

The symbols used for the diagrammatic representation of nystagmus are shown in Fig. 23.3, while Fig. 23.4 is a diagrammatic representation of a patient with congenital nystagmus.

Detailed waveform characteristics

A diagrammatic eye movement recording of the five main types of nystagmus is shown in Fig. 23.5. The variation in the nystagmus on right and left gaze is shown. In jerk nystagmus, the fast phase returns the eye to its original gaze direction. The examples of

the five types depicted in Fig. 23.5(a) are described as follows.

• Congenital nystagmus: the nystagmus is right-beating in the primary position. The intensity increases on extreme right and left gaze, and is least at 10° left gaze in this example (null region). The nystagmus is right-beating on right gaze, changing to left-beating beyond the null region. The slow phase has an accelerating velocity waveform shown as a curved line (increasing exponential), in which the drift is initially slow but increases exponentially until the fast phase intervenes (breaking saccade). It has been suggested that the accelerating velocity waveform is due to an inappropriate feedback loop between the brainstem and cerebellum, and represents high gain instability within this closed loop system (gain > 1).

• Manifest latent/latent nystagmus: these two forms of nystagmus have identical waveforms. The tracing from the right fixating eye is shown. The fast phase is directed towards the fixing eye (right-beating). The

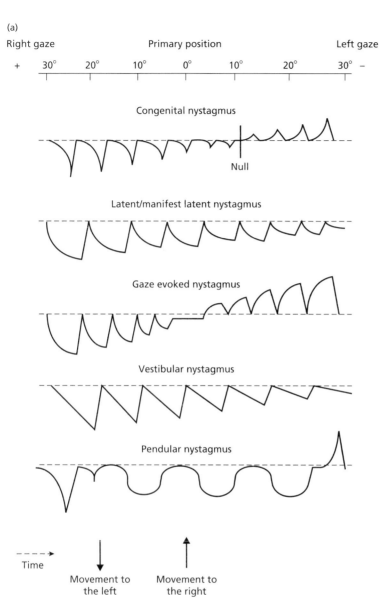

(a)

Right gaze   Primary position   Left gaze

+   30°   20°   10°   0°   10°   20°   30°   –

Congenital nystagmus

Null

Latent/manifest latent nystagmus

Gaze evoked nystagmus

Vestibular nystagmus

Pendular nystagmus

Time

Movement to the left

Movement to the right

(b)

1   2   3

Fig. 23.5 (a) Detailed waveform characteristics. A diagrammatic representation of the five main types of nystagmus. (b) 1 = oblique trajectory; 2 = circular trajectory; 3 = eliptical trajectory.

intensity of the nystagmus is maximum on right gaze in the direction of the fast phase and minimum on left gaze. The slow phase has a decelerating velocity waveform (decreasing exponential). A characteristic of this type of nystagmus is the response to covering one eye. Patients with manifest latent nystagmus will show either an increase in intensity of the nystagmus if the nonfixing eye is covered or a dampening or reversal of direction if the fixing eye is covered. Latent nystagmus becomes apparent on covering one eye, with the fast phase in the direction of the uncovered eye.

• Gaze-dependent nystagmus: gaze-evoked nystagmus is used as an example. There is no nystagmus in the primary position; the intensity increases on right and left gaze. The nystagmus is right-beating on right gaze and left-beating on left gaze; the intensity increases on eccentric gaze. The slow phase has a decelerating velocity waveform (decreasing exponential), in which the drift is initially fast but slows as the eyes move towards the primary position. The decelerating waveform is explained by a decrease in the pull exerted by the orbital viscosity as the eye moves away from the eccentric gaze position.

• Vestibular nystagmus: the nystagmus tracing illustrates the effect of a right peripheral vestibular lesion. There is a right-beating nystagmus in the primary position that increases in intensity on right gaze towards the side of the lesion, and decreases in intensity on left gaze. The slow phase has a linear velocity waveform giving it a sawtooth appearance.

• Pendular nystagmus: the waveform is of equal velocity in both directions. The oscillations are to the left of fixation with the region of minimum velocity located at fixation, where the direction of pendular nystagmus reverses. A jerk waveform is seen on lateral gaze, and is a common finding.

Trajectories of nystagmus

Not infrequently patients with nystagmus show a waveform that has vertical, horizontal and rotary components. When a horizontal and vertical component coexist and are superimposed on each other, three characteristic nystagmus trajectories can be observed (Fig. 23.5b).

• Vertical and horizontal components of equal frequency and amplitude and in phase with each other (oblique trajectory).

• Vertical and horizontal components of equal frequency and amplitude and 90° out of phase with each other (circular trajectory).

• Vertical and horizontal components of equal frequency but unequal amplitudes and 90° out of phase with each other (eliptical trajectory).

Approach to the patient with nystagmus

History

Age of onset

An onset within the first 3 months of life should reliably differentiate congenital nystagmus from other forms.

Visual function

This is expected to be below normal in congenital nystagmus, and the visual handicap may result in limited achievement at school, inability to drive, and disappointing occupational attainment.

It is useful to determine how the presence of the nystagmus was brought to the patient's attention:

• Present for as long as he can remember: typical of congenital nystagmus.

• Incidental finding by an optician, i.e. no visual symptoms: this is a feature of congenital nystagmus but is also seen in acquired down-beat and up-beat (central vestibular) nystagmus.

• Visual symptoms of oscillopsia: oscillopsia is the illusion of rhythmical movement of stationary objects. This symptom is often volunteered in acquired nystagmus, but not in congenital nystagmus.

• Visual symptoms of diplopia combined with nystagmus, suggesting brainstem involvement:

1 horizontal diplopia is a feature of internuclear ophthalmoplegia, Arnold–Chiari malformation, syringobulbia and sixth nerve palsy with multiple sclerosis;

2 vertical diplopia is a feature of skew deviation with down-beat nystagmus, and of cavernous sinus spread from a local tumour, which can be associated with see-saw nystagmus.

• Additional systemic symptoms:

1 vertigo, dizziness, nausea, deafness, suggesting vestibular dysfunction;

2 vertigo, dysarthria, dysphagia, diplopia, suggesting a ponto-medullary lesion;

3 ataxia and coordination difficulty are features of a cerebellar syndrome.

Medication history

Drugs which can cause nystagmus, such as phenytoin and alcohol, more frequently result in a gaze-evoked nystagmus, but can lead to a primary position nystagmus in some instances.

Relevant medical history

Relevant features of the medical history include:

• Previous treatment for spina bifida is associated with an increased incidence of Arnold–Chiari malformations; the first manifestation of this condition may be down-beat nystagmus in adult life.

• Severe head trauma or brainstem stroke can result in a delayed appearance of an unusual type of nystagmus termed ocular-palatal myoclonus; sometimes there is a delay of 3 months or longer before the nystagmus appears. This is a pendular and usually vertical nystagmus associated with rhythmical movements of the palate, diaphragm and other structures, and is frequently associated with severe oscillopsia (see below).

Family history

A number of conditions associated with congenital nystagmus are inherited, including albinism, Leber's amaurosis and idiopathic congenital nystagmus. Consanguinity is an important risk factor, especially for those conditions with an autosomal recessive form of inheritance.

Examination

Significant features with particular reference to the nystagmus include:

• Presence of a head posture: an abnormal head posture is a feature of congenital nystagmus. It is adopted to improve visual acuity by utilizing the null region, and may only be observed when the visual task involves fine detail: for example, it can be seen as the patient approaches the limit of his visual acuity on a Snellen chart. The head posture is frequently more marked on distance fixation. Most commonly it consists of a face turn, but may involve a chin elevation or depression and a head tilt.

• Nystagmus in the primary position: the nystagmus should be observed in the primary position for 2–3 min to look for any change in the characteristics, such as a reversal of the waveform or a transient change from a horizontal to a vertical direction, both features of periodic alternating nystagmus.

• Diagrammatic record of the nystagmus: the pattern of the nystagmus should be recorded in the primary position and in each position of gaze showing the waveform (jerk/pendular), direction (horizontal, vertical, rotary) and the amplitude and frequency (Fig. 23.4).

• Nystagmus characteristics on distance and near fixation and on convergence: congenital nystagmus characteristically dampens on near fixation and with convergence. Subtle forms of see-saw nystagmus may be easier to observe on distance fixation.

• Effect of covering one eye (i.e. cover test): patients with manifest latent nystagmus will show either an increase in the intensity of the nystagmus if the non-fixing eye is covered or a dampening or reversal of direction if the fixing eye is covered. Latent nystagmus can be identified on cover test. Congenital nystagmus may be associated with latent nystagmus, and the effect of the latent component on the overall waveform can be observed.

• Effect of removing fixation (see below): peripheral vestibular nystagmus characteristically increases when fixation is removed, whereas congenital nystagmus may reduce in intensity. Central vestibular nystagmus shows no change. Techniques of removing fixation are described below.

• Optokinetic testing: this is important in assessing the pursuit and saccadic eye movement systems. Convergence retraction nystagmus can often best be demonstrated by using a downward rotating optokinetic drum. In approximately two-thirds of cases of congenital nystagmus, a horizontal rotating optokinetic drum will show an inverted response. For example, a patient with a right-beating horizontal nystagmus will continue to show a right-beating nystagmus when the drum is rotated to his right.

• The presence of rhythmical movement of the eyelids and soft palate. This is seen in ocular-palatal myoclonus.

• Head nodding is frequently seen in congenital nystagmus. The presence of a largely unilateral nystagmus, head nodding and a head posture are features of spasmus nutans.

Other important aspects to note on examination include the following:

• Visual acuity: this should be recorded with and without any head posture. It should be measured not only uniocularly but also with both eyes open for near and distance. Visual acuity with both eyes open is often significantly better in patients with congenital nystagmus.

• Refraction: even small amounts of refractive error should be corrected. Patients often report an improvement in visual acuity that may not be measurable on Snellen testing. Patients with retinal dystrophies commonly have high levels of refractive error and astigmatism.

- Stereoacuity: a near-normal level of stereoacuity on TNO testing virtually excludes albinism as the cause of congenital nystagmus.

All patients should have a full ocular examination, and those patients suspected of acquired nystagmus should undergo a general medical and neurological examination. Family members should be examined for evidence of the condition or features of the carrier state in X-linked disorders. Relevant further investigations are discussed under the specific conditions.

Observing and recording nystagmus

Nystagmus may be observed and recorded using various techniques.

- Unaided.
- Local magnification with +10 DS lenses or with Fresnel lenses, which have the advantage of removing fixation and accentuating certain types of nystagmus.
- Slit lamp: observation of the conjunctival or iris vessels facilitates the detection of very small amplitude movements.
- Ophthalmoscope: the use of the ophthalmoscope to observe the optic disc can detect very small amplitude nystagmus. The direction of the nystagmus is opposite to the movement of the disc. Asking the patient to occlude one eye while the examiner observes the optic disc in the other eye can readily assess the effect of removing fixation.
- Video recording.
- Eye movement recording (see Chapter 6).

The best facilities combine video and eye movement recording techniques so that an eye movement recording signal is superimposed on a real-time video recording of the eye movement.

Techniques of removing fixation

- Spielmann translucent occluder: this type of occluder prevents fixation of a nonilluminated target while still allowing observation of the eye behind the occluder.
- Fresnel lenses: powers of +10 DS and greater are suitable.
- Eye movement recording in the dark or with the eyes closed.

Childhood nystagmus

Classification

The classification of childhood nystagmus is shown in Table 23.2.

Congenital forms

Congenital nystagmus

Congenital nystagmus has an onset during the first 3 months of life. It can be classified as shown in Table 23.3.

Description

Congenital nystagmus is present in the primary position. It characteristically has a symmetrical jerk and pendular waveform.

It is probably true to say that congenital nystagmus represents a primary motor instability of eye movement control, resulting in a 'fixation nystagmus'; it can exist with or without a bilateral defect of the anterior visual pathway. The typical waveform characteristics of congenital nystagmus can occasionally be seen following bilateral visual loss in an adult; this suggests that postnatal environmental factors in combination with the maturing visual system have an

Table 23.2 Classification of childhood nystagmus.

Congenital forms
Congenital nystagmus
  Sensory
    Visual loss
      Media opacities
      Retinal abnormalities
      Anterior visual pathway disorders
  Idiopathic
Latent/manifest latent
Others

Acquired forms
Spasmus nutans
Intracranial disease
Ipsilateral visual loss

Table 23.3 Classification of congenital nystagmus.

Sensory
  Media
    Ptosis
    Corneal dystrophy
    Cataracts
    Persistent hyperplastic primary vitreous (PHPV)
  Retina
    Foveal hypoplasia
      Albinism
      Aniridia
    Leber's amaurosis
    Rod monochromatism
    Congenital stationary night blindness (CSNB)
  Anterior visual pathway
    Optic nerve hypoplasia

Idiopathic

---

important part to play in its development. If one assumes that not all patients with the propensity to develop congenital nystagmus actually go on to develop it, then one can go some way to explaining the condition on the basis of:

• Congenital idiopathic nystagmus (no anterior visual pathway defect) occurs when the propensity to develop nystagmus is already unmasked at birth; the mechanism by which unmasking occurs probably resides in a yet-to-be discovered defect in the anterior visual pathways or ocular motor circuitry in the brainstem.

• Congenital nystagmus with sensory loss occurs when poor vision either adversely influences postnatal development of ocular stabilization or increases the demand on visual fixation in an attempt to see clearly. Congenital nystagmus is unmasked in some patients and not in others.

• Sensory loss in childhood may or may not result in nystagmus, and this somewhat variable effect can be explained by the age at which the visual loss occurs:

  1 visual loss from birth to 2 years of age: nearly all cases show nystagmus;

  2 visual loss from 2 to 4 years of age: some will develop nystagmus;

  3 visual loss after 4 years of age: it is rare to develop nystagmus.

The cause and severity of the visual loss are also influential:

1 Albinism is almost invariably associated with congenital nystagmus, irrespective of the level of visual acuity. This suggests that the unmasking of congenital nystagmus in this group of patients may be related either to the miswiring of the visual pathways that is characteristic of albinism or to an unidentified brainstem abnormality.

2 Bilateral congenital cataracts result in congenital nystagmus, which can be prevented and occasionally reversed by early surgical removal of the cataracts, thus confirming the influence of postnatal developmental factors in the pathogenesis of congenital nystagmus.

3 Only bilateral moderate to severe forms of optic nerve hypoplasia result in congenital nystagmus, supporting the finding that the development of nystagmus is influenced by the severity of the anterior pathway dysfunction.

The maturing visual system is clearly very sensitive to loss of vision. Most individuals probably have the potential to develop congenital nystagmus if sufficiently severe visual loss occurs early enough. Presumably patients with anterior visual pathway disease who do not develop congenital nystagmus have more stable eye movement control.

Features

• In congenital nystagmus patients with a sensory defect outnumber those without a sensory defect by a factor of around 9 : 1 (Gelbart & Hoyt 1988).

• A bilateral horizontal and symmetrical jerk and pendular waveform is typically seen. Idiopathic congenital nystagmus usually remains horizontal in all gaze positions; a poorly sustained rotary component is occasionally apparent on extreme lateral gaze (Fig. 23.6). When congenital nystagmus is associated with sensory loss, a vertical or rotary component is often present in the primary position; a gaze-evoked component on vertical gaze is also common and probably reflects the influence of poor vision on the developing gaze control mechanism (neural integrator).

• The nystagmus characteristics frequently change as the visual system matures. A roving eye movement pattern is sometimes present in the early stages of congenital nystagmus with sensory loss associated with

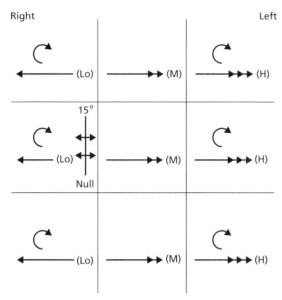

Fig. 23.6 Congenital nystagmus shows a medium amplitude and moderate frequency left-beating jerk nystagmus in the primary position which increases in intensity on left gaze and decreases in intensity on right gaze. There is a null region in right gaze where the waveform is pendular. The nystagmus is bilateral and symmetrical and remains horizontal in all gaze positions.

Leber's amaurosis and severe bilateral optic nerve hypoplasia (see later); in time these patients develop a more typical congenital nystagmus waveform. A grossly asymmetrical pattern may later become symmetrical. An initial pendular pattern (Fig. 23.5) may develop a jerk component or change to a jerk waveform.

• Visual attention and anxiety accentuate the nystagmus. It is usually damped on convergence and with lid closure and is abolished during sleep.

• A null region can often be identified but not all patients make use of it. The visual potential in patients with congenital idiopathic nystagmus is related to the duration of any foveating period (Figs 23.1 & 23.2). The longer the duration the better the visual acuity.

• Compensatory mechanisms adopted to minimize the nystagmus and improve vision comprise:

  1 a face turn to centralize the null region;

  2 voluntary convergence;

  3 head shaking;

  4 involuntary convergence and the development of an esotropia (nystagmus blockage syndrome; see Chapter 14).

• The optokinetic response is typically inverted in two-thirds of patients with congenital nystagmus. If, for example, the patient has a right-beating nystagmus, movement of the stripes to the left, which normally induces a fast phase to the right, should increase the intensity of the nystagmus by a process of summation. However, damping or even reversal to a left-beating nystagmus occurs. The optokinetic response is normal when the stripes are moved vertically.

• Patients do not complain of oscillopsia or are not troubled by it; however, it may occur in certain environments, for example when viewing a brightly lit object in a dark room.

• A superimposed latent nystagmus can be identified by observing the waveform when either eye is covered; the underlying congenital nystagmus will be seen either to increase or decrease in intensity or even change direction.

Pathogenesis

The pathogenesis of congenital nystagmus has been attributed to an abnormality of the ocular stabilization systems. These systems comprise the visual fixation and pursuit systems, which function to stabilize the image on the fovea; the vestibular and optokinetic systems help to maintain foveal fixation during head movement. It is possible that an abnormality in the ocular stabilization systems contributes to or causes congenital nystagmus.

• Visual fixation: congenital nystagmus increases with visual attention and anxiety and is abolished during sleep. These characteristics suggest that it arises from an inherent abnormality of the fixation reflex; it has been referred to as a 'fixation nystagmus'. There is, however, no real evidence to support this hypothesis; indeed there is good evidence from the waveform characteristics of congenital nystagmus that these patients have a strong visual fixation reflex. A unique characteristic of congenital nystagmus is the foveating period, which represents an area in the waveform where eye velocity is at a minimum and visual acuity is maximal (see Figs 23.1 & 23.2). The presence of regular foveating periods in both sensory and idiopathic congenital nystagmus supports a strong visual fixation drive and refutes the notion that these patients have a primary disturbance of the visual fixation reflex. (Dell'Osso *et al.* 1992).

• Pursuit system: eye movement recording during visual tracking of a slow-moving target (pursuit) in patients with congenital nystagmus shows a congenital nystagmus waveform superimposed upon the sinusoidal smooth pursuit movement. In some patients the foveating periods precisely match the target position, suggesting that the pursuit system is functioning surprisingly accurately despite the congenital nystagmus oscillations. In others, the pursuit system does not appear to be functioning normally, perhaps related to associated visual loss.

• Vestibular ocular reflex: intermittent head shaking associated with visual attention frequently occurs in congenital nystagmus. Two types are seen:

  1 an involuntary head shake that does not appear to affect visual acuity;

  2 a synchronous compensatory head shake opposite to the direction of the fast phase of the nystagmus, which improves visual acuity (Gresty & Halmagy 1979).

When the head rotates during visual fixation, the eyes normally rotate in the opposite direction by the same amount to maintain fixation. If the vestibular ocular reflex is functioning normally, head shaking will result in no net change in gaze position and it therefore has no net influence on the nystagmus. If the vestibular ocular reflex is deficient, head shaking will result in a change in gaze position: for example, when the head moves to the right, the eyes move only partly to the left, resulting in a net right gaze movement. If this is opposite to the direction of the nystagmus, it can result in lower velocity and therefore improved visual acuity.

• Optokinetic system: the optokinetic control system prevents the shift of the image across the retina. Lack of visual input can impede the development of this system. Its failure to develop is believed to allow the formation of permanent opportunistic abnormal nystagmus generators (Kommerell 1984). These generators develop in a random fashion which could explain the varied wave forms seen in the sensory form of congenital nystagmus.

In summary there is little scientific evidence to support a primary abnormality in the ocular stabilization systems in congenital nystagmus.

Investigation

A history should be taken and examination carried out as described earlier. Any child suspected of having a visual handicap should ideally be assessed by a multidisciplinary team, led by the ophthalmologist. The ophthalmologist should direct investigations towards identifying a cause for the nystagmus in the anterior visual pathway. Neuro-imaging and other invasive tests should not be carried out routinely unless indicated by the clinical features of the individual case. Access to genetic advice is also important. All cases of congenital nystagmus should be assumed to be due to a disorder affecting the anterior visual pathway until proven otherwise.

Examination

OCULAR EXAMINATION

Particular attention should be paid to:

• The refractive error: high levels of refractive error with astigmatism are commonly associated with retinal dystrophies.

• The size of the cornea, which is enlarged in congenital glaucoma.

• The clarity of the media (e.g. cataracts).

• The presence of iris transillumination defects, which are associated with albinism, or iris hypoplasia, which is seen in aniridia.

• The pupil reaction, which may show a paradoxical response, especially in cases of retinal dystrophy when the pupil dilates in the light and constricts in the dark. Sluggish pupil reactions are a feature of severe Leber's amaurosis and optic nerve hypoplasia.

• The retina, looking for retinopathy of prematurity, retinal folds or the presence of colobomas.

• The presence of the fovea, which may, for example, be hypoplastic in albinism. The foveal architecture is often poorly developed from birth to 6 months of age, making the diagnosis of foveal hypoplasia difficult in this age group.

• The optic nerves (e.g. optic nerve hypoplasia).

OCULAR EXAMINATION OF PARENTS AND SIBLINGS

• Close relatives may show the same signs as the patient or, in the case of X-linked ocular albinism, the mother often shows carrier-state characteristics of the disease (Gillespie & Covelli 1963).

- An electroretinogram (ERG) is essential in the overall investigation.
- We also find the visual-evoked potential (VEP) useful in confirming the presence of crossed asymmetry in albinism. A markedly attenuated response is obtained in the presence of significant optic nerve hypoplasia (see Chapter 4 for further details on electrodiagnosis).

In the absence of any evidence of ocular disease and a normal ERG and VEP, the likely diagnosis is congenital idiopathic nystagmus. This diagnosis should not be ascribed to cases which have an atypical waveform or other abnormalities until neuro-imaging has excluded the presence of intracranial disease.

Differential diagnosis of the ocular cause

In the absence of an obvious media or retinal abnormality, most cases of congenital nystagmus are related to a bilateral sensory abnormality affecting the anterior visual pathway. Causes include:

- ocular albinism;
- oculocutaneous albinism;
- Leber's congenital amaurosis;
- optic nerve hypoplasia;
- rod monochromatism;
- congenital stationary night blindness;
- congenital idiopathic nystagmus.

Latent nystagmus and manifest latent nystagmus
Description

- Latent nystagmus is a horizontal jerk nystagmus that is absent when both eyes are open but is present when the light stimulus to one eye is reduced.
- Manifest latent nystagmus is apparent (manifest) with both eyes open; the amplitude increases when the light stimulus to the nonfixing eye is reduced and decreases or even changes direction when the stimulus to the fixing eye is reduced (Fig. 23.7). Otherwise, it has the same characteristics as latent nystagmus.

Dell'Osso *et al.* (1979) have shown that patients with apparent latent nystagmus frequently demonstrate a subclinical nystagmus on electronystagmography when both eyes are viewing, and that true latent nystagmus is very rare.

Features

The features of latent and manifest latent nystagmus

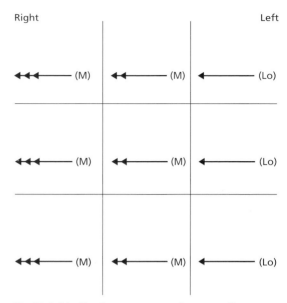

Fig. 23.7 Manifest latent nystagmus shows a medium amplitude and moderate frequency jerk nystagmus beating towards the fixing right eye. The intensity increases to the right and decreases to the left. The nystagmus remains horizontal in all gaze directions.

are the same and any difference between them can be considered quantitative. There is a bilateral, horizontal jerk nystagmus, which is usually symmetrical.

- The fast phase is always directed towards the viewing (fixating) eye.
- Reducing the light stimulus to one eye results in latent nystagmus becoming manifest.
- One eye is used for fixation when both eyes are open in manifest latent nystagmus.
- The amplitude increases on covering either eye.
- The intensity increases on abduction and decreases on adduction.
- The slow phase of the nystagmus shows a decelerating velocity waveform (Fig. 23.5).
- A face turn to the side of the fixing eye is commonly seen, particularly when testing visual acuity.
- Manifest latent nystagmus has been reported in the good or remaining eye in some patients who have had unilateral blindness since birth or have had an eye removed in early childhood (Harcourt & Spencer 1985).
- Binocular single vision is absent or poor in most patients.

• Manifest latent nystagmus is commonly found in infantile esotropia and in association with DVD.

Pathogenesis

The pathogenesis remains unknown. Four theories have been proposed to explain the phenomenon:

• Cortical motion processing defect: this is said to be responsible for the horizontal asymmetry of the opto-kinetic nystagmus (OKN) response, temporal to nasal pursuit movement being of larger amplitude than nasal to temporal movement.

• Subcortical optokinetic system imbalance.

• Extraocular proprioception disorder.

• Defective egocentric localization: this theory is supported by a patient who was blind in one eye and could change the direction of the nystagmus by simply trying to look out of his blind eye.

Neither latent nor manifest latent nystagmus requires further investigation.

Congenital forms of adult nystagmus

Typical or atypical forms of adult nystagmus are sometimes congenital. We have seen cases of periodic alternating nystagmus, see-saw nystagmus, up-beat and down-beat nystagmus which were of congenital origin. Investigation as described under the adult form is required.

Acquired forms

Acquired forms of childhood nystagmus comprise:

• spasmus nutans;

• nystagmus with intracranial disease;

• nystagmus with ipsilateral visual loss.

Spasmus nutans

Description

Spasmus nutans is a combination of an asymmetrical nystagmus, involuntary head movements and an abnormal head posture (the triad of spasmus nutans).

Features

• Onset is usually between 3 and 18 months of age.

• The nystagmus is of low amplitude and fast frequency with a horizontal, vertical or torsional pendular waveform. It often appears unilateral but on close inspection the other eye is seen to be involved to a lesser extent in most cases.

• The nystagmus varies considerably in different positions of gaze and if head nodding is present, the intensity increases if the head is immobilized.

• The head movement often precedes the onset of the nystagmus. It consists of an involuntary nodding or shaking movement. The head movement is in the opposite phase to the eye movement. The head movements do not appear to compensate for the nystagmus as they are of different frequency. They disappear during sleep.

• Spasmus nutans may last from a few weeks to several years.

Investigation

If all three components of the triad are present and the visual pathways show no abnormality in an otherwise normal child, we believe that further investigation is not required apart from regular monitoring. If all components of the triad are not present or there is evidence of visual or general abnormality, then neuro-imaging should be used to exclude the presence of intracranial disease.

Nystagmus with intracranial disease

Acquired nystagmus during childhood can be the presenting sign of an intracranial tumour. The nystagmus seen with such tumours is frequently asymmetrical, and is not associated with head nodding or an abnormal head posture (Farmer & Hoyt 1984; Lavery *et al.* 1984). Optic atrophy is often present. Some of these cases were initially diagnosed as spasmus nutans, a term which should be reserved for those showing all three components of the triad described earlier. We recommend that all patients presenting with acquired nystagmus in childhood which does not conform to the diagnostic criteria of spasmus nutans should undergo a full neurological examination, including neuro-imaging.

Nystagmus with ipsilateral visual loss

See under 'Acquired pendular nystagmus' below.

Adult nystagmus

The classification used for adult nystagmus is based on:

• the principal waveform characteristics (jerk or pendular);

Table 23.4 Classification of adult nystagmus.

Jerk nystagmus
Primary positional
   Conjugate
      Vestibular
         Peripheral
         Central
            Down-beat
            Up-beat
      Periodic alternating nystagmus
      Others
         Brun's
   Disjugate
      See-saw
      Convergence retraction
Gaze-dependent
   Gaze-evoked
   Gaze-paretic
   Dissociated

Pendular nystagmus
Horizontal
Vertical

- whether there is spontaneous nystagmus in the primary position (primary positional) or only with gaze (gaze-dependent);
- whether the nystagmus is conjugate or disjugate;
- the presence of vestibular symptoms and signs.

Classification

The classification of adult nystagmus is summarized in Table 23.4.

Acquired jerk nystagmus

Acquired jerk nystagmus can be primary positional or gaze-dependent.

Primary positional jerk nystagmus

Both conjugate and disjugate primary positional nystagmus are seen.

Conjugate nystagmus

Primary positional conjugate nystagmus is classified as vestibular nystagmus, periodic alternating nystagmus and other forms of conjugate nystagmus.

Vestibular nystagmus

Vestibular nystagmus can result from lesions involving the peripheral or central vestibular system.

Vestibular nystagmus has a linear velocity jerk waveform (Fig. 23.5) which is conjugate and present in the primary position. It may be unidirectional (down-beat, up-beat, etc.) or multidirectional: the intensity usually increases in the direction of the fast phase.

Other symptoms of vestibular dysfunction are frequently present and may overshadow the visual symptoms, explaining why many of these patients present first to ear, nose and throat or neurological specialists. Vestibular nystagmus can be due to disease affecting the peripheral or central parts of the vestibular system.

PERIPHERAL VESTIBULAR NYSTAGMUS
The peripheral vestibular system is made up of the membranous labyrinth in the inner ear and the eighth cranial nerve. Disorders affecting this part of the vestibular system are nearly always associated with severe vertigo and as such infrequently present first to the ophthalmologist.

Features (Fig. 23.8)
- The nystagmus is typically a mixed horizontal and rotary waveform which is present in the primary position. A vertical and rotary waveform is also common. The overall amplitude of the nystagmus is small. The intensity increases in the direction of the fast phase and decreases in the direction of the slow phase. The nystagmus beats in the same direction irrespective of the position of gaze.
- The fast phase is directed away from the side of the lesion.
- The frequency of the nystagmus is always high, giving the nystagmus a shimmering quality.
- In mild cases or in those that are long-standing the nystagmus may not be present in the primary position. Preventing fixation invariably uncovers the nystagmus, or accentuates it if already present.
- Oscillopsia, tinnitus and deafness are common symptoms.
- The nystagmus is relatively transient as central

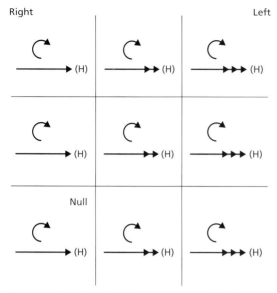

Right   Left

Null

Fig. 23.8 Peripheral vestibular nystagmus resulting from a right-sided lesion showing a mixed horizontal jerk and rotary waveform which beats away from the site of the lesion. The intensity increases to the left and decreases to the right.

compensation mechanisms act to reduce its intensity after a few weeks.

Pathogenesis of peripheral nystagmus

Common causes of peripheral vestibular dysfunction include:

- infections;
- toxic reactions;
- trauma;
- inflammation.

Each semicircular canal primarily excites two extraocular muscles, one in each eye. The anterior and posterior canals excite a pair of cyclovertical muscles, for example the ipsilateral superior oblique and the contralateral inferior rectus, and the horizontal canal excites the ipsilateral medial rectus and contralateral lateral rectus. Most lesions involving the membranous labyrinth result in nonselective damage to the semicircular canals and therefore result in a mixed waveform nystagmus.

In the resting state the vestibular system of both sides exerts an equal and opposite tonic innervation on the ocular motor system. The effect of the innerva-tion from one side is to produce a slow drift of the eyes towards the opposite side. Loss of innervation from one side because of dysfunction therefore causes a slow drift of the eyes towards the side of the lesion followed by a fast movement to the opposite side. Lesions affecting the peripheral vestibular system result in a jerk nystagmus with the direction of the fast phase opposite to the side of the lesion.

The ocular stabilization systems of visual fixation and smooth pursuit have their final common pathway through the central vestibular nuclei and their connections. Peripheral vestibular dysfunction leaves the ocular stabilization systems intact to dampen the nystagmus. Removal of fixation results in an accentuation of the nystagmus, and may even uncover the presence of a primary positional nystagmus. Vestibular nystagmus is one of the few forms of nystagmus to be accentuated by closing the eyelids.

Investigation

A number of tests can easily be performed in the clinic without the need for specialized equipment. These tests are based on stimulating the vestibular system to uncover any imbalance between the two sides; the tests are generally referred to as the dynamic assessment of vestibular dysfunction.

- The patient is asked to read down a distance Snellen test type with both eyes open; the examiner stands behind the patient and rotates his head from side to side at between 2 and 3 cycles per second while the patient reads down the chart again. Vestibular imbalance reflected in abnormal gain (eye velocity and head velocity) will result in failure to maintain fixation as the eyes repeatedly drift off target, requiring small saccades to recover fixation. In the presence of an abnormal vestibular gain, visual acuity will deteriorate by 1–2 lines when tested with the head rotating. The procedure is repeated, this time rotating the head in the vertical plane.

- A similar test to the one described above involves asking the patient to shake his head in the horizontal plane for 10–20 s. At the end of this period a transient nystagmus indicates a vestibular imbalance. The test can then be repeated with the head shaking in the vertical plane, when a transient vertical nystagmus may be seen.

- Positional testing is useful in patients complaining

of vertigo associated with a change of posture. The patient is seated on a suitable couch with his head central. He is rapidly placed supine on the couch, with his neck extended, resulting in the head hanging 30° below the horizontal. After 30 s, the patient is rapidly returned to the upright position. The procedure is repeated with the head turned both to the right and left shoulders. Transient nystagmus produced during these manoeuvres, often in association with vertigo, is strongly suggestive of a condition termed benign paroxysmal positional vertigo.

• Caloric testing is useful in determining the side of a peripheral vestibular lesion. The examiner should first check that the ears are free of significant wax and that the tympanic membranes are intact. The test relies on using warm and cold water to set up temperature gradients across the semicircular canals; the resulting convection currents in the endolymph bend the cupula, so stimulating the hair cells. The patient's head is positioned 30° from supine, which places the lateral canal in the vertical plane, maximizing the effect from the convection currents. Cold water (30°C) is irrigated into the external auditory meatus of first one side then the other. The procedure is then repeated using warm water (44°C). A normal response is for cold water to produce nystagmus with a fast phase directed to the opposite side. With warm water the fast phase is to the same side. An asymmetry in the response of greater than 25% suggests peripheral vestibular imbalance. Ideally, the patient should be alert during the test, with fixation disrupted either with a Fresnel lens or by performing the test in darkness while recording the eye movements.

Management
Patients with evidence of peripheral vestibular dysfunction should be referred to the appropriate subspecialty for further management.

CENTRAL VESTIBULAR NYSTAGMUS
Damage to the central vestibular nuclei can occur acutely because of:
• infarction;
• inflammation (demyelination);
• trauma.
Acute dysfunction is likely to be associated with other vestibular symptoms of vertigo and nausea.

Chronic damage to the vestibular nuclei can arise from:
• structural abnormalities (e.g. Arnold–Chiari malformations);
• slow-growing tumours;
• degenerative conditions.
In these slowly progressive conditions central vestibular adaptation takes place, making vertigo and nausea uncommon symptoms. Patients with chronic damage to the vestibular nuclei frequently present to the ophthalmologist with an isolated vertical nystagmus.

Features
• Unidirectional waveforms that are vertical, but can also be horizontal or rotary, are typical of central vestibular damage.
• Mixed waveforms also occur which are indistinguishable from those seen with peripheral vestibular lesions.
• The amplitude of the nystagmus can be quite variable and at times large. The intensity usually increases in the direction of the fast phase and decreases in the direction of the slow phase. The nystagmus may reverse direction on changing gaze.
• Removing fixation does not have any effect on the intensity of the nystagmus.
• A gaze-evoked nystagmus may also be present (see later).
• Oscillopsia is common; tinnitus and deafness are rare.
• When the cause is chronic, the nystagmus tends to be long-standing.

Two important types of central vestibular nystagmus are down-beat and up-beat nystagmus. These will be discussed in more detail.

DOWN-BEAT NYSTAGMUS
Description
This is a primary positional vertical jerk nystagmus in which the fast phase is downwards.

Features (Fig. 23.9)
• The nystagmus can occasionally be accentuated by tilting the patient to one side or by convergence.
• On rare occasions down-beat nystagmus increases in intensity on up-gaze.

Right   Left

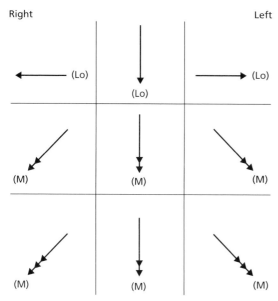

Fig. 23.9 Primary position down-beat nystagmus with a superimposed horizontal gaze-evoked nystagmus. The intensity of down-beat nystagmus increases on down-gaze and laterally. The frequency of the nystagmus tends to be lower and the amplitude larger than that seen in peripheral vestibular nystagmus. The superimposed gaze-evoked nystagmus produces a horizontal vector to the waveform on side-gaze, shown as an oblique trajectory. The down-beat nystagmus dampens on up-gaze; only gaze-evoked nystagmus is present on up-gaze and laterally.

• The vertical vestibular ocular reflex is often abnormal.
• Impaired horizontal gaze-holding and combined eye-head tracking are also commonly seen.
• The down-beat nystagmus may be asymmetrical and on occasions unilateral. An incomitant skew deviation may be associated (Baker & Ansons 1996).

UP-BEAT NYSTAGMUS
Description
This is a primary positional vertical jerk nystagmus in which the fast phase is upwards.

Features
The features of up-beat nystagmus are similar to those described for down-beat nystagmus with the exception that:

• up-beat nystagmus does not usually increase on lateral gaze;
• convergence has a variable effect on the intensity;
• a rare form of up-beat nystagmus called bow-tie nystagmus may occur, consisting of obliquely directed up-beat components which alternate to the right and left.

PATHOGENESIS OF DOWN-BEAT AND UP-BEAT NYSTAGMUS
The pathogenesis of down-beat and up-beat nystagmus remains unknown. Four main ocular motor centres have been implicated in central vestibular nystagmus.
• Vestibular ocular reflex: central connections from the anterior and posterior semicircular canals synapse in the medial vestibular nucleus before projecting to other structures. Experimental lesions involving the central projections of the semicircular canals result in down-beat nystagmus when the lesion affects the posterior canals and up-beat nystagmus when it affects the anterior canals (Fig. 23.10).
• Otoliths: tilting the head can occasionally accentuate the intensity of central vestibular nystagmus, which suggests otolith involvement.
• Smooth pursuit: vertical smooth pursuit movements are frequently impaired in patients with up- and down-beat nystagmus, suggesting this ocular motor control system may be involved.
• Gaze-holding mechanism: damage to the horizontal neural integrator in the medulla may result in some imbalance in vertical gaze-holding and also in a central shift in the perceived position of primary gaze. If this shift is upward, then the eyes will drift upwards from the primary position and will show a down-beat nystagmus.

Down-beat nystagmus is most frequently seen in association with disease affecting the cerebellum and medulla, and can be a sign of drug toxicity. Up-beat nystagmus is most often associated with lesions affecting the medulla. Lesions include the Arnold–Chiari malformation, syringobulbia, cerebellar degeneration and multiple sclerosis.

INVESTIGATION
In the absence of a causative factor, patients suspected of a central vestibular nystagmus require magnetic resonance (MR) neuro-imaging of the lower brain-

Fig. 23.10 Pathogenesis of down-beat and up-beat nystagmus. Central connections from the posterior and anterior semicircular canals synapse in the medial vestibular nucleus before projecting to other structures. Experimental lesions involving the dorsal medulla result in down-beat nystagmus, while lesions of the brachium conjunctivum and ventral tegmentum produce up-beat nystagmus.

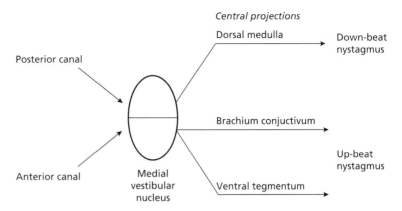

stem and cerebellum. Particular importance should be paid to identifying structural abnormalities in this region, such as the Arnold–Chiari malformation, for which surgical treatment is available.

Periodic alternating nystagmus

DESCRIPTION

Periodic alternating nystagmus is a horizontal jerk nystagmus in which the oscillations in the primary position change direction every few minutes.

FEATURES

• Each cycle lasts between 3 and 4 min, starting with an increased intensity of a unidirectional jerk nystagmus, followed by a decreasing intensity lasting 1–2 min. There is then a short period when there is either no movement or a down-beat nystagmus. The horizontal jerk nystagmus then begins again following the same pattern but beating in the opposite direction.

• Smooth pursuit movement is also impaired.

The condition is usually acquired in association with disease of the medulla and cerebellum. A less well-defined form of periodic alternating nystagmus can be seen in patients with albinism.

INVESTIGATION

The investigations are the same as for central vestibular nystagmus.

Other types of conjugate nystagmus

BRUNS' NYSTAGMUS

Description

Bruns' nystagmus is a combination of a fine peripheral vestibular nystagmus and a coarse gaze-evoked nystagmus.

Features (Fig. 23.11)

• Bruns' nystagmus consists of a fine peripheral vestibular nystagmus and a coarse gaze-evoked nystagmus.

• Fine vestibular nystagmus is seen in the primary position and on gaze to the side opposite the lesion.

• Coarse gaze-evoked nystagmus is seen on gaze towards the side of the lesion.

• It is seen in association with cerebellar pontine angle tumours, which can affect other cranial nerves (fifth, sixth, seventh and eighth cranial nerves).

Investigation

Neuro-imaging should be arranged to detect the presence of a mass lesion in the cerebellar pontine angle.

Disjugate nystagmus

The two manifestations of disjugate nystagmus are see-saw nystagmus and convergence retraction nystagmus.

See-saw nystagmus

DESCRIPTION

The nystagmus consists of a conjugate rotary component with a disjugate vertical component.

FEATURES (Fig. 23.12)

• The vertical component of the nystagmus usually has a pendular waveform, although jerk waveforms have been reported.

Right   Left

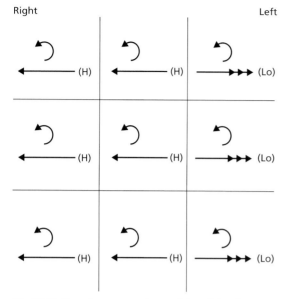

Fig. 23.11 Bruns' nystagmus shows a left peripheral vestibular nystagmus with a small-amplitude, high-frequency right-beating horizontal and rotary waveform. This is seen in the primary position and in right gaze and results from the tumour compressing the left eighth cranial nerve. As the tumour enlarges, it compresses the brainstem and damages the ipsilateral neural integrator, resulting in large-amplitude, low-frequency gaze-evoked nystagmus on left gaze.

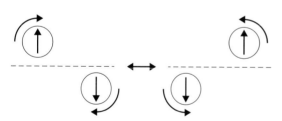

Fig. 23.12 See-saw nystagmus consists of a conjugate rotary component and a disjugate vertical component. There is a synchronous intorsion of the elevating eye and extorsion of the depressing eye.

- The movement consists of a synchronous intorsion of the elevating eye and an extorsion of the depressing eye.
- One eye remains fixing on the target.
- One component of the nystagmus may predominate depending on the position of gaze.

- The commonest association is with large parasellar tumours and bitemporal hemianopia, although it can also follow trauma and brainstem stroke.

PATHOGENESIS

The pathogenesis of see-saw nystagmus is probably related to damage of the interstitial nucleus of Cajal, which is located in the midbrain: discrete lesions to this nucleus have resulted in see-saw nystagmus. Stimulation of the nucleus has resulted in the ocular tilt reaction (Westheimer & Blair 1975), which is similar to one half-cycle of see-saw nystagmus.

INVESTIGATION

All patients presenting with see-saw nystagmus should undergo neuro-imaging to the region of the optic chiasm.

Convergence retraction nystagmus

DESCRIPTION

Convergence retraction nystagmus is really a saccadic disorder consisting of intermittent periods of opposing adducting saccades, which are usually elicited by attempted upward saccades.

FEATURES

- The nystagmus can usually be elicited by making the patient attempt an upward gaze movement. This is best demonstrated by using a downward rotating optokinetic drum.
- Mild cases may only show the characteristic movements in the upper field of gaze.
- Convergence and retraction of the globe occurs on attempting up-gaze.
- The nystagmus is part of the dorsal midbrain syndrome (see Chapter 22).

INVESTIGATION

The investigation and management are discussed in Chapter 22.

Gaze-dependent nystagmus

Description

This is a jerk nystagmus that only becomes manifest when gaze is directed away from the primary position.

Gaze-dependent nystagmus can be unilateral, bilateral, horizontal or vertical, or a combination of these features.

Classification

Three main types can be differentiated on the basis of whether or not the range of extraocular movement is affected and whether the nystagmus is symmetrical or asymmetrical between the two eyes:

- Gaze-evoked nystagmus is the term used to describe any nystagmus that is manifest only on eccentric gaze. Excluded are those cases that demonstrate gaze-paretic or dissociated nystagmus.
- Gaze-paretic nystagmus is a type of gaze-evoked nystagmus which is associated with either a partial gaze palsy or a paralytic or mechanical disorder of eye movement. There can be limited extraocular movement or fatiguable extraocular muscles.
- Dissociated nystagmus is a type of gaze-evoked nystagmus in which the nystagmus is markedly asymmetrical between the two eyes. The most common example is the nystagmus seen in patients with internuclear ophthalmoplegia.

Features (Fig. 23.13)

- A jerk nystagmus that is absent in the primary position and is manifest on eccentric gaze.
- The fast phase is always in the direction of eccentric gaze.
- The frequency is usually low to medium.
- The nystagmus shows a decelerating velocity waveform (Fig. 23.5).
- The same disease process often affects the central pursuit and visual fixation systems; there is frequently saccadic pursuit.
- If these systems are unaffected, the nystagmus is accentuated when fixation is removed.

Pathogenesis

Gaze-evoked nystagmus is due to a deficient eye position signal that results in failure to maintain the eyes in an eccentric position of gaze. The eyes drift back towards the primary position until fixation is re-established by a saccade.

The brainstem system responsible for coding eye position is the neural integrator. Eye position signals are coded for saccadic, pursuit and vestibular ocular

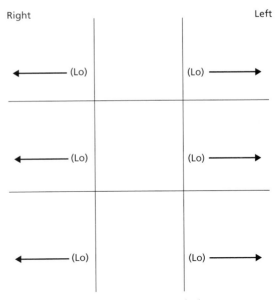

Fig. 23.13 Bilateral horizontal gaze-evoked nystagmus. There is a small-amplitude, low-frequency horizontal nystagmus; the fast phase is in the direction of gaze.

movements. The neural integrator responsible for horizontal gaze consists of:

- part of the cerebellum;
- the perihypoglossal nuclei in the brainstem;
- the medial vestibular nucleus.

A lesion affecting any one of these three areas results in a horizontal gaze-evoked nystagmus.

For ocular movement to take place passive forces must be overcome to start the movement and to hold the eyes in place once they are in the new gaze position. In all eccentric positions of gaze, passive orbital forces tend to return the eye to the primary position. To prevent this happening there must be steady contraction of the extraocular muscles. The amount of contraction required to maintain the eyes in eccentric gaze will increase the further the eyes move from the primary position. This sustained level of muscle contraction arises from a step increase in neural activity. Taking the saccadic system as an example, a saccadic eye movement is generated by a pulse and a step of neural activity (see Chapter 22). The saccadic step is generated by the neural integrator, which synthesizes in the mathematical sense the eye velocity command (pulse) into the appropriate position-coded information (step) for the ocular motor neurones (Fig. 23.14).

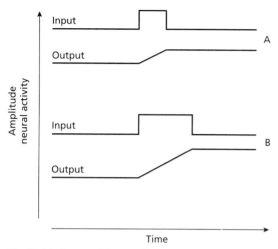

Fig. 23.14 Output of the neural integrator. Mathematical integration basically means the area under the curve. In example A the integration of the input pulse produces a step increase in output. In example B a large pulse signal, corresponding to a larger velocity and amplitude movement, generates an appropriately large step output.

The deficient step or position command in gaze-evoked nystagmus probably represents an early decay of the step signal rather than a true reduction in the signal. The decay has been attributed to a leaky neural integrator.

Neural integrator dysfunction can be:
• Primary: in association with cerebellar and brain-stem disease and as a result of drug toxicity.
• Secondary: as an adaptive change to pathological nystagmus (usually vestibular nystagmus).

The mechanism for vertical gaze-holding is less well understood. The mesencephalic nuclei, in particular the interstitial nucleus of Cajal, appear to be important.

Gaze-paretic nystagmus

In a partial horizontal supranuclear gaze palsy there is reduced drive to the neural integrator on one side. Eye movement to that side and the ability to hold the eyes in a position of eccentric gaze are both impaired: consequently the eyes tend to drift back towards the primary position until the movement is corrected by a saccade to the side of the gaze palsy.

An asymmetric form of gaze-paretic nystagmus is seen in association with paralytic and mechanical strabismus.

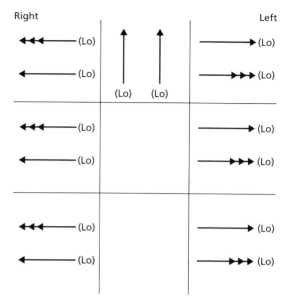

Fig. 23.15 Bilateral internuclear ophthalmoplegia with bilateral dissociated nystagmus on lateral gaze. The amplitude of the nystagmus in the abducting eye is larger than in the adducting eye. There is also a gaze-evoked up-beating nystagmus on extreme up-gaze due to mild dysfunction of the vertical neural integrator.

Dissociated nystagmus

Dissociated nystagmus is most frequently seen in inter-nuclear ophthalmoplegia in which the low-frequency moderate-amplitude nystagmus in the abducting eye contrasts with no movement or a small-amplitude nystagmus in the adducting eye.

Features (Fig. 23.15)

The features of dissociated nystagmus are fully covered in Chapter 22.

Acquired pendular nystagmus

Description

This nystagmus is characterized by oscillations that have similar velocity and amplitude in both directions.

Acquired pendular nystagmus may be horizontal or vertical or a combination of the two; it may be symmetrical or asymmetrical.

Classification

The classification of acquired pendular nystagmus is summarized in Table 23.5.

Table 23.5 Classification of acquired pendular nystagmus.

Horizontal
    Multiple sclerosis

Vertical
    Symmetrical
        Ocular myoclonus
    Asymmetrical
        Monocular visual loss

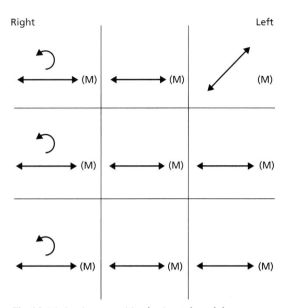

Right   Left

Fig. 23.16 A primary position horizontal pendular nystagmus of low amplitude and moderate frequency. A rotary component occurs on right gaze and the waveform takes on an oblique trajectory on elevation in left gaze.

Horizontal pendular nystagmus of multiple sclerosis

Multiple sclerosis is one of the few causes of an acquired purely horizontal pendular nystagmus. In a number of cases, however, the trajectory of the nystagmus is oblique or elliptical (see 'Trajectories of nystagmus' above) because of a superimposed vertical component; a rotary component is also seen.

Features (Fig. 23.16)
• The frequency of the oscillation tends to be around 3–5 Hz and remains fairly constant in any one patient.
• Oscillopsia is common.
• Vision may be reduced from previous episodes of optic neuritis.
• Other brainstem involvement from multiple sclerosis is common.

Vertical pendular nystagmus (ocular-palatal myoclonus)
Description
This is a pendular nystagmus, usually vertical, associated with rhythmical movement of the palate, diaphragm and other structures.

Features
• A symmetrical oscillation with a frequency of 3–5 Hz.
• Rhythmical movement of the palate and diaphragm are common; the eye movements are usually synchronous with the palatal movements.
• Oscillopsia is present and is often very disturbing
• The cause is usually trauma or a brainstem stroke. The nystagmus and oscillopsia typically start 3 months or more after the causative event. Ocular-palatal myoclonus does not usually show spontaneous improvement.

Pathogenesis
Ocular-palatal myoclonus follows damage to the: inferior olivary nucleus (medulla); dentate nucleus (cerebellum); red nucleus (midbrain); or the pathways which connect these structures (the myoclonic triangle) (Fig. 23.17). Pathological examination shows hypertrophy of the inferior olivary nucleus.

Investigation
Close liaison with the neurologists is important in managing these patients.

Nystagmus associated with monocular visual loss
Description
This is a unilateral vertical pendular nystagmus seen in association with monocular visual loss.
    The visual loss may be:
• congenital;
• acquired during early childhood;
• acquired during adulthood.

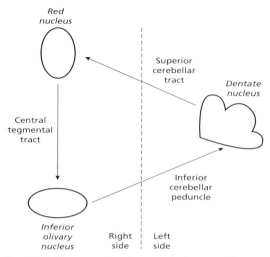

Fig. 23.17 The connections between the dentate nucleus in the cerebellum, the red nucleus in the midbrain and the inferior olivary nucleus in the medulla make up the myoclonic triangle. A lesion involving any part of the myoclonic triangle can result in ocular-palatal myoclonus.

Features
- The nystagmus is primarily vertical, although small horizontal components can be present.
- The waveform is pendular with a low frequency, ranging from 0.12 to 5 Hz, and variable amplitude that is usually less than 10° (Pritchard *et al.* 1988).
- It is not infrequently seen in adults following acute cataract formation, and in young adults with uncorrected unilateral aphakia. Oscillopsia is often present when viewing through the affected eye.
- The nystagmus is generally associated with loss of fusion. Removal of a cataract with the implantation of an intraocular lens can result in intractable diplopia. Surgery should initially involve removal of the cataract and correction with a contact lens to assess if fusion is present prior to implanting an intraocular lens. The nystagmus rarely disappears following removal of the cataract and correction of the aphakia (Yee *et al.* 1979).
- The aetiology remains unknown.

Investigation
Further investigation, including neuro-imaging of the anterior visual pathway, is indicated in both children and adults with unexplained visual loss.

Nystagmus-like oscillations

Inappropriate saccades

Description
These consist of rhythmical and nonrhythmical eye movements resulting from voluntary or involuntary saccades (Fig. 23.18). They differ from nystagmus in that the movement-breaking fixation is a saccade, whereas it is a slow drift in nystagmus.

Inappropriate saccades can be classified as follows:
- Involuntary:
  1 Intrusions, which break and then resume fixation.
  2 Oscillations, which oscillate across fixation.
- Voluntary saccadic oscillations.

Involuntary
Saccadic intrusions (Fig. 23.18)
Saccadic intrusions are transient breaks in fixation. They appear as small jerky movements to one or other side of fixation, giving the impression that the patient will not hold his fixation steady.

- Square-wave jerks are usually small-amplitude conjugate saccades (< 5°) which move the eyes away from fixation and back again, with a latency of around 250 ms between saccades, which occur singly or in bursts. These small-amplitude movements are best observed with the aid of magnification or by using an eye movement recorder. Square-wave jerks are a common finding, especially in the elderly.
- Square-wave pulses (macro square-wave jerks) usually have a larger amplitude (> 5°) and a shorter intersaccadic latency (100–150 ms) than square-wave jerks. They are less common than square-wave jerks and are usually an indication of neurological malfunction.

Saccadic oscillations
Saccadic oscillations usually have amplitudes larger than 5°. The oscillations cross fixation and the episodes occur in bursts. Macro saccadic oscillations can be reliably distinguished from ocular flutter only by eye movement recording.

- Macro saccadic oscillations appear as shimmering movements during fixation. They have a similar intersaccadic latency to square-wave jerks.

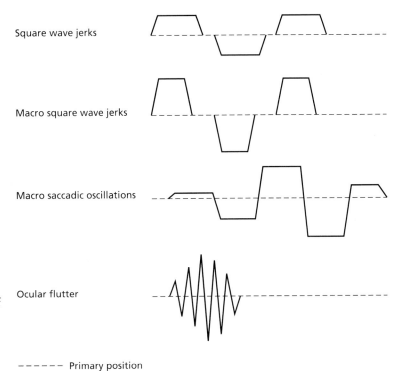

Square wave jerks

Macro square wave jerks

Macro saccadic oscillations

Ocular flutter

– – – – – – Primary position

Fig. 23.18 Inappropriate saccades are rhythmical and nonrhythmical eye movements resulting from involuntary saccades. The absence of a slow drift differentiates these eye movements from nystagmus. The diagrammatic characteristics of inappropriate saccades are shown.

• Ocular flutter represents back-to-back horizontal saccades without any intersaccadic latency.
• Opsoclonus has a similar waveform to ocular flutter but is multidirectional and associated with oscillopsia.

Pathogenesis
• The pathogenesis of inappropriate saccades remains unknown.
• Opsoclonus, ocular flutter and saccadic dysmetria probably represent a continuum of dysfunction. Opsoclonus is seen to change to ocular flutter before it finally resolves, and saccadic dysmetria is closely associated with opsoclonus and ocular flutter. These inappropriate saccadic movements are said to be associated with cerebellar disease, although opsoclonus and flutter may represent dysfunction affecting the pause cells of the brainstem gaze centres (see Chapter 6).

Investigation
Opsoclonus is associated with occult neuroblastoma in childhood and neoplasia in adults; further investigation is always required.

The other types of inappropriate saccades are less specific in terms of diagnostic value. They can be seen in a wide range of conditions which affect the brainstem and cerebellum; these include:
• multiple sclerosis;
• Parkinson's disease;
• progressive supranuclear palsy;
• cerebellar disease.

Superior oblique myokymia
This is a rare unilateral condition which may occasionally follow an acquired superior oblique palsy.

Aetiology
Hoyt and Keane (1970) have compared this disorder with facial muscle myokymia, which occasionally follows facial nerve palsies, and suggest that there is acquired alteration in the membrane threshold of neurones in the fourth cranial nerve nucleus. Kommerell and Schaubele (1980) carried out electromyographic studies and concluded that in the case reported there was inadequate supranuclear control of regenerated

fourth nerve neurones. Lee (1984) described two cases in which the phenomenon developed following superior oblique palsy, and suggested that this disorder should be grouped with cyclic oculomotor palsy, cyclic esotropia and the aberrant regeneration syndrome as rather ill-determined cyclical or recurrent phenomena which may be associated with previous ocular motor palsies. It has also been reported in association with a posterior fossa tumour (Morrow *et al.* 1990), although in most cases no central nervous system disease can be found.

Features

• Recurrent episodes of involuntary rapid eye movements of small amplitude, which may be vertical, torsional or oblique. The fine movements are most easily seen by direct ophthalmoscopy or slit-lamp examination.

• Between attacks there may be a superior oblique palsy or rarely the muscle may overact, simulating a palsy of the contralateral inferior rectus (Heaven *et al.* 1995).

• Uniocular oscillopsia, which is usually the presenting symptom.

• Attacks are often precipitated by reading.

Management

Superior oblique myokymia is often self-limiting and the patient should be reassured about the generally benign nature of the condition. Further investigations are generally not required unless the case history or examination uncovers underlying central nervous system disease. No treatment is required if symptoms are slight or infrequent, a period of observation is recommended to document the natural history of the condition.

MEDICAL TREATMENT

We prefer to start treatment with oral beta-blockers such as propanolol, gradually increasing the dose until a response is noted or side-effects occur (Tyler & Ruiz 1990). If beta-blockers are not effective some success has been reported following treatment by oral carbamazepine (Tegretol) (Rosenberg & Glaser 1983). Improvement may be explained by the neurone membrane-stabilizing properties of this drug.

SURGICAL TREATMENT

If the oscillopsia is persistent and very disturbing to the patient, it can be relieved by superior oblique tenotomy. The resulting superior oblique palsy causes other symptoms that may be only partly relieved by ipsilateral inferior oblique weakening and/or contralateral inferior rectus recession. Surgery is not without significant side-effects and is therefore not recommended.

Voluntary saccadic oscillations 'nystagmus'

Description

This is a voluntary, poorly sustained conjugate oscillation of the eyes consisting of rapidly alternating small-amplitude saccades.

Features

• The oscillations are conjugate, usually horizontal and symmetrical, and consist of back-to-back saccades (Shults *et al.* 1977).

• The oscillations can be sustained only for a matter of seconds; convergence is usually associated with either the initiation or the maintenance of the oscillation.

• The amplitude of the movement is small and the frequency high.

• There may be a familial basis for the ability to initiate voluntary 'nystagmus' or it may be learned.

Voluntary 'nystagmus' can be readily differentiated from acquired nystagmus and does not require further investigation.

Roving eye movements

Description

Roving eye movements consist of conjugate large-amplitude low-frequency horizontal pendular-like movements.

The movement is apparent soon after birth and is generally associated with severe anterior visual pathway disease. We have mainly seen roving eye movements in association with Leber's congenital amaurosis and severe forms of bilateral optic nerve hypoplasia. With time the amplitude becomes smaller and a congenital nystagmus waveform may become superimposed on the roving pattern or may replace it.

Physiological nystagmus

Following vestibular stimulation

• Caloric testing: the labyrinth can be stimulated by irrigating one ear with warm or cold water. The convection currents created in the horizontal semi-circular canal cause an imbalance of tone between the labyrinths, resulting in peripheral vestibular nystagmus.
• Rotational: if a normal subject is rotated in the Barany chair (or more commonly at a fun fair!), the currents set up in the semicircular canals cause a horizontal deviation of the eyes to match the direction of spin. If the rotation suddenly ceases, the stimulus from the semicircular canals continues for a few seconds. During this time the visual fixation system is opposed by the now inappropriate stimulation from the semicircular canals, inducing transient nystagmus.

Following optokinetic/pursuit stimulation

• Optokinetic nystagmus: the term 'nystagmus' is a misnomer and this phenomenon is more correctly described as the optokinetic response. Smooth pursuit movement is used to fixate on the moving object of regard, followed by a saccade to refixate on the next object entering the visual field.

Gaze-dependent

• End-point nystagmus: when a normal subject adopts extreme eccentric gaze, the eyes may drift back towards the primary position, requiring small correct-ive saccades to maintain gaze. The drift ceases after a few oscillations. End-point nystagmus must be differentiated from the more prolonged oscillations seen in gaze-evoked and gaze-paretic nystagmus.

Management of nystagmus

Ophthalmic management of congenital nystagmus

The aims of treatment in patients with congenital nystagmus are:

• to improve visual acuity;
• to reduce any abnormal head posture;
• to improve the appearance of any strabismus.
  A small group of patients may respond to treatment aimed at diminishing the intensity of the nystagmus.

Management
The management options for congential nystagmus can be summarized thus:
• Refraction and equalization of vision.
• Reduction of nystagmus intensity, using:
  1 prisms;
  2 surgery.
• Reduction of abnormal head posture.
• Treatment of nystagmus blockage esotropia.

Improvement in visual acuity
Improvement in visual acuity can result from:
• correction of refractive error;
• treatment of amblyopia;
• reduction in the intensity of the nystagmus.

Correction of refractive error
A cycloplegic refraction is essential in all children with congenital nystagmus. High levels of both myopic and hypermetropic astigmatism are common, especially when there is sensory loss.

Refractive errors should be corrected; correcting even trivial refractive errors can result in improved visual performance, or can provide a subjective improvement or enhance the child's visual awareness. Correction of the refractive error may also result in the reduction of an abnormal head posture. Spectacle use may be less than ideal in the presence of an abnormal head posture because of the need to use an eccentric position of the lens. Contact lenses can result in better visual acuity compared with spectacles in congenital nystagmus (Allen & Davies 1983). This visual improvement may be due to:
• improved correction of corneal astigmatism;
• since the contact lens moves with the eye, the patient looks through the optical centre of the lens for most of the wearing time, even in the presence of an abnormal head posture;
• a reduction of the intensity of the nystagmus possibly arising from extra vergence and accommodative effort generated by contact lenses (Abadi 1979);

• a form of sensory feedback caused by the edges of the contact lenses rubbing on the eyelids, making the patient aware of the intensity of the nystagmus.

Restoration of visual acuity

Amblyopia may be caused by:

• strabismus;
• anisometropia;
• deprivation—this is an important factor in congenital nystagmus associated with bilateral congenital cataracts (see Chapter 10 for details of amblyopia management in this group of patients).

Amblyopia should be managed using total occlusion of the nonamblyopic eye.

Reduction in the intensity of the nystagmus

CONSERVATIVE TREATMENT

Base-out prisms

The patient must have binocular single vision to benefit from the use of prisms to stimulate convergence. If there is a significant reduction in the intensity of the nystagmus for near, stimulating fusional convergence by using base-out prisms can improve visual acuity at distance fixation (Dell'Osso *et al.* 1974). It is our experience that patients rarely persevere with this form of treatment unless very well motivated.

SURGICAL TREATMENT

Surgery to reduce the intensity of the nystagmus usually involves recessing all four horizontal rectus muscles to behind the equator of the eye. Recessions of 10–12 mm are required; the medial rectus is recessed 2 mm less than the lateral rectus to reduce the risk of postoperative consecutive divergence. Most patients have binocular single vision and are therefore able to compensate for minor degrees of postoperative misalignment. We tend to restrict such surgery to those patients who require improved visual acuity for occupational reasons or to obtain a driving licence. Any improvement in visual acuity is small, therefore the patient's preoperative level of visual acuity must be close to that required.

Reduction of abnormal head posture

An abnormal head posture is adopted to improve visual function by utilizing an eccentric null region where the intensity of the nystagmus is least. The

Table 23.6 Summary of the management of abnormal head posture.

Refraction and equalization of vision
Abnormal head posture with BSV
Horizontal
Prism
Surgery on horizontal muscles
Vertical
Prism
Surgery on vertical muscles
Tilt
Prism
Surgery on vertical muscles
Abnormal head posture and strabismus
Surgery on horizontal muscles to correct both conditions
Correction of strabismus followed by surgery on the fixing eye for the head posture

direction of the nystagmus determines the type of head posture. There may be three components:

• a face turn, seen with horizontal nystagmus;
• a chin elevation or depression, seen with vertical nystagmus;
• a head tilt seen with rotary nystagmus.

These components may be combined when there is more than one trajectory.

An abnormal head posture may exist with or without strabismus.

Before considering treatment of an abnormal head posture any refractive error should be corrected and amblyopia treated in children under 8 years of age. Even the correction of minor degrees of refractive error can result in a significant improvement in an abnormal head posture.

Any surgical intervention aimed at correcting the abnormal head posture should be delayed until its characteristics have been fully assessed and it has been shown to be stable. We usually wait until the child is 5 years or older before undertaking surgery.

The management of abnormal head posture is summarized in Table 23.6.

Conservative management

Prisms are the mainstay of conservative management of abnormal head postures. The prism is orientated so that:

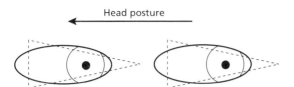

Fig. 23.19 A diagrammatic representation of a patient with a right face-turn with the eyes deviated towards the null region in left gaze. To correct the head posture a prism is positioned base-out before the right eye and base-in before the left eye.

- the apex points towards the null region or;
- the base is in the direction of the head posture.

For example, if the patient has a right face turn with the eyes deviated towards a null region in left gaze, the prism before the right eye is positioned base-out and that before the left eye base-in (Fig. 23.19). The opposite would apply in a patient with a left face turn.

If there is a chin elevation or depression then the prisms are positioned:
- base-down in front of both eyes for chin-down head postures;
- base-up in front of both eyes for chin-up head postures.

Most abnormal head postures associated with congenital nystagmus that require treatment exceed 20°. The long-term use of prisms is therefore impractical because of the high prism strength required. Prisms are useful preoperatively to confirm that the head posture will respond to the planned operation. We find them particularly valuable in patients whose head posture has more than one component, or in those requiring further surgery for a residual head posture.

Surgical management
- Surgery is indicated if there is a constant cosmetically poor or uncomfortable compensatory head posture that is being used to centralize the null region.
- Surgery is usually only required for head postures larger than 20°. Lesser degrees of head posture are not treated unless they are causing social problems.
- Surgery is not usually performed before the age of 5 years unless there is a very marked cosmetic defect. Before this age it is difficult to be certain that the head posture is consistent.

- The aims of surgery are to reduce the head posture without disturbing the ocular balance. This is achieved by moving the eyes in the direction of the head posture.

TECHNIQUES IN PATIENTS WITH BINOCULAR SINGLE VISION
In all techniques both eyes are rotated an equal amount to maintain parallelism of the visual axes.

Horizontal head posture
There are three main techniques:
- Kestenbaum procedure: surgery is performed on all four horizontal rectus muscles.
- Anderson procedure: surgical recession to two horizontal rectus muscles.
- Goto procedure: surgical resection to two horizontal rectus muscles.
The Kestenbaum procedure is the one we generally recommend.

Kestenbaum procedure: Surgery is performed on all four horizontal recti; in a patient with a right face turn the left lateral rectus and the right medial rectus are recessed and the left medial rectus and right lateral rectus are resected (Fig. 23.20).

Head postures up to 30° can be effectively corrected using the 5,6,7,8 formula described by Marshall Parks (Parks 1973), who advocated a total amount of surgery to each eye of 13 mm; his formula takes into account the greater effect of surgery on a medial rectus compared to a lateral rectus muscle. In general, to obtain the same change in alignment 2 mm

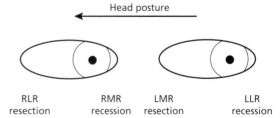

Fig. 23.20 A diagrammatic representation of a patient with a right face-turn with the eyes deviated towards the null region in left gaze. The Kestenbaum procedure to correct the head posture consists of a left lateral rectus and right medial rectus recession and right lateral rectus and left medial rectus resection.

more surgery needs to be performed on the lateral rectus than on the medial rectus. In the above example this would result in:

• right medial rectus recession 5 mm;
• left medial rectus resection 6 mm;
• left lateral rectus recession 7 mm;
• right lateral rectus resection 8 mm.

Head postures larger than 30° often remain undercorrected using Park's formula. A modification of the Kestenbaum procedure has been proposed in which the amount of surgery is augmented by 40% or 60% for large head postures (Nelson *et al.* 1984).

A 40% augmentation of Park's formula results in 7 mm, 8.4 mm, 9.8 mm and 11.2 mm.

A 60% augmentation of Park's formula results in 8 mm, 9.6 mm, 11.2 mm and 12.8 mm.

A limitation of gaze contralateral to the face turn is seen following augmented surgery. The eyes may only just cross the mid-line following a 60% augmented procedure. The patient and family need to be aware of this side-effect of surgery.

Vertical head posture

Chin elevation or depression is much less common than a horizontal head posture. Surgery involves either bilateral recession or bilateral recession and resection of the vertical rectus muscles, depending on the size of the head posture.

For a chin-up head posture:

• a recession of both inferior rectus muscles;
• a recession of the inferior rectus and a resection of the superior rectus on both eyes.

For a chin-down head posture:

• a recession of both superior rectus muscles;
• a recession of the superior rectus and a resection of the inferior rectus on both eyes.

Head tilt

It is important to exclude all other possible causes of a head tilt before attributing it to congenital nystagmus. The nystagmus causing the head tilt can be of a very low intensity and identification may require magnification.

A number of surgical options have been described to correct the head tilt, including:

• surgery to all four oblique muscles (Conrad & de Decker 1984).

• vertical transposition of the horizontal rectus muscles;
• slanting the insertions of all eight rectus muscles;
• horizontal transposition of all four vertical rectus muscles (von Noorden *et al.* 1993).

We prefer to use the transposition approach described by von Noorden *et al.* In a patient with a right head tilt:

• the right superior rectus is transposed nasally;
• the right inferior rectus is transposed temporally;
• the left superior rectus is transposed temporally;
• the left inferior rectus is transposed nasally.

Residual abnormal head postures

The initial postoperative improvement may not be maintained in all cases and the head posture may recur. Further surgery can usually be performed in patients who show a significant residual head posture. If the patient has previously undergone a Kestenbaum procedure using Park's formula, surgery could comprise:

• a further recession of 2 mm and a posterior fixation suture to the previously recessed muscles;
• a further resection of 4 mm to the previously resected muscles.

The patient and family need to be informed that gaze will be restricted in the direction opposite to the head posture following this procedure, and diplopia may occur.

Abnormal head posture and strabismus

A special situation arises where strabismus and an abnormal head posture coexist. Both congenital nystagmus and manifest latent nystagmus can be associated with strabismus.

In congenital nystagmus with strabismus:

• the esotropia is usually unilateral, with a face turn to the side of the fixing eye;
• surgery is aimed at correcting both the esotropia and the abnormal head posture either with a single operation or by correcting the esotropia first, followed by treatment for the abnormal head posture;
• surgery aimed at improving the head posture must be directed at the fixing eye.

In manifest latent nystagmus with strabismus:

• alternating esotropia is frequently seen;
• there is a face turn towards the side of the fixing eye (fixation in adduction preference);

- if the esotropia is alternating the face turn changes with the change in fixation;
- surgery involves recession of the medial rectus muscles with or without posterior fixation sutures (see Chapters 9 and 14).

Treatment of nystagmus blockage syndrome

Adelstein and Cüppers (1966) first described this condition to explain an esotropia that results from the use of the convergence mechanism to block or abolish manifest nystagmus and improve visual acuity. This condition is rare compared with essential infantile esotropia; management is discussed in Chapter 14.

Ophthalmic management of acquired nystagmus

The aims of treatment in patients with acquired nystagmus are:
- improvement in visual acuity;
- relief of diplopia.
  Management can be summarized as follows:
- Improve visual acuity:
  1 Head posture: improve using prisms.
  2 Oscillopsia: treat using drugs, botulinum toxin or surgery.
- Relieve diplopia: using prisms, botulinum toxin or surgery.

Improvement of visual acuity

- All patients must be wearing an up-to-date and accurate refractive correction if needed.
- Bifocal and multifocal lenses restrict the patient's direction of gaze and should generally be avoided.
- Single focal lenses allow the patient to use a region of gaze where oscillopsia is least.

Head posture

- In patients with down-beat nystagmus the intensity of the nystagmus and the oscillopsia in most cases is maximal on down-gaze, leading to a chin-down head posture. The use of single focal reading spectacles is helpful if there is a consistent or uncomfortable head posture; base-down prisms are occasionally effective.

Oscillopsia

Oscillopsia is the illusion of rhythmical movement of stationary objects. It is a feature of acquired nystagmus and is not a complaint of patients with congenital nystagmus. It can be unilateral or bilateral and may be present only in certain gaze directions. It is seen with:
- Acquired pendular nystagmus: oscillopsia can be a debilitating symptom in both ocular-palatal myoclonus and the horizontal pendular nystagmus seen in multiple sclerosis. The environment is perceived to be moving continuously back and forth.
- Acquired jerk nystagmus: vestibular nystagmus is frequently associated with oscillopsia. In down-beat nystagmus the oscillopsia is worst on down-gaze. Patients with gaze-evoked nystagmus occasionally complain of oscillopsia that is gaze-dependent. The environment is perceived as moving in the opposite direction to the slow phase; no movement is perceived during the fast phase as saccadic suppression occurs.
- Superior oblique myokymia: the environment appears to shimmer or become blurred; the phenomenon is intermittent and unilateral.

MEDICAL TREATMENT

Medical treatment for acquired nystagmus has not been very effective. Baclofen has been used successfully in a patient with periodic alternating nystagmus (Halmagyi *et al.* 1980). The use of clonazepam has also been proposed for the treatment of nystagmus-induced oscillopsia (Currie & Matsuo 1986).

Down-beat nystagmus can be a side-effect of anti-convulsant medication; reducing the dose can lead to resolution of the nystagmus (Chrousos *et al.* 1987).

BOTULINUM TOXIN

Botulinum toxin has proved to be effective in dampening the oscillations of acquired nystagmus, leading to an improvement in visual acuity (Helveston & Pogrebniak 1988). There are certain constraints on this form of therapy:
- binocular single vision is sacrificed for improved monocular visual acuity;
- the reduced range of eye movement which follows injection demands that the patient makes compensatory head movements;
- the resultant muscle paralysis upsets coordination and balance; we have found that patients who are wheelchair bound gain most benefit from the injection;
- repeat injections are required.

A unilateral injection of botulinum toxin can be administered into:

- selected extraocular muscles; this method is used mainly in nystagmus with horizontal waveforms, for example acquired pendular nystagmus;
- the retrobulbar space; this method is effective in ocular-palatal myoclonus.

SURGICAL TREATMENT

Down-beat nystagmus associated with the Arnold–Chiari malformation may improve following posterior fossa decompression. Surgery is, however, rarely justifiable if the only symptoms are ocular.

Relief of diplopia

Brainstem disease that results in acquired nystagmus may also involve the ocular motor nerves. Resultant diplopia should be managed in the same way as in patients with acquired palsies without nystagmus (see Chapter 19). Patients with unstable or progressive disease affecting the brainstem should be managed conservatively, using prisms or botulinum toxin when necessary.

References

Abadi, R.V. (1979) Visual performance with contact lenses and congenital idiopathic nystagmus. *British Journal of Physiological Optics* **33**(3), 32–37.

Adelstein, F.E. & Cüppers, C. (1966) Zum problem der echten und scheibaren Abducenslahmung (das sogenannte 'Blockierungs syndrom'). In: *Buch der Augenarzt*, pp. 271–278. Enke, Stuttgart.

Allen, E.D. & Davies, P.D. (1983) Role of contact lenses in the management of congenital nystagmus. *British Journal of Ophthalmology* **67**, 834–836.

Baker, L. & Ansons, A.M. (1996) Incomitant skew deviation in association with Arnold–Chiari malformation. In: *Transactions of the 23rd Meeting of the European Strabismological Association, Nancy* (ed. M. Spiritus) pp. 375–380. Aeolus Press, The Netherlands.

Chrousos, G.A., Codry, R., Schuelein, M., Abdul-Rahim, A.S., Matsuo, V. & Currie, J.N. (1987) Two cases of down-beat nystagmus and oscillopsia associated with carbamazepine. *American Journal of Ophthalmology* **103**, 221–224.

Conrad, H.G. & de Decker, W. (1984) Torsional Kestenbaum procedure: evolution of a surgical concept.

In: *Strabismus 11* (ed. R.D. Reinecke), pp. 301–314. Grune & Stratton, Orlando, Fla.

Currie, J.N. & Matsuo, V. (1986) The use of clonazepam in the treatment of nystagmus induced oscillopsia. *Ophthalmology* **93**, 924–931.

Dell'Osso, L.F., Flynn, J.T. & Daroff, R.B. (1974) Hereditary congenital nystagmus; an infrafamilial study. *Archives of Ophthalmology* **92**, 366–374.

Dell'Osso, L.F., Schmidt, J.P. & Daroff, R.B. (1979) Latent, manifest latent and congenital nystagmus. *Archives of Ophthalmology* **97**, 1877–1885.

Dell'Osso, L.F., Van der Steen, J., Steinman, R.M. & Collewijn, H. (1992) Foveating dynamics in congenital nystagmus 1: Fixation. *Documenta Ophthalmologica* **79**, 1–23.

Farmer, J. & Hoyt, C.S. (1984) Monocular nystagmus in infancy and early childhood. *American Journal of Ophthalmology* **98**, 504–509.

Gelbart, S.S. & Hoyt, C.S. (1988) Congenital nystagmus: a clinical perspective in infancy. *Graefe's Archives of Clinical Experimental Ophthalmology* **22**, 178–180.

Gillespie, F.D. & Covelli, B. (1963) Carriers of ocular albinism with and without ocular changes. *Archives of Ophthalmology* **70**, 121–125.

Gresty, M.A. & Halmagyi, G.M. (1979) Abnormal head movements. *Journal of Neurology, Neurosurgery and Psychiatry* **42**, 705–714.

Halmagyi, G.M., Rudge, P., Gresty, M.A. *et al.* (1980) Treatment of periodic alternating nystagmus. *Annals of Neurology* **8**(6), 609–611.

Harcourt, B. & Spencer, F. (1985) Manifest latent nystagmus affecting patients with uniocular congenital blindness. In: *Transactions of the 14th Meeting of the European Strabismological Association* (ed. E. Gregerson), pp. 259–264. APS, Copenhagen.

Heaven, C.J., Ansons, A.M. & Casson, S. (1995) Superior oblique myokymia masquerading as an inferior rectus palsy. *Eye* **9**, 382–383.

Helveston, E.M. & Pogrebniak, A.E. (1988) Treatment of acquired nystagmus with botulinum A toxin. *American Journal of Ophthalmology* **106**, 585–586.

Hoyt, W.F. & Keane, J.R. (1970) Superior oblique myokymia. *Archives of Ophthalmology* **84**, 461–467.

Kommerell, G. (1984) Congenital nystagmus, characteristics and pathophysiology. In: *Transactions of the Fifth International Orthoptic Congress, Cannes* (eds A.P. Ravault & M. Lenk), pp. 345–351. LIPS, Lyon.

Kommerell, G. & Schaubele, G. (1980) Superior oblique myokymia: an electromyographic analysis. *Transactions of the Ophthalmological Society of the United Kingdom* **100**, 504–506.

Lavery, M.A., O'Neill, J.F., Chu, F.C. & Martyn, L.J. (1984) Acquired nystagmus in early childhood: a presenting sign of intracranial tumour. *Ophthalmology* **91**, 425–434.

Lee, J.P. (1984) Superior oblique myokymia: a possible etiologic factor. *Archives of Ophthalmology* **102**, 1178–1179.

Morrow, M.J., Sharpe, J.A. & Ranalli, P.J. (1990) Superior oblique myokymia associated with a posterior fossa tumor: oculographic correlation with an idiopathic case. *Neurology* **40**, 367–370.

Nelson, L.B., Ervin-Mulvey, L.D., Calhoun, J.H., Harley, R.D. & Keisler, M.S. (1984) Surgical management for abnormal head position in nystagmus: the augmented modified Kestenbaum procedure. *British Journal of Ophthalmology* **68**, 796–800.

von Noorden, G.K., Jenkins, R. & Rosenbaum, A. (1993) Horizontal transposition of the vertical rectus muscles for treatment of ocular torticollis. *Journal of Pediatric Ophthalmology and Strabismus* **30**, 8–14.

Parks, M.M. (1973) Congenital nystagmus surgery. *American Orthoptic Journal* **23**, 35–39.

Pritchard, C., Flynn, J.T. & Smith, J.L. (1988) Waveform characteristics of vertical oscillations in longstanding vision loss. *Journal of Paediatric Ophthalmology and Strabismus* **25**, 233–236.

Rosenberg, M.L. & Glaser, J.S. (1983) Superior oblique myokymia. *Annals of Neurology* **13**, 667–669.

Shults, W.T., Stark, L., Hoyt, W.F. & Ochs, A.L. (1977) Normal saccadic structure of voluntary nystagmus. *Archives of Ophthalmology* **95**, 1399–1404.

Tyler, T.D. & Ruiz, R.S. (1990) Propanolol in the treatment of superior oblique myokymia (letter). *Archives of Ophthalmology* **108**, 175–176.

Westheimer, G. & Blair, S.M. (1975) The ocular tilt reaction: a brain stem oculomotor routine. *Investigative Ophthalmology* **14**(11), 833–839.

Yee, R.D., Jelks, G.W., Baloh, R.W. & Honrubia, V. (1979) Uniocular nystagmus in monocular visual loss. *Ophthalmology* 511–518.

Index